I0644169

A Dream Interpreted Within a Dream

A Dream Interpreted Within a Dream

Oneiropoiesis and the Prism of Imagination

Elliot R. Wolfson

ZONE BOOKS · NEW YORK

2011

© 2011 Elliot R. Wolfson
ZONE BOOKS
1226 Prospect Avenue
Brooklyn, NY 11218
All rights reserved.

No part of this book may be reproduced, stored in a retrieval system, or transmitted in any form or by any means, including electronic, mechanical, photocopying, microfilming, recording, or otherwise (except for that copying permitted by Sections 107 and 108 of the U.S. Copyright Law and except by reviewers for the public press), without written permission from the Publisher.

References to Internet Web sites (URLs) were accurate at the time of writing. Neither the author nor Zone Books is responsible for Web sites that may have expired or changed since the book was prepared.
Printed in the United States of America.

Distributed by The MIT Press,
Cambridge, Massachusetts, and London, England

Library of Congress Cataloging-in-Publication Data

Wolfson, Elliot R.
A dream interpreted within a dream : oneiropoiesis and the prism of imagination / Elliot R. Wolfson.
p. cm.
Includes bibliographical references and index.
ISBN 978-1-935408-14-7
1. Dreams. 2. Dreams—Religious aspects—Judaism. 3. Mysticism—Judaism. 4. Dream interpretation. 5. Sleep. 6. Wakefulness. 7. Imagination. I. Title.

BF1078.W574 2011
154.6'3–DC22

2011000122

To the memory of
Edith Wyschogrod,
for showing me the way
to the way of nonshowing

Somnium somnia quasi semper vives.
Vive quasi hodie moriebar.

Contents

While one is dreaming one does not know it is a dream, and in one's dream one may even try to interpret a dream. Only after one wakes does one know it was a dream. And someday there will be a great awakening when we know that this is all a great dream.

—Chuang Tzu

All that we see or seem
Is but a dream within a dream

—Edgar Allan Poe

Acknowledgments

I would like to thank Daniel Boyarin, Aaron Hughes, and Jeffrey Kripal, who read an earlier version of this book and made invaluable suggestions for revision. Daniel, in particular, was instrumental in pushing me to expand my discussion of Maimonides, which eventually evolved into a separate chapter wherein I explore his reflections on prophecy and the oneiric vision in conversation with Michel Foucault's sustained meditation on Ludwig Binswanger's theory of the dream phenomenon. I also want to express my sincere gratitude to Ramona Naddaff, one of the editors of Zone Books, who offered many important recommendations to improve the manuscript both substantively and stylistically. Her discerning editorial eye is greatly appreciated. I am also grateful to Ramona and to Daniel for inviting me to participate in the seminar "Old Things": Classical Studies and Contemporary Humanities, sponsored by the Doreen B. Townsend Center for the Humanities at the University of California, Berkeley. I benefited from the responses and queries I received from the participants in the seminar when I visited the campus on March 9, 2010. Versions of the final chapter were read as the Scholars without Borders lecture sponsored by the Department of Near and Middle Eastern Civilizations, University of Toronto, February 11, 2010, and as a paper delivered in the Humanities Seminar at Muhlenberg College, February 24, 2010. The audiences at both events helped me sharpen my argument. Finally, I want to express my deepest indebtedness to Virginia Burrus, who selflessly read through the entire manuscript in her characteristically gracious manner. As her own scholarly work attests, Virginia is an exemplary hermeneut, one who approaches the text with the rare combination of poetic sensitivity and analytic incisiveness. Her ability to intervene critically by listening so attentively is truly admirable.

May 24, 2010

Preface

> The hermit does not believe that any philosopher—assuming that every philosopher was first of all a hermit—ever expressed his real and ultimate opinions in books: does one not write books precisely to conceal what one harbors?... Every philosophy also conceals a philosophy, every opinion is also a hideout, every word also a mask.
> —Friedrich Nietzsche, *Beyond Good and Evil*

Dreams have attracted the curiosity of humankind for millennia. Even a cursory glance in any good library demonstrates how many authors from a wide range of disciplinary approaches have dedicated their attention to this phenomenon. And still, something is withheld from comprehension, something remains mysterious, lending credence to the ancient sentiment that enigma is the natural language of dreams.[1] If I may be allowed a generalization at the outset, albeit a generalization that by definition safeguards the exception, the allusive and elusive place that dreaming occupies in the panorama of human experience can be explained by the fact that the dream distinctively marks an imaginal excessiveness that expresses itself in each occurrence as foreseeable, but unprecedented. The imaginative faculty is obviously not limited to *Homo sapiens*, and yet, when compared with other sentient beings, human dreaming appears to be an unrivaled form of mental activity, both whimsical and inexorable,[2] that bears a mythologic—a term that should not be construed as privileging either logical or mythical patterns of discourse, rendering one subordinate to the other—that extends beyond itself in the indeterminate determining of the bounds of its unbinding.[3] The dream, we might say, incarnates the mental characteristic of intensity described by Michel Foucault (1926–1984) as the *pure difference* that precedes the "space of representation"—constituted by the triadic web of sensation, image, and memory—wherein perceptual resemblances are sorted out by the polarizing impulses of "quantitative equalization" and "qualitative variation." The intensity of consciousness exemplifies, prior to the gradation by representation, a "difference that displaces and repeats itself, contracts and expands; a singular point that constricts and slackens the indefinite repetitions in an acute event. One must give rise to thought as intensive irregularity. Dissolution of the Me."[4] The language of oneiropoiesis, which is both private and shared, doggedly peculiar and eerily common, is uniquely suited to express the intensiveness of our spatiotemporal distension in the world, the genuine iteration that fosters the perpetuation of self in the eventfulness of its ongoing extinction.

In these pages, I set out to ruminate on some aspects of the oneiropoetic phenomenon. Obviously, the offerings that I will lay before the reader bear the influence of a chorus of voices that have inspired me on the path these many years. This has been the case in all my monographs and essays, but this book must be set apart from previous studies, insofar as it is not an exegetical work on the history of Jewish mysticism or on any other clearly defined element of Jewish thought. To be sure, in these pages the reader will encounter citations from biblical, rabbinic, kabbalistic, and philosophical texts that have been the sustenance of my spiritual and intellectual diet for several decades. Nonetheless, I will not attempt to construct an architectonic of the dream imagination based on them. In lieu of the scholarly endeavor to excavate literary corpora in accord with the canons of philological and historical analysis, which has been my customary praxis, my goal here is to produce a polyphonic sketch, at once restorative and innovative, but ultimately a sketch of what is necessarily fragmentary. Encapsulating an archaic wisdom, Michel Henry (1922–2002) insightfully noted that *the thought of movement is not movement*.[5] The dream, quintessentially, is movement—attested, for instance, in the common use of the dream to denote the experience of something that passes swiftly—and hence one can think the dream, but it is never the dream one has thought. The determination of the dream presupposes the anterior manifestation of the dream; the manifestation of the dream, however, comes into view only posteriorly to the determination of the dream.

Approaching my fiftieth birthday, I decided to compose a different kind of book, a dreambook, doubly so—that is, a book about dreams inscripted in the pattern of a dream in which one dreams about compiling a book on dreams. Other intervening obligations have delayed the writing and publication of this study, but I have tried to remain faithful to the initial aspiration throughout the laborious process of textual production that demands citation and organizing thoughts in a coherent and logical sequence. In the ruminations that follow, I endeavor to think the matter of the dream from inside the contours of the dream, so that it would not be unfair to depict the work I have produced as itself a dream interpreted within a dream, a "tireless labyrinth," in the language of Jorge Luis Borges (1899–1986),[6] that occasions and is occasioned by the act of speaking and, even more profoundly, writing about the dream. In setting out to accomplish just this, I have found it impractical to extricate myself from the very act that I have sought to explicate in virtue of having been extricated therefrom. The poetically inspired words of Gaston Bachelard (1884–1962) are worth citing here:

> How can one not dream while writing? It is the pen that dreams. The blank page gives the right to dream. How hard is the destiny of a maker of books! He has to cut and sew up in order to make ideas follow logically. But when one writes a book on reverie, has the time not come to let the pen run, to let reverie speak, and better yet to dream the reverie at the same time one believes he is transcribing it?[7]

Beautifully stated and seemingly not too onerous to achieve—to just *let the pen run*, to let reverie speak. Bachelard juxtaposes writing and dreaming such that the former is understood in terms of the latter, but we could surely reverse the order and argue that dreaming can be appreciated by pondering the mission of writing. To some extent, all creative writing partakes of the reverie of dreaming, but writing a phenomenological exposé of the dream—or, to be more precise, an exposé of several crucial features of the dream—does so in an especially poignant way. Can the author of such a book—I consent to the authorial status, provided it is understood that the subjectivity therein affirmed, as will be argued from the example of the dream, is one in which the identity of the self is constituted by the identity of the others that are constituted by the self—be constricted to making a logical argument? To write of the dream from within the dream presupposes the experience of the very reverie that one believes one is transcribing. The mind is thus ensnared in a uroboric state that puts into question the bivalent logic of a linear reason, the function typically lateralized in neuroanatomy to the left hemisphere of the brain.

This mode of thinking, moreover, is a form of inferential judgment predicated on the disparity between truth and untruth that is problematized by the dream imagination, which, as will become apparent at various junctures in the course of this book, is characterized by the inability to disentangle true and untrue—the truth of the dream, if one wishes to keep speaking in this fashion, consists veritably of its being false. This is not to discard the assumption that many cultures throughout history have upheld the distinction between true and false dreams. It is not sufficient, however, simply to delineate this distinction ethnographically,[8] for it is justified conceptually only on the basis of beliefs—whether theological, cosmological, anthropological, or psychological—that are extraneous to the dreams. Nothing in the narrative yarn of the dream validates unraveling the threads of veracity from deception. To be clear, let me emphasize that I am not repudiating the widely held view that the dream experience, like other human experiences, is conditioned by suppositions that a particular individual shares with others in the community to which he or she belongs. Nevertheless, the assertion is warranted, inasmuch as the notion that experience is hermeneutically shaped by a preexperiential interpretive scheme affords us the opportunity to discern the extent to which the dream exemplifies the paradox of the oxymoron *fictional truth*, a truth whose authenticity can be gauged only from the standpoint of its artificiality.[9] In a Platonic reversal, therefore, we can speak of the dream as the *semblance of the simulacrum* par excellence, wherein truth is not opposed epistemically to error, since the appearance of truthfulness cannot be determined independently of the truthfulness of appearance.[10]

I surmise that this quality of the oneiropoetic is related to a manner of behavior that some primatologists have even explained as the factor that accounts for the ascendancy of human beings in the evolutionary chain: while other species exhibit activities that we classify as play or sport, and even as tactical deception—indeed, trickery and cunning have been flagged as key aspects in the development of social cognition amongst primates—the hominid with the largest neocortex has the greatest facility to deceive.[11] What likely began as a congenital propensity to lie in order to maximize reproductive opportunities and the potential for survival mutates at the top of the biopyschosocial tree into the fanciful art of combining the credible and incredible, the willful effort to deceive the other by concealing truth in the shroud of lie, without any discernible utilitarian benefit or pragmatic advantage. This process, as Friedrich Nietzsche (1844–1900) well understood and painstakingly documented in his poetic aphorisms, is elemental to our aesthetic sensibility and the valorization of the figurative nature of truth as a mask. Particularly in the domain of literature, in the words of Maurice Blanchot (1907–2003), "deceit and mystification are not only inevitable but constitute the writer's honesty."[12] In the province of the fictive, duplicity is the very condition that facilitates sincerity.[13] With respect to this matter, we note again a crucial affinity between dreaming and writing.

The relationship between these two activities is spelled out in another comment by Blanchot on the "exactness of relation between the dreamed state and the written state": "It is not a matter of making a literary work out of nocturnal elements that have been transformed, embellished, or mimed by poetic resources.... Writing takes hold of the dream in its exteriority; the present of the dream coincides with the non-presence of writing. At least, this is the postulate of the enterprise that one could formulate in this way: I dream, therefore it is written."[14]

In Chapter 1, I will discuss this dimension of Blanchot's thought in more detail; suffice it here to record that for both Bachelard and Blanchot, the kinship between dreams and writing underscores that the texture of the latter is potentially available to all through the experience of the former. A key feature of this affiliation is brought to light by the observation of Blanchot that *the present of the dream coincides with the nonpresence of writing.*

Prima facie, this asymmetry would seem to indicate lack of coincidence. But it is precisely from the vantage point of the non-presence of the present, "the infinite presence of what remains radically absent, a presence in its presence always infinitely other, presence of the other in its alterity,"[15] that the temporal sway of the dream—the caesura of anarchic temporality, the countertime of the infinitive that is, at all times, the time of absence—is to be contemplated.[16] Thus, we can speak of the "inaccessible proximity of the image," of "pure resemblance," of "an apparition that transforms all other presents into appearances,"[17] and the time assigned to the dream—the "refusal to sleep at the heart of sleep"[18]—is a "present without duration, a presence without person, the non-presence in which no being ever arises."[19] This phenomenon, to which I refer as the *undoing of time*, will be the subject matter of the final chapter.

The directive of Bachelard is not only stylistically viable, but eminently reasonable: to write of the dream, one must just let the pen run. To follow this mandate, however, is precarious; the temptation to allow thoughts to flow unimpeded has the potential to result in idiosyncratic, if not incoherent, prose. Would the words that materialize in this manner not be, ipso facto, maximally distinctive? Would they not articulate an eccentricity that defies generalization and therefore strive to communicate what is inherently incommunicable?[20] Indeed, are they not like the dream images themselves, inimitable and uncertain meanderings amenable to metaphoric decoding, but not to systematic categorization or taxonomic classification? This denial of axiom we will accept as axiomatic.

It is worth recalling the confession of Artemidorus of Daldis (second century) in the commencement of the fourth book of the *Oneirocritica*: "I collected as many noteworthy examples as I could find and put them down in a rather random arrangement. For it was completely impossible to create a perfect whole from things so disparate in their nature or to unite them in a single entity."[21] Needless to say, what is herewith produced does not measure to the magnitude of this classic, but my own inquiry is marked similarly by a sense of randomness and indeterminacy,[22] insofar as I do not adhere to one theory or explanatory model, nor do I pretend to present a morphology of the dream phenomenon that avers to be comprehensive.[23] In his recently published *The Secret History of Dreaming*, Robert Moss coins the expression "dream archeologist" to designate

> the kind of investigator who is able to read all the clues from a scene in another time, *enter* that scene, and then bring back new discoveries that will stand up to cross-examination. While archeology is often understood to be the science of unearthing and studying antiquities, the root meaning of the word takes us deeper: it is the study of the *arche*, the first and the primal, chief and essential, things.

Moss goes on to delineate three requirements for the dream archaeologist: mastery of a panoply of sources; the ability to locate dreaming in its physical, social, and cultural contexts; and the ability to enter a different reality and experience it from inside.[24] Utilizing these criteria, what I offer in this book can be classified as a linguistic archaeology of the dream, a philosophically inflected excavation of a psychobiological phenomenon that celebrates the contingent and ambiguous as signifiers of truth that is conceived of as proportionate to, but not prescribed by nature. The dream provides an interpretive algorithm to assess the relationship of word to being that conforms neither to the familiar paradigm of idealism nor to that of realism.

I do postulate, however, that dreams have a logic of their own, a mythologic, to be exact, as I noted, and from this assumption a critical hermeneutical rule can be inferred: dreams display the concurrence of purportedly contradictory or incongruent images. Consequently, to heed the cadence of the dream, we do well to appropriate a calculus of the noncalculable, embracing the paradox (reiterated often in my work) that opposites are the same in virtue of being opposite. The flexibility and variability of this tenet ought to blunt the criticism of those who would ascribe to me some form of essentializing or totalizing. The strategy I endorse is one whose general applicability is expressed in the divergence of each particular instantiation. Following Alain Badiou, we can speak meaningfully of a universal singularity—as opposed to a singular universality—a universal that enjoins indefinite specification and is thus recurrently determined by the *infinite generic multiple* induced by the idiosyncrasies of any given situation.[25] The task of the thinker is to frame the predicative description of the singular in terms of the descriptive predication of the universal, but in such a way that the equivocal and implicative capriciousness of the former is not sublated by the univocal and deductive inescapability of the latter.

I will side with those who detect in the dream a mythopoeic propensity that cannot be subsumed under the stamp of scientific explanation, no matter how broadly the criterion of empirical data is conceived. This is not to say that I deny that the contents of the dream can be explained as neural correlates of consciousness. On the contrary, in my way of thinking, the cerebral activity of dreaming should be considered exemplary of the increased aptitude for abstraction and ratiocination that developed in the hominid brain as a consequence of the multimodal sensory integration. Through a process of evolutionary selection, this augmented apperception, enhanced intelligence, and the ensuing refinement of the nervous system formed what has legitimately been called the *numinous mind*,[26] a degree of mentation typified above all by the symbolic cognition that has endowed us with myriad incomparable traits, including the proclivity to imagine the unimaginable. The emblematic language of dreaming, likely to have originated as a mechanism of social organization aimed at the preservation of the species, becomes a pivotal feature that distinguishes apelike mentality from humanlike consciousness. The hominization of primates eventuated in increasingly complex biopsychological adaptations that bestowed on humans the mental capacity to have eidetic dreams.[27] Hence, the challenge in this book to the reduction of mindfulness to biochemical structures and electromagnetic fields emerges from the findings of neuroscience itself. The penchant to think the unthinkable should be granted as much integrity as other acts of human imagination conventionally judged to be nonpathological. The dream, it is safe to conjecture, is a "normal" psychic state—however we are to chart the parameters of normalcy—through which we gain access to the paranormal, a term that does not imply a realm outside the universe, but its edge (a theoretical, rather than a topographical taxonomy, since it is unintelligible to continue to suppose that there is a cosmic perimeter) that is apprehended apophatically through the imaginary confabulation of the margin at the center. On this score, dreams may be considered semiotic signposts that delineate the limit of semiosis; like poems, they point the way to the parting of the way.[28]

Let me conclude with a personal anecdote. In his lifetime, my father was wont to say *ḥalom ḥalamti*, "I dreamt a dream," when some anticipated celebration or commemoration would come to an end. For decades, I have mulled over the meaning of this rhetorically simple, but poetically vibrant, verbal gesture, coerced by it to contemplate the juxtaposition of passing away and the dream. What does closure disclose to us about the prospect of dreaming and the prospect of dreaming about closure? The sense of having been ensconced in a dream is enunciated from experiencing acutely the passing standstill of time and the vanishing of an incident to come that had been projected in the imagination. This sense, in turn, informs us that the time of dreaming is to be ascertained from the dreaming of time, but the dreaming of time can be calibrated only in the time of dreaming. The squaring away of this circularity, as it were, sheds light on a fundamental obscurity of the dreamtime, a perplexity that will become more palpable in the succeeding discussions.

Ḥalom ḥalamti—words that conveyed to me as a child, and even more so now as a middle-aged man, a sigh of disappointment, an intoning of the interminable termination of ambition, the end of expectation, the facet of waiting for what we cannot (and therefore, paradoxically, have no choice but to) await.[29] Recently, it occurred to me that my father's signature valediction resonates with the remark in the philosophic aside in the concluding section of the hymn *u-netanneh toqef*, attributed to the tenth-century German-Jewish martyr Amnon of Mainz,[30] recited in the solemn moment of the traditional High Holiday liturgy when God is said to arbitrate the fate of every person for the upcoming year:

adam yesodo me-afar
we-sofo le-afar
be-nafsho yavi laḥmo
mashul ke-ḥeres ha-nishbar
ke-ḥaṣir yavesh
ukhe-ṣiṣ novel
ke-ṣel over
ukhe-anan kaleh
ukhe-ruaḥ noshavet

ukhe-avaq poreaḥ
we-kha-ḥalom ya'uf
we-attah hu melekh
el ḥai we-qayyam[31]

One's foundation is from dust,
and one's end is to dust,
with one's life one brings one's bread,
one is like the pottery that is broken,
like the harvest that has dried,
like the spark that is extinguished,
like the shadow that passes,
like the cloud that vanishes,
like the wind that blows,
like the sand that is scattered,
like the dream that flies,
but you are king,
the living and everlasting God.

The fleeting nature of the dream (described in the diction of Job 20:8) is the last in a litany of allegorical tropes deployed to distinguish the transience of human life from the eternality of the divine. Bracketing the (to my ear dissonant) theocentric gist of the poem, from its majestic lyric about the evanescence of the dream we may yet elicit the insight that discerning the end is vital to fathoming the beginning. This is not to imply a closed circle wherein the one is adducible from the other in a reversible and predictable design; it presumes rather that the circle is open at both termini, revolving irreversibly and unpredictably in the steadfastness of its irresolution. But, we are left to wonder, must the dream always comport in the stipulation of what is to come? Is this provision necessary to write about dreams? And if so, is it inevitable that the hope imparted by the dream renews itself sporadically as the hope deferred perpetually? Is the possibility of a future, in other words, linked invariably to the impossibility of there being a future?

INTRODUCTION

Transcending Transcendence and the Specter of Invisibility

> The historical situation of a philosopher delimits what he can think about with certitude, but not what he can try to think about.
> —Maurice Merleau-Ponty, *The Incarnate Subject: Malebranche, Biran, and Bergson on the Union of Body and Soul*

In his philosophic exposition of the psychoanalytic hermeneutic on dreams, Paul Ricoeur (1913–2005) observed that essential to the project of Sigmund Freud (1856–1939) was the belief that "the interpretation of culture will be the great detour that will reveal the dream model in its universal significance."[1] Inverting this statement, I begin my exposé of the dreamscape with the assertion that the interpretation of dreams is a great detour that has the capacity to reveal a particular cultural model in its universal significance.[2] The manner in which the act of dreaming is interpreted may illuminate the way the interpreter comprehends human nature and being more generally. The fluctuation in our understanding of dreams and their interpretation serves as a barometer to gauge changing perceptions of the nature of reality refracted through the oneiric prism.[3] My contention is meant to contest the binary polarization of the particular and the universal, because it seems to me that the only way to avoid the equally problematic methodological extremes of essentializing contexts or contextualizing essences is to situate oneself in the middle routinely excluded by the law of the excluded middle. Political correctness notwithstanding, to declare absolutely that there are no absolutes smacks of a self-contradictory posture that is no less dogmatic in its alleged dismissal of dogmatism than the evidently dogmatic claim that there are absolutes available to human discernment. Lest there be any misunderstanding, let me state unequivocally that I am not advocating for a foundationalism of either an ontological or an epistemological sort. My point, rather, is that perspectivism—in any of its forms—cannot be cogently affirmed without negating itself, since the truth that there is no truth but from a particular perspective should itself be subject to the very criterion of perspective. As philosophers have long noted, the relativist position ensnares one in the ironic trap of pyrrhonian skepticism: to state categorically that truth is unattainable can be true only if it is false.

In the ensuing chapters, we are guided by the premise that the dream may yet persist as one of the enduring and most effective ways of defending against the ubiquity of the materialistic bias that has dominated psychophysiology and neuroscience. In his celebrated introduction to the French translation of Ludwig Binswanger's *Traum und Existenz*,[4] which appeared in 1954,[5] Foucault positions the analysis of the dream offered by Binswanger in terms of the "classical theme of the relations between imagination and transcendence" that reappears in Baruch Spinoza (1632–1677) and Nicolas Malebranche (1638–1715):

> the notion that the imagination, in its mysterious ciphers, in the imperfection of understanding, in its half-light, in the presence which it always shows forth elusively, points beyond the content of human experience, beyond even the discursive knowledge we can master, to the existence of a truth which surpasses man in all sides, yet bends towards him and offers itself to his mind in concrete species of images. The dream, like every imaginary experience, is thus a specific form of experience which cannot be wholly reconstituted by psychological analysis, one whose content points to man as transcended being. The imaginary, sign of transcendence; the dream, experience of this transcendence under the sign of the imaginary.[6]

In a second passage from the same text, Foucault remarks that "the dream, like every imaginary experience, is an anthropological index of transcendence; and in this transcendence it announces the world to man by making itself into a world.... In its anthropological significance, the history of the dream teaches us that it both reveals the world in its transcendence and modulates the world in its substance, playing on its material character."[7] Finally, in a third passage, Foucault clarifies that the transcendence of which he speaks cannot be defined in terms of the classical dichotomy of objectivity and subjectivity; it is rather the aspect in and through which the "dream discloses the original movement by which existence, in its irreducible solitude, projects itself toward a world which constitutes itself as the setting of its history."[8] I will elaborate Foucault's position in subsequent chapters, but suffice it here to stress that my consent to the portrayal of the dream as the *experience of transcendence under the sign of the imaginary* likewise does not comprise imploring the supernatural in order to flee the cognitive implications of the aforementioned naturalistic approaches to the human predicament.[9] The transcendence I associate with the dream is intertwined with the configuration of the world (and not merely in the negative sense as the otherwise than being), and hence I will not revert to the ancient view—even if it be clothed in some contemporary garb—that the dream provides a medium by which we may access an archetypal image, symbolic form, or immutable and trans-empirical essence presumed to be impervious to spatiotemporal contingencies.[10]

Traditionally, as Edith Wyschogrod (1930–2009) reminded us, spatial exteriority has been central to the notion of transcendence: "Whatever transcends, whether conceived as unlimited in the absolute sense or as unsurpassable by any other being, acquires its meaning by virtue of its elusiveness. For if the object has been attained, a limit has been transgressed. What is exterior has been incorporated into a totality and what transcends now lies elsewhere."[11] In my understanding of transcendence, I retain the qualities of elusiveness and exteriority, but reject the possibility of incorporation into a totality. Indeed, transcendence, as I regard it, precludes that possibility. There is nothing beyond nature that is not already part of nature. In the Deleuzian sense, beholden in no small measure to Spinoza,[12] we are prepared to affirm that the transcendental field, which "eludes all transcendence of the subject and of the object," is to be relocated on the "pure plane of immanence," the life that is the "immanence of immanence, absolute immanence."[13] Thus, we can think of *transcendence within the immanent*, which would preclude circumscribing immanence as *immanent to a transcendent*, that is, an "encompassing" that "is no more than a reservoir for eruptions of transcendence."[14] Since we do not accept the positing of ontologically external entities or relations, what we can assent to, at best, is a *metaphysics within physics*.[15] To speak meaningfully of transliminal experience, therefore, is to retrieve the immanent transcendence, that is, the transcendence in immanence, affirmed by Edmund Husserl (1859–1938), the periphery in virtue of which the exteriority of the immanent is configured noematically as the interiority of the transcendent,[16] the mode of belonging wherein bestowing constitutes reception,[17] the ecstatic horizon enveloped in the nonappearance of what appears within its purview as the appearance that is manifest by not appearing,[18] the essence beyond being and nonbeing in virtue of which we can appraise the engenderment of nonbeing that is, concomitantly, the denegation of being. We seem to harbor an unrivaled ability amongst sentient beings to reach with the mind the insentient fringe that exceeds conceptualization and linguistification and yet must be thought and declaimed—indeed incarnated[19]—from within the border of the conceptual and linguistic,[20] an ability that is realized peculiarly in our dreams.[21] Neurophysiologically speaking, this phenomenological surplus is both less and more than the contents of what is circumscribed at any given interval within the confines of consciousness.[22]

It may strike some readers that the notion of imaginal superfluity I am putting forward is consonant with the *saturated phenomenon* advanced by Jean-Luc Marion.[23] Undoubtedly, the former, like the latter, rests on the Husserlian distinction between an object whose intuition is contained in the concept and an event whose intuition extends beyond the concept. However, my own sense of transcendence eludes the theological import that continues to haunt Marion's thought, despite his insistence that the ontotheological conceptions of God are all idolatrous insofar as they embroil one in the false appearance of the unapparent.[24] A similar critique of Marion was offered by Calvin O. Schrag. After summarizing Marion's thought and comparing it to the negative theology of Pseudo-Dionysius, Schrag notes: "A more robust and radical notion of alterity and transcendence is thus required if one is to proceed beyond the inherent limitations in classical theism, a more radical probing of the very grammar about God, about the divine, about the holy."[25] The transcendence I affirm transcends the idea of transcendence that unfailingly entails recourse to the theopoetic imagination,[26] the figural iconization of the invisible in anthropomorphic and anthropopathic imagery.[27]

I hasten to add that the transcendence I avow should also not be interpreted atheistically, as the ineffable abyss one confronts in acknowledging that there is no God outside the cosmos, a stance that is the obverse of the theistic portrayal. Others have argued that the property of ineffability can equally describe the respective experiences of the atheist and the theist, although the experiences plainly must be differentiated—for the former, the ineffable is linked to the void, for the latter, to the plenitude of being.[28] In my estimation, there is no need to bifurcate the two; even the locution "beyond the beyond" is inappropriate,[29] since it still implies a boundary—albeit the boundary demarcated as being outside all boundaries—that must be breached. Transcendence neither is nor is not this boundary, and consequently, the theist's sense of plentitude and the atheist's sense of void need not be set in opposition. Logically, the transcendent is what is not, but this is only so because it is not what is. Metaphorically, we may construe it as the plenitudinal vacuum, swarming with the fullness of being's nothingness, the intrinsic reality that intrinsically lacks reality, the ultimate emptiness that is itself empty, even of its own emptiness, and thus the space of nonlocality that resists the reification of nothing as something or of something as nothing.[30]

To sharpen my viewpoint, let us consider the following formulation of Catherine Keller:

> it is the rhetoric of God as omnipotent Creator/Governor that belies the personal relationship with God. The language of that personal relationship—of covenant, faithfulness, and love—has borne the cross of a later language, that of the immutable omnipotence of an extrinsic transcendence. Might theology be starting to reimagine this personal relationship—not to a Superperson but to *a mystery that encompasses the personal and the impersonal*, an honest transcendence, to which we can only relate *as persons*?

Keller goes on to assert that such a "personal relationship" is not "an anthropomorphic person-to-person relationship," in which we fantasize about the divine in what she regards (focusing on some of the major symbols that have colored Christian faith and practice) as "dishonest deployments of the rhetoric of divine transcendence." The "pseudo-transcendence" of thinking about a personal relationship with the "mystery of life" in these "all-too-human images" lacks coherence, since "that which is transcendent in God is truly that which we must leave to negative theology, to the unspeakable alterity."[31] It is difficult to continue to think of *that which is transcendent in God*, and it is equally problematic to imagine a personal relationship to the mystery of life that is not an act of anthropomorphizing. Keller does emphasize that the mystery comprises the personal and impersonal. Indeed, the latter is a modality of the former. More importantly, philosophically speaking, there seems to be no reason to personalize a mystery that is described as an "unspeakable alterity." If that mystery is not personalized, I do not see how it is feasible to have a personal relationship to it. Keller seems aware of the very point I raise here when she asserts that "if we are going to go ahead and speak—as all apophatic theologians have done—then our kataphatic affirmations will need to come from the best metaphors of relationship, not the worst (the dominative, the oppressive, the patriarchal). And those metaphors, drawn from human and nonhuman life, will intensify relationship in difference and difference in relation." The alternative rhetoric of this "affirmative God-talk" is supported by a "process ontology of radical relationality."[32]

I certainly concur with much of this approach, both intellectually and morally—in my own work on the dimensions of negative theology in Jewish esotericism, I have noted the commingling of apophasis and kataphasis, the verbal acts of negation (speaking-away) and affirmation (speaking-with).[33] However, it seems difficult to validate any appeal to the "best metaphors of relationship" on the basis of an assumed divine transcendence. In the absence of such validation, it may be best to suspend all god talk, to stand nakedly (dis)embodied, stripped of word and image, before the desolateness of a nothing that is neither good nor evil because both good and evil, neither loving nor vengeful because both loving and vengeful, neither caring nor indifferent because both caring and indifferent.[34] Of the transcendent, all we can (un)say is that it is because it is not and it is not because it is. As Keller herself commented in another publication: "The only proper name for God, from the perspective of negative theology, is the infinite: a purely negative term. Theology, however, whether in scholastic sophistication or in popular religion, is perpetually tempted to mistake the infinite for the finite names and images in which we clothe it. And this is idolatry. Idolatry of a most deceptive kind, the truth made lie: we might call it *theolatry*."[35]

Along similar lines, David L. Miller has written, "Theological discourse tends to be one-sided, unambivalent, unimaginative, not poetic. It wants to aim at historical clarity and certainty. It is theistic when speaking about God and christocentric when speaking about Jesus, tending thereby, if taken literally, to be Theolatry or Jesusolatry."[36] Miller, following the lead of Stanley Hopper,[37] has emphasized that the theopoetic is a radical form of poeticizing indebted to the Heideggerian notion of truth as the unveiling (*aletheia*) that lets that which is appear as that which is. Language, the house of being, is ineluctably metaphorical. This must be thought as well from the perspective of Nietzsche's death of God, which in its most exacting sense means the subversion of any logical reasoning about God, that is, any theology. Theopoiesis thus avoids the ontotheological by deobjectifying all discourse about the divine in a manner that coheres to some degree with the apophatic tradition of naming the unnameable, the gesture of speaking-not, which is to be distinguished from not-speaking. Theology, however, always runs the risk of literalizing the metaphor and turning the figurative trope into a reified idol of veneration.

There are interesting affinities between the claims of Keller, Miller, and myself—and several other thinkers that could have been mentioned—on the place accorded the imagination in theological (mis)representation. These affinities reflect a shared understanding of idolatry as the false imaginings by which the human mind constricts the imageless one. This perspective, which in the history of Jewish thought Moses Maimonides (1138–1204) notoriously affirmed, is corroborated in Jean-Luc Nancy's observation that the true legacy of monotheism is "the fact that divine unicity is the correlate of a presence that can no longer be given in this world but rather must be sought beyond it (the presence in this world being that of an 'idol,' the rejection of which is no doubt the great generation and federating motif of the threefold Abrahamic traditions)."[38] Viewing the matter in this way leads to the disquieting claim that "monotheism is in truth atheism," which is to say, the aniconic ramification of the monotheistic creed is the undoing and demythologization of theism.[39] As Nancy puts it elsewhere:

> the unique *thēos*, deprived of appearance [*figure*] and name, really represents an invention, even the invention, of "god" in general. There is neither "the god" nor "the divine," not even perhaps "the gods": these do not come first or, again, they do not quite exist so long as there are the people or the species of immortal figures.... We must therefore suppose that the invention of "atheism" is contemporaneous and correlative with the invention of "theism." Both terms, in effect, have their unity in the principal paradigm or premise [*paradigme principiel*].[40]

A comparable point seems to underlie Miller's more recent attempt to distinguish "theopoetry" from "theopoetics" on the grounds that the former is the "poeticizing of an extant religious faith or theological knowledge," whereas the latter refers to "strategies of human signification in the absence of fixed or ultimate meanings accessible to knowledge or faith," a "reflection on poiesis, a formal thinking about the nature of the making of meaning" that is "severed from any dependencies on transcendental referents," a "radicalized poetics in the face of nothingness, i.e., the no-thingness of ultimate reality."[41] The epochal duty before us is not to expand the analogical imagination in envisioning transcendence—in Freudian terms, we must cease idealizing the father in the image of ourselves, to which we might add that the problem has only been amplified by idealizing the mother in an incontestably noble effort to redress gender imbalance by positing images of the feminine to signify the heterogeneity intended to liberate transcendence from a dominative and homogenous masculinity[42]—but to overcome it, to rid monotheism not only of the psychological tug to personify the impersonal, but also of what Henry Corbin (1903–1978) called the "pious illusion of negative theology" and the pitfall of "metaphysical idolatry."[43]

The exigency of the moment—to subjugate the theistic personification of God and the corresponding egoistic depiction of self[44]—demands a sweeping and uncompromising purification of the idea of the infinite from all predication, including the ecological tendency to deify the cosmos in incarnational language as the embodiment of the transcendent. If, as Miller argues, theopoetics begins at the terminus where theology ends, then the term can still be meaningful, but it seems to me that it is prone to its own idolization, insofar as a radical poeticizing remains dialectically entwined with theological pronouncements. The power of the theopoetic as an apophatic utterance, an appraisal of allegorical dissimilarity, derives from the assertion of nothing-to-assert, but it is an assertion, nonetheless. What is necessary, although by no means easy, is the termination of all modes of representation, even the representation of the nonrepresentable, a heeding of silence that outstrips the atheological as much as the theological, the saying of an unsaying that thinks transcendence as the other beyond theism and atheism.[45] I concur with the gloss of Maurice Merleau-Ponty (1908–1961) on the assertion of Jean-Paul Sartre (1905–1980), "the foundation of the negation is negation of negation,"[46] that "nothingness hollows itself out and fills itself. A philosophy that really thinks negation, that is, that thinks it as what is not through and through, is also a philosophy of Being."[47] Inasmuch as negation constitutes itself as lack, we escape the binary of being and nothingness, "because dualism has been pushed so far that the opposites, no longer in competition, are at rest the one against the other, coextensive with one another."[48] And yet, to poeticize from this spot of "absolute negativity" that is at the same time "absolute positivity"—what Nietzsche called the "deeper cave" within the cave, the "abysmally deep ground behind every ground"[49] that undermines any attempt to substantiate the beliefs we hold to be true—is itself a manner of figuration that should be subject to iconoclastic revision. In the judicious assessment of Ludwig Wittgenstein (1889–1951), "All that philosophy can do is to destroy idols. And that means not creating a new one—say on the 'absence of an idol.'"[50] And here we do well to recall the observation of Gilles Deleuze (1925–1995) that negative theology "combines the negative method with the affirmative, and claims to go beyond both.... Negative theology can therefore only be defined by its dynamics: one goes beyond affirmations in negations, and beyond both affirmations and negations in a shadowy eminence."[51] Beyond affirmation and negation, even the affirmation in negation—this is the mandate before us, to rebuff the atheological as well as the theological, to implement the apophasis of apophasis by not speaking about that of which we cannot speak, not even our inability not to speak, because this, too, has become quite tiresome.

The postheistic orientation I affirm may also be branded *postmetaphysical* and *postfoundational*.[52] I do not assume a transcendental subjectivity, an ipseity unattainable in its hyperessentiality, but somehow superintending the creation and looking over the affairs of humanity, a being beyond being that is the ground of all beings, no *parousia* of which to speak,[53] no metaphysical presence—even the presence of absence, the absent presence—that is deemed necessary to account for the appearance of what is designated "reality."[54] Thinking in the wake of Nietzsche's critique of metaphysical substantialism, Wyschogrod astutely noted that transcendence can no longer connote a "referring term—that is, the notion that 'something' transcends or that this 'something' can be interpreted as having causal efficacy." Rather it is a "*post hoc* constitution," and thus can be labeled—in the sense used by Martin Heidegger (1889–1976), Emmanuel Levinas (1906–1995), and Jacques Derrida (1930–2004)—as a trace that portends "the disappearance of the origin through a reciprocal, back-and-forth oscillation which permits the emergence of both trace and origin. . . . [I]n the dialectic of trace and origin the moment of reciprocal constitution is a non-event . . . as such it can never become the object of thought."[55] There is no need, therefore, to posit a gift of a pure and simple bestowal (the given-being of the being-given)[56] issuing from an invisible source hypothetically crossing the domain of the visible, an ontic irruption of the atemporal and aspatial that is cast theologically as an epiphany.[57] The force of life (for want of a more suitable term) must be assigned the quality of givenness that involves—by the being of its logic and the logic of its being—the reciprocity of the given and the giving.[58] Nonetheless, exactly because this is the case, there can be no compelling reason to deduce that there is a gift, and in the absence of a gift, there is no need to posit one who gives, even if it be admitted that the giver is freed from the constraints of being. No rationale dictates that we speak of this givenness as the gift of divine creation, and surely no justification exists to postulate an experience of revelation by means of which one could chance upon a transcendent being in the phenomenal sphere of becoming.[59]

I acquiesce to the phenomenological truism that perceptual experience consists of the apprehension of things in the *manner of their givenness*—an "epistemological category," as Wilfrid Sellars (1912–1989) critically noted, invoked "to explicate the idea that empirical knowledge rests on a 'foundation' of noninferential knowledge of matter of fact."[60] For if things were not so given, how could we experience or know them? Nevertheless, this self-presenting of what there is (not that there is either a "self" or a "what" of which to speak outside the parameters of human cogitation) is better left nameless, not because it is something beyond language, but because it is neither being nor nothing and therefore not susceptible to being named or interrogated.[61] The "indeterminateness of being" is the "impersonal anonymous residue" that wells up in the occlusion of all beings, akin to the *es gibt* of Heidegger or the *il y a* of Levinas,[62] the unconcealment of the concealed in the revealing of what is destined to be other than what is,[63] the withholding-projection of existence without existents,[64] the saying that cannot be absorbed by the said or the non-said.[65] The infinitation of transcendence is expressive of a "nonintentional intentionality" that is generative of intentional consciousness, but is itself without intentional correlate,[66] and therefore it does not sanction—indeed, it stubbornly spurns—the showing of the face in the world of phenomena, unless we think of this showing as an a/theophany or a disfiguration, the nonappearing of the aniconic, utterly singular, alterity or radical otherness.[67] In line with the longstanding aniconism of the Jewish tradition, Levinas privileges the auditory over the ocular, and hence, in language that overtly vilifies the incarnational foundation of Christian logocentrism, he notes that "the real presence of the other... is fulfilled in the act of hearing, and derives its meaning from the role of transcendent origin played by the word that is offered. It is to the extent that the word refuses to become flesh that it assumes a presence amongst us."[68] The face of the other, which is manifest in the voice that comes from "another shore," teaches about transcendence, the "presence of infinity breaking the closed circle of totality."[69] Transcendence, therefore, is a "total alterity" that "does not shine forth in the *form* by which things are given to us," and as such, it is "the vision of the very openness of being" (*la vision de l'ouverture elle-même de l'être*) that "cuts across the vision of forms and can be stated neither in terms of contemplation nor in terms of practice. It is the face; its revelation is speech" (*Elle est visage; sa révélation est parole*)."[70] Whereas vision is "essentially an adequation of exteriority with interiority," the "exteriority of discourse cannot be converted into interiority. The interlocutor can have no place in an inwardness; he is forever outside."[71]

I do not think it is either obligatory or justified to conceive of this face in ethical terms so that the "unknown God" might be severed from a "wordless, negative theology."[72] Levinas insists that the "original ethical signifying of the face," which is embodied in the twin commandments of the love of God and the love of one's neighbor, is "without any metaphor or figure of speech, in its rigorously proper meaning—the transcendence of a God not objectified in the face in which he speaks; a God who does not 'take on body,' but who approaches precisely through this relay to the neighbor—binding men among one another with obligation, each one answering for the loves of all the others."[73] Despite the lofty ambition underlying Levinas's plea, the correlation of alterity and transcendence in the manner he conceives it is already too much of an effacement of the nonphenomenalizable, too much figuring of the unfigurable, too much of a risk of making the anti-idolatry of formlessness into a form of idolatry[74] by incarnating the disincarnate[75] and ascribing interest to the disinterestedness of what is ostensibly beyond being.[76] That Levinas was aware of this possible pitfall is most strikingly attested in the section called "The Metaphysical and the Human" in *Totality and Infinity*:

> To relate to the absolute as an atheist is to welcome the absolute purified of the violence of the sacred. . . . Only an atheist being can relate himself to the other and already *absolve himself* from this relation. Transcendence is to be distinguished from a union with the transcendent by participation. The metaphysical relation, the idea of infinity, connects with the noumenon which is not a numen. This noumenon is to be distinguished from the concept of God possessed by the believers of positive religions ill disengaged from the bonds

> of participation, who accept being immersed in a myth unbeknown to themselves. The idea of infinity, the metaphysical relation, is the dawn of a humanity without myths. But faith purged of myths, the monotheist faith, itself implies metaphysical atheism.[77]

In a manner similar to the view of Nancy mentioned above, Levinas asserts that the "monotheist faith" (*la foi monothéiste*), if truly faithful, must eradicate all vestiges of myth, and hence, ironically enough, it implies a metaphysical atheism (*l'athéisme métaphysique*).[78] In what strikes the ear as utopian enthusiasm,[79] Levinas characterizes the idea of infinity, the underpinning for the metaphysical relation, which is contrasted with the God of positive religions, as the *dawn of a humanity without myths*. Following the correlative dialogic of Hermann Cohen (1842–1918), Martin Buber (1878–1965), and Franz Rosenzweig (1887–1929), moreover, Levinas writes that revelation is "discourse," which requires a "separated being" as the interlocutor. "To hear the divine word," accordingly, "does not amount to knowing an object; it is to be in relation with a substance overflowing its own idea in me.... Discourse, which is at the same time foreign and present, suspends participation and, beyond object-cognition, institutes the pure experience of the social relation, where a being does not draw its existence from its contact with the other." The emphasis on the social relation is meant to highlight that the "dimension of the divine opens forth from the human face," and thus it is a "relation with the Transcendent free from all captivation by the Transcendent" (*Une relation avec le Transcendant—cependant libre de toute emprise du Transcendant*).[80]

With this turn to the ethical, we can appreciate better the link between monotheism and atheism: "The atheism of the metaphysician means, positively, that our relationship with the Metaphysical is an ethical behavior and not theology, not a thematization, be it a knowledge by analogy, of the attributes of God." Levinas is willing, therefore, to depict the "total Transcendence of the other" as "the invisible but personal God" (*le Dieu invisible, mais personnel*).[81] The possibility of an invisible being is plausible, but it is not easy to conjure the notion of a personal being that is invisible unless one resorts to the spiritual entities in the Neoplatonic cosmology that would embroil Levinas in an ontotheological conception of the Infinite he sought to avoid in affirming an inapparent illeity, the "event of being" (*l'événement d'être*) that "passes over to what is other than being" (*l'autre de l'être*), "being's other," the "otherwise than being" (*autrement qu'être*), which is the "very difference of the *beyond*, the difference of transcendence," the "third" that is no longer subject to the polarity of being and not-being because it is "beyond the opposition of ipseity and alterity."[82]

I understand full well that the trope of invisibility is used by Levinas, as he writes in *Otherwise Than Being*, to depict the nonpresence and unrepresentable nature of the Good[83] and to enunciate the fact that subjectivity—the incomparable unicity of self that withdraws from essence and thus is without the identity of an ego coinciding with itself[84]—is irreducible to consciousness and to thematization. Proximity, therefore, is "the relationship with the other, who cannot be resolved into 'images' or be exposed in a theme.... Not able to stay in a theme, not able to appear, this invisibility which becomes contact and obsession is due not to the nonsignifyingness of what is approached, but to a way of signifying quite different from that which connects exposition to sight." Signification, accordingly, relates to the characteristic of transcendence beyond visibility, which is expressed in the "surplus of responsibility" that one must bear for the other, the "very signifyingness of signification, which signifies in saying before showing itself in the said" (*la significance meme de la signification laquelle signifie dans le Dire avant de se montrer dans le Dit*).[85] While I appreciate that the other cannot be "tamed" or "domesticated" thematically, I am not convinced that this notion of invisible subjectivity—the face of the neighbor always "escapes representation" inasmuch as it "is the very collapse of phenomenality" (*la defection meme de la phénoménalité*) and hence the disclosing thereof is an abandoning of self (*abandon de soi*) that is "more naked than nudity," the caressing of the skin that is the "divergency between the visible and the invisible, quasi-transparent, thinner than that which would still justify an expression of the invisible by the visible"[86]—is sustainable as a foundation for the ethical relationship as described by Levinas. The "glory of the Infinite" to be staged in the social domain implies that transcendence, the beyond essence, is concurrently a being-in-the-world (*A la transcendance—à l'au-delà de l'essence qui est aussi être-au-monde*),[87] but the diachronic nature of transcendence nevertheless necessitates that it "is not convertible into immanence."[88] Analogously, the *invisible, but personal God* is separate from and yet cannot be approached outside of "human presence"—indeed, the divine is accessible only in the pursuit of justice, the "uprightness of the face to face," and hence ethics is identified as the "spiritual optics"—and yet it cannot be reduced to a fabrication of human consciousness. It is from this standpoint that Levinas claims that the "Transcendent, infinitely Other, solicits us and appeals to us.... The Other is not the incarnation of God, but precisely by his face, in which he is disincarnate, is the manifestation of the height in which God is revealed."[89]

The insistence that God is inextricably bound to the interhuman makes it difficult, if not well-nigh implausible, to separate the theocentric and anthropocentric dimensions of the Levinasian project. Thus, Levinas speculates about "an invisible, unthematizable God, who expresses himself in this face and for whom my responsibility for the other bears witness without referring to a previous perception." The invisible God cannot be considered a term in a relationship, since it is Infinite, but Levinas is nonetheless willing to say that one is "destined" to this God "by a non-intentional thought which no preposition in our language—not even the *à* [unto] to which we resort here—could translate the devotion."[90] The tension of which I speak comes to a head in Levinas's contention that the Infinite "speaks" (*il parle*), followed by the disclaimer that "he does not have the mythical format that is impossible to confront."[91] In my judgment, to allege that the Infinite speaks,[92] let alone solicits and appeals to human beings, is to implicate the Infinite in the very myth making that Levinas tries to avoid. And surely, even though the image of the face, to which I alluded above, is meant to intimate—based exegetically on Levinas's reading of the exchange between God and Moses in Exodus 33:20–23—an alterity that cannot be known or named, the "wholly open" that "is in the trace of illeity,"[93] that which "is beyond the visible that offers itself to our gaze, or to the power of representation,"[94] it is nevertheless a mode of personifying infinity that assaults the neutrality and incommensurability of otherness. Simply put, the disclosure of the transcendence in any form of revelatory giving[95] suggests that the mind submits in the end to imaging the unimaginable, rather than remaining silent in apophatic unknowing and aporetic suspension.[96]

In contrast to Levinas, therefore, we will entertain in our analyses of the dream the notion of a transcended transcendence dis(en)closed as pure immanence within the visual field, whence everything in its nothingness manifests the nothingness that is everything.[97] The transcending of transcendence endorsed here is also to be distinguished from the similar expression used by Jean Wahl, an important source of inspiration for Levinas.[98] According to Wahl, there is a form of transcendence (or, to be more precise, *transdescendence*, as opposed to *transascendence*) that is a movement "directed toward immanence, whereby the transcendence transcends itself [*lorsque la transcendance se transcende elle-même*]. Perhaps the greatest transcendence is that which consists of transcending the transcendence, that is to say, of falling back into immanence [*Peut-être la plus grande transcendance est-elle celle qui consiste à transcender la transcendance, c'est-à-dire à retomber dans l'immanence*]." To transcend transcendence, paradoxically, affirms and negates transcendence, indeed affirms it by negating it and negates it by affirming it. The attainment of the "second immanence" appears "after the destroyed transcendence" (*après la transcendance détruite*), but that transcendence "is never completely destroyed, never completely transcended," and hence it is described as resting in the "background of spirit like the idea of a lost paradise," the bereavement for which generates the hope and longing for a presence that constitutes the "value of our attachment to the here-below."[99] Immanence in the here-below is valorized as something positive, therefore, only insofar as it points to the absolute, nameless one, the mystery that transcends all existing realities in the world. Utilizing another terminological distinction made by Wahl, we can differentiate between the "transcendent immanence of perception" (*l'immanence transcendante de la perception*) and the "immanent transcendence of ecstasy" (*la transcendance immanente de l'extase*). The former is correlated with the silence of positive ontology "in which the mind is nourished by things," and the latter with the silence of negative ontology, the "mystical event," wherein the "mind achieves union with its own highest point, which is at the same time the highest point of the world."[100] This highest point, wherein objectivity and subjectivity converge in their mutual dissolution, leads one dialectically to the self-transcending transcendence, the transcendence that transcends and thereby preserves itself in the immanence that is the web of interrelational entities. As Deleuze and Guattari correctly observed, the immanence in Wahl's thinking, as in that of religious authority more generally, can be compared to a "terraced fountain where water can briefly immanate on each level but on condition that it comes from a higher source and falls lower down."[101] Conversely, when I speak of transcending transcendence, there is a full embrace of immanence that has no recourse to any trace of an unknowable transcendence from a higher source. This does not require an agency of gifting, only an event of giving that yields apperception of the energy streams or wave packets (in the current quantum idiom) cohering extensively in space and intensively in time.[102] To be divested of the fideism that has triggered the return to religiosity in contemporary philosophy is, as Quentin Meillassoux has observed, to think the eventual in its absoluteness, that is, etymologically speaking, to conceive of the event absolved from all dependency, to ponder the plausibility of "a world without the givenness of the world," "to break with the ontological requisite... according to which *to be is to be a correlate*." The task, accordingly, would consist "in trying to understand how thought is able to access the uncorrelated, which is to say, a world capable of subsisting without being given."[103]

An equivalent approach can be detected in Badiou's claim that "appearance" denotes the being-there of beings "caught in a situated relational network," whereas "transcendental" is to be applied to the "operational set which allows us to give meaning to the 'more or less' of identities and differences in a determinate world."[104] It is not philosophically requisite to posit a consciousness or subject "in order to testify that beings are obliged to appear—to be there—under the logic of a world." Appearance is "imposed upon beings to guarantee their being once it is acknowledged that the Whole is impossible: beings must always manifest themselves locally, and there can be no possibility of subsuming the innumerable worlds of this manifestation. The logic of a world is what regulates this necessity, by affecting a being with a variable degree of identity (and therefore of difference) relative to the other beings of the same world." There must be a "scale"—the *transcendental of the situation*—that allows for an evaluation of identities and differences, and thus, "a being can only exist in a world in so far as it is indexed to this transcendental." We can speak, therefore, of the "transcendental organization" that "fixes the moving singularity of the being-there of a being in a determinate world."[105] One can argue, moreover, that the thought of being-there necessarily includes the possibility of not-being-there, and this implies that "the consistency of appearance requires there to be a transcendental marking, or a logical mark, of non-appearance. The possibility of thinking non-appearance rests on this marking, which is the intra-worldly index of the not-there of a being."[106] Badiou promotes an atheist ontology according to which transcendence is the semantic tag to name the groundwork for a radical this-worldliness.[107]

Aligning Badiou with the description of Derridean deconstruction, we can speak of the "movement of 'transcendence'... a passion for transgression, a passion for trespassing the horizons of possibility... provoked by the promise, impregnated by the impossible, hoping in a certain messianic promise of the impossible."[108] Instead of treating the possible and impossible as antinomical, we must be attuned to the possibility of the impossible, the possibility that is in no other way possible but as impossible, an unconditional opening to a future that is inherently undecidable and indeterminate, a future that issues from the negative infinity of time. Contrary to the attempts to discern a religious turn in Derrida's thinking or to utilize his thought to buttress a religion beyond religion, the promise of the messianic without messianism that he affirms is by his own admission a decidedly "atheological heritage";[109] the hope connected to the promise stems structurally from the infinite negativity of time, the impossible possibility that makes it always possible that the future that is coming (*à-venir*) threatens not to be that for which one has hoped.[110]

Together with Merleau-Ponty, the invisible of which I speak is not to be understood as "an object hidden behind another, and not an absolute invisible, which would have nothing to do with the visible. Rather it is the invisible *of* this world, that which inhabits this world, sustains it, and renders it visible, its own and interior possibility, the Being of this being."[111] Following this computation, the universe can be envisaged chiasmically as the invisibly visible specter of the visibly invisible, provided that invisibility is not construed in substantialist terms,[112] whether understood innately or relationally. For it is not a something (or, for that matter, a nothing) with or without essential or accidental properties, but rather the nonphenomenalizability that is the epistemic condition of all phenomenality, the unseeing that enframes every act of seeing, the negative ideal of irreducibility that positivizes the recurrent patterns and perspectival mutations that shape the sensible world of human experience reckoned quantifiable by natural sciences in an effort to compress the flux of our synergic and synthetic perceptions into a "monocular image" of a "focused whole."[113] Analogous to the revision of the Lacanian idea of the Real proffered by Slavoj Žižek, or what he calls the *parallax Real*,[114] the invisible does not signify a transcendent reality, but the principle of falsification of any such reality:

> the disavowed X on account of which our vision of reality is anamorphically distorted; it is simultaneously the Thing to which direct access is not possible *and* the obstacle which prevents this direct access, the Thing which alludes our grasp *and* the distorting screen which makes us miss the Thing.... What this means, ultimately, is that the status of the Real is purely parallactic and, as such, nonsubstantial: it has no substantial density in itself, it is just a gap between two points of perspective, perceptible only in the shift from the one to the other.[115]

The invisible, accordingly, is not an excess of the real, the limitless positivity of the possible impossibility positioned outside the symbolic, but rather the signifier of lack, the delimited negativity of the impossible possibility inherent in the symbolic.[116] The real, if we continue to avail ourselves of this nomenclature, is sustained by the multitude of appearances it maintains by disrupting them repeatedly, rendering them visible in their invisibility and invisible in their visibility, without, however, professing the existence of a noumenal core that persists as the same beneath the semblance of the phenomenal—no face behind the mask that is not itself a mask.[117] By the same logic, there is no summoning of the supranatural or metaphysically transcendent in the elucidation of dreams presented in this book.

CHAPTER ONE

Imagining Otherwise: Oneiropoiesis and the Randomness of Mind

> But the time comes when dream must be measured by dream and revelation by revelation, and all tested by a total human experience.
> —Amos Wilder, *Theopoetic: Theology and the Religious Imagination*

In the opening section of *The Birth of Tragedy* (1871), Nietzsche asserts that the continuous development of art is dependent on the "perpetual strife" and periodic "intervening reconciliation" of the dual impulses of order and chaos, which are linked respectively to the dreaming of Apollo and the intoxication of Dionysius. Building on the ideas of previous thinkers as diverse as Lucretius (ca. 99 b.c.–55 b.c.), Arthur Schopenhauer (1788–1860), and Richard Wagner (1813–1883), Nietzsche emphasizes the connection between the creative inclination (manifest paradigmatically in poetry) and the dream imagination. It is in virtue of the "illusion" (*Schein*) of the dreamworlds—a quality accentuated both by the etymology of the name Apollo as the "shining one" (*der Scheinende*)[1] and by the image of the Apollonian mask through which the appearance (*Erscheinung*) of the Sophoclean hero was projected unto a dark wall[2]—that every person can be considered an artist. "In our dreams we delight in the immediate understanding of figures; all forms speak to us; there is nothing unimportant or superfluous. But even when this dream reality is most intense, we still have ... the sensation that it is *mere appearance* ... and for its frequency—indeed, normality—I could adduce many proofs, including the saying of the poets."[3] Just as a criterion of the philosophical presentiment is to view reality as appearance, so a mark of the aesthetic sensibility is to consider dreams a key to interpreting life. The emphasis on the dream, moreover, is meant to overcome the traditional metaphysical hierarchy, to accord primacy to the image over the real, to unsettle the all-too-typical preference for the waking state by depicting the dream as the vehicle that gives us access to the "mysterious ground of our being."[4] The dreamer, like the poet, views metaphor not simply as a "rhetorical figure" to depict an inaccessible reality that lies beneath or beyond appearance, but as the "vicarious image" through which reality is exposed as the (dis)semblance that it really is;[5] the dream, exemplified by Apollo—the "deity of light," who "rules over the beautiful illusion of the inner world of fantasy," the "glorious divine image of the *principium individuationis*"[6]—is the experience of knowing that one's experience is not metaphysically real, since there is nothing but appearance.[7] The point is conveyed by Nietzsche's account of the phenomenon that is currently referred to as "lucid dreaming":

> Let us imagine the dreamer: in the midst of the illusion of the dream world and without dreaming it, he calls out to himself: "It is a dream, I will dream on." What must we infer? That he experiences a deep inner joy in dream contemplation; on the other hand, to be at all able to dream with this inner joy in contemplation, he must have completely lost sight of the waking reality and its ominous obtrusiveness.[8]

The desire to keep the dream going signals "an ardent longing for illusion," the human yearning for "redemption through illusion" by which one is "impelled to the metaphysical assumption that the truly existent primal unity, eternally suffering and contradictory, also needs the rapturous vision, the pleasurable illusion, for its continuous redemption." Inasmuch as the phenomenal world is perceived "as a continuously manifested representation of the primal unity," the dream will be looked upon "as a *mere appearance of mere appearance*," and thus it is "a still higher appeasement of the primordial desire for mere appearance."[9] The doubling of illusion constitutes as well the "ineffable joy" experienced by the artist.

In the aphorism "Dreams and culture" from *Human, All Too Human* (1878), Nietzsche elaborates on the matter of the dream:

> The brain function most impaired by sleep is memory: not that it completely pauses—but it is returned to a state of imperfection, as

> may have been the case for everyone in primeval times of humanity, even during the day and while awake. Capricious and confused as it is, it continually mistakes things on the basis of the most fleeting similarities: but with the same caprice and confusion peoples composed their mythologies.... But in dreaming we all resemble this savage; failing to recognize things and erroneously equating them are the reasons for the bad inferences that we are guilty of making in dreams; so that whenever we call a dream clearly to mind, we frighten ourselves, because so much folly lies hidden within us.—The perfect clarity of all dream representations, which presupposes an unconditional belief in their reality, reminds us again of the conditions of an earlier humanity, in whom hallucination was exceptionally frequent and sometimes seized upon whole communities, whole peoples at the same time. Therefore: in sleep and dreams we go through the lessons of earlier humanity once again.[10]

Significantly, for Nietzsche, the clarity of dream images, which is computed by an unconditional belief in their reality, is reminiscent of, and in fact provides the mechanism to retrieve, a more primitive layer of human existence, the savage state, wherein hallucinations were accorded the same unassailability as sense perceptions. The "origin of all metaphysics" lies in this ability of people living in the "ages of raw, primordial culture" to believe that "in dreams they came to know a *second real world*." For without dreams, "there would have been no reason to divide the world. The separation into soul and body is also connected to the oldest view of dreams, just like the assumption that the soul can appear in bodily form, hence the origin of all belief in ghosts, and probably also the belief in gods."[11] With predictable brilliance, Nietzsche goes on to say that the *logic of dreams*, whence the distinction between the being of invisible reality and the image of visible appearance came about, persists as the primal mode of thinking that undergirds what he considers to be the more chronologically advanced forms of reasoning: "While we are dreaming, this primeval piece of humanity continues to exercise itself in us, for it is the foundation upon which a higher reason was developed and is still developing in every human being: dreams take us back to the distant circumstances of human culture and give us the means for understanding them better."[12]

Dreaming and the Irreality of the Real

Freud, it will be recalled, gave credit to Nietzsche's depiction of the dream as a path leading to knowledge of humanity's archaic heritage when discussing his own conception of the regressive potential of dreams and neuroses.[13] Moreover, Freud also seems to have appropriated Nietzsche's insight that this primitive mental state, wherein fiction and fact merge, is central to the poet and to the artist. The link between dream and poiesis will be discussed in greater detail below, but suffice it here to note that Freud's genealogy of culture is indebted to the naturalistic and demystifying hermeneutics of Nietzsche[14] and that for both men, dreaming occupies the psychogenic space wherein it becomes epistemologically difficult, if not impossible, to distinguish fantasy from reality: the real is ascertained by the image of what is conceived to be real, and thus the susceptibility for hallucination is sanctioned as the possibility of there being consciousness of the irreal (*irréel*) without any ontology of the unreal, since an ontology of the unreal would perforce be unreal and thus lacking consciousness of anything but the reality of its unreality.[15] Alternatively expressed, the unreal is a negation of the real, that is, the determinate particularity that may be real, but is presently not so, whereas the irreal is the inchoate particularity that is at no time either real or unreal—this is the philosophical import of Nietzsche's depiction of Apollo as the principle of individuation.

We can distinguish between a "real" dream and an "imagined" one, that is, a dream that I have imagined in fact and a dream that I have only imagined to have imagined, but the veracity of the former is not substantively different from the duplicity of the latter.[16] Thus, Jennifer Windt and Thomas Metzinger, responding to Norman Malcolm's well-known challenge concerning the experiential character of dreams,[17] remarked:

> dreams are conscious experiences because they can be described as the appearance of an integrated, global model of reality within a virtual window of presence. From a purely phenomenological perspective, dreams are simply the *presence of a world*.... And even though it is a model constructed by the dreaming brain, it is not recognized as a model but is experienced as reality itself. Put in philosophical terms, one can say that the reality model created by the dreaming

> brain is phenomenally transparent; the fact that it is a model is invisible to the experiential subject.[18]

Truth and falsehood are retroactive value judgments that apply respectively to what we consider to be real and unreal, but they are irrelevant with regard to the immediacy of the irreal as such.

A similar sentiment, albeit in a different linguistic attire, was expressed by Søren Kierkegaard (1813–1855) in his enunciation, based on the account of the certainty of sensuous knowledge discussed in the first part of the *Phenomenology of Spirit* by Georg Wilhelm Friedrich Hegel (1770–1831),[19] of the inherent contradiction of the consciousness of doubt in the pseudonymous treatise *Johannes Climacus, or De omnibus dubitandum est*:

> *Immediacy* is precisely *indeterminateness*. In immediacy there is no relation, for as soon as there is a relation, immediacy is canceled. *Immediately, therefore, everything is true*, but this truth is untruth the very next moment, *for in immediacy everything is untrue*. If consciousness can remain in immediacy, then the question of truth is canceled. How does the question of truth arise? By way of untruth, because the moment I ask about truth, I have already asked about untruth. In the question of truth, consciousness is brought into relation with something else, and what makes this relation possible is untruth.[20]

In the continuation of this discussion, Kierkegaard correlates immediacy with reality, mediacy with the word, and consciousness with the contradiction that necessarily arises from the relationship between them. "The moment I make a statement about reality, contradiction is present, for what I say is ideality. The possibility of doubt, then, lies in consciousness, whose nature is a contradiction that is produced by a duplexity [*Dupplicitet*] that itself produces a duplexity."[21] What the nineteenth-century Danish thinker called "reality" as opposed to "ideality"—related to the Hegelian distinction[22] between particularity and universality—corresponds to what I have designated (on the basis of the phenomenological lexicon) "irreality." Overlooking the semantic disparity, the common point is that human language is a form of mediation that cancels the immediacy of our sense experience—by presupposing and giving expression to it—and thus guarantees that what I will say is necessarily something different from what I intended to say;[23] any venture toward verbalization occasions a clash between the real and the ideal, the particular and the universal, and, ipso facto, transposes every statement of truth into an untruth. The dream, by contrast, is a manner of consciousness that perpetually stays open to the immediate because the duplexity of which it singularly partakes, *the duplexity that produces duplexity*, precludes any friction between actual and fantastical. Dreaming, therefore, can be thought of as a genre of imaginality in which the image is manifest by concealing its character as image.[24]

Apropos of this discussion, it is germane to bear in mind that in *An Essay Concerning Human Understanding*, John Locke (1632–1704) articulated what may still be considered the commonsensical view as support of his empiricist contention that we can distinguish between an idea revived in our minds through memory and an idea received in our minds on the basis of sense experience:

> If any one say, "A dream may do the same thing, and all these ideas may be produced in us without any external objects," he may please to dream that I make him this answer: (1.) That it is no great matter whether I remove his scruple or no: where all is but dream, reasoning and arguments are of no use, truth and knowledge nothing. (2.) That I believe he will allow a very manifest difference between dreaming of being in the fire, and being actually in it. But yet if he be resolved to appear so skeptical as to maintain, that what I call "being actually in the fire" is nothing but a dream; and that we cannot thereby certainly know that any such thing as fire actually exists without us; I answer that, we certainly finding that pleasure or pain follows upon the application of certain objects to us, whose existence we perceive, or dream that we perceive, by our senses: this certainty is as great as our happiness or misery, beyond which we have no concernment to know or to be.[25]

Acknowledging that some individuals would reject the privileging of sentient experience based on the presence of external objects impinging on the senses by appeal to the fact that similar sensations accrue in the dream, Locke offers a two-pronged argument to defend the empirical perspective: first, if all is but a dream, then reason is of no avail and the very criteria to establish truth and knowledge are undermined; second, the skepticism that would deny the difference, for instance, between dreaming that one is in a fire and the experience of actually being in a fire is itself weakened by the fact that the measure of our judgment is determined ultimately by the pleasure or pain consequent to our experiences. Returning to this point in another passage of the same book, Locke once more makes an appeal to the alleged certainty of our sense experience as contrasted to the images of the dream:

> But yet, if after all this any one will be so skeptical as to distrust his senses, and to affirm that all we see and hear, feel and taste, think and do, during our whole being, is but the series and deluding appearances of a long dream whereof there is no reality, and therefore will question the existence of all things or our knowledge of any thing; I must desire him to consider, that if all be a dream, then he doth but dream that he makes the question; and so it is not much matter that a waking man should answer him. But yet, if he pleases, he may dream that I make him this answer, that the certainty of things existing in *rerum natura*, when we have the testimony of our senses for it, is not only as great as our frame can attain to, but as our condition needs.[26]

For Locke, the skeptical position subverts itself: if one asserts that all is a dream, then this assertion is itself subject to the possibility that it is nothing more than a dream utterance. In the end, the human condition is such that the nature of things imposes the facticity of being upon us. The skeptic may contend that this, too, is a matter that is dreamt, but the certainty of the testimony of our senses is not diminished by this disbelief.

The plausibility of Locke's empiricism notwithstanding, the epistemological challenge of skepticism cannot be discarded. Commenting on the first passage of Locke cited above, Gottfried Wilhelm Leibniz (1646–1716) already observed that while the skeptic would acknowledge a difference between sensations and imaginings, "a difference in degree does not create a difference in kind." Moreover, even if we concede that "sensations are ordinarily livelier than imaginings, still we know that sometimes imaginative people are as much impressed by their imaginings as others are by the truth of things, and perhaps more so." Leibniz goes on to say that the "true criterion" for determining the efficacy of the senses is the "linking together of phenomena, i.e. the connectedness of what happens at different times and places and in the experience of different men.... And the linking of phenomena which warrants the *truths of fact* about sensible things outside us is itself verified by means of *truths of reason*, just as optical appearances are explained by geometry." Based on this criterion, Leibniz concludes that "it is not impossible, metaphysically speaking, for a dream to be as coherent and prolonged as a man's life." While this may be as "contrary to reason" as the assumption that a book of fiction is produced by the chance jumbling together of the printer's type, it is nevertheless the case that "so long as the phenomena are linked together it doesn't matter whether we call them dreams or not, since experience shows that we do not go wrong in the practical steps we take on the basis of phenomena, so long as we take them in accordance with the truths of reason."[27] As far-fetched as it may seem from the sense of reality that dominates our everydayness, dream images betray a cogency and vibrancy equivalent to, if not greater than, empirical data, a point also entertained by Thomas Hobbes (1588–1679), although he ultimately insists on the asymmetry between dreaming and waking, since while awake, one knows with certainty that one is not dreaming, but when dreaming, one may very well think that one is awake.[28]

In my judgment, this insight is not phenomenologically defensible, for a symmetrical relation between dream and wakefulness is more likely to pertain, as is attested most poignantly by the hypnagogic state that precedes sleep and the hypnopompic state that follows awakening; even so, it has been affirmed by Hobbes and others, and not limited to Western philosophy. Here I will offer an interesting illustration from the *Maggid Mesharim*, the revelatory diary of Joseph Karo (1488–1675), Safedian kabbalist, exegete, and legalist. In the introductory section, Karo's angelic mentor, the *maggid*, who is also portrayed in the same work as the personified *Mishnah* or the textually incarnate *Shekhinah*,[29] raises the following query:

> It must be asked why does a man suffer more concerning something that happens in a dream than if he saw it while awake? This is because when he is awake, the soul is clad in the body, and he does

not feel the intensity [*doḥaq*] as much, for the body is protective; but in a dream, it is naked, and the damage inflicts him and he suffers more. And thus one can comprehend in the section of *Miqqeṣ* the verse "his spirit was agitated" (Genesis 41:8).[30]

The remark is predicated on a conception well attested in, but hardly unique to, medieval kabbalistic sources—the soul is enclothed in the body. Based on older rabbinic sources,[31] moreover, kabbalists (especially conspicuous in the zoharic anthology) widely believed that nocturnal dreams could be explained by the fact that in sleep, the spirit is stripped of it corporeal armor and ascends to the divine pleroma in accord with its earthly demeanor,[32] a theme that has resonance with ancient conceptions of the dream as the means by which the soul makes contact with the incorporeal realm, such as we find in Pythagorean, Stoic, and Neoplatonic philosophies, so that the truth may be revealed.[33] Sleep, accordingly, is depicted as a partial simulation of the separation of body and soul,[34] an idea that expanded the rabbinic tradition that sleep is one-sixtieth of death.[35] On account of the nakedness associated with sleep, the pain endured in the nocturnal dream is greater than in waking reality. The scriptural proof text mentioned at the end of the citation relates that Pharaoh's spirit was agitated on the morning after he dreamt about the seven lean cows devouring the seven hefty cows on the bank of the Nile—the *spirit* was agitated, for the anguish concerns the psychic condition, and not the physical. If we were to pitch Karo's maggidic teaching in an electrophysiological tone, we could say that the decreased arousal by external sensory stimuli during sleep and the consequent inhibition and suppression of the release of thalamocortical relay neurons occasion the incitement of internal sources of stored sensorial information, and this, in turn, triggers a neuronal sensitization that allows the brain to access a more subtle level of consciousness,[36] the *realm of the imaginal*, a psychic province where, paradoxically enough, the somatic tangibility intensifies, even as the coarse materiality is eviscerated and the mental acuity grows more vivid in the muting of the empirical apparatus.

Carl Gustav Jung (1875–1961) articulated a similar sentiment, albeit without employing the technical terminology of the imaginal, the elocution made popular by Corbin,[37] that has been applied to him by various interpreters (especially due to the influence of James Hillman) based on his description of archetypes as constructs of the active imagination.[38] The unconscious, Jung argued, can be considered a speculum that "mirrors the totality of the world—a world of reflex images. Looked at from the standpoint of the conscious, this world is the reality and that the reflex. But the reflex is just as living and real, just as big and complicated. There is even the standpoint that the external world is a reflex of the unconscious."[39] In an overstated and what may strike the contemporary ear as a tendentious manner, Jung goes on to differentiate the Western (with the notable exclusion of Plato) and Eastern perspectives on the grounds that the former believes the sensible world is reality and the world of images a mirage, whereas the latter believes that the images are real, and thus what we call reality is naught but a "degenerate phantasmagoria," the "veil of Maya."[40]

In previous work, I have discussed this possibility from a varied and far more moderate hermeneutical perspective, resisting the allure of universalization and limiting my comments to what may be detected in particular textual archives. In an effort to unearth the philosophical underpinnings of the archaic mythopoeic correlation of the celestial and the terrestrial temples in ancient and medieval forms of Jewish esotericism,[41] I argued that contemporary scholars are apt to assume that those who subscribed to this belief maintained that the space above mirrors the space below, but it is not impossible logically—I would add empirically, as well, but that would demand verification using both textual and archaeological means—to invert this correspondence. Better yet would be the discernment that there is a double mirroring, a reciprocal reciprocity by which the lower appears in the image of the upper apperceived through the prism of the upper (dis)appearing as the image of the lower. Accordingly, any investigation of the phenomenon would have to be set on grounds where the binary of upper and lower, and the closely allied binary of inner and outer, are no longer presumed to be the sole arbiters of truth.

Here I wish to apply this argument to the question of the status of the image and the imagined relative to the dream. The dream image is imagined as the imagined within the strictures of the imagination. To catch the dream, as it were, we will need to go through this revolving door, entering as we exit our entering. Reversing the sequence to which we are accustomed, events brought to light in the phenomenal spacetime of the physical realm may be viewed as the effect, rather than the cause of what is experienced imaginally in the timespace of the internal drama that is the dream world. To be sure, as Homer speculated, not only are dreams hopelessly puzzling, but most people do not believe that the bulk of them have a purpose (*teleietai*). Still, he distinguished between deceptive dreams that pass through the ivory gate and veridical dreams that pass through the horn gate; the former are unfulfilled (*akraanta*), whereas the latter accomplish the truth (*etuma krainousin*).[42] The Homeric distinction, which influenced Virgil and a plethora of other pagan and Christian authors in Late Antiquity and the Middle Ages, may no longer be hermeneutically viable, but contemporary philosophical and scientific literature has affirmed this ancient notion of the dream as prognostication, if this is understood not merely as foretelling the future, but as giving shape to the reality that will come to pass.

From the perspective of a phenomenological psychology, which I still find to be a viable tool to appraise human experience, even though I cannot embrace the delineation of phenomenology as an eidetic science that deals with essential structures of intentional consciousness, it is not significant if the experienced datum is determined to be real or imaginary. The transcendental attitude is consequent to the suspension (*epochē*) of the ontological presuppositions of the natural attitude; the habitual belief in the world as an existing totality is bracketed so that the grounds for positing it may be interrogated.[43] "From the beginning," writes Husserl in a section from *The Crisis of European Sciences and Transcendental Phenomenology*, "the phenomenologist lives in the paradox of having to look upon the obvious as questionable, as enigmatic, and of henceforth being unable to have any other scientific theme than that of transforming the universal obviousness of the being of the world—for him the greatest of all enigmas—into something intelligible."[44] Restating this essential belief of transcendental phenomenology, Eugen Fink (1905–1975) noted that "the phenomenological epoché is not a method for delimiting

(*Einschränkung*) an area within the world, but is rather a method for going beyond the world by *removing limits* (*Entschränkung über die Welt hinaus*): the totality of beings signified by the title 'world' is made a problem by viewing the world as a unity of acceptances lying within the life of the reductively disclosed transcendental subjectivity."[45] When phenomena are examined from within the reduction, the very fact that something is imaginable is what matters; its ontological status as an externally existing object is completely beside the point in gauging the authenticity of what is imagined by human subjectivity.[46] In a crucial passage from the first book of *Ideas Pertaining to a Pure Phenomenology and to a Phenomenological Philosophy*, Husserl put the matter as follows:

> In the natural attitude, the apple tree is for us something existing in the transcendent realm of spatial actuality, and the perception, as well as the liking, is for us a psychical state belonging to real people.... In such situations characterizing mental processes, it may be in certain cases that perception is "mere hallucination," the perceived, this apple tree before us, does not exist in "actual" reality.... Only the perception remains, but there is nothing actual there to which it is related. Let us now go to the <transcendental> phenomenological attitude. The transcendent world receives its 'parenthesis,' we exercise the epoχή in relation to <positing> its actual being.... With the whole physical and psychical world, the actual existence of the real relation between perceiving and perceived is excluded; and, nonetheless, a relation between perceiving and perceived (as well as between liking and liked) remains left over, a relation which becomes given essentially in 'pure immanence,' namely purely on the ground of the phenomenologically reduced mental processes of perceiving and liking precisely as they fit into the transcendental stream of mental processes.... Concerning hallucinations, illusions and perceptual deception of whatever sort, it may be that phenomenology has something to say, and perhaps even a great deal; but it is evident that here, in the role which they played in the natural attitude, they undergo exclusion. Here, in the case of perception and also in the case of any progressive concatenation of perceptions whatever... there is no question to be raised of the sort whether or not something corresponds to it in "the" actuality. This posited actuality is indeed not there for us in consequence of judging.[47]

Reiterating the point in *The Crisis*, Husserl commented: "By virtue of our present method of epochē, everything objective is transformed into something subjective.... Through the radical epochē every interest in the actuality or nonactuality of the world (in all modalities, thus including the possibility and conceivability, as well as the decidability of this sort of thing) is put out of play."[48] The psychic formation, the image in consciousness, to which irreality is properly ascribed, may in fact be nonexistent.[49] The (ultimately Kantian) conviction that the "real entities" in the world are phenomena constituted as "object-poles" (*Gegenstandspole*) by the "correlative intentionalities" of a transcendental subjectivity, the intentive activity through which they attain "ontic meaning" (*Seinssinn*),[50] challenges the naïve representationalism of modern epistemology, not by affirming an antirepresentationalism, but by postulating a more subtle and sophisticated conception of the idealized construction of the essences that inform the "constituted pole" (*konstituierten Pol*) of the lifeworld (*Lebenswelt*) we inhabit as psychophysical beings.[51] As Husserl famously proclaimed, "Thus if one is fond of paradoxical phrases... one can say in strict truth, that 'feigning' [*Fiktion*] *makes up the vital element of phenomenology as of every other eidetic science*, that feigning is the source from which the cognition of 'eternal truths' is fed."[52]

The claim that *fiction* is the source whence cognition of eternal truths ensues has intensely influenced my analysis of the dream world, particularly the attentiveness to the convergence of truth and untruth—the truth of the dream cannot be isolated from its untruth, since it is true to the extent that it is not true. The matter of eternal truths holds no truth for me, but the insight of Husserl (and, more generally, the compliance to the transcendental tradition of German philosophy) still seems relevant to this limited, but significant point, as I have already noted in the Preface and to which I will return below. True existence is not determined by the correspondence of things to the intellect, but by an ongoing approximation—what Husserl intends by the "principle of correlation" (*Korrelationsprinzip*)—of the subject that constructs the object in its mode of givenness to the object constructed by the subject in its mode of bestowing. The reality of truth is thus equal to an infinite series of appearances or imaginative presentations (*Phantasievorstellungen*) that are potentially available, but never actualized, since even if one were to mount a successive viewing of the manifold perspectives, each one would reflect only one side or profile (*Aschattung*) at any given time.[53]

In more technical terms, we must distinguish noesis and noema; the former is the concrete psychic act and the latter the meaning that is assigned to it.[54] Sartre rightfully noted that the noematic correlate of our perceptual experiences is an "ideal existence" that can be depicted as "an irreality."[55] Utilizing Husserl's categories, he speaks of dream imagination in terms of the irrealizing function of noetic consciousness and of the imaginary as its noematic correlate.[56] If one insists, as Husserl did, that the structure of consciousness is intentional—to be conscious always entails being conscious of something, even if, or especially if, the latter is nothing other than the fact of being conscious—then the mental images, whether conceived on the basis of sentient experience or envisaged on the basis of imaginary confabulation, are presumed to relate to objects in the world, a process of irrealization that imposes the binary of presence and absence even within the parenthesizing of the phenomenological reduction. The irreal—in the fabrication of the oneiric situation and in the factuality of the sensory condition—can be said to be determinative of what is perceived to be real.[57]

Foucault expressed a similar conception when he noted, explicating the view of Binswanger, that "one finds, at the origin of the theme of the dream as manifestation of the soul in its inwardness, the Heraclitean principle:[58] We share a world when we are awake; each sleeper is in a world of his own."[59] The dictum of Heraclitus conveys the paradox that the world of experience is solely one's own, but still not merely subjective. In sleep, by contrast, one enters into a private sphere shaped by unique personal experiences expressive of the solitude that reinforces the elemental freedom of the human subject, a freedom that is expressed in the delimitation of the objective world:

> What constitutes the *idios kosmos* of the dreamer is not the absence of perceptual contents but their elaboration into an isolated universe. The dream world is a world of its own, not in the sense of subjective experience defying the norms of objectivity, but in the sense that it is constituted in the original mode of a world which belongs to me, which at the same time exhibiting my solitude.... The dream

> unveils, in its very principle, that ambiguity of the world which at one and the same time designates the existence projected into it and outlines itself objectively in experience. By breaking with the objectivity which fascinates waking consciousness and by reinstating the human subject in its radical freedom, the dream discloses paradoxically the movement of freedom toward the world, the point of origins from which freedom makes itself world.[60]

Extrapolating Husserl's undermining of the representational theory of perception, Foucault maintains that the dream is a way of freely being-in-the-world that is constituted necessarily as the eventual that transcends the confines of an immanent subjectivism. The dream is not, as Freud insisted, primarily about the "libidinal instinct," but rather signifies "the originative movement of freedom, the birth of the world in the very movement of existence."[61] Referring to Johann Gottfried Herder (1744–1803) and Novalis, the pseudonym of Georg Phillip Friedrich Freiherr von Hardenberg (1772–1801), Foucault further characterizes the dream as the "original moment of genesis" and thus the "primary image of poetry," the "maternal language," the excessive subjectivity that is "at the very center of becoming and objectivity."[62] In the dream, therefore, the dreamer meets "a world of his own... because he can recognize there the fact of his own destiny";[63] he "encounters what he is and what he will be, what he has done and what he is going to do, discovering there the knot that ties his freedom to the necessity of the world."[64] The supreme contradiction between freedom and necessity accounts for the juxtaposition of dream and death. Like death, the dream "at once realizes itself and denies itself as destiny," and thus it "exhibits the fullness of being which existence has now attained."[65] Rendering the matter in comparatively less forbidding terms, Roger Caillois writes: "The revelation that comes from a dream is a double that precedes and shackles reality. Dream fixes reality as it ought to take place.... This is the power of the dream: to twist reality after itself."[66]

Dreaming That One Is Dreaming

On this accord, dreaming that one is waking from the dream may be the most subtle facet of the dream, pointing to the difficulty of discriminating between one who dreams to be awake and one whose wakefulness is a dream. Synesius of Cyrene, the bishop of Ptolemais appointed by Theodorus, already expressed the point in his treatise *On Dreams*, written in Alexandria in the early part of the fifth century: "And yet, all this is the waking reality of the dreamer and the dream of one who has awakened, for both are engaged in the same underlying state, the imaginative nature." Synesius goes on to distinguish the two states by noting that when awake, the *phantasia* enable us to make mental images as we wish, whereas in sleep, these images are formed spontaneously as a pledge from the god.[67] If we disregard the divine element, we can translate this hoary insight into a more current psychoanalytic idiom: the dreamer dwells—always, it seems, as a transient alien, rather than a permanent citizen[68]—in the place between the unconscious and preconscious, where the difference between dreaming and wakefulness cannot be distinguished clearly.[69] "We are close to waking," wrote Novalis, "when we dream that we are dreaming."[70] Phenomenologically, and I suspect neuroanatomically, there is no way to decide between the possibility that one is awake when dreaming or that one is dreaming when awake. As A. Graham Cairns-Smith put it, "the process of waking shows us each morning that there are no sharp distinctions between dreams and other forms of our conscious being." We traverse from "dreaming asleep" to "dreaming awake," and finally to "dreaming aware," whence we move on to higher levels of wakefulness in which the "conscious experiences" are connected with the "structure of our surroundings." The perception of the external world is itself a byproduct of the inner perceptual world of which dreams and hallucinations may be considered "half-baked perceptions." The dreaming brain, therefore, can be thought of as "practising parts of its main activity of building a perceptual world."[71] In comparison with dreams, these "higher" brain activities exhibit a greater correspondence between interior psychic states and exterior physical things. Notwithstanding this difference, the gap between the respective forms of representation in dreaming and wakeful consciousness is significantly narrower than common sense and even many learned explanations may presume. To quote Caillois again:

> Someone, in a dream, wakes up—or rather believes that he has awakened, although he continues to dream—and now lies expecting

> another awakening, which this time may be real but may also be as illusionary as the first. In this way he will be transported from one dream to another, from one awakening to another, without ever being absolutely certain whether he has finally arrived at the true awakening, the one that will restore him to the world of reality.... Since, at every moment of the dream, the sleeper is unaware of the fact that he is dreaming, and is even convinced that he is awake, it is clear that there can never be a moment in which a person who believes himself to be awake does not have to entertain the suspicion of a doubt that he might perhaps at that time actually be dreaming.... It may happen that one dreams in a dream that one has wakened from a dream while in actual fact the same dream continues to unfold. The sleeper draws from this peripety but a misleading assurance that he is now awake. He generally passes through a state in which his reason so mingles with illusion that both soon become inextricable from each other.[72]

The dream and the hallucination attest to a mode of consciousness wherein the imaginary is believed to be real to the one who dreams and/or hallucinates because of the vivid sensory quality of its content, even as it is at the same time deemed to be unreal and devoid of sensual depth by one standing outside the experience. The divergence between imaginary and real is no longer viable; both dream and hallucination consist of perceiving the nonperceptual,[73] and thus the image does not become more objective if it becomes more real. On the contrary, the "objectivity" of the image is not determined by its correspondence to an external object, nor does the dearth of such correspondence necessarily render the perceiver delusional, a pathology that may, in fact, be associated with chronic hallucination combined with psychotic behavior. Consider the assessment of Jason Brown, a clinical professor of neurology:

> The hallucination is not accepted as a real object because it looks like an object, it is accepted as real because it is the only object the person has. There is no other object or image that is truer to reality to which the person can appeal.... When hallucination replaces perception, there is no real world left in that modality.... In dream, or in wakefulness, there is a conspiracy of the senses so the individual cannot disconfirm the imaginary nature of his images. The world is

> accepted as real when its reality is not disproven by one of its modes of representation.[74]

The insights expressed by Caillois and Brown (and numerous others whom I could have cited) have deep roots in the Western philosophical tradition. One thinks, for instance, of the observation of Aristotle that "the faculty by which, in waking hours, we are subject to illusion when affected by disease, is identical with that which produces illusory effects in sleep."[75] Aristotle goes on to identify dreaming as an activity that belongs to the faculty of sense perception, albeit qua the imagination.[76] More specifically, he insists that the dream is a sort of image that occurs in sleep due to the "imaginative movement" based on impressions derived from and residually left behind in each of the sense organs. This movement

> causes an image to present itself, and makes the dreamer think, owing to the effects borne in from the organ of sight, that he actually sees, and owing to those which come from the organ of hearing, that he really hears; and so on with those also which proceed from the other sensory organs. In every case an appearance presents itself, but what appears does not in every case seem real, unless when the deciding faculty is inhibited, or does not move with its proper motion.

Aristotle readily admits the affinity between one who is subject to illusions when awake and one who dreams when asleep; in both instances, "what has little similarity to something appears to be the thing itself."[77] The dream image and the wakeful illusion can be both traced to the residuary movements that exist within the soul potentially, the remnants of sense impressions that actualize themselves without any external stimulus. What the soul sees during sleep are appearances (*phantasmata*) produced in the imagination (*to phantastikon*) that mimic images based on ordinary perception. These simulacra are basically a "replay of previous waking experience, sometimes bizarrely scrambled as a result of physiological experience."[78] Phenomenally, the dream and the hallucination are to be differentiated, but with regard to ontological status, they are not, since neither provides epistemic certitude beyond the fact that some image coheres in the mind (we might say the neural cortex) that itself presumes a corresponding reality. I do not think it exaggerated to say that this lives on as the prosaic perspective adopted by most people, or what Husserl called the *natural attitude*, for if one were to let go of it, the distinction between veritable and specious reasoning would be compromised. Imagine if soundness of judgment could no longer be determined by appeal to something "real" external to the mind. I assume the reader would readily agree that without such an appeal, havoc would ensue, certainly in the precinct of thought, but also likely in the arena of behavior.

The insight of Aristotle conforms to what was expressed at a much later date by Sartre in response to the question *how can the patient believe in the reality of an image that is essentially given as an irreality*? "We therefore arrive at this first conclusion: in hallucination, in the dream, nothing can destroy the irreality of the object as imaged as immediate correlate of the imaging consciousness."[79] The human imagination, whether expressed in the production of hallucinatory images or dream images, has the capacity to create an imaginary whose noetic status is determined by a reality that is imaginatively devised in the duration of the event—as opposed to the reflection stimulated by the reminiscence of the sensorily experienced event—as unreal. The Sartrean view resonates as well with the position articulated centuries before by René Descartes (1596–1650) regarding the inability to distinguish cognitively between the content of a dream and a waking episode with respect to both thoughts and sensations.[80] Sartre's depiction of the hallucinatory object is applied without qualification to the dream object:

> But in all likelihood the object is not given in memory as irreal; in fact there was no *positing* of irreality during the event; the production of the irreal object was simply accompanied by nonthetic consciousness of irreality. This nonthetic consciousness does not pass into the memory since ... the memory of the perceived object delivers us an irreality in the same way as a reality and, in order that one may be distinguished from the other in recollection, it is necessary that at the moment of their appearance they must have been the objects of explicit positings of reality or irreality.[81]

The dream, therefore, "closely resembles error in Spinozism: error can be given as truth, but to possess the truth is sufficient for the error to dissipate itself."[82] The error may fade when divulged in the light of truth, but in the moment of erring, the error appears as truth and thus it is truly an error. A dreamer likewise really dreams and does not merely dream that she or he dreams, although there may be a type of dream in which one dreams that one is dreaming or a dream in which one realizes that one is dreaming—the two are phenomenologically and neurophysiologically on a par, even if in the latter, unlike in the former, the judgment is not itself part of the dream[83]—but in these scenarios, too, one is really dreaming that one is dreaming, and hence the irreality of the dream is real because the reality of the dream is irreal.

The antiquity of this insight is attested in a remark of the second-century philosopher Alexander of Aphrodisias in his commentary on book 5 of Aristotle's *Metaphysics*:

> But it is another way that things of the following type are false: those that, although they are beings, are nevertheless the source of a false appearance because they appear either not to be the *kind* of thing that they are, or to be things that *are not*.... Similarly, the images (*phantasmata*) in dreams are also something (for certain movements take place in those who see the dream-images), but these images are not the kind of thing that they appear to be.

Dream images, like images in a mirror, are false appearances not because they are "completely non-existent," but "because they appear either not to be the *kind* of thing that they are, or to be things that *are not*."[84] The images of dreams are true because they exist, but they exist as false; they are not what they appear to be and thus appear not to be what they are. It is well-nigh logically impossible, therefore, to rule out the possibility that what we estimate to be wakefulness is naught but a dream, perhaps a dream that one is waking from a dream.

Wittgenstein seems to have been acutely aware of the dilemma when he considered the following hypothetical: Upon being aroused from slumber, someone remembers the utterance "I believe I am now dreaming," a verbal gesticulation that signifies that one has dreamt that one said that one was dreaming. "Might it not actually happen that a dreamer, as it were emerging from the dream, said in his sleep, 'I am dreaming?' It is quite imaginable that there should be such a language-game."[85] That one may utter the proposition "I am dreaming" in the context of the dream points to the difficulty of distinguishing "true" and "false" with respect to a dream,[86] even if we grant that if one does indeed dream that one is dreaming or one makes a judgment that one is dreaming, one would likely still be aware of the contents of the dream and not just dreaming that one is aware of them.[87] Or could it be that even this distinction is not warranted? Not only is the line dividing fiction and reality nebulous, but the notion of a "fictional" dream as opposed to one that is real also seems untenable.[88] In any given cultural context, a particular dream vision may be deemed illusory and another real, but this estimation does not rest exclusively on a consideration of the phenomenal stuff of the dream; it reflects instead the wider set of beliefs that inform the community with which the dreamer is associated. The philosophical insight has been confirmed by more recent psychological studies of human cognition that dispute any substantial variation in the manner that we judge imagined or perceived beings to be real. The estimative process by which we ascribe veridicality to objects of perception is not substantially different from the process by which we ascribe veridicality to objects of imagination. Everything in the dream *seems* real and also *feels* real, and thus with respect to both sensorial and emotional detail, there is no basis to discriminate the imaginary and the actual.[89]

The longevity of this philosophical impasse is attested by the fact that Plato had Socrates inquire of Theaetetus to what evidence one could appeal to determine if one were awake or asleep or if the conversation one is having is actually taking place or is simply something that one is dreaming. Theaetetus replied, "Indeed, Socrates, I do not see by what evidence it is to be proved, for the two conditions correspond in every circumstance like exact counterparts. The conversation we have just had might equally well be one that we merely think we are carrying on in our sleep, and when it comes to thinking in a dream that we are telling other dreams, the two states are extraordinarily alike." As Socrates rightly infers, if we cannot confidently decide whether we are asleep or awake, this leaves "plenty of room for doubt."[90] Astonishingly, with all the progress in time and the refinement of technological tools and investigational skills, there is still no satisfactory way to adjudicate such a rudimentary point concerning our experience of the world. In her study of dreams and illusions in Indian mythology, Wendy Doniger O'Flaherty noted that if the only reasonable criterion to differentiate the real and unreal is the Popperian principle of falsification, then we must confront the counterintuitive fact that we can verify that we are dreaming by waking up, but we cannot verify that we are awake by falling asleep. Consequently, "the hypothesis 'This is real' can be falsified (when we wake up) but not verified, while the hypothesis 'This is a dream' can be verified (again, when we awaken) but not falsified."[91] Following this trajectory to its logical consequence, the mind arrives at a point where lucidity would of necessity comprise the feasibility of its opposite: to think clearly, one would have to assume the pretense of all that is experienceable, rendering dubious the claim to any truth, including the assertion regarding the pretense of all that is experienceable, divested of every modicum of untruth. Paradoxically, the very ground that allows us to distinguish madness from sanity renders the distinction indefensible.

The Collusion of Opposites and the Illusion of Allusion

To grasp the import of this philosophical claim, which has been substantiated in more recent times by neuroanatomical evidence and the claims of evolutionary biologists regarding the pressures of the selection process to forge correspondences between the inner world and the presumed external environment,[92] let us remember the attitude expressed by Freud in *The Interpretation of Dreams* that the "dreams of neuropaths . . . do not allow any conclusions to be drawn about the dreams of those of sound mind."[93] This is contradicted to some extent by Freud's own focus on the dream as a primary (though surely not exclusive) tactic to base psychopathological evaluations on psychological inferences. Thus, in another noteworthy passage from this work, he writes:

> dreams prove to us *that what is suppressed continues to exist in normal persons too, and remains capable of psychical functioning*. The dream itself is one of the expressions of what is suppressed; in theory, this is so in all cases; palpably and empirically it is so at least in a great number of instances, and these, in fact, display the striking characteristics of the dream-life at their clearest. In waking life, what is suppressed in the psyche is thwarted in its attempts at expression by

> the *removal of contradictions by their opposite* and cut off from internal perception; at night, and in the power of compromise-formations, it finds ways and means of forcing its way into consciousness.[94]

I will return in Chapter 4 to the insight regarding the augmented capability of the dream to allow contradictory sensibilities to coexist, a notion that Freud links exegetically to the statement in Virgil's *Aeneid* (vii.313), which also serves as the epigraph of his book: *Flectere si nequeo superos, Acheronta movebo*, "If Heaven I cannot bend, then Hell I will arouse." Suffice it for now to say that the dream facilitates a coincidence of opposites, so that it is not only the case that the dreamer can concomitantly bend heaven and arouse hell, but, even more profoundly, the bending of heaven is itself the arousing of hell. In Freud's thinking, the fusion of antinomies in the dream alludes to the blurring of the boundary between psychological well-being and neurotic or psychotic malady. Freud himself noted that the property of a dream to express a sentiment through its opposite—the example he gives is the exhibiting of the desire for solitude, which is related to the issue of secrecy surrounding the compulsion to masturbate, in the image of being in the presence of many strangers—is also discernible in paranoia.[95] In an early work that marked his departure from Freud, Jung properly gave credit to his older colleague for this insight:

> Since the dream is unconcerned with the real condition of things, it brings the most heterogeneous matter together, and a world of impossibilities takes the place of realities. Freud finds progression characteristic of thinking when awake, that is to say, the advancement of the thought excitation from the system of the inner or outer perception through the endopsychic work of association, conscious and unconscious, to the motor end; that is to say, toward innervation. In the dream he finds the reverse, namely, regression of the thought excitation from the pre-conscious or unconscious to the system of perception, by means of which the dream receives its ordinary impression of sensuous distinctness, which can rise to an almost hallucinating clearness.[96]

The severing of the dream from the real condition of things allows for the possibility of maximal heterogeneity, the amalgamation of discordant images that replace the familiar "realities" of mundane experience with the exotic "world of impossibilities." Consequently, the *sensuous distinctness* associated with the oneiric rises to the level of *hallucinating clearness*. Reflecting the language of Nietzsche cited at the beginning of this chapter, Jung's provocative and counterintuitive expression is worthy of sustained reflection and relates, I suspect, to his appropriation of the Platonic theme of divine madness, to which he also refers as "divine delusion."[97] Madness should not be despised or feared, but accepted, since through it, we can be in touch with the incomprehensible mystery of life.[98] That clarity is linked to hallucination bespeaks the fact that a mind-set judged by societal mores as anomalous may actually divulge a greater degree of perceptual acuity, and hence what is conventionally considered to be clarity is, in truth, obfuscation, a point that lamentably we see too often in political discourse. In the lecture "On the Psychogenesis of Schizophrenia" (1939), Jung commented that the dream is "functional disturbance" insofar as it "can manifest all stages of personal disintegration," and hence, "it is no exaggeration to say that the dreamer is normally insane, or that insanity is a dream which has replaced normal consciousness. To say that insanity is a dream which has become real is no metaphor." Jung concludes, therefore, that the phenomenology of the dream and of schizophrenia are "almost identical," the critical difference being that the former normally occurs during sleep and the latter upsets the waking or conscious state.[99]

Surely one can appreciate the far-reaching implications of Jung's assertion that the dream is a form of *normal insanity*. One may not want to go to this extreme, but the decisive and incontestable point is that the Freudian enterprise itself rests on the assumption that dreams can teach us about the functionality of mental illness, a claim that is rendered hyperbolically in the oft-cited statement, which was added to one of the later editions of *The Interpretation of Dreams*, "*The interpretation of dreams is the royal road to a knowledge of the unconscious activities of the mind.*"[100] Even more poignant is the comment of Hughlings Jackson that Freud added (presumably on the authority of Ernest Jones) in a footnote from 1914 to his observation that the proposition that the dream is to be regarded as a fulfillment of unconscious wishes makes it "only the first member of a class which is of the greatest significance to psychiatrists and an understanding of which implies the solution of the purely psychological side of the problem of psychiatry":[101] "Find out all about dreams and you will have found out all about insanity."[102] Pertinent as well is the remark of Freud in *An Outline of Psychoanalysis*: "A dream is a psychosis with all the absurdities, delusions and illusions of a psychosis."[103] In a letter to Wilhelm Fliess from May 31, 1897, Freud appended a draft of some remarks in which was included a section entitled "Fiction and Fine Frenzy," a title (the last two words appeared in English in the original) derived from the fifth act of Shakespeare's *Midsummer Night's Dream*:

> The poet's eye, in a fine frenzy rolling
> Doth glance from heaven to earth, from earth to heaven,
> And, as imagination bodies forth
> The forms of things unknown, the poet's pen
> Turns them to shapes, and gives to airy nothing
> A local habitation and a name.[104]

Freud noted that the "mechanism of fiction is the same as that of hysterical fantasies.... So Shakespeare was right in juxtaposing fiction and madness (fine frenzy)."[105] In another letter from January 4, 1899, Freud surmised that "the key to hysteria as well really lies in dreams."[106] If we combine these statements, we can see that, in Freud's thinking, creativity in writing is a form of hysteria that is known as well from the activity of dreaming.[107] Simply put, dreams exemplify the characteristics of mental illness to the degree that, like hallucinogenic experiences, they concoct an unreal world that we regard as real.

The psychoanalytic orientation has been criticized on this very point. Jacques Lacan (1901–1981), for example, protested sharply to the aforecited comment of Jackson: we can find analogies between dreams and derangement, since they work with the "same elements" and the "same symbols," but we cannot identify them. On the contrary, our task is to clarify how the "defining mechanism" of madness "has got nothing to with what happens every night in dreams.... And don't let go of the idea that the problem of the dream leaves all the economic problems of psychosis completely unresolved."[108] A similar critique was offered by the anthropologist Murray Wax:

> As formulated by Sigmund Freud, psychoanalysis fitted dreams (and relative activities) onto a biomedical template and so made their investigation respectable, but at the cost of severe distortion. Worse yet, the cultic orthodoxy of the Freudian movement foreclosed the possibility of moving beyond naïve scientism, while the biomedical identification confirmed the authoritarianism within and without the consulting chamber. Dreams were assimilated to neurotic symptoms, and valuable human potentialities were labeled as "psychopathologies."[109]

The legitimacy of this condemnation notwithstanding, Freud's insight has sweeping implications for the possibility of domesticating the deviant. In accord with Foucault's depiction of Freud's contribution to the understanding of madness, we might say that in his interpretation of dreams, as well, he sought to restore "the possibility of a dialogue with unreason."[110] The Freudian perspective has to be seen as part of the larger post-Cartesian project of modern thought in which doubt is no longer sustained in order to ascertain an innate idea that signals an indubitable truth, an ontological and epistemological bedrock for our sense of self and the world:

> After Descartes, it is no longer necessary to traverse courageously the uncertainties of delirium, dreams and illusions, and it is no longer necessary to overcome once and for all the perils of unreason: rather, it is from the depths of unreason that reason can be interrogated, and what appears once more is the possibility of regaining the essence of the world in the dizzying spin of a unifying delirium, in an illusion equivalent to the truth, that brings together the being and non-being of the real as one.[111]

In the essay "Nietzsche, Freud, Marx" (1967), Foucault compared the experience of madness to the "disappearance of the interpreter" that occurs at the spot where one discerns that the "absolute point of interpretation would be at the same time that of a point of rupture," the "convergence of interpretation on a point that renders it impossible."[112] To the degree that the dream exemplarily ensues from this junction where impossible and possible are no longer distinguishable, it calls into question the rigorous boundaries of self and other that are typically presumed in the delineation of mental instability and the consequent remedial interventions. I am reminded here as well of Hillman's clever transposition of Jung's statement that in interpreting the archetypes of the collective unconscious, the "most we can do is to *dream the myth onwards*"[113] to the conjecture that analysis consists of "pathologizing the myth onward," which implies that "therapy for the abnormal would have to be abnormal.... By following pathologizing onward we are attempting to discover precisely the methods and laws of the imaginal in distinction to the rational and the physical. Madness teaches the method."[114] There is sublime wisdom in the potentially perilous insight that madness itself instructs us about the method to treat madness, going back, as Hillman himself acknowledges, to the ancient Greek principle of "like has affinity with like."

Parallels between dreaming and psychopathological tendencies have been suggested by more recent neuroscientific research. For instance, J. Allan Hobson, who has studied and written copiously about dreams, endeavoring to integrate neural science and psychoanalysis,[115] has argued that there is an electrochemical similarity between our dream life and the demented state associated with psychosis, a likeness that would, to some degree at least, blur the diagnostic discrepancy between aberrant and normal.[116] I am in no position to judge such a claim, but its underlying logic strikes me as cogent, resonating, as it does, with a sensibility attested in much older sources in which dreaming is viewed as an upsurge of imagination—at once lucid and disorienting—bordering on lunacy. Paraphrasing Norman O. Brown, we could say that resisting this madness might be the maddest way of being mad.[117] What the dreamer and the madman share is the propensity to accept the false image as true and to be transported thereby into an imaginary realm where the *dizzying spin of a unifying delirium* destabilizes the ability to distinguish with precision between the apparent and the real. The dream, in short, is the virtual reality that instantiates the reality of the virtual.

Calculating the Incalculable: The Algorithm of Reverie

Let me continue with a reflection that may be elementary for some readers. A major contribution to dream study on the part of neuroscience has been to argue that sleep activity can be recorded through electrodes implanted in the brain and muscles, and hence, the information of the dream can be tallied mathematically, which affords the possibility that corresponding states of consciousness with accompanying patterns of somnambulistic behavior may be detected or induced in other mammals.[118] To state what is perhaps obvious, the theoretical underpinning of this perspective is the belief that the brain mechanism for imagery in humans and animals can be studied from perspectives that are subject to objective methods of exploration and quantitative analysis.[119] In some measure, this stance complies with the *oneirological materialism* affirmed in ancient times by Aristotle, who maintained that, given the link between dreaming and sense perception, only animals can dream, and while humans dream the most, dreaming is not exclusive to this species.[120] But the question still begs to be asked, what makes the dream a dream? Are neurobiological and psychophysiological criteria to be favored taxonomically, or are they even determinate in the determination that may turn out to be indeterminate?[121] As explanatory models, do they not betray the limits of their suitability at the very point they lay bare the suitability of their limits? Consider the following appraisal of two acclaimed scientists:

> The fact that not only humans but *all mammals* display the REM[122] state made it possible for neuroscientists to go one step further: they could identify the *brain mechanisms* underlying the REM state (read: dream state) by means of animal experiments that were ethically unacceptable in humans. This is where the slippery slope began, for no matter how close the homologue may be between the REM state in humans and other mammals, we have no way of knowing whether the same applies to their *dreams*. The moment investigators switched from studying humans to other animals, the monitoring of their subjects' dreams (as such) was perforce abandoned.[123]

It may be unwarranted to relegate dreams to the fulfillments of repressed childhood wishes lodged in the unconscious, as Freud notoriously argued, or to see them as symbolic expressions of archetypal images, presumed to be universal and yet linked peculiarly to the process of individuation, as Jung maintained, but it seems to me equally reductive to view dreams as nothing more than random and idle side effects of the nervous system, chance synaptic firings produced by a neural network configured in different areas of the forebrain.[124] It is worth recalling Jung's own warning to patients, "who imitate the technical and theoretical jargon of the doctor, and do this even in their dreams, in accordance with the old tag, *Canis panem somniat, piscator pisces*."[125] Although I do not know the source of the Latin proverb cited by Jung and thus cannot be certain of its contextual import, I can safely say that it is patently far from the intellectual universe of contemporary neurobiology.[126] Yet the intent that he extracts therefrom falls prey to a similar reductionism—the dog invariably will dream of bread and the fisherman of fish, for dreams are naught but mental projections of instinctual needs. In the current scientific environment, such a computational approach to hypnagogic images is a particular instantiation of a more general presumption regarding the material nature of consciousness, a perspective that has achieved prominence not only in the sphere of theoretical science (including, but not limited to neurophysiology, evolutionary biology, and behavioral psychology), but also in the realm of therapeutic practice.[127] The viewpoint is framed incisively by Edward Kelly in the introduction to the book *Irreducible Mind*, which challenges the prevailing paradigm:

> We human beings are nothing but extremely complicated biological machines. Everything we are and do is in principle causally explainable from the bottom up in terms of our biology, chemistry, and physics—ultimately, that is, in terms of local contact interactions among bits of matter moving in strict accordance with mechanical laws under the influence of fields of force. . . . Mind and consciousness are entirely generated by—or perhaps in some mysterious way identical with—neurophysiological events and processes in the brain. Mental causation, volition, and the "self" do not really exist: they are mere illusions, by-products of the grinding of our neural machinery. And of course because one's mind and personality are entirely products of the bodily machinery, they will necessarily be extinguished, totally and finally, by the demise and dissolution of that body.[128]

Even if we grant that "there is a physical substrate of the dream experience," we need not yield to the "more general assertion that all states of mind are states of the brain."[129] The inadequacy of the neural reductionism is brought to the fore in the following account of the process of dreaming: "Universal in occurrence among humans and other mammals, it stems from a nonsymbolic surge of arousal from the brainstem that splays the cerebrum with fireworks. In humans these random fireworks are interpreted by the neocortex and given symbolic shape, in both idiosyncratic and culturally shared patterns."[130] I would counter that the presumed gap between the "nonsymbolic surge" of "random fireworks" in the brain stem and their symbolic interpretation in the neocortex is not merely a quantifiable difference. To claim that all mammals potentially can experience the former, but that only humans attest to the latter raises the question of whether or not we should speak of a "dream" indiscriminately in humans and in other mammals.

What's in the name "dream," one might ask? Not everything that some neuroscientists are prepared to call a dream. The issue is not simply a matter of semantic quibbling. There may very well be a biochemical link between arousal (a term that is used to name the different levels of human brain activation related to dreaming)[131] and mammalian patterns (especially in the cultivation of social practices in the hominid consciousness)[132] that precede the evolutionary growth of a cerebral cortex, but the meaningful application of the term "dream" to certain forms of consciousness and their attending modes of conduct is a hermeneutical decision that depends on an indispensable element that is thought to be present in humans, but absent in other mammals,[133] namely, the manner in which the phantasmagoria (primarily visual and aural, though potentially also tactile, odorous, and oral) are cast symbolically by the narratological framing of—or, better, that is—the dreamer.[134] As Wax observed, "it is plausible that other animal species experience dreams. However, when we discuss and interpret human dreams, we are dealing with phenomena narrated in *language*. Human group life is based on natural language, which has the potentiality for complex intercommunication beyond bodily gesture and response."[135] Wax is critical of the psychoanalytic emphasis on interpretation and the language of dreams, a slogan that he borrows from Erich Fromm, but what is essential to underline is his own recognition that human dreams must be treated as qualitatively different in kind from brain activity attested in other animal species that we may refer to as dreaming.

I see no compelling reason to presume a shift from nonsymbolic to symbolic, as if the latter were a cognitive-linguistic web superimposed on the phenomena—what one might be tempted to call the uninterpreted statistics of experience. But the prospect of the latter is highly suspect; the external world, scientists and philosophers have long agreed, is mediated by our sensory organs and brain processes. With respect to this matter, there is no appreciable difference between dreaming and wakefulness.[136] It seems to me, therefore, legitimate to think of dreaming as a biopsychological process that chemically prompts in the electromagnetic lattice of the brain an event of symbolization at the level of experience. The symbolic intent, consequently, would be attested in the manufacture of dream images, and not only in the postexperiential interpretation of them.[137] By this criterion, there is a significant chasm separating the human from other mammals. We may assume, for that reason, that the intent of the dreamer, both in configuring the dream visually in imagination and in communicating it verbally through memory, is to impart something of the psychic landscape, however we construe the contours of (inter)subjectivity.

It would be ludicrous to deny the validity of the neuronal elements of dreaming. Indeed, even the criterion of narratological reframing that I have invoked can and perhaps ought to be examined through this lens, because it is itself a mental function that is the product of rather sophisticated brain activity.[138] I have no reason to oppose the assumption that the term "dream" can be explained by a theorem based on empirical evidence elicited systematically from the measuring and classifying of neurons thought to discharge randomly in the brain. In fact, it seems reasonable to accept the view that the dream experience, like other forms of consciousness, requires a "whole body explanation" that links the hypothalamus with the cortex through neural projections and the endocrine system responsible for the multifaceted human emotions and desires.[139] But perhaps not without some sense of irony, the very criterion of randomness, which I would link to the related, but independent quality of bizarreness that several thinkers have referred to as a distinctive trait of the dream phenomenon,[140] poses a philosophical challenge to the neuroscientific quest to determine the indeterminable, an aspiration that is reminiscent of the effort to provide a theory of the quantization of chaos, a concept inherently applicable to classical dynamic systems, but one that is articulated as well by some proponents of quantum mechanics who still maintain, in defiance of Heisenberg's uncertainty principle,[141] that nonreckonable physical laws can have predictive value.[142] One can conceivably discern in the dominant neuropsychological approach an implied rejection of the blend of psychic determinism and the category of the uncanny associated especially with Freudian psychoanalysis,[143] but the emphasis on the arbitrary and fantastic nature of dream activity creates its own form of constricting human consciousness, even as it sets it free of the constraints of a psychological determinacy.

Oneiropoetic Duplicity and the Dissolution of the Dreamer

To forestall such a pitfall, I would assent to the approach recently hailed by Kelly Bulkeley (on the basis of a technical expression coined by Henry P. Stapp)[144] as *interactive dualism*, "a view that focuses on the dynamic interplay between the sleeping brain and the dreaming mind, leaving open . . . the question of their ultimate metaphysical connection."[145] Moreover, I concur with a number of thinkers who have argued that the neurological approach should be combined with a more literary perspective, one that views dreaming from the slant of the poetic or the metaphorical, the duplicitous play of manifest and latent, all features that, incidentally, one can find in the scope of Freud's vision, a point to which I will return. At this juncture, I wish to emphasize that by speaking of duplicity, I intend pairing the calculating sway of the scientific and the incalculable drift of the symbolic in such a way that the two are preserved in their integrity, even as they collude to inform and transform each other reciprocally. From this integrative angle, the computable dimension of dream making may be cataloged as a form of oneiropoiesis,[146] or a kind of "involuntary poetry,"[147] assuming, as I do,[148] that the fusion of images that one typically encounters in poetry—the linking of metaphors that may be compared metaphorically to the stringing of pearls on a necklace,[149] a doubling of singularity endemic to the metaphor—bears a phenomenological similarity with the symbols that coalesce (in the manner of concurrence rather than confluence) in the pageant of the dream theatre.[150]

In this matter, I follow other thinkers, but especially Bachelard, for whom "dreams take on coherence precisely because of their poetic qualities. Poetry forms the dreamer and his world at the same time."[151] Elaborating the kinship between poem and dream, Bachelard writes: "The poet's room is full of words, words which move about in the shadows. Sometimes the words are unfaithful to the things. They try to establish oneiric synonymies between things. The phantomalization of objects is always expressed in the language of visual hallucinations. But for a word dreamer there are phantomalizations through language. In order to go to those oneiric depths words must be given the time to dream."[152]

The basic elements whence the dream is crafted are metaphoric images produced by and in the brain of the dreamer. I have just written of "the dream" and "the dreamer," but I do not think it advantageous to view the dreamer as an entity that can be surgically severed from the event of the dream that is dreamt. The images are confabulated in the very consciousness that is confabulated by the images. Considering this conundrum, Bachelard wondered if the dreamer "who crosses the madness of the night" is sure of being the one who is dreaming the dream. Boldly, he concludes, the "night dreamer cannot articulate a *cogito*. The night dream is a dream without a dreamer."[153] If we are to uphold an identity of a dreamer, it is enfolded within the folds of the dream unfolded in its being retold, whether in word, image, or deed. The dream may very well be a "phenomenological descent into the self,"[154] but the self that is exposed thereby would be better conceived (contra Freud) as an impersonal, nonegological consciousness, the disbanding of the individual in a transpersonal unconscious.[155] We can speak, therefore, of the dreaming self as constituted dialectically by the confrontation with an alterity that is both indigenous and alien to itself.[156] Hegel had already discerned that in the chaos, confusion, and flux of dreaming, the fixed boundaries of subjectivity are dissolved: "In the dream state one allows everything to run through one's mind without connection, without purpose, and without understanding.... In dream I do not relate to myself as the concrete center. In dreams everything is ordered without reference to this concrete center-point that constitutes actuality, the rationality of my representing, the most concentrated point of the nexus, that in turn constitutes objectivity."[157] Contrasting wakefulness and sleep, Hegel characterizes the former as the division of oneself from oneself, whereas the latter is the covering of oneself in oneself. In the absence of any opposition between the interior and exterior, the I withdraws and sinks within itself, immersed "in substantiality, which is the power of the individual." Ironically, however, this inundation—the touchstone of Hegel's understanding of madness, which in some respects prefigures Freud's explanation of neurosis—is a blurring of individuality in the disruption and alteration of identity, a being different in relation to oneself.[158] Hegel thus lumps dreams together with the ravings of the priestess, the inhuman shape of witches, and the voices of trees and birds, insofar as these paranormal phenomena "are not ways in which truth manifests itself," but rather "warning signs of deception, of an absence of self-possession, of the singularity and contingency of the knowing."[159]

The point seems to have been grasped as well by Schopenhauer, who argued that in the "state of pure contemplation" one is momentarily elevated above all willing and all desire, such that the forms of life "merely float before him as a fleeting phenomenon, as a light morning dream to one half-awake, through which reality already shines, and which can no longer deceive; and, like this morning dream, they too finally vanish without any violent transition."[160] As the locution intimates, the morning dream comes just as one is waking up, and hence it is subject to retrieval by memory, stirred either by external or internal impressions,[161] and in that sense, it serves as an intermediary between the unconscious and conscious mind.[162] What is most important for our present discussion is the fact that the oneiric phenomenon, according to Schopenhauer, denotes a psychic state wherein the will that binds one to the physical world is overcome, and the lines that demarcate the identity of the self become indistinct.

Even more proximate to my view is the opinion expressed by Foucault in his exposition of Binswanger: "the subject of the dream is not so much the personage who says 'I' . . . as the whole dream in the entirety of its dream content. . . . The subject of the dream, the first person of the dream, is the dream itself, the whole dream." Everything imagined in this state, even the image of empty space, is expressive of the "I" of the dreamer, but, at the same time, that "I" is itself constituted by the phantasmagoria that become visible in the dream. Foucault resorts to an impassioned poetic flourish to describe this state of consciousness: "The dream is an existence carving itself out in barren space, shattering chaotically, exploding noisily, netting itself, a scarcely breathing animal, in the webs of death. It is the world at the dawn of its first explosion when the world is still existence itself and is not yet the universe of objectivity." Insofar as the dreamer is the dream, we could also say that this world is not yet the universe of subjectivity. To dream, then, is a "radical way" that the dreaming subject experiences its own world, a world in which existence has not pronounced itself as world. "The dream is situated in that ultimate moment in which existence still is its world; once beyond, at the dawn of wakefulness, already it is no longer its world."[163]

Anthony Damiani has expressed a similar point in a somewhat more digestible form:

> Think of a dream. We have a series of thoughts one after the other, but they all revolve around the unknown center—the person who's having the dream. The entity in the dream has the feeling that he or she has or is real being... [but] the reality is coming from the person. The congeries of thought is what the dream is all about. And they revolve around the reality of the person. But if you look at the congeries of thought and you expect to find a real ego there, all you'll find is one thought after the other. In other words, there's a level of higher being which we're equating with the person, and there's a lesser level or lower level of being and we are saying that's the dream. The person is immanent in the dream. That immanence gives the ego the feeling that it is *some* thing. That's a misconstruction, a misunderstanding.... It is only the immanence in the dream of the person having the dream that... makes it possible for a dream ego to arise. The center of the vortex is not neutral. The center of the vortex is the presence of the "I AM" in the matrix of possibilities.[164]

Dreams are threaded from an individual's life experience encoded in the brain stem and then projected outward during sleep. It can be said, therefore, that characters in the dream are generated internally by a mind isolated from external sensory stimuli. Yet the suggested incongruity between "person" and "dream ego" seems to me erroneous. The dreamer—the *real person* dreaming—is a figure in the dream that is dreamt. Any clear demarcation between subjectivity and objectivity is severely called into question by the blurring of self and other that occurs within the boundaries of the dream. I thus accede to the proposition that it is

> empirically plausible to assume that the phenomenal dynamics of dreaming result from self-organizational processes in the underlying neurodynamics that unfold when the brain is confronted with a strong internal stimulus source. The complex confabulatory narrative of the dream is the brain's way of interpreting this strong internal stimulus source, which in turn results from massive shifts in the internal chemical landscape and the neuroanatomical architecture of REM sleep. At the same time as this internal fairytale unfolds, the sleeping subject is functionally decoupled from the outer world and unable to perceive and interact with her current environment.[165]

Dreamer and dream should not be conceived as binarily quantized entities, as when we speak commonly of one *having* the dream, as if the persona of the dreamer could be determined independently of the dream, a view epitomized in Freud's contention that dreams are "absolutely self-centered" and hence every figure that appears in a dream should be decoded as a mask that conceals (and thereby reveals) the self.[166] As I will argue below, the notion of the mask will prove to be paramount for grasping the poetic comportment of the dream, but I see no reason to brand the images that appear in the dream as masks donned by a dreamer—to speak of a mask, one must suppose the existence of a face, but within the phenomenal constellation of the dream, there is no face of which to speak that is not a mask. The Freudian perspective is repeated in Hobson's contention that the "one orientational anchor that is never lost in dreams is the self, the 'I' who dreams.... True, some dreamers see themselves as dream actors (rather than being the centre of the action), but the self is always there. It is the construct of constructs, the organizational unity of consciousness. I dream, therefore, I am."[167] The playful paraphrase of the well-known Cartesian maxim may indeed touch upon a fundamental truth, but what it conveys is not that there is some permanent self that is the organizational unity of consciousness, the dreamer to which the dream is attributed, but rather that the self of the dreamer is constantly being shaped by the dream experiences. The relationship should be conceptualized nondualistically, whereby the two phenomenological poles, rendered distinct in the mind's eye, are perceived reciprocally as the dream engendering the dreamer engendering the dream. Nietzsche had already expressed this outlook: "The human being in the world actually could conceive himself as a character in a dream that itself is part of a dream."[168]

The dissolution of self characteristic of the dream can be appreciated from the example of the writer for whom the different persona created are veils through which one is revealed to the extent that one is hidden. Explicating this affinity between dreaming and creative writing, Blanchot offered the following:

> In the dream, who is dreaming? Who is the "I" of the dream? Who is the person to whom one attributes this "I," admitting that there is one? Between the one who sleeps and the one who is the subject of the dream's plot, there is a fissure, the hint of an interval and a difference of structure; of course it is not truly another, another person, but what is it? And if, upon awakening, we hastily and greedily take possession of the night's adventures, as if they belonged to us, is it not with a certain feeling of usurpation (of gratitude as well)? Do we not preserve the memory of an irreducible distance, a distance of a peculiar sort, the distance between me and myself, but also the distance between each of the characters and the identities—even certain—that we lend them, a distance without distance, illumination and fascinating, which is like the proximity of the remote or contact with faraway? An intrigue and a questioning that refer us to an experience often described of late: the experience of the writer when, in a narrative, poetic, or dramatic work, he writes "I," not knowing who says it or what relation he maintains to himself. In this sense, the dream is perhaps close to literature, at least to its enigmas, its glamour, and its illusions.[169]

The recording of dreams is not primarily for the sake of deciphering them according to some theoretical scheme; rather, the purpose is to allow them to be received in their own light, "as traces of a literary affirmation that is not psychoanalytic or autobiographical. They were dreams; they are signs of poetry."[170] Identifying dreams as *signs of poetry* insinuates that just as the poet's identity is both constricted and expanded by the poem—the poet's sense of self is created by the poem that could have only been created by this poet—so the dream is woven from the cloth whence the dreamer, too, is woven. And just as the poet (or artists of other aesthetic media) would both take pride in his or her creation and yet refuse to aver ownership—the work of art is thus often depicted as having come unintentionally by way of an external fount of inspiration—the dreamer both lays claim to and disowns the content of the dream.[171] Oneirically, we configure the configuration that configures us. Hence, the dream may be compared to "a presence that would disregard or forget our capacity to be present in it." We are permanently in the status of strangers vis-à-vis our own dreams, because, as Blanchot puts it,

> the I of the dreamer does not have the meaning of a real I. One could even say that there is no one in the dream and therefore, in some sense, no one to dream it; whence the suspicion that when we are dreaming, it is just as easily someone else who is dreaming and who dreams us, someone who in turn, in dreaming us, is being dreamed by someone else, a premonition of the dream without dreamer, which would be the dream of the night itself.[172]

In the *game of resemblance* that is the dream, the self of the dreamer is an image of the self that is dreamt, "no more subject than object and rather the shadow of itself, a sparkling shadow that frees itself of us like a truer copy because it is at once more resemblant and less familiar." Accordingly, in the depth of the dream—a "depth that is all surface"—lies "an allusion to a possibility of being that is anonymous, such that to dream would be to accept this invitation to exist almost anonymously, outside of oneself, under the spell of this outside and with the enigmatic assurance of semblance: a self without self, incapable of recognizing itself as such because it cannot be the subject of itself."[173] When the phenomenon of the dream—and under this rubric I include both the dream experience and the recounting thereof, which can take on many aesthetic forms—is specularized from this perspective, which Michael Talbot (on the basis of David Bohm's taxonomy) called the *omnijective nature of the dream*,[174] that is, the assumption that the subjective and objective, mind and matter, are inextricably linked in a correlationality that is called *omnipresence*, we can discern that the consciousness of the dreamer is intricately embedded in the labyrinth of dreaming, and hence the self of the dreamer is itself constituted by the very selves that are constituted by the dreamer.

Depersonalization and the Incarnate Fold of the Dream

There is no dream of which it cannot be said that the dreamer is both cause and effect of what is dreamt. From the dream, then, we can find support for a non-narcissistic psychology informed by a quantum understanding of self as a multifarious grid of relationality.[175] Here it is beneficial to adduce an extraordinary passage in Merleau-Ponty's *Phenomenology of Perception* wherein he asserts that metaphysics—the "coming to light of something beyond nature"—is "not localized at the level of knowledge; it begins with the opening out upon 'another', and is to be found everywhere, and already, in the specific development of sexuality."[176] The correlation of metaphysics and sexuality naturally brings to mind Freud, and especially his ascribing to the sexual the function of primary metaphor, the activity vis-à-vis which all other human activities are interpreted metaphorically, a conjecture that is particularly prominent in his interpretation of dreams. Consider the précis of the Freudian perspective offered by Ricoeur: "all dream-symbolism is found to be related to an activity of language, but the enigma of this activity is simply disguised by the supposition of an original verbal identity where the same words denote the sexual and the nonsexual. The hypothesis of these ancient ambiguous roots is simply an expedient whereby one solves the problem by projecting it into a 'basic language' in which similarity would already be identity."[177] From another theoretical perspective, Žižek has offered a similar observation:

> The ultimate properly Freudian lesson is that the explosion of human symbolic capacities does not merely expand the metaphoric scope of sexuality (activities that are in themselves thoroughly asexual can become 'sexualized,' everything can be 'eroticized' and start to 'mean that'), but, much more importantly, this explosion *sexualizes*

> *sexuality itself*: the specific quality of human sexuality has nothing to do with the immediate, rather stupid, reality of copulation, including the preparatory mating rituals; it is only when animal coupling gets caught in the self-referential vicious circle of the drive, in the protracted repetition of its failure to reach the impossible Thing, that we have what we call sexuality, that is, that sexual activity itself becomes sexualized.[178]

Merleau-Ponty seemed to be expressing a view akin to this in juxtaposing the sexual and the metaphysical, even though he was quick to distinguish it from the psychoanalytic precedent.[179] Mulling over the Freudian postulation that sexuality is a phenomenon that "conceals itself from itself beneath a mask of generality, and continually tries to escape from the tension and drama that it sets up," Merleau-Ponty counters that it is more suitable to speak of sexuality as a matter that is "transcended and submerged in the more general drama of existence." By shifting the focus in this way, two conceptual mistakes may be avoided: the first, which is associated with the "philosophies of consciousness," is to fail to recognize in existence any content but the overt forms of "distinct representation," and the second, which is linked to the "psychologies of the unconscious," is to treat the latent as "consisting of representations" in the manner of the obvious. For Merleau-Ponty, the sexual is not a product of unconscious representation, but rather a part of the omnipresent atmospheric conditions of the embodiment of nature—the knitting of the human and non-human bodies in the intersubjective mesh that he eventually calls "intercorporeity"—that precedes the separation into subject and object, the cogito and the world.[180] Body and mind are "abstract moments" of an "incarnate significance,"[181] a "primary process of signification in which the thing expressed does not exist apart from the expression, and in which the signs themselves induce their significance externally." In this signifying mode, which is anterior to conventional means of expression,

> the body expresses total existence, not because it is an external accompaniment to that existence, but because existence comes into its own in the body. Understood in this way, the relation of expression to thing expressed, or of sign to meaning is not a one-way relationship like that between original text and translation. Neither

> body *nor existence* can be regarded as the original of the human being, since they presuppose each other, and because the body is solidified or generalized existence, and existence is a perpetual incarnation.

Merleau-Ponty singles out the matter of sexuality as the specific example that illustrates more generally the nature of our embodied being in the world:

> When we say that sexuality has an existential significance or that it expresses existence, this is not to be understood as meaning that the sexual drama is in the last analysis *only* a manifestation or a symptom of an existential drama. The same reason that prevents us from "reducing" existence to the body or to sexuality, prevents us also from "reducing" sexuality to existence: the fact is that existence is not a set of facts... capable of being reduced to others or to which they can reduce themselves, but the ambiguous setting of their intercommunication, the point at which their boundaries run into each other, or... their woven fabric.[182]

Merleau-Ponty's surmise is elucidated further by appeal to the dream:

> The dreamer does not first visualize the latent content of his dream, the one, that is, which is to be revealed with the help of suitable images by the "second account"; he does not first perceive "in clear" the stimuli of genital origin as being genital, only subsequently translating the text into figurative language. For the dreamer, indeed, who is far removed from the language of the waking state, this or that genital excitation or sexual drive *is* without more ado this image of a wall being climbed or cliff-face being scaled, which are seen as the obvious content.... The dreamer's penis *becomes* the serpent which appears in the obvious content. What we have just said about the dreamer applies equally to that ever slumbering part of ourselves which we feel to be anterior to our representations, to that individual haze through which we perceive the world.[183]

From the dream phenomenon a more comprehensive claim may be inferred about perceptual experience.[184] The chiasmic quality of our enfleshment is such that we are not simply perceiving subjects placed as observers in an otherwise incalcitrant objective world; on the contrary, we look through visual fields at objects that exercise control over us, a condition of consciousness that has been designated *referential transcendence*.[185] The structuring of our intentionality, therefore, entails a relationship that is reciprocal—the mind bestows upon the sensible entity what the sensible entity yields to the mind:

> The sentiment and the sensible do not stand in relation to each other as two mutually exclusive terms, and sensation is not an invasion of the sentiment by the sensible. It is my gaze which subtends colour, and the movement of my hand which subtends the object's form, or rather my gaze pairs off with colour, and my hand with hardness and softness, and in this transaction between the subject of sensation and the sensible it cannot be held that one acts while the other suffers the action, or that one confers significance on the other.... The sensible gives back to me what I lent to it, but this is only what I took from it in the first place. As I contemplate the blue of the sky I am not *set over against* it as an acosmic subject; I do not possess it in thought, or spread out towards it some idea of blue such as might reveal the secret of it, I abandon myself to it and plunge into this mystery, it "thinks itself within me", I am the sky itself as it is drawn together and unified, and as it begins to exist for itself; my consciousness is saturated with this limitless blue.[186]

Depicting perception as the openness of a saturated mind to a world subtended by the gaze of a living body—the "hollow" or "fold" as opposed to the Hegelian notion of a "hole" in being—undermines the dichotomy of inside and outside, the *for itself* and the *in itself*, the binary associated with the structure of the "constituting consciousness."[187] Combating this sort of intentionality, Merleau-Ponty presumes that the perception of the world is an expansion of the temporal-spatial "field of presence" (*Präsenzfeld*),[188] a pivotal concept he appropriates from Husserl,[189] who anticipated the overcoming of the binary between subjectivity and objectivity by noting that the world is constitutive of consciousness to the same degree that consciousness is constitutive of the world; the constituting subject, in other words, is constituted by the very objects it constitutes.[190] Husserl referred to this dilemma as the "paradox of our doubling [*Verdoppelung*].... We are fated as human beings to be the psychophysical subjects of a mental life in the real world and, at the same time, transcendentally to be subjects of a transcendental, world-constituting life-process."[191] The point was well understood by Fink, who mused that "phenomenological cognition has to rely upon the mundane situation of outward manifestation. This means that all transcendental self-cognition, which is realized in regressive inquiry into constitution, does not merely move out from the natural attitude but remains also referred back to it."[192] Relating to the same issue, James Dodd wrote:

> the unfolding of the history of the empirical subject is part and parcel of the ongoing idealization of the world. One must thus speak of a *double translation*: it is only *via* the constitution of the empirical subject that the apprehension of the material world is possible; and it is only *via* the apprehension of the material world that the development, or coming to be, of the empirical subject is possible.[193]

The phenomenological reduction, accordingly, can be depicted as a turning to look

> at its own movement as the movement of self and world, which is as such a movement of mutual obliviousness, precisely in order to be what it is.... Which is exactly what the epoche does—it is an activity that, turning towards the most fundamental possibility of life itself as the double movement of self-accomplishment and world-accomplishment, *seeks to hold this accomplishment still*, i.e., seeks to arrest its forward motion in the space of a "turning back."[194]

In Merleau-Ponty's formulation of this double translation, the human being is an "incarnate subject... through which an object perceived can concentrate in itself a whole scene or become the imago of a whole segment of life. Sense experience is that vital communication with the world which makes it present as a familiar setting of our life. It is to it that the perceived object and the perceiving subject owe their thickness."[195] The line dividing empirical reality and dreaming, and, by extension, the variation between healthy and pathological states of imagining,[196] are blurred on account of this saturation: "Every sensation carries within it the germ of a dream or depersonalization such as we experience in that quasi-stupor to which we are reduced when we try to live at the level of sensation."[197] The dream calls attention to the fact that the "real" is not based solely on a coherence of representation indicative of a substantialist ontology and the reified demarcation of truth and falsehood,[198] but it arises from a "closely woven fabric" constituted by the "subject destined to the world."[199] The dream provides a "striking experience of unreality" wherein "I hold the world present in order to keep it at a distance, and I revert to the subjective sources of my existence. The phantasms of dreams reveal still more effectively that general spatiality within which clear space and observable objects are embedded." Merleau-Ponty illustrates the point by the experience of rising and falling: the physical movements in "objective space" can be interpreted as referring to respiratory or sexual events, but in the oneiric space, these events, which assume symbolic significance by appearing in the guise of images such as the flight and descent of a great bird, "settle in a different theatre." But this we cannot comprehend unless "we endow the body, even in the waking state, with an emblematic value." The representation of "our bodily emotions, desires, and bodily attitudes" in this figurative way—in waking consciousness and in the dreamscape—implies "not only a contingent connection or even an analogical relationship," but a "mutually symbolic" character, "because both express the same essential structure of our being, being situated in relation to an environment, of which we have already stated that this structure alone gives significance to the directions up and down in the physical world."[200]

Influenced by Binswanger's *Dream and Existence*, which is explicitly cited in this context,[201] Merleau-Ponty remarks that the "phantasms of dreaming," as mythological and poetic imagery,

> are not linked to their meaning by a relation of sign to significance... they really contain their meaning, which is not a notional meaning, but a direction of our existence. When I dream that I am flying or falling, the whole significance of the dream is contained in the flight or the fall, as long as I do not reduce them to their physical appearance in the waking world, and so long as I take them with all their existential implications.[202]

The full intent of this comment will become clearer in the next chapter when I discuss Binswanger's view as it was interpreted by Foucault. In this context, it is only necessary to highlight Merleau-Ponty's rendering of Binswanger's existential understanding of the dream and its application to our state of embodiment in the world. Just as Binswanger argued that the symbolic import of the dream images must be elicited from an environment that precedes the division into subject and object—from one perspective everything is comprised in the subjectivity of the dreamer, but from another perspective, the dreamer is shaped by what manifests itself in the dream—so Merleau-Ponty writes about the "emblematic value" of the body, which is to say, the essential structure of being that is shared by consciousness and the world. For Merleau-Ponty, there should be "no occasion to ask ourselves why the thinking subject or consciousness perceives itself as a man, or an incarnate or historical subject, nor must we treat this apperception as a second order operation which it somehow performs starting from its absolute existence; the absolute flow takes shape beneath its own gaze as '*a* consciousness', or a man, or an incarnate subject, because it is a field of presence—to itself, to others and to the world—and because the presence throws it into the natural and cultural world from which it arrives at an understanding of itself."[203]

As he expressed the matter elsewhere,

> it is necessary that there be mediation between the pure For Itself and that which consciousness poses In Itself in the presence of itself, that there be a connivance between the For Itself and the In Itself.... In order to get beyond this alternative, it would be necessary not to consider pure consciousness first, but to return to the perception itself: to take consciousness already at work, already situated, and not to put our trust in a schematic notion of consciousness.[204]

The domain of the dream, in particular, gives us access to the experiential flux—the originating ground of the primordial presence (*Urpräsenz*), the "original and fundamental presentability" (*Urpräsentierbarkeit*) of the world and the body as one flesh—whence the differentiation between subject and object materializes.[205]

One might protest that when an individual depicts the dream, either to oneself or to another, the dreamer is claiming some sense of identity separate from the dream. Prima facie, this objection is reasonable enough, but, upon closer inspection, it becomes clear that it neglects to consider one critical (even if tautological) fact: in recalling the dream, the dreamer cannot remember being apart from the dream, that is, there is no memory of having had the dream but as one who has had the dream. In any recollection of the dream, the dreaming self is construed from the vantage point of having been the dreamer of the very dream in which one is an agent within the dream. The dreaming self is a form that emerges from—and almost as immediately disappears within—the mist of the dream vision.[206] The dream phenomenon thus typifies the larger philosophical problem that Husserl referred to as the "paradox of human subjectivity: being a subject for the world and at the same time being an object in the world."[207] As I noted above, for Husserl, the phenomenological attitude is to be contrasted with the natural on the basis that the external world is no longer assumed to be the indisputably existing ground of being, but is transformed into a "transcendental phenomenon," that is, within the brackets of the reduction, everything presumed to be objective becomes subjective. But if this is so, then it would seem to foster a pansubjectivism, or in Husserl's own language, "a universal concept of the subjective encompasses everything: ego-pole and universe of ego-poles, multiplicities of appearance or object-poles and the universe of object-poles."[208] The world is thought to be constituted by consciousness, but the latter is itself an event constituted within the world.[209] Husserl raises the obvious question: "How can a component part of the world, its human subjectivity, constitute the whole world, namely, constitute it as its intentional formation...? The subjective part of the world swallows up, so to speak, the whole world and thus itself too. What an absurdity!"[210]

Can we reconcile the contradictory juxtaposition of the claims that the human being is a "conscious subject *for* the world" and at the same time a "subjectivity *in* the world as object," that humanity must be viewed "as world-constituting subjectivity and yet as incorporated in the world itself?"[211] Or is the constituting subject, whose synthetic activities provide the conditions for objectivity, simply incapable of itself being given as an object? Husserl attempts to resolve the perplexity by denying that human subjectivity, the "ego-pole" that is the intentional correlate to the "object-pole," is involved in the constitution of the world. Within the phenomenological reduction,

> nothing human is to be found, neither the soul nor psychic life nor real psychophysical human beings; all this belongs to the "phenomenon," to the world as constituted pole.... The "I" that I attain in the epochē...is actually called "I" only by equivocation—though it is an essential equivocation since, when I name it in reflection, I can say nothing other than: it is I who practice the epochē, I who interrogate, as phenomenon, the world which is now valid for me according to its being and being-such, with all its human beings, of whom I am so fully conscious; it is I who stand above all natural existence that has meaning for me, who am the ego-pole of this transcendental life, in which, at first, the world has meaning for me purely as world.[212]

What we refer to as the human subject, consequently, is not the constituting agent, but itself a constituted entity. In spite of Husserl's confidence that he has discovered a way out of the quandary of the metaphysical presuppositions regarding the construction of subjectivity, he has, in truth, only embellished it in a new garb.[213] The constituting consciousness consists of the constituting stream of experiences through which temporal objects appear, but that consciousness is one of these objects, indeed the "self-objectification of transcendental subjectivity" (*Selbstobjektivation der transzendentalen Subjektivität*).[214]

To summon the argument of Sartre, which is based on an assumption made by Descartes, the dreaming consciousness perforce entails consciousness of itself dreaming, a particular application of the more general phenomenological assertion that human consciousness is inexorably self-consciousness: to think, one must be thinking that one thinks. The self of which I speak, therefore, is not a durable substance that can be amputated from the ever-changing maze of feelings, sensations, thoughts, fantasies, and memories. The apposite image to grasp the nature of this self-consciousness—consciousness of self that is the self of consciousness—would be ripples in the lake; beyond the encircling of the concentric circles there is no thing presumed to be going around in circles, nothing but the seething effulgence, the bubbling-up of an ecstatic intensity that creates the semblance of the sensuous field in which all things phenomenal become visible.[215] If, however, dream consciousness, like other forms of consciousness, is innately reflexive and refractive, then logically, this implies the awareness that one is aware that one is aware of being aware, and so on ad infinitum. From this infinite regress it follows that consciousness of dreaming includes within its purview consciousness of the dreamer dreaming the dream.[216] This would imply that, to some degree, every dream partakes of the much-discussed and notionally captivating phenomenon of lucid dreaming, a mode of metacognition attained through the consciousness in which one has full knowledge that one is experiencing a dream.[217]

The inescapable web wherein the identity of the dreamer is configured precisely in its dissolution is well expressed in the following words of Blanchot:

> The one who dreams turns away from the one who sleeps; the dreamer is not the sleeper; sometimes dreaming that he is not dreaming and therefore that he is not sleeping; at other times dreaming that he is dreaming and thus, through this flight into a more inner dream, persuading himself that the first dream is not a dream, or else knowing that he is dreaming and then awakening into a very similar dream that is nothing other than an endless flight outside the dream, a flight that is an eternal fall in a similar dream (and so it is through other twists and turns).[218]

To be aware that one is dreaming during the dream hardly divests one of the role of dreamer. Quite the reverse; this only sharpens the perspicuity of doubling at play in the mirror of self-reflection: the dreamer's subjectivity is shaped as part of the very dream that the dreamer dreams on the basis of images stored in the visual cortex, or, perhaps more accurately, the replayed memories of those images, which reside in a cerebral cortex that supersedes the visual, because the dream is not, technically speaking, a sensory experience,[219] a judgment made already by Freud.[220]

Mythopoiesis of the Dream

The replication sheds further light on the mythopoeic nature of the dream,[221] a trait that I would proffer as one of the "formal properties" of dreaming.[222] As Ricoeur put it,

> dreams attest that we constantly mean something other than what we say; in dreams the manifest meaning endlessly refers to hidden meaning; that is what makes every dreamer a poet. From this point of view, dreams express the private archeology of the dreamer,

> which at times coincides with that of entire peoples.... But even when they do not coincide, the mythical and the oneiric have in common this structure of double meaning.[223]

Needless to say, the affiliation between dreamer and poet was not ignored by Freud; indeed, this aesthetic link is well attested in many writers, as we see, for example, in the statement of Cicero (106–43 B.C.) put into the mouth of his brother, Quintus, in *On Divination* (I.xxi.42) regarding the imaginary recounting of a dream in the *Annales* of Ennius (ca. 239–ca. 169 B.C.): "Although these words are the creations of a poet, nonetheless they are not alien to the regular experience of dreams."[224] In spite of the exceptional quality of the poetic words, they are congruent with regular oneiric experiences. In the 1908 essay "The Poet and Day-Dreaming," Freud explicitly discussed the relation of poetic production to daydreaming,[225] but even prior to the publication of that study, in the *Interpretation of Dreams*, he had already noted the connection between poetry and dreams: "Most of the artificial dreams invented by the poets are intended for this kind of symbolic interpretation, for they render the author's thoughts in a disguise found to match those characteristics of our dreaming familiar to us from experience."[226] This statement, which immediately succeeds the reference to the scriptural account of Joseph's interpretation of Pharaoh's dream, implies that the poem and dream are unvaryingly open to symbolic interpretation, since, rhetorically, both are forms of dissimilitude, the masking of one's intent through a condensation of images that demand a hermeneutical decoding, a rending of the veil to reverse the process and thereby convert the manifest dream images back to the latent dream thoughts.[227] The kinship of the conscious creativity of poetic fantasy and the unconscious productivity of dream imagery is elaborated in a second passage from this work: "The relationships of our typical dreams to fairy-tales and other poetic materials are certainly neither isolated nor accidental. The poet is normally the instrument of the transformation process, but on occasion the keen poet's eye has understood it analytically and pursued it backwards, tracing the poem back to the dream."[228]

Although Freud surely recognized the relationship between poetry and dreaming, credit is to be given to his interpreters for drawing out the full implications of his contribution to aesthetic theory.[229] As Ella Freeman Sharpe proffered, we can trace the origin of both dreams and poetry to the unconscious experience, especially of bodily states. "The laws of poetic diction, evolved by the critics of great poetry and the laws of dream formation as discovered by Freud, spring from the same unconscious sources and have many mechanisms in common."[230] The mental construction of dreams, therefore, can be understood from a comparison with the creation of poetry. In a parallel vein, Hanns Sachs (1881–1947) noted the connection between these two creative exploits,[231] but he also differentiated the two:

> The Unconscious is the basis underlying each of these three phenomena: dreams, daydreams, and poetic creation; but it works in a different way in each of them. The same material, or rather the same source of energy, is used and shaped and finally represented in every one of them in the characteristic manner which belongs to it. . . . The dream has its poetic moments as poetry has its dreamlike aspects. But, on the whole, the dream belongs to another world or, what is the same thing, to another state of our mind, and the doors which lead to it are opened only by sleep. This makes such a vast difference that we can, for the present, give our attention only to the differences in daydreams and poetry, both of which are fashioned by what we consider our normal, waking, work-a-day mind.[232]

One may well counter that the undertaking of Sachs to categorize dreams and poetry separately rests on distinguishing waking and sleeping mentation in a manner that is not supported by physiological data, according to which the process of imagining shared by poet and dreamer proceeds from a state of "quasi-wakeful non-consciousness."[233] Granting the legitimacy of this critique, it is still important to note the inference that the dream has its poetic moment and the poem its dreamlike aspect. This insight can well serve as the methodological foundation not only for a literary approach to understanding the dream imagination, but to seeking a scientific explanation that takes into account this property of the human brain. Sachs, after all, insisted that the "tangible diversities and dissimilarities" between dream and poetry had to be cogitated before one could "enter the study of the hidden identity."[234] Continuing this line of speculation, Kenneth Burke remarked that the "psychoanalysis of Freud and of the schools stemming from Freud has brought forward an astoundingly fertile range of observations that give us insight into the poem as dream. There is opened up before us a sometimes almost terrifying glimpse into the ways in which we may, while overtly doing one thing, be covertly doing another."[235] The application of Freud's dream analysis to poetry relates to the

> ways in which grammatical rules are violated... the dream's ways of enacting conjunctions, of solving arguments by club offers of mutually contradictory assertions; the importance of both concomitances and discontinuities for interpretative purposes (the phenomena of either association or dissociation... revealed with greatest clarity in the *lapsus linguae*); the conversion of an expression into its corresponding act... and, above all, the notion that the optative is in dreams, as often in poetry and essay, presented in the indicative.[236]

The poetic quality of the dream and the dreamlike quality of the poem revolve about two Freudian terms, *condensation* and *displacement*, which may be viewed as complementary approaches to the same phenomenon; in the case of each, one event becomes the synecdochic representative of some other event, albeit from an opposite direction,[237] that is, condensation points to the manner in which a word image is more and hence less than what it is and displacement to the manner in which it is less and hence more than what it is—the two correspond respectively to the linguistic operations of metaphor and metonymy.[238] Along similar lines, Ricoeur noted that the twofold depiction of the nighttime dream as manifest and hidden alludes to a structure that is prevalent in dreaming and in the making of poetry.[239] Elaborating the point in a second passage, he writes that the function of dreams "stems from the fact that they reveal all that is nocturnal in man, the nocturnal of his waking life as well as of his sleep."[240] The assertion that dreams reveal what is nocturnal for the human psyche, irrespective of whether one is awake or asleep, signifies that nocturnality should be understood principally as a figurative trope to denote a state of mind, rather than a period of time, a mental condition that revolves about the translucency of the obscure, illumined in the dimness of its transparency, the open secret, manifestly hidden from sight. Lacan proposed a comparable reading of Freud: "The work on the dream makes it possible—through a pretty turnaround of its initial aspect, as memory—for the subject to evoke what is manifest. But what makes up the dream is something which we must look for, and which truly belongs to the unconscious. This desire, we find or we don't find it, but we only ever see it silhouetted at the back."[241] The manifest content of the dream, therefore, is like a mirage, an optical illusion, revealing the unconscious desire of the dreamer by hiding it, hiding it by revealing it, a desire that comes to light only in the silhouette of the night vision. Freud's understanding of the dream sets up the symbolic—predominantly disclosed in language—as a shield that protects us from the real. The real, accordingly, is absented from the symbolic, or, alternatively expressed, through the prism of the symbolic, the real is relegated to it own impossibility. It follows that the symbolic includes the "negation of what it is not," the "surplus element of negation."[242] What there is to see of this nonexistence, which is the unconscious desire, is to see that there is nothing to see, a theme that Lacan himself will later connect to the phallus. To transmute the matter psychosemiotically, every symptom of the unconscious is a translation of an essentially untranslatable foreign language.[243] The link between the dream and the nocturnal, therefore, brings to light the inherently symbolic function of the former, disclosing the concealed in a manner that the concealed is disclosed as concealed and the disclosed concealed as disclosed.

Oneiric Mask and the Navel of the Dream

The allusive and elusive feature of the dream is related to its being a state of consciousness hovering between the light of alertness and the darkness of comatosity. From that angle of vision, we can think of the dream as a vehicle of dissimulation, comporting an intent that is both hidden in and uncovered through the shadow of sentient images, chiefly visual and auditory. Hence, the dream can be compared to the phenomenon of the esoteric, which proffers the notion of mystery whose depth must be disclosed by proper interpretative decoding, though the secret, like the dream, is positioned between concealment and disclosure, concealed in the disclosure of its concealment, disclosed in the concealment of its disclosure. In the dream, manifest and latent are opposites that coincide in the dialectical surpassing of the dialectic, and hence they are no longer opposite but in the coincidence of their opposition; one's inner wishes are disclosed, and thereby realized, in Ricoeur's formulation, "in the mode of disguise, regression, and stereotyped symbolization." Exactly with regard to these "masks of desire," veiled in the unveiling of what is veiled, does the Freudian *Traumdeutung* provide a prototype to delineate the parameters of a "hermeneutics of culture" in oneiropoietic terms: "Psychoanalysis is of value insofar as art, morality, and religion are analogous figures or variants of the oneiric mask. The entire drama of dreams is thus found to be generalized to the dimensions of a universal poetics."[244] The "object of psychoanalysis," consequently, "is not simply to *accept* the difference between the sterility of dreams and the creativity of art but rather to treat it as a difference that *poses a problem* within a single problematic of desire. Psychoanalysis thereby rejoins Plato's view on the deep-seated unity of poetry and love, Aristotle's view on the continuity of purgation with purification, and Goethe's view on demonism."[245]

The interface of the dream and poetics can be regarded from the standpoint of the oneiric mask. Phenomenologically, the mask is an artifact that conceals by revealing and reveals by concealing, a duplicity that is reminiscent of the secret and the hermeneutic play of esotericism.[246] Freud first introduces this topos in a note in the analysis of his own dream that occurred on July 23–24 1895: "I have the feeling that the interpretation of this part is not taken far enough to follow all its hidden meaning. If I were to pursue the comparison of the three women, I would digress too far. Every dream has at least one place where it is unfathomable, the navel, as it were, by which it is connected to the unknown."[247] In the section on forgetting dreams, Freud elaborates the point in language that is decidedly more poetic:

> The best-interpreted dreams often have a passage that has to be left in the dark, because we notice in the course of interpretation that a knot of dream-thoughts shows itself just there, refusing to be unravelled, but also making no further contribution to the dream-content. This is the dream's navel, and the place beneath which lies the Unknown. Indeed, the dream-thoughts we come upon as we interpret cannot in general but remain without closure, spinning out on all sides into the web-like fabric of our thoughts. Out of a denser path in this tissue the dream-wish then arises like a mushroom from its mycelium.[248]

Freud's comment appears after he acknowledges with remarkable candor that it is not possible to interpret every dream, since the interpreter must combat the very "psychical powers that are responsible for the distortion in the dream. In this way it becomes a contest of relative strength whether one's intellectual interest, capacity for self-overcoming, psychological insight, and practice in the interpretation of dreams can master the internal resistances."[249] But even if one were able to overcome these obstacles, there would still be a dimension of the dream that exceeds the limits of analysis, an inherent impenetrability, the vagueness and opaqueness that is elusive, equivocal, and indefinite,[250] the knot of the dream thoughts (*ein Knäuel von Traumgedanken*) that cannot be disentangled, an inscrutable factor that is marked linguistically as the navel of the dream (*der Nabel des Traums*), a figure of speech that draws Freud's thinking close to a mystical sensibility,[251] as the image of the umbilicus, the scar that circumscribes the place where the end of the umbilical cord was tied after being cut—a metaphorical trope that Freud endorsed to articulate the inherently metaphorical nature of the dream—connotes the twofold bind, to be bound and unbound, connected to and yet separate from the origin in the unconscious cloaked in its interpretive disrobing. Beneath the place of the dream's navel lies that which can be known only as unknown (*Unerkannten*), a vestige of the absurd and erratic dimensions of the dream activity that are transformed through a "secondary revision" into more coherent and orderly dream thoughts,[252] a resounding and abounding silence, forever exceeding the reach of language.[253] The interpretation of the dream, according to Freud, embraces the concept of *Verneinung*, which can be translated as "negation" or "denial," but which I would render as the (un)saying of one thing through its opposite, revealing by means of concealing, concealing by means of revealing.[254] The creation of metaphor, of which the dream is a particular manifestation, stems from this capacity, the self-deception that engenders the contrived similarities of the dissimilar, the unmasking of the mask in masking the unmasked.

Wittgenstein criticized Freud for transforming the essentially silent nature of dream images into a dream language that bears a "certain resemblance to the signs of a language."[255] The Austrian philosopher insisted that the inherently unsayable constituent of the dream is its aesthetic component, a component that could not be addressed in any analytic regimen, including Freudian psychoanalysis.[256] There is merit to Wittgenstein's critique, but there is a reading of Freud that could entertain the possibility that in his own mind, the dream dissembles in a language of silence that is incompatible with the syntactical and grammatical rules of ordinary language. A repercussion of this possibility can be discerned in the following aporetic admonition of Jung: "In dream-analysis we must never forget, even for a moment, that we move on treacherous ground where nothing is certain but uncertainty." The predilection, therefore, is to instruct the dream interpreter, "Do anything you like, only don't try to understand!"[257] Jung's approach to the dream is reflective of a more systemic paradox that colors his understanding of the human psyche: unveiling the mystery of the unconscious would require it becoming part of consciousness, which it cannot become without ceasing to be unconscious, and thus the more one plumbs the depths of the self, the greater the mystery one becomes to oneself.[258] The roots for this epistemological agnosticism can be traced to Plato, who skeptically viewed the dream, in contrast to waking, as a kind of apprehension that falls short of knowledge—like the fables that poets fabricate to serve as a "useful drug" (*pharmakon chrēsimon*) in allowing us to speak of ancient events that we do not know by likening falsehood to truth as much as is possible[259]—since one cannot give an account of judgments based on it.[260] In the *Theaetetus*, Plato, through the persona of Socrates, proffers that the dream, much like the method employed by mathematicians, presumes the existence of "first things" or "elements" that are unknowable. While these unanalyzable elements can be named, they are nonetheless beyond discourse.[261] The metaphor of the dream's navel in Freud is meant, correspondingly, to communicate the sense that, semiotically, the dream strives to express the inexpressible, that is, to express what is beyond expressibility and thus subject to incessant expression. As Lacan observed, "It is not without effect that, even in a public speech, one directs one's attention at subjects, touching them at what Freud calls the navel—*the navel of the dreams*, he writes, to designate their ultimately unknown centre—which is simply, like the same anatomical navel that represents it, that gap of which I have already spoken."[262]

Elsewhere, Lacan refers to this gap as that which "constitutes awakening," that is, the temporal fissure in which the phenomenon of the "emergence of the represented reality" that awakens one from the dream is dreamt as part of the dream.[263] By attending to the fact that the "noise" that arouses the dreamer from sleep is itself the final gesture of the dream, Lacan marks the spot where the border between wakefulness and dreaming is both clarified and obfuscated. Resolutely from that site, the "place of the real, which stretches from the trauma to the phantasy,"[264] does he issue the rhetorical queries that illumine the nature of the dream:

> Is not the dream essentially, one might say, an act of homage to the missed reality—the reality that can no longer produce itself except by repeating itself endlessly, in some never attained awakening? What encounter can there be henceforth with that forever inert being—even now being devoured by the flames—if not the encounter that occurs precisely at the moment when, by accident, as if by chance, the flames come to meet him?[265]

Turning Freud's analysis against itself, Lacan concludes that the dream cannot be considered a wish fulfillment. If need is the operative term, then the desire that the dream truly satisfies is to prolong sleep, for by prolonging the somnolent state, the "unique encounter" with the underlying traumatic event is endlessly commemorated in the hiatus wherein the dream summons the constituted phenomenal reality that exposes the nonrepresentational Real beyond, but still enveloped within, the dream imagery.[266] In Lacan's paradoxical language, "Thus the encounter, forever missed, has occurred between dream and awakening, between the person who is still asleep and whose dream we will not know and the person who has dreamt merely in order not to wake up."[267] What is essential to the dream is the role Freud assigned to the unconscious, the *Vorstellungsrepräsentanz*, which Lacan renders as "that which takes the place of representation" (*le tenant-lieu de la representation*). The phantasy of the dream, accordingly,

> is never anything more than the screen that conceals something quite primary, something determinant in the function of repetition.... This, indeed, is what, for us, explains both the ambiguity of the function of awakening and of the function of the real in

> this awakening. The real may be represented by the accident, the noise, the small element of reality, which is evidence that we are not dreaming. But, on the other hand, this reality is not so small, for what wakes us is the other reality hidden behind the lack of that which takes the place of representation—this, says Freud is the *Trieb*.

The drive of which Freud spoke is thus interpreted by Lacan as the "real" that "has to be sought beyond the dream—in what the dream has enveloped, hidden from us, behind the lack of representation of which there is only one representative," the "real that governs our activities more than any other."[268] From the dream, then, we awaken to be resituated in a "constituted and represented reality," but that reality is itself a fanciful covering of the Real that is beyond the dream imagery, indeed, the representative surfeit that repudiates any and every shot at representation.

Even more effusive in its repudiation of the dream's imagistic representability according to Freud is the reflection proposed by Derrida:

> Such a proposition, this time, no longer concerns a provisional limit, a reserve of meaning that still awaits us; it concerns rather a night, an absolute unknown that is originarily, congenitally bound or tied (but also in itself unbound because ab-solute) to the essence and to the birth of the dream, attached to the place from which it departs and of which it keeps the birthmark: the umbilicus, the omphalic place is the place of a *tie*, a knot-scar that keeps the memory of a cut and even of a severed thread at birth. And the *general* proposition, the assertion in the form of an unconditionally posed law, which is itself cut off from its context and detached from the fragment of the dream that gives its pretext, is the assertion according to which *every* dream, *always*, carries within it at least one place (*eine Stelle*), one marked *topos* that situates it as *unergründlich, gleichsam einen Nabel*: impenetrable, unfathomable, unanalyzable, like a navel, an *omphalos*.[269]

We can, on this basis, refer to the dream as the spectacle of what cannot be specularized, not a something that cannot be envisioned, but the absence of vision that makes vision of any sort possible. The images of the dream (in whatever sentient form they are experienced) point beyond themselves to that place that lies deeper still within, what Derrida calls the *trace*, the metaphor that is, metaphorically speaking, the metaphor of metaphoricity. As is well known, for Derrida, the trace is not a trace of some presence that has withdrawn and hence has the potential to be represented, but a trace of a trace, a trace that is from the beginning a retrace, originally a copy, the first that is second, a simulacrum of the simulacrum. In this retrace, the withdrawal of withdrawal (*re-trait*), is the opening of the impossible possibility, possibly impossible, the opening of opening, and thus it is compared allegorically to the "matrix, womb, or receptacle that is never and nowhere offered up in the form of presence, or in the presence of form."[270] Derrida rightly notes that Plato had already juxtaposed the image of the dream and space (*khōra*), the interval between (*metaxy*) things perceptible to the senses and the Forms, appearance and reality, becoming and being, time and eternity. Recourse is made to the dream, therefore, to articulate a kind of seeing that "cannot simply be conceived in terms of the opposition between sensible and intelligible."[271] For Plato, this space is a "third nature," that which

> admits not of destruction and provides a home for all created beings, and is apprehended, when all sense is absent, by a kind of spurious reason, and is hardly real—which we, beholding as in a dream, say of all existence that it must of necessity be in some place and occupy a space, but that what is neither in heaven nor in earth has no existence. Of these and other things of the same kind, relating to the true and waking reality of nature, we have only this dreamlike sense, and we are unable to cast off sleep and determine the truth about them.[272]

The cadence of the dream may be heeded from this breach between what is imagined to be real and what is really imagined, the spectral of the spectral, as it were, whence we see the unseeable as the invisible cause of visibility and the seeable as the visible effect of invisibility. Plato's conception of the *khōra* provides a model to grasp the intricate nexus of the poetic and the oneiric: the poem, as a dream, is a nonspatial space, a space that is neither celestial nor terrestrial, an opening of the imagination where the invisible is envisioned as the absence that is present as the presence that is absent. The implications of this conception are made explicit in the following rumination of Bachelard:

"Primal poetry, poetry that allows us a taste for our inner destiny, is an adherence to the invisible.... True poetry is a function of awakening."[273] I would add—by way of amplification, and not alteration—that this awakening is a *waking to* rather than from the dream, that is, awakening to dream the dream of awakening.

Sign Language and Visual Metaphoricity

The homology between the dream and poetry is enhanced by the fact that the former provides examples of what Ralph Waldo Emerson (1803–1882) called *picture-language*,[274] or, in the more recent phrase of Ernest Hartmann, *picture metaphors*,[275] expressions that imply that the sharp contrast between the verbal and visual is not particularly appropriate or useful.[276] It seems, rather, that we should seek the formation of dream images in a space of the brain, as it were, where the sensory lines crisscross, a neural netting that would likely account for the experience of synesthesia, a looping of the two epistemic modes, an optical allusion, the seeing of what is heard that is concomitantly the hearing of what is seen. Some people, apparently, are more prone to this phenomenon, but, to a degree, it is present potentially in each of us, and it finds a more or less attenuated instantiation in the terrain of dreams. Every dream image is, in fact, an image of an image, a reiteration that calls to mind the twofold meaning enfolded in the fold of metaphor, a literal skin enveloping a figurative body. Furthermore, the duality of the dream vision, which can be framed more generally as a specific instance of representational seeing,[277] renders fluid the boundary between inner and outer, and thus it would be equally plausible to speak of a literal body enveloping a figurative skin. Indeed, a distinctive, though by no means exclusive, contribution of rabbinic oneiromancy is the emphasis placed on the hermeneutical dimension of dream interpretation as a practice of interpreting sentient forms as linguistic pointers.[278] I will explore this insight in greater detail in Chapter 3, but suffice it here to translate it into a more contemporary neuroanatomical register: the dream can be considered a type of brain activity in which the image at the level of its confabulation is a semiotic doubling, a simulacrum that puts on the (dis)appearance of a simulacrum, the duplexity of the duplexity, to which we referred previously. I approve of the nicely formulated conclusion of Hartmann that "the dream is doing (in pictures) something very similar to what we do when we speak of life metaphorically as a road, a plant, a tree, or a fire, or speak of love metaphorically as a journey. We try to explain something important but difficult or problematic in terms of something simpler; we especially try to explain it in terms of a visual image."[279]

A dream may be likened to the narration of a story, not in a secondary sense, but as part of the experience that is primarily being recounted, that is, a story about telling a story.[280] I would resist the attempt to distinguish experience and the postexperiential report, as we find in the following remarks of Patricia A. Kilroe:

> The dream while it is being dreamed is experience, not text. Our memory of that experience, whether we report it or not, is the text of the dream. So there is something between the initial experience of the dream and the dream report, just as there is something between waking experience and our report of that experience. The report in both cases is a text; the experience itself is not.[281]

The distinction enunciated in this passage is hermeneutically flawed, and consequently, the attribution of the label "text" exclusively to the memory or account of a dream that is no longer experienced is also questionable. Closer to the mark is a second comment by Kilroe, which expresses her own perspective more faithfully:

> We can hardly produce a dream report, moreover, if the experienced dream is not already a unit of text.... So it is necessary to begin, at least, by examining dream *reports* for evidence of textuality and narrativity in the experienced dream.... In addition to positing that experienced dreams are texts, I consider the verbal dream report to be a particular form of text which transforms the experienced-dream text into an objective product, analogously to the way a given story can be told through different media.[282]

The dream, on this score, may be considered continuous with states of wakeful consciousness wherein the line between experience and interpretation is not easily drawn. Even from a strictly neurophysiological approach to consciousness, it has been argued with respect to what is technically called the *subjective referrals of cerebral sensory responses*: "Subjective experiences of mental events, generally, are not reducible to or describable by the activities of the nerve cells that give rise to the experiences."[283] From this it follows that "a complete knowledge of the neuron activities would tell you nothing about the subjective experiences they may elicit. To get at the latter, you must ask for an introspective report of the experience by the individual, who alone has 'access' to his conscious functions."[284] The scientific contention that the nature and content of conscious experiences are not isomorphic with the nerve cell activities that produced them bolsters the hermeneutic sense that the experiential and interpretive radii intersect in the phenomenological vector of human subjectivity. I would, therefore, reject the notion that "interpretation always writes over the dream," a deduction that is based on the additional faulty assumption that there is an inherent "struggle between the word and the image."[285] On the contrary, the dream phenomenon underscores that word and image are two facets of one imaginal reality; the verbal and the visual converge in such a way that we cannot envision the image without the word or heed the word without the image. In the matter of the dream, we might say, retelling itself is part of the texture of the tale that is told inceptually; there is no trace of origin or origin of the trace, but only an original trace, a trace that is itself a trace. Each dream, therefore, is a text,[286] or a hypertext, a palimpsest, inscripted by the dreamer in the poiesis of dreaming, an activity that is referred to psychoanalytically as the dreamwork.[287]

The composite relation between dream and dreamer tied to the mythopoeic production of images can be compared fruitfully to the relation between observer and field articulated in quantum mechanics, the principle of complementarity that bridges the seeming incommensurability between the psychic and physical by maintaining that the knowability and measurability of a phenomenon depend on the circumstances under which one attempts to measure its properties.[288] As Anders Karlsson put it, "information encoded on quantum systems, which we can call quantum information, can sometimes be as subtle and fragile as a dream. When you describe a dream to someone else, your memory of it changes, and you can never convey the complete picture. In the quantum world, if you interact with a quantum system, inevitably, you are also changing it."[289] Expressed rudimentarily, the nature of a quantum entity has a dual potential; it can be either particles or waves; its "actual" nature is dependent on the observational bias of the physicist. For some, this constructivist stance entails, in the language of Christopher Norris, the "flight from realism" and the "logic of an anti-realism."[290] The summation of his view is worth citing:

> Moreover, as I have said, it is often the case that quantum mechanics is invoked in support of various anti-realist positions. What suits it for this role is the way that it inverts the realist order of priority between ontology and epistemology by transferring the burden of unresolved doubts, paradoxes, uncertainties, etc., from our restricted *knowledge* of whatever transpires in the quantum-physical domain to the *very nature* of quantum "reality" construed—in vaguely Kantian terms—as a noumenal thing-in-itself. Whence the idea (congenial to some) that physics has itself at last come around to the kind of anti-realist or constructivist outlook that is something like the default philosophy of many thinkers in the present-day social and human sciences.[291]

Even if we were not to go so far as to repudiate the existence of an empirical reality independent of mind, we would be hard-pressed to disavow the valuation of Bernard d'Espagnat that such a reality, while knowable on the basis of experiential data, remains veiled, indeed, veiled precisely because our routine assumptions are enshrouded by the theoretical models through which it is known.[292] To be more precise, d'Espagnat, who distinguishes between the common-sense view or "conventional realism" and "idealism" or "phenomenism" as two leading explanations of the claim that "physics is an experimental science,"[293] reaches the following conclusion:

> To sum up: some aspects of idealism, and especially of Kantianism, are definitely obsolete, including in particular the main motivations Kant had for developing his ideas. But on the other hand, and contrary to appearances, the realist's firm belief that the primary qualities are possessed by the objects ("really" are, on the whole, as we see them to be) and that space (or, nowadays, space-time) is an independently existing arena where the things (nowadays, events) *are*, does not seem to be well grounded either in logic (pure reason)

> or in factual knowledge. Or, to put it less bluntly, if, after all, it *is* somehow grounded in the latter, the way it is is by far not as obvious as it would seem, and the extent to which it is must be analyzed and discussed.[294]

The author embarks on a detailed analysis of the clash between "open realism" or "strong objectivity" and "weak objectivity," the belief that there is no independent reality in ordinary space and time,[295] but from his perspective, it is not feasible to entertain a theory that would be both ontologically interpretable and scientifically convincing.[296] Avoiding further discussion of these philosophical intricacies, we can assert confidently that the rejection of a scientific approach that draws a firm line between subject and object, mind and matter, epistemology and ontology, would seem to well fit the porous and ostensibly illogical nature of the dream reality, which I relate more generally to what some phenomenologists call the indeterminacy of the imagination.[297] The presumption that quantum physics is "based on a mathematical framework of nonobservable entities" and the further assumption that the quantum wave function, perceptible at the microscopic level, necessarily consists of both real and imaginary parts, that is, "a part that could be pictured as a real physical wave and a part that only exists in our imagination," provide a reasonable scientific standard to serve as a "metaphorical basis" to explain the convoluted neural events that we classify as dream states.[298] As Terrence McKenna observed, "the major quantum mechanical phenomena that we all experience, aside from waking consciousness itself, are dreams and hallucinations. These states ... occur when large amounts of various sorts of radiation conveyed in the body by the senses are restricted. Then we see interior processes that are psychophysical."[299]

To delve into the dream, one must adopt a logic that purports the probability of the counterfactual,[300] that is, a logic that is not predicated on the partition of truth and fallacy on the basis of a simple correspondence model. The veracity of the dream rests on the disjunctive compossibility between interior and exterior. Moreover, the intonation of temporality that we experience, or imagine that we do, in the dream is commensurate with the reversibility of time affirmed by some quantum physicists and the related notion of a retroactive causality—the belief that the causal arrow may be inverted, such that the present is determinative of the past as much as the past is determinative of the present.[301] This vantage point lends credence to the comment of McKenna that the dream is "an example of telekinesis," that is, of mind causing matter to move.[302] Or, in the related articulation of Talbot:

> The omnijective continuum of a dream provides an adequate explanation for a causal phenomenon. For instance, I can dream that I gaze at a flower and cause it to bloom. In a dream this is perfectly normal. I do not wonder why the flower bloomed in accordance with my whim. No psychokinetic energies or interaction need pass between the flower and myself to explain this cause and effect. The consciousness of the dreamer generates the space-time of the dream.[303]

Extending the matter beyond the dream, we can say that mindfulness, or whatever word one may educe, is itself part of the warp and woof of the material world configured in and by consciousness, whether imagined as real or realized as imagined, a distinction that makes little difference if the impact of what occurs is gauged from the effect on the nervous system. How substantial is the quantitative deviation in the psychoelectrical activity of my brain between actually seeing a beautiful object or simply imagining one to be so?

Brain waves move matter in the same patterns in both networks, and, hence, it is not logically objectionable to accord mind the status of first cause. Mind and matter are still the basic coordinates by which we orient ourselves in the phenomenal realm and in virtue of which we would be justified to speak in quantum terms, as I noted above, of an interactive dualism, that is, a theory of being that preserves the autonomy of the mental and physical, even as it insists on their constant and inevitable interweaving.[304] Viewing things from a psychophysical as opposed to the (similarly reductive) panpsychic[305] or panmaterialist perspectives inverts the anticipated temporal alignment of cause and effect. I will return to this matter in the final chapter, but let me here state unequivocally, lest there be any misunderstanding, that I do not intend to enforce upon the dream a structure or a process that presumes a clearly defined subject-object division or even the *noesis-noema* classification of Husserlian phenomenology; nevertheless, I do think we must attribute intentionality to every state of consciousness, even that of a dream;[306] indeed, the claim is necessitated by the eminently credible hypothesis that consciousness is dependent on intentionality, rather than vice versa.[307] However, in consonance with the venerable apophatic tradition, I would argue that there is a type of intentionality that can be demarcated only as the nonintentional—humans are capable, and I suggest uniquely so, of thinking about the unthinkable and speaking about the unspeakable—the mental affixing of a linguistic sign to the signpost to which no sign can be affixed. Consider the following remark of Wittgenstein: "By 'intention' I mean here what uses a sign in a thought. The intention seems to interpret, to give the final interpretation; which is not a further sign or picture, but something else, the thing that cannot be further interpreted. But what we have reached is a psychological, not a logical terminus."[308]

Wittgenstein encourages the reader to perform a thought experiment, to translate the "sign-language" into "an unambiguous picture-language, a language consisting of pictures painted in perspective."[309] The former yields different interpretations of an "intended picture," whereas the latter marks the end of the possibility of interpretation, because the picture itself allegedly represents the likeness of the reality to which the similarity corresponds.

> It is as if at first we looked at a picture so as to enter into it and the objects in it surrounded like real ones; and then we stepped back, and were now outside it; we saw the frame, and the picture was a painted surface. In this way, when we intend, we are surrounded by our intention's pictures and we are inside them. But when we step outside intention, they are mere patches on a canvas, without life and of no interest to us.[310]

The interpretative process, as the matter of intention more generally, unfolds to the extent that one is inside the pictorial enframing as part of the picture, rather than standing outside as someone gazing upon it. As Wittgenstein recapitulated the matter:

> It's beginning to look somehow as if intention could never be recognized as *intention* from outside; as if one must be doing the meaning

> of it oneself in order to understand it as meaning. That would amount to considering it not as a phenomenon or fact but as something intentional which has a direction to it. What this direction is, we do not know; it is something which is absent from the phenomenon as such.[311]

Intention cannot be grasped from outside a phenomenon, but it is also not integral to the phenomenon. Wittgenstein tenders the particular example of the dream to illustrate this more general phenomenological predicament: "In dreams it sometimes happens that we first read a story and then are ourselves participants in it. And after waking up after a dream it is sometimes as if we had stepped back out of the dream and now see it before us as an alien picture."[312]

Not only is the dream not inimitable, but it is illustrative of the problem of intentionality more generally, which is related to a psychological need to bridge the spatial-temporal chasms that separate images linked together in family resemblances. To speak of intentionality requires that one is situated inside what needs to be viewed as outside. In this (non)locality, future and past crisscross, not as lines converging from opposite ends of the spectrum, but as a wave, bending back on itself, in the recollection of expectation and the expectation of recollection. Foucault insisted, against the explanation of Freud, that the dream cannot be understood simply as the obsessive repetition of an original trauma, a reliving of the primal scene. The dream is the retrieval of the "originative movement of the imagination"—the "bringing forth" of that "which in *Existenz* is most irreducible to history"—wherein the "fundamental forms of existence" are restored.[313] This temporal inception, which is impervious to historical calibration, is as much looking forward as it is looking backward.[314] The dreamer is always in and of the moment of the dream, abiding boundlessly in the bounded space we call time and lingering immeasurably in the measured time we call space, the interim beyond subjectification, the stipulation beyond objectification. Still, we must ponder, how does one speak of intentionality in the dream? How does one explain nocturnal vision, this seeing in the dark?

CHAPTER TWO

Seeing-Not: Nocturnality and the Dream Vision

O little root of a dream
you hold me here
undermined by blood,
no longer visible to anyone,
property of death.
—Paul Celan, *Glottal Stop*

In the previous chapter, we marshaled a significant amount of phenomenological evidence, punctuated by neuroscientific data, to substantiate the claim that nonintentional intentionality may be singled out as the distinctive characteristic of the dream that accounts concurrently for uniformity and variation. To probe this dimension, it is necessary to contemplate the *nocturnality of the oneiric*, a term that denotes not a temporal demarcation, but an epistemic condition, that is, the nocturnal is not limited to nighttime, but can relate as well to dream visions that occur diurnally. We will be guided on this path by the truism that there can be no seeing in the dark that is not also a seeing of the dark. But what is it to see the dark from within the dark, to envision the depth of a surface that is the surface of a depth not offered to the ocular gaze? The task before us is to explore the paradox that dreaming is a genre of maximal imaginality revealed in the image concealing its character as image. The dream, on this score, fosters the appearance of the inapparent, disclosing thereby the limit delimited and yet breached by the imagination in unveiling the image whence it is disclosed that the substance of the dream can be phenomenally present only in being absent from being either ontically present or absent.

To advance this understanding of presence-to-being as absence-from-being, I turn first to the thought of Moses Maimonides, rabbinic authority, physician, and philosopher. It is no exaggeration to say that no figure in the history of Jewish thought from any period has been discussed and analyzed as much as Maimonides. Needless to say, the burden of previous scholarship must weigh heavily on anyone who seeks to contribute something novel on any discrete topic in the body of his thought. It would be imprudent to rehearse the plethora of opinions regarding the dream expressed by this seminal thinker. My aim, therefore, is not to provide such a survey or to offer a comprehensive analysis; rather, extrapolating from the Maimonidean discourse, I will present a model for looking at the dream as the imagistic resistance to the reification of image through the profusion of image. The dream, in other words, is the phantasm that allows us to see the chimerical nature of the phantasm, the speculum through which we perceive the speculum as that through which we perceive the speculum. In piercing through this prism, we discern the invariable and unsettling truth that the image is true to the degree that it is false and false to the degree that it is true. The veracity of this truth breaks with the law of the excluded middle (P or not-P) and the corollary principle of noncontradiction (a thing cannot be both P and not-P in the same respect and at the same time) to which Maimonides indefatigably adhered as the logical foundations of humanity's ontological experience in the world, determined primarily by the yearning to cultivate knowledge—as Aristotle notoriously put in the opening lines of the *Metaphysics*—much as the conventional distinction between good and evil serves as the axiological foundation for humanity's political experience and the social behavior necessary for its promotion.[1] To treat truth and deception as indistinguishable is a sign of foolishness and weak-mindedness.[2] The exception, however, is the dream, about which it can be said, in the accepted parlance deployed in some medieval Jewish thinkers and more expansively in later texts, that it is "one substratum that bears two opposites" (*shenei hafakhim be-nose eḥad*), a motif that will figure prominently in Chapter 4.[3] In my judgment, the core of Maimonides' thinking about the dream and human imagination can and should be specularized from the standpoint of this paradox, the dimension that exceeds the perimeter of his own vision, a process that may be called *demarcating the center from the margin.*

Indeed, there is at least one critical passage wherein Maimonides seems to edge himself toward stepping over the line and subverting what he considered to be the elemental basis for any logical calculus. In describing the manifestation of truth as a sudden flash of light—perhaps influenced by the language of Ibn Bājja (1085–1139)—he notes that for most people, this occurs intermittently, so that the obscure and dark night will appear momentarily to be bright as day. But there is an individual, he admits, "for whom the lightning flashes time and again, so that he is always, as it were, in unceasing light. Thus night appears to him as day."[4] The individual to whom Maimonides refers is Moses, the greatest of prophets, who attained the permanent state of conjunction, encoded in the scriptural image of standing with the divine (Deuteronomy 5:28),[5] and thus, for him, there was no more opposition between diurnal and nocturnal.[6] Maimonides may fall short of explicitly saying that the principle of noncontradiction does not apply to the infinity of God, as one finds, for instance, in the thought of Nicholas of Cusa (1401–1464),[7] but his characterization of one knowing the secret wisdom surely lends weight to the argument that the object of that wisdom would itself validate the overcoming of the binary. The conflation that is usually ascribed to the blind person—the inability to discern the difference between light and dark[8]—is here applied to the maximum vision that was realized by only one human being. Thinking in the footsteps of Maimonides, I will make such a claim for the dream state more generally, a move that is justified by the fact that he, like many of the medieval philosophers and theologians who articulated the rudimentary tenets of scriptural monotheism, catalogued dreams as an integral aspect of prophecy.

The account of the oneiric and prophetic imagination to be elicited from Maimonides will be interrogated further by a return to the critical text by Foucault explicating the views of Binswanger. The bringing together of these thinkers may strike one as a curious harnessing of disparate figures separated not only by the chasm of time, but also by vast and seemingly unbridgeable cultural differences. The juxtaposition, however, is justified not only by an affinity of thought, but by the fact that at a decisive moment in the presentation of his argument, Foucault refers to Spinoza,[9] whose views on dreams and prophecy unequivocally exhibit the influence of Maimonides.[10] The thematic and historical rationalization aside, the pairing of Maimonides and Foucault conceptually casts a vivid light on the inherent nocturnality of the dream vision, a light that does not dispel, but deepens the darkness of our oneiric capability to imagine what cannot be imagined, a seeing when there is nothing to be seen, a configuration of the disfigured that opens the possibility of the disfiguration of the configured.

Prophecy and the Dream

In the Hebrew biblical canon, we find various views on the relation of prophetic revelation and dreams, although a common denominator seems to be the privilege accorded the ocularcentric dimension of both phenomena.[11] What is significant about the dream is that it is a mode of seeing in the present about the future based on the past, and similarly, prophecy is a preview of what will transpire, often envisioned in parabolic images that call for interpretation. Thus, the Deuteronomist warns against the "prophet or dreamer of dreams" (*navi o ḥolem ḥalom*), who wishes to entice the Israelites to worship other gods (Deuteronomy 13:2–6). The coupling of dream and prophecy in this setting has a pejorative connotation; there are those who use prophetic vision to promote erroneous beliefs. Jeremiah, too, distinguishes false and honorable prophets on the grounds that the former proffer their dreams to legitimate their message and the latter receive the word of God faithfully (Jeremiah 14:14, 23:25–29, 27:9–10, 29:8–9). This should be set in opposition to the priestly oracle (Numbers 12:6) placed in the mouth of the divine addressing Aaron and Miriam at the opening to the Tent of Meeting: YHWH appears to the prophet in a vision (*mar'ah*) and speaks to him in a dream (*ḥalom*). Prophetic vision and dream are acknowledged as the means by which God communicates to human beings.[12] The legitimacy of the oneiric as an oracular source is underscored by the combination of prophecy and dreams in the case of Saul (1 Samuel 28:6, 15). Correspondingly, the words "dreams" (*ḥalomot*) and "visions" (*ḥezyonot*) are used interchangeably in the apocalyptic hope for the return of prophetic inspiration expressed as an eschatological prediction "I will pour out my spirit on all flesh; your sons and daughters shall prophesy; your old men shall dream dreams, and your young men shall see visions" (Joel 3:1).

The divergent views chronicled in the scriptural canon have served as fodder for the Jewish exegetical imagination across time, some interpreters (possibly visionaries in their own right) emphasizing the prophetic propensity of the dream and others making a point of noting that dreams are a less direct and inferior means of revelation.[13] It has even been suggested that the increase of dreams in postbiblical literature, which includes textual reports of dreams, as well as documentation concerning dreams that result from incubation oracles,[14] may be related to the presumption that prophecy ceased as an official institution.[15] Let us evoke the observation of Philip Alexander that *all* the aphorisms included in the rabbinic dreambook, which is redacted in the ninth chapter of the tractate of Berakhot in the Babylonian Talmud, "circle round one burning question, viz., Are dreams—the dreams of the Rabbis and their contemporaries—prophetic? That is to say, do they contain authoritative messages from God—instructions as to how to act, or predictions of the future?"[16]

Support for this contention can be drawn from a number of dicta scattered about the vast rabbinic corpus, for instance, the exegetical gloss of Rava on the verse "I will keep my countenance hidden on that day" (Deuteronomy 31:18): "The blessed holy One said, Even though I have concealed my countenance from them, 'I will speak to him in a dream' (Numbers 12:6)."[17] The ostensibly simplistic comment betrays a very complex exegesis that simultaneously undermines and upholds the intent of the scriptural proof text. According to the literal sense, divine speech in a dream is a form of prophetic theophany; the rabbinic reading presumes that God's auditory appearance in a dream occurs in the moment of withdrawal of the visual. Hence, with a touch of more than a little irony, the dream turns out to be a mode of prophecy that is still available in the time of the hiding of the divine face; indeed, if we are bold enough to read between the lines, we can detect that it is the very concealment that occasions the disclosure, that is, God's word is heard in the dream because the face is occluded from sight. The narrowing of the gap between ordinary dreaming and prophecy[18] is epitomized as well in the statement of R. Yoḥanan that if a scriptural text occurs to a person upon waking, it is a "minor kind of prophecy" (*nevu'ah qeṭannah*),[19] and even more so in the anonymous pronouncement that "a dream is one-sixtieth of prophecy"[20] or in Ḥanina bar Yiṣḥaq's proverbial quip that the dream is the unripe fruit of prophecy (*novelet nevu'ah ḥalom*).[21]

The premonitory perspective on the dream continued to evolve in the course of time, as is confirmed by the widespread practice in medieval Jewish magical, mystical, and even halakhic sources—the two best-known examples are Moses ben Jacob of Coucy's introduction to *Sefer Miṣwot Gedolot* (*Book of the Great Commandments*) and Jacob of Marvège's *She'elot u-Teshuvot min ha-Shamayim* (*Responsa from Heaven*)[22]—of inducing a revelation of the divine through the dream inquiry (*she'elat ḥalom*), which is thought to be on a par with prophecy.[23] In the case of some kabbalists—for example, Isaac of Acre[24]—it is even linked to letter permutation, the meditational technique that facilitates conjunction with God.[25] Furthermore, the impressionistic dicta of the rabbinic sages (at least as may be gathered from how they have been conserved) on the relationship of the oneiric and the prophetic were thematized in a more coherent fashion by later medieval commentators. The importance of this issue, which is discussed in diverse cultural contexts, is attested especially by the place it occupies in the work of Christian and Islamic thinkers, who were conversant with and likely influenced by Jewish doctrines, just as we can reasonably assume the reverse to be true. In the history of Judaism, the most significant voice in this regard was Maimonides, for not only does he provide a valuable revisioning of the earlier texts, but he articulates, albeit in the idiom contemporary to his time, the speculative underpinning of some of the older aphorisms on the nexus between divination and the dream.[26] My reading of the Maimonidean material will focus principally on his understanding of the dream imagination as an apophatic effacement of the imagistic. The discussion of the dream in Maimonides accentuates that the imagination, unfettered by the impediment of logical verification or empirical corroboration, is the path that leads to the annihilation of the image. When applied to the matter of prophecy, the theological implications of this apophasis remain as startling today as in his own time: theism in its extreme gives way to atheism, the rejection of a theistic conception of the divine and a rendering of all God language as an analogical discourse about a being that is fundamentally dissimilar to all other beings but itself.

Dream Imagination and Envisioning What Is Not

In *The Guide of the Perplexed* (*Dalālat al-ḥā'irīn*), Maimonides sets the elucidation of the dream in a prophetology informed by cosmological and epistemological assumptions well attested in medieval science, indebted to the Arabic translations and amplifications of the *Corpus Aristotelicum*. Without denying the many nuances and variations of the description of prophecy, dreams, and divination that can be culled from the rich literature of Islamic philosophy, it is fair to say that there is, generally speaking, a reemergence of the ancient figure of the "scientific prophet," the divinely inspired sage to whom knowledge has been entrusted.[27] In particular, Maimonides appropriates the view of Abū Naṣr al-Fārābī (ca. 870–950) on the dynamics of revelatory experience. In *The Political Regime* (*al-Siyāsa al-Madaniyya*), al-Fārābī states that prophetic illumination is explained by the mechanics of the process of intellection related to the quadripartite division of the intellect—delineated in greater detail in his *Epistle on the Intellect* (*Risāla fī al-'Aql*)—with the major exception that the soul worthy of revelation is said to progress through the stages of actualization by its own effort and with the aid of divine power, but without the instruction of an external source. The intellectual overflow issues from God through the Active Intellect (*al-'aql al-fa''āl*)—the last of the ten separate intellects correlated with the heavenly spheres—to the individual's potential intellect (*al-'aql bil-quwwa*), and as a consequence, one obtains knowledge of the universals or intelligible forms. Once the potential intellect is so realized, it becomes the actual intellect (*al-'aql bil-fi'l*), and when the latter becomes self-intelligible, it is called the acquired intellect (*al-'aql mustafād*). The prophetic experience entails a supplementary efflux to the imagination of the soul that has attained the rank of self-intellection wherein there is no intermediary separating itself and the Active Intellect. Prophecy, so understood, consists of the imaginative translation of rational truths into allegorical images.[28] Analogously, in his chapter called

"Representation and Divination" in *On the Perfect State* (*Mabādi' Ârā' Ahl al-Madīnat al-Fāḍilah*), al-Fārābī, in part following the lead of al-Kindī (ca. 801–870) in the treatise *On Sleep and Dream* (*Risālah fī Māhīyat an-Naum war-Ru'yā*),[29] states that objects of the dream perception consist of the symbols that are confabulated in the imagination when it is "free from the fresh imprints of the sensible which are provided again and again by the sense, and is relieved of the service of the rational and appetitive faculties."[30] The Arabic version of Aristotle's explanation of veridical dreams, transmitted principally through the *Parva Naturalia* (*Kitāb al-Ḥiss wal-Maḥsūs*), included one crucial modification that had a major impact on Islamic and Jewish approaches to dreams and prophecy. Whereas Aristotle explained these dreams as arising on account of coincidences or because of purely naturalistic causes (either physiological or psychological), the altered text, inspired by the Stoic doctrine of divination, maintained that the dreams result from providence operating through the Active Intellect.[31] According to al-Fārābī, dream visions and prophetic revelations occur through the same procedure, but with another major difference: the former arise when the Active Intellect imparts its effulgence upon the faculty of imagination as it relates to practical reason, whereas the latter concern theoretical reason.[32]

It is against this backdrop that we have to understand Maimonides' insistence that the intellectual overflow connected to prophecy perfects imagination as well as reason. Maimonides offers a concise formulation of the al-Fārābīan perspective:

> Know that the true reality and quiddity of prophecy consist in its being an overflow from God... through the intermediation of the Active Intellect, toward the rational faculty in the first place and thereafter toward the imaginative faculty. This is the highest degree of man and the ultimate term of perfection that can exist for his species; and this state is the ultimate term of perfection for the imaginative faculty.[33]

Implicit in the above description is the contrast of the traditional stance on prophecy with the philosophical on the grounds that the former insists that this phenomenon depends solely on divine volition, whereas the latter depicts it as chiefly a natural process. Lest one think that this is Maimonides' esoteric position, it should be noted that this explanation of prophecy is embraced even in his patently more exoteric legal works. Consider the sixth of the thirteen principles of faith enunciated in his *Commentary on the Mishnah* in the introduction to the tenth chapter of the tractate Sanhedrin: "The sixth principle—prophecy. That is, one should know that there are human beings possessing a superior nature and great perfection. They prepare their souls till they receive the form of the intellect. The human intellect then conjoins with the Active Intellect. From it a noble emanation emanates upon them. These are the prophets; this is prophecy and this is its essence."[34]

Similarly, we read in the account of prophecy in the laws delineating the foundations of Torah at the beginning of Maimonides' *Mishneh Torah*, the code of rabbinic ritual and jurisprudence:

> One of the principles of the Law is to know that God prophecies to human beings. Prophecy comes only to a sage of exceptional wisdom, valiant in moral traits. His evil inclination never subdues him in any matter. By virtue of his intellect he always subdues his evil inclination. He possesses an exceptionally expansive mind. A person who possesses all these traits and is whole of body, when he enters the orchard [*pardes*] and deliberates upon those great and obscure matters, has an adequate mind to understand and to apprehend, sanctifies himself and separates from the ways of the masses, who walk in the darkness of the temporal, and he goes and incites himself and he trains his soul not to think at all about the idle things or the vanities of time and its conceits, but his mind is always open to what is above, bound to what is beneath the throne of glory, to comprehend those holy and pure forms, and to contemplate the wisdom of the blessed holy One, in its entirety, from the first form to the navel of the earth, and from these he knows his greatness—immediately the holy spirit dwells upon him. When the spirit rests on him, his soul is conjoined with the rank of angels called *ishim*, and he is transformed into a different individual. He understands in his mind that he is not as he was, but rather he is elevated above the rank of the rest of the sages.[35]

The prophet attains a state of conjunction with the Active Intellect, referred to as *ishim* (the plural of *ish*, which means "man"), so called because the last of the ten angelic beings is directly responsible for actualizing each human being's potency as the rational animal. That this state of conjunction is to be distinguished from what is experienced by the philosopher is made clear at the end of the passage, where it is asserted that the prophet "is elevated above the rank of the rest of the sages." Even so, there is no indication that prophecy is anything but a natural condition to be realized by one of exceptional theoretical and moral perfection.

This is not to deny that Maimonides invokes the will of God as a causal agent to explain the production of prophetic visions. Indeed, this is the very criterion that distinguishes the view on prophecy that Maimonides labels the "opinion of our Law and the foundation of our doctrine" from the opinion of the multitude of pagans and the masses of those who profess adherence to the Law, on the one hand, and from the opinion of the philosophers, on the other. The belief of the vulgar is such that God chooses whom he wishes and turns that person into a prophet; the intellectual merits of the individual are irrelevant, although it is presumed that the person possesses a "certain goodness and sound morality." The more sophisticated philosophical perspective maintains that prophecy is consequent to an individual's ethical and cognitive worth, which also comprises perfection of the imagination. The stance of the Law—or, more specifically, the conviction held by informed practitioners—is identical with the philosophical view, with the exception that it may happen that one who is fit for prophecy will not become a prophet on account of the divine will; the ultimate agency is the volition of God.[36] The implications of Maimonides' words were stated lucidly by the Andalusian thinker Isaac Ibn Laṭif (ca. 1210–1280) when he remarked that "every prophet is a philosophical sage, but not every philosopher is a prophet." The one worthy of prophetic inspiration must achieve the requisite perfections of the soul associated with the philosopher, but the holy spirit will not dwell in such a person unless it is so decreed by the volition of God (*ḥefeṣ elohi*).[37] The question that needs to be confronted is what is the divine will? Has Ibn Laṭif interpreted Maimonides correctly, or is it possible that the references of the latter to this notion are dissimulating figures of speech employed to hide a more radical and perhaps even nontheistic view in the language of the accepted theological dogma? Is the divine will nothing more than a poetic way of speaking about the order in nature?[38] At the very least, Maimonides' uncompromising denial of attributing human characteristics to God and his insistence on the utter dissimilarity between the divine and all other beings would preclude the likelihood of interpreting these anthropomorphic statements literally.[39]

However one is to decide on this issue, it follows that to assess Maimonides' statements about prophecy properly, and by extension his understanding of dreams, it is necessary to investigate his idea of providence, particularly in light of the conflict between the supernaturalistic and naturalistic conceptions of divine agency implied by his linking divine governance to the intellect.[40] Such an undertaking, however, would take us too far afield, and for our immediate concerns, what is more crucial to emphasize is Maimonides' insistence on the dreamlike status of the prophetic vision as mediated through the imagination (*al-khayāl*). In a manner consonant with al-Fārābī's position, the perfection of the imaginative faculty (*mutakhayyila*) on the part of the prophet leads Maimonides to distinguish prophecy from ordinary wisdom. That is, the prophet may possess the same knowledge as the philosopher, but it comes about in a way that defies philosophical understanding:

> Know that the true prophets indubitably grasp speculative matters; by means of his speculation alone, man is unable to grasp the causes from which what a prophet has come to know necessarily follows.... For the very overflow that affects the imaginative faculty...is also the overflow that renders perfect the act of the rational faculty.... For the overflow of the Active Intellect goes in its true reality only to it [that is, to the rational faculty], causing it to pass from potentiality to actuality.[41]

On the basis of this epistemological claim, Maimonides distinguished three types of human attainment: the men of science, for whom the influx reaches only the intellect; the prophets, for whom it reaches the intellect and the imagination; and the legislators, for whom it reaches only the imagination.[42] The greatest and noblest action of the imagination occurs during sleep, when the senses rest, and it receives an outpouring that results in a dream that is true. The same inundation occurs during prophecy, and thus we can speak of a difference in "degree" and not in "kind." To cite his words again, "it is known and established as a principle that no prophecy and no prophetic revelation come in any other way except *in a dream* or *in a vision* and through the agency of an angel."[43] That the reference to an "angel" is a figurative trope for the imagination may be gathered from a second passage that describes a similar process in the formation of dreams that occur during sleep:

> For every force charged by God . . . with some business is an angel put in charge of that thing. Accordingly, *Midrash Qoheleth* has the following text: When man sleeps, his soul speaks to the angel, and the angel to the cherub.[44] Thereby they have stated plainly to him who understands and cognizes intellectually that the imaginative faculty is likewise called an *angel* and that the intellect is called a *cherub*.[45]

The datum of both the prophetic and the oneiric vision is considered as if it were a sensory image prompted by stimuli external to the mind exactly when the senses are weakened.[46] Significantly, insofar as prophecy is classified as a species of the genus of veridical dreams, we must view it in the al-Fārābīan sense as the imagination seeing the interior psychological state as if it was an exterior reality,[47] rather than as a similitude (*mithāl*) of the unseen, spiritual reality as al-Ghazālī (1058–1111)[48] and, in his wake, Ibn Khaldūn (1332–1406) argued.[49] Commenting on the midrashic interpretation that the scriptural description of the "ever-turning fiery sword" (*lahaṭ ha-ḥerev ha-mithappekhet*) that was placed at the entrance to the Garden of Eden (Genesis 3:24) signifies that "sometimes they turn into men, sometimes into women, sometimes into spirits, and sometimes into angels,"[50] Maimonides remarked: "Through this dictum they have made clear that the angels are not endowed with matter and that outside the mind they have no fixed corporeal shape, but that all such shapes are only to be perceived in the *vision of prophecy* in consequence of the imaginative capacity."[51] Maimonides is mindful that for most people, it is difficult to apprehend an existence that is "pure of matter and absolutely devoid of corporeality." Only after "strenuous training" in the art of discursive reasoning can one differentiate between "that which is cognized by the intellect and that which is imagined." Even for the majority of those engaged in speculation existence and nonexistence are determined by whether or not something can be caught within the net of imagination.[52]

To comprehend Maimonides' deliberations on the ontic status of the dream, we must take stock of the views articulated by two other Muslim philosophers, Avicenna (Ibn Sīnā, c. 980–1037) and Averroës (Ibn Rushd, 1126–1198). For Avicenna, the dream experience is an illustration of his theory of intellectual prophecy or intuition (*ḥads*), which he proffered as a legitimate way that one can gain knowledge of the intelligible world through conjunction of the Active Intellect with the "holy" or "angelic intellect" (*ʿaql qudsī*, *ʿaql malakī*), terms that he used to name the special type of the *intellectus in habitu* (*ʿaql bi-l-malaka*), the terminology coined by Alexander of Aphrodisias to designate the state between the pure potentiality of a person prior to acquiring universal knowledge and the full actuality of one engaged in intelligible thought.[53] The conjunction brings about the effortless reception of the forms contained in the Active Intellect without resorting to the usual process of cogitation and the gradual acquisition of axiomatic truths by way of deduction and propositional logic. In addition to intellectual prophecy, Avicenna maintained the possibility of a lower form that involved the conjunction of the compositive imaginative faculty (*mutakhayyila*) with the supernal region (*malakūt*), which includes the souls of the celestial spheres, the incorporeal intellects, and perhaps the First Cause (*al-sabab al-awwal*), the First Existent (*al-mawjūd al-awwal*), or the necessary of existence (*wājib al-wujūd*).[54] In this case, theoretical knowledge, which includes prognostication, is recast into sensible images, and thus, scientific truths are depicted figuratively in a manner that will demand exegesis (*ta'wīl*) or interpretation (*taʿbīr*). Avicenna similarly related in his autobiography that philosophical problems presented themselves and were unraveled in his dreams.[55] In the *Epistle Concerning Dreams* (*Risāla al-Manāmiyya*), which is attributed to Avicenna, and, some scholars think, justifiably so, the view of Aristotle is presented as affirming that the paramount source for a "true spiritual dream-vision" consists of a "representation" (*taṣawwur*) of the Universal Intellect (*al-ʿaql al-kullī*) from God, who informs the intellect of an individual through this intermediary in the course of sleep "of what will happen in the future to himself and of what will happen to the whole world."[56]

On the opposite end of the spectrum, in the *Epitome of Parva Naturalia* (*Talkhīṣ Kitāb al-Ḥiss wal-Maḥsūs*), Averroës maintained that dreams do not deal with theoretical matters or the apprehension of universals, but only with forecasting particular events. Dreams are grouped together with divination and prophecy, the common denominator of the three types of perception being the acquisition of foreknowledge. The prevalent view is that dreams come from angels, divination from demons, and prophecy from God. The discussion of Averroës turns on his making explicit the distinction implicit in Aristotle between true and false dreams. Both kinds of dream are related to the activity of the imaginative faculty producing images without the presence of sense objects outside the soul. During waking hours, external objects move the senses, and then the images stored in the common sense (*sensus communis*; *al-ḥiss al-mushtarak*) move the imaginative faculty, but in sleep, the imaginative faculty receives the images internally from the faculty of memory, and these, in turn, move the common sense. The movement of the imagination in extrasensory perception is excessive because in sleep, it is no longer subject to the control of the cogitative faculty, but precisely because this is so, it is more perfect and more spiritual. True dreams (*al-ru'yā al-ṣādiqa*), which occur through the agency of the intellect in actuality,[57] endow one with knowledge, albeit in a manner that foregoes the usual way that this acquisition occurs. The interpreter of dreams well knows that oneiric images are the imitation of corporal things on the part of spiritual entities. To decode dreams properly, one must be of a temperate nature, abandoning the pursuit of physical pleasure.[58] Averroës thus famously defended Aristotelian philosophers, the Peripatetics, by asserting that they accepted that people are capable of having a "spiritual perception" during sleep in which God communicates to them about future predictions,[59] but he insisted that they do not deal with theoretical things, since scientific comprehension demands the method of rational investigation leading to demonstrative knowledge of universal principles, and it cannot be ascertained instantaneously on the basis of intuition or vision, even if it is of the most noble sort, related to the divine element in the human soul.[60]

It seems, on balance, that Maimonides' adaptation of the notion of *ḥads* from al-Fārābī and Avicenna was colored by a critique similar to that of Averroës.[61] Thus, he assumed that the content of the veridical dream, like that of the prophetic vision, is without tangible referentiality apart from the parabolic confabulation. In the case of the dream, the exoteric meaning (*ẓāhir*) cannot be disentangled from the esoteric (*bāṭin*) and hence, Maimonides would have surely assented to the formulation of the Provençal exegete, grammarian, and philosopher David Kimḥi (1160–1235), employing a commonly used hendiadys, that scriptural dreams appear by way of "parable and riddle [*mashal we-ḥiddah*]."[62] Indeed, Maimonides uses this very language in a section in the *Mishneh Torah* wherein he distinguishes the prophecy of Moses from that of the other prophets: the former received the divine message without an angelic intermediary, and thus he saw what he saw clearly, without parable or riddle (*be-lo ḥiddah uve-lo mashal*), whereas the latter received the message through the medium of an angel, and thus they saw through "parable and riddle" (*be-mashal we-ḥiddah*). The angelic vehicle, as we have already seen, is a figurative reference to the imagination, the cognitive instrument of prophecy. Therefore, the prophets saw God in a "dream" (*ḥalom*) or in a "vision" (*mar'ah*), but Moses, who spoke to God mouth to mouth—the biblical expression for an unmediated encounter—"beheld the likeness of God" (*temunat yhwh yabiṭ*) plainly and without any riddle (Numbers 12:6–8).[63]

Ironically, to behold the divine image is to have an intellectual vision without recourse to images, a mode of sight that is completely untethered to the imagination, a seeing that is, in effect, unseeing, seeing that there is nothing to be seen. Describing the inherently metaphoric nature of prophetic vision (*mar'eh ha-nevu'ah*), Maimonides notes that some prophets spoke of the parable (*mashal*) and its interpretation (*pitron*), whereas others spoke of one or the other. The common denominator, however, is that all the prophets "prophesied through parable and by way of riddle [*we-khullan be-mashal we-derekh ḥiddah hem mitnabbe'im*]."[64] Elaborating on this theme in the *Guide*, Maimonides avails himself of the talmudic notion of the dream interpreted within the dream[65] to explain how the prophet receives the parable and its clarification in the vision:

> For sometimes a prophet sees a thing under the aspect of a parable, the meaning of that parable being sometimes interpreted to him in that very same *vision of prophecy*—just as a man may see a dream and imagine in that dream that he has already awakened and that he has related the dream to somebody else and has interpreted its meaning to him, all this taking place in a dream. This is what they call *a dream solved in a dream.*[66]

The mentioning of the dream here is not merely for the sake of comparison; the dream and vision, whatever their differences, are the two ways by which the prophet receives the word of God. Maimonides emphasizes that both forms of communication entail the use of figurative images to divulge in a sensible medium the imageless that is beyond sense experience. It is for this reason that the prophet, to whom the parable and its meaning are disclosed, resembles the dreamer, who dreams of the interpretation of the dream as part of the dream, a duplication that underscores that awakening consists of apprehending that there is no escape from dreaming, that there is no access to truth but through the guise of untruth, no way to reveal reality that is not concomitantly its concealment. This insight underlies Maimonides' assertion that the utilization of hyperbole in the prophetic books confirms the maxim attributed to R. Ammi that the "Torah speaks in exaggerated language."[67] On the face of it, the intent of this comment is to clarify that if one interprets the metaphorical tropes according to their standard meaning, then incongruities will arise inevitably. But from a more nuanced perspective, the remark of Maimonides that the prophetic idiom is of necessity hyperbolical indicates that there is no hermeneutical basis to differentiate the exoteric and esoteric—the text is figuratively literal because it is literally figurative.

Close in spirit to Maimonides is the comment of Isaac Ibn Laṭif, "The totality of prophecies are a parable [*mashal*] without doubt... for the prophetic vision is a simple spiritual entity [*pashuṭ ruḥani*] that is not comprehended at all by the senses, and all the more so if it is in a dream."[68] In a second passage, in which the author is explicit about his indebtedness to al-Fārābī and Maimonides, he elaborates that the vision (*mar'eh*) or the dream (*ḥalom*)—terms that "comprise all the gradations of prophecy" (*kolelim kol ma'alot ha-nevu'ah*)—are distinguished to the extent that the influx of light from the Active Intellect comes to the rational faculty when the senses cease, and from there to the imaginative faculty, so that the latter is perfected, resulting in the impression that the internal perception is a matter coming from the outside impinging on the external senses.[69] Inasmuch as the parable enclothes the rational truth in an imaginary reality that has no autonomous existence, it seems to fit with the last of the four types of speech delineated by Ibn Laṭif: entirely true, entirely false, both true and false, neither true nor false.[70] The thirteenth-century kabbalist Abraham Abulafia, who wrote no fewer than three mystical commentaries on the *Guide*, reached the same conclusion in his assessment of the "substance of the form of the images" (*mahut ṣiyyur ha-dimyonot*) that are psychically constellated in the prophetic vision:

> Thus all the prophets, sages, and philosophers explained ... that the imaginary form [*ha-ṣiyyur ha-dimyoni*] is very physical [*gufani me'od*], and thus it is not possible to imagine [*leṣayyer*] anything of the intelligible matters [*ha-devarim ha-muskalim*], except by means of participation with comprehension of a corporeal form [*hassagah ṣiyyurit gashmit*]. Thus, even with respect to the prophet, in the moment that he comprehends the prophetic word that emanates from God, blessed be he and blessed be his name, through the intermediary of the Active Intellect in man by means of the permutation of letters contemplated in the heart, it is not possible that he will not imagine [*yeṣayyer*] what he has comprehended in the form of a body speaking a certain matter ... on account of the reality of the imaginative faculty that is in him. But the prophet knows in truth that the body imagined by him [*ha-guf ha-mitdammeh lo*] in the moment of prophecy has no physical existence [*meṣi'ut gufanit*] at all, but it is an intelligible entity, entirely spiritual [*davar sikhli kullo ruḥani*], and it materializes in relation to him [*hitgashem eṣlo*] in the moment of his comprehension, since the prophet is a body that contemplates the truth in his spiritual intellect [*heyot ha-navi guf ha-maskil ha-emet be-sikhlo ha-ruḥani*] that is actualized in that moment.[71]

Abulafia obviously follows the philosophical approach, with the crucial difference that the means to attain prophecy is identified by him as the meditative technique of letter permutation, something very far from the purview of Maimonides. The content of the experience, however, is identical; prophecy consists of configuring the intelligible in a corporeal form as it is mediated through the imagination. The prophet knows that this form has no actual physical existence outside the mind; it is a spiritual entity—in other passages identified more specifically with the angelic Metatron—that materializes as a human form in the imaginative faculty of the enlightened prophet, whose body has been transfigured in light of comprehending the truth in the state of intellectual conjunction.[72]

That the vision is interpreted in this way underscores the considerable challenge that the philosophical perspective adopted by Maimonides imposes on a literal reading of the biblical accounts of prophecy and the traditional assumptions regarding their objective validity. The distinction between literary fiction and historical facticity is blurred considerably, for even if we were to accept that God is the implied author of the scriptural text—a belief that cannot be literally true on Maimonidean grounds—we still would be compelled to say that the historiographical truth of prophetic narratives, in their rhetorical artifice and syntactical emplotment, is fictional.[73] Consider the blunt assessment on the part of Maimonides in his delineation of the eleventh and highest degree of prophecy (excluding the level attained by Moses):

> Inasmuch as I found scriptural texts attesting that prophets heard speech—it having been made clear that this was *in a vision*—I said by way of conjecture that it is possible that the speech that is heard *in a dream* and the like of which may not occur *in a vision*, is that regarding which it is imagined by the prophet that God addresses him; all this is said in following the external sense of the verse. One could also say that every vision in which you find the prophet hearing speech was in its beginning a vision, but ended in a state of submersion and became a dream.... All speech that is heard, whatever the way may be in which it is heard, is heard only *in a dream*.... On the other hand, in a *vision of prophecy* only parables or intellectual unifications are apprehended that give actual cognition of scientific matters similar to those, knowledge of which is obtained through speculation.[74]

Maimonides here reverses a predilection for privileging the auditory over the ocular that, as we will see, he demonstrates in an exegesis of Exodus 33:11, ascribing a higher status to the prophets who see in a vision, as opposed to those who hear a voice in a dream. The prophets heed the speech of God through the intermediary of the imagination, and thus they envisage that the divine is conversing with them as one person in dialogical exchange with another, when in fact, there is no personal other of whom and with whom to speak. Mention should be made here of another passage where Maimonides entertains both a figurative reading, according to which the hearing of the voice connotes apprehension, and a literal reading, according to which the voice is a created entity, an idea that resonates with the notion of the "created word" (*dibbur nivra*) elaborated by Saadya Gaon (892–942).[75] More poignantly, in another chapter, Maimonides states that after one has attained the true knowledge that God exists not in virtue of existence and that God is one not in virtue of oneness, it is necessary to comprehend "the denial of the attribute of speech" with reference to God. In no uncertain terms, Maimonides writes that the rabbinic belief that the Torah was created "is meant to signify that His speech that is ascribed to Him is created. It was ascribed to Him only because the words heard by Moses were created and brought into being by God.... The intention here is to indicate that predicating speech of Him is similar to predicating of Him all the actions resembling ours."[76] When the words "saying" or "speaking" are applied to God, they

> denote either will and volition or a notion that has been grasped by the understanding having come from God, in which case it is indifferent whether it has become known by means of a created voice or through one of the ways of prophecy.... The terms in question never signify that He, may He be exalted, spoke using the sounds of letters and a voice, nor that He, may He be exalted, possesses a soul into which notions are impressed so that there would subsist in His essence a notion superadded to that essence.[77]

The gesture of divine speech serves a pedagogical purpose when understood figuratively as a denotation of divine volition or of an act of human comprehension, but to interpret it literally is no less equivocal than attributing to God any other human quality. In the moment that the prophet imagines that he is hearing the word of God, he is in a dream state, conjuring something that is not factually true, since God has no body and therefore no tongue or voice to converse verbally.

The vision granted the prophets is also to be understood as a parabolic representation of intellectual apprehension.[78] This is the import of the aggadic dictum (transmitted in the name of R. Yudan) "Great is the power of prophets, for they liken the form to its creator" (*gadol koḥan shel nevi'im she-medammin et ha-ṣurah le-yoṣrah*).[79] Defending the rabbis against the charge of anthropomorphism, Maimonides emphasized that this proclamation

> makes clear and manifest that all the forms apprehended by the prophets in the *vision of prophecy* are created forms of which God is the Creator. And this is correct, for every imagined form is created.... They have thus made clear and manifest, as far as they themselves are concerned, that they were innocent of the belief in the corporeality of God; and furthermore, that all the shapes and figures that are seen *in the vision of prophecy* are created things.[80]

The theistic language of God creating the forms beheld by the prophet is an attempt to avoid an epistemological idealism that would reduce these forms to nothing more than subjective fantasies. It should be fairly obvious, however, that to speak of the divine creating these forms is a verbalization that anthropomorphizes the supposedly amorphous and incompossible being. From the Maimonidean standpoint, the rabbinic sage was instructing us in the prophetic act of poiesis through which the immaterial and disembodied essence of God, which is beyond all representational form, is represented in the likeness of the sensible entities of the natural world, which is identified as the "back" (*aḥor*) of the glory beheld by Moses (Exodus 33:23), expressed theologically as "all the things created" by God or, philosophically, as that which "follows necessarily" from the divine will.[81] We may conclude, therefore, that the images of the dream—even the prophetic dream—are figuratively true, but literally false, since there is nothing corporeal outside the mind to which they correspond. The visions of the night connote the "relation of what was said," and not a "relation of what took place within matters having existence."[82] The events communicated by prophetic parables take "place only *in a vision of prophecy*, they are not real actions, actions that exist for the external senses."[83] The imaginal phantasms that one envisions in the dream have no concrete reality, but they are nevertheless experienced with the immediacy and certainty that characterizes waking, intentional perception.[84]

Rending the Veil of the Dream in Seeing the Unseen

From the preceding discussion, we may conclude that, for Maimonides, dream apparitions are imaginary pictures compounded from experiences stored in memory; they do not refer to divinely ordained events or objects outside the mind, even though the dreamer apperceives them with the same certainty and clarity as sense perceptions, nor are they to be understood as subtle "imaginative forms" perceived by the common sense, also identified as the faculty of fantasy (*fanṭāsiya*), thought to be lodged in the anterior ventricle of the brain, as intermediate between the spiritual and the corporeal, an idea explicated by al-Kindī and Isaac Israeli (ca. 832–932), although its roots presumably go back to earlier commentaries on Aristotle such as pseudo-John Philoponus,[85] and it is reaffirmed in later sources such as Solomon Ibn Gabirol (ca. 1021–ca. 1058)[86] and Ibn Khaldūn.[87] Just as prophecy is understood as the spectral representation of rational truths, which are ascertainable through deductive-syllogistic logic, so dreams are viewed as the vestibule to a realm of fantasy uninhibited by the habitual restrictions of the phenomenal world. We have seen, moreover, that in the case of the prophets, the imagination undermines itself in fabricating images of what cannot be imaged except as the unimaginable. Does the dream similarly comport the possibility of constricting the image through its expansion? Before we can respond to this inquiry, we will have to explore in more detail the example of Moses, who will provide us (through the interpretive lens of Maimonides) the paradigm of the prophet who sees most clearly because he sees nothing at all but the translucency of his own unseeing.

The supremacy of Mosaic prophecy is explained by the fact that his vision is not dependent on the intermediary of the imagination, or, in the talmudic lingo, he saw through a translucent speculum, whereas all other prophets saw through an opaque speculum.[88] In spite of the qualitative distinction that separates Moses from all other prophets, his rank serves as the measure by which all prophetic visions are to be judged and, consequently, the nature of dreams, since the latter, as we have seen, provide the psychological framework by which the former are explained. The example of Moses provides the paradigm by which we can apprehend the theological merit of the dream as that which prefigures the seeing of what is not seeable, the perceiving of the imperceptible, the blindness that is at the heart of visualizing the invisible.

Expounding the ideal of intellectual worship in a chapter toward the end of the *Guide*, Maimonides even goes so far as to intimate that Moses attained a state of angelic perfection insofar as his apprehension was completely devoid of the senses, and the gross operations of his body ceased to exist,[89] a postrational experiential state (described by technical Ṣūfi terminology)[90] that is alluded to in God's directive to Moses to stand with God, *we-attah poh amod immadi* (Deuteronomy 5:28),[91] a posture that distinctively denotes the quality of immutability associated with God and the angels or incorporeal intellects.[92] This understanding of Mosaic prophecy is attested elsewhere in Maimonides' oeuvre, for example, in the *Mishneh Torah*,[93] the seventh of the thirteen principles from the *Commentary on the Mishnah*,[94] and the seventh chapter of his introduction to the tractate Avot, known as the *Shemonah Peraqim*.[95] There is a clash, however, between the depiction of Moses in the first and second of these sources and the third, a matter into which it is worth delving, because it sheds light on Maimonides' understanding of the potential of human nature, a topic that has a direct bearing on the question of the apparently obstinate need of the imagination to anthropomorphize ultimate reality (even if we construe that reality nonanthropomorphically as the no-thing that neither and therefore both is what it is not and is not what it is). In the passage from the *Mishneh Torah* and the seventh principle from the *Commentary on the Mishnah*, Maimonides endorses the possibility that Moses rent all the veils of corporeality[96] and, as a consequence, joined the rank of the angels, that is, he became an acquired intellect, separate from all matter, and was conjoined with the Active Intellect. In the seventh of the *Shemonah Peraqim*, he begins by saying that for Moses, there was no more veil, but then proceeds to say that even he could not apprehend the divine essence, which is expressed scripturally as God's denying him a vision of the face, since qua human, Moses is inescapably embodied and thus incapable of apprehending the incorporeal.[97]

This view is also found in Maimonides' *Guide*. For example, in one chapter, Maimonides asserts that it is impossible for humans to apprehend clearly the deity or the intellects because they are immaterial, and thus, matter is portrayed figuratively as a veil that always shrouds our vision.[98] In the chapter dedicated to the exposition of the term "face" (*panim*), Maimonides provides an exegesis of the scriptural dialogue between Moses and God, centered on his request to see the glory of God and the response that he could see the back, but not the face (Exodus 33:18–21). Maimonides is attentive to the fact that in the same context, there is a verse that states explicitly that God spoke to Moses face to face (Exodus 33:11), which he aligns with two other verses that describe the Israelites' experience of God at Sinai, "Face to face the Lord spoke to you on the mountain out of the fire" (Deuteronomy 5:4) and "The Lord spoke to you out of the fire; you heard the sound of words but perceived no shape—nothing but a voice" (Deuteronomy 4:12). Juxtaposing these three verses, Maimonides comes to the conclusion that the expression "face to face" (*panim el panim*) denotes the "kind of speaking and hearing" that has no image, an aural address that lacks an ocular component, "the hearing of a speech without the intermediary of an angel." In this case, too, "angel" stands metaphorically for the imaginative faculty. Maimonides' point, then, is that Moses spoke to God from behind a curtain, as it were, without the intervention of an image.

Technically, attributing this notion of speaking to God should be no less problematic for Maimonides than theorizing about the possibility of seeing God; both equally embrace a form of anthropomorphization that is idolatrous when literalized or ontologized as real. However, reflecting a long-standing bias, he viewed the visual as more dangerous than the auditory, and hence, he could conceive of Moses speaking to God face to face, a figurative denotation of the dialogical relationality that can have no recourse to figurative representation, a matter that still proves difficult for the human mind to comprehend. For Maimonides, this was possible, but he nevertheless insisted that in spite of being capable of this experience, Moses could not apprehend the divine essence as such. This is the meaning of God's declaration that his face will not be seen, "the true reality of My existence as it veritably is cannot be grasped."[99]

Significantly, Maimonides does not end the discussion with this apophatic utterance. He goes on to say that the word *panim* functions adverbially in a semantic mode that resonates with two Arabic terms, *amāmaka* and *bayna yadayka*, "in front of thee" and "in thy presence," or literally, "between your hands."[100] This leads him to consider the Aramaic translation of the Hebrew *u-fanay lo yera'u*, "My face cannot be seen" (Exodus 33:23), by Onkelos as *we-teḥezei yat de-vatray we-diqadamay lo yitḥazun*, "you shall see those behind Me but those in front of Me shall not be seen." Maimonides zeroes in on the expression "those in front of Me shall not be seen," and concludes that it "indicates that there are likewise great created beings whom man cannot apprehend as they really are. These are the separate intellects." What can be seen are the things behind the divine, that is, the "things endowed with matter and form," which are "beneath the separate intellects"; these can be grasped "in their true reality . . . with respect to their rank in that which exists."[101] If taken at face value, this passage would suggest a serious obstacle to human knowledge and the possibility of prophetic experience understood as intellectual conjunction, since not even Moses, and therefore, by implication, no human, can apprehend the true reality of anything incorporeal, whether God or the separate intellects.

This perspective is avowed as well in another chapter of the *Guide* in which Maimonides writes of the two requests made by Moses, to see God's face and to know God's ways. The former is the request to know God's essence, which is denied, and the latter is the request to know the things of nature, the attributes of action, or the rabbinic conception of the thirteen characteristics of divine mercy (derived exegetically from Exodus 34:6–8), which are called collectively God's goodness.

> The meaning here is not that He possesses moral qualities, but that He performs actions resembling the actions that in us proceed from moral qualities—I mean from aptitudes of the soul; the meaning is not that He . . . possesses aptitudes of the soul. Scripture has restricted itself to mentioning only those thirteen characteristics, although [Moses] apprehended all his goodness—I mean to say all His actions—because these are the actions proceeding from

> Him...in respect of giving existence to the Adamites and governing them.[102]

The specific governance of Israel by Moses is dependent on his knowledge of the order of the divine governance through the angels or separate intellects.[103] This *imitatio dei* is the model for all political leadership.[104]

In some contexts, pursuant to the aforementioned view of al-Fārābī that the supreme perfection of the human is described as the acquired intellect, a state of comprehension wherein the act, subject, and object of intellection are indistinguishable,[105] Maimonides thought that Moses was capable of the maximum union with the Active Intellect.[106] In this state, one can cognize without any somatic faculty, since, in concurrence with the Aristotelian principle that the intellect becomes identical with the object it cognizes (based on the belief that the sensible object and the act of sensation are one and the same), it would not be possible for a human intellect to know a form separate from matter if it did not itself have the capacity to immaterialize.[107] Maimonides retains the Aristotelian principle and accepts the earlier view of al-Fārābī that it is possible for the human intellect to apprehend the Active Intellect, and indeed, the immortality of the soul is linked to this apprehension; the traditional notion is thus understood philosophically in terms of the immateriality that ensues from the conjunction of the acquired intellect with the Active Intellect. As we have seen, this grade is attained to some degree by all prophets, and not just by Moses, although the level achieved by the latter is unique. In one passage in the *Guide*, Maimonides describes divine intellection as the union of intellect, intellectually cognizing subject, and intellectually cognizing object, a triadic unity that is applied to human intellection, as well. Hence, in the act of knowing, when one becomes an actualized intellect, the knower is identical with what is known.[108] Also noteworthy is another passage, where Maimonides refers to and accepts the doctrine of the unity of the intellect expounded by Ibn Bājja: with respect to the immaterial, there can be no multiplicity or complexity (that is, no divisibility), and therefore nothing individually differentiated can survive after the death of the body. In the state of cognitive attainment that is marked as intellect *in actu*, there can be no difference between one mind and another, contrary to the opinion of those who professes an individual afterlife, for instance, al-Kindī and Ibn Sīnā.[109] In other passages, however, Maimonides seems to deny this very possibility and follows the view of al-Fārābī in his later work by insisting that insofar as the human intellect cannot divest itself of its corporeal encasement, it cannot apprehend something immaterial.[110]

With respect to the indigenous potential of human nature, a key factor in understanding the capacity for prophecy and, by extension, oneiric experience, we conclude that Maimonides offers conflicting perspectives. The contradictions in this instance cannot be resolved by any of the seven criteria that Maimonides lays out in the introduction to the *Guide* to "account for the contradictory or contrary statements found in any book or compilation."[111] In the end, we are as confounded as we were at the beginning. Diane Lobel has suggested that the notion of perplexity (*ḥayra*) in the *Guide*—signposted in the title itself—may reflect the idea of learned ignorance (in the celebrated locution of Nicholas of Cusa) found in a number of Ṣūfi sayings, that is, the notion that the culmination of knowledge consists of knowing that one does not know.[112] Specifically, she surmises that Maimonides may have been influenced by the eleventh-century rabbinic and philosophical sage Baḥya Ibn Paquda. In one passage, Baḥya refers to a dictum of the "knowers," *ʿārifīn*, a technical term for one who has knowledge of God (*maʿrifat Allāh*) by way of experiential or intuitive gnosis: "One of the knowers [of God] said, 'The one who is most knowing of God (*ʿāraf al-nās bi-llāhi*) is most perplexed (*taḥayyuran*) by him.'"[113] Lobel traces this statement to al-Miṣri as cited by Qushayrī. I agree that Maimonides' depictions of the *via negativa* are close to the Ṣūfi embrace of bewilderment. Yet when Maimonides describes this state, he does not use any term related to perplexity. At best, he speaks of "all the philosophers" saying that the mind is dazzled by the divine beauty, which is hidden from us on account of the intensity with which it is manifest, just as the sun is hidden from eyes too weak to glimpse it.[114] It is better to assume, as Joel Kraemer has argued, that Maimonides' use of the term reflects the Arabic translation of the Greek *aporia* as *ḥayra* or *taḥayyur*.[115] As he put it in his recently published intellectual biography of the great eagle, as Maimonides was known:

> The Guide is a *dalala*, a pointing, guidance, indication, pathmarker for the *ḥa'irun*, those who are disconcerted, perplexed, confused, straying, and astray. It shows the path, the Sacred Way, to those who search for God if they march toward him and do not go astray. The words *ḥayra* and *taḥayyur* often render Greek *aporia* (*aporein*). An *aporia* is an impasse, literally meaning that "no passage" (*poros*) has been found to the solution of a puzzle. The word *ḥayra* has to do with being dazzled and unable to see one's way, to lose one's course, go astray, wander about lost in the desert, confused and dismayed. The implied reader, then, is a person who has come to an impasse and needs to be shown the way. The impasse is cognitive and existential, affecting mind and body.[116]

The issue, then, is not the Ṣūfi notion of bemusement when encountering the divine in its unknowability, but the sense of aporia discussed by Aristotle in book 3 of the *Metaphysics*, 995a30–31, the standstill to which the path of discursive analysis inevitably leads, an epistemological knot that paradoxically impels the process of thinking and yet prevents that process from going forward. Particularly relevant is the explication of this concept on the part of Alexander of Aphrodisias in his commentary on the *Metaphysics*:

> If the discovery and establishment of the objects of the inquiry depends on the solution of the points of aporia, and it is not possible for people to untie a knot unless they first know it, i.e. how it has been tied...and if the aporia of thought is the knot in the matters under inquiry...it is necessary first of all to face the aporia concerning the matters under inquiry, the matters that are to be proven—given that discovery comes from solving the points of aporia, and only those who know how the aporia has developed can solve the points of aporia.[117]

What Maimonides intends, therefore, is the state of logical befuddlement (*aporein*) that Socrates applies to himself in Plato's *Meno* (80c) or in the view attributed to Socrates in Plato's *Theaetetus* (155d3) that philosophy commences in an act of wondering (*thaumazein*), an idea echoed in the observation in Aristotle's *Metaphysics*, 982b12–13, which has had an enduring impact on Western thought, notably in the work of Heidegger.[118] For Maimonides, this is not only the starting point, but it is the end point, as well. Surely, this is the case with regard to the question whether human beings are capable of apprehending incorporeal entities without the medium of images.

Dream Images and Delimiting the Imagination

From Maimonides' discussions about prophecy and dreams, the following paradox may be elicited: the very phenomena that express the imagination most exorbitantly also hint at its dissolution. In the excess of imagination, the imagination imagines more than can be imagined to be real. The images conjured by the imaginative faculty at the limits of its capability cannot be deciphered imaginatively; they are nothing more than the phantoms whose ontic status is that of privation or nonbeing.[119] Appropriating the words of Blanchot, we can say the dream is

> the place of similitude, an environment saturated with resemblances where a neutral power of resembling, which exists prior to any particular designation, is ceaselessly in search of some figure that it elicits, if need be, in order to settle on it. It is Faust's mirror, and what Faust sees is neither the young girl nor something resembling her face, but resemblance itself, the indefinite power to resemble, the innumerable scintillations of reflection.[120]

The dream may be likened to the mirror of Faust, a mirror that mirrors not a reality external to it, but the mirror of the mind gazing upon nothing but its own proclivity to dissemble indeterminately and deficiently. The oneiric seeing is thus a vision of nocturnality gleaming forth at the heart of nocturnality—even when the dream occurs in daylight—a beholding of the darkness too incandescent to behold. For Blanchot, as for Maimonides, components of the dream are necessarily drawn from the pool of one's previous sense experience; the reproductive prowess of the dreamer, however, is not constrained by the reservoirs of the memory bank, because the dream elementally is a mimesis of the irrepresentable, a "fictionality without props," a world of make-believe whose truthfulness "can be construed as a matter of what is to be imagined rather than what actually is imagined."[121] In this section, I will explore a parallel argument proffered by Foucault.

In his introduction to Binswanger's *Traum und Existenz*, to which I have already referred on several occasions, Foucault frames his discussion of the dream in the broader context of calling for an anthropology of imagination that would be based on a new understanding of the relation of meaning and symbol, image and expression. Pushing against Freud, Foucault notes that the "presence of meaning in the dream is not meaning making itself fully evident. The dream betrays the meaning even as it effects it, offering it only while ephemeralizing it."[122] If the dream is understood as a fulfillment of desire, it is so "precisely because the dream also answers to all the 'counter desires' which oppose the desire itself." From this example a general principle is adduced: "The dream is a functional composite, and if the meaning is invested in images, this is by way of a surplus, a multiplication of meanings which override and contradict each other. The imaginative plasticity of the dream is, for the meaning which comes to light in it, but the form of its contradictoriness."[123] The morphology of the dreamspace, accordingly, is not to be determined by the overdetermination of the psychoanalytic interpretation of symbols and the hermeneutic principle that the "meanings exhaust the reality of the world which displays that reality," but by the "free, luminous space" in which the images are unbound and viewed solely from the perspective of the laws and structures of the imaginary world.[124] Relying on Husserl's distinction between sign and index, Foucault argues that "the authentic sign, to be significant, does not need to rest on any objective situation," and hence, the "phenomenology of the dream, to be rigorous, must not fail to distinguish between indicative elements, which may designate for the analyst an objective situation they betoken, and significant contents which constitute, from within, the dream experience."[125] But what are we to make of this act of signification? Its essence, writes Foucault, "must be sought beyond, and even before, the verbal expression or the image structure in which it may be embodied."[126] The dream, quintessentially, is an act of signification that precedes both image and word, an act of imagining the veracity of which makes no appeal to an objectivity independent of the images. What might seem a liability is turned into an asset by Foucault in his assertion that the meaningfulness of the dream is to be determined from "the poverty of its objective content. It is all the more valid in that it has the less reason for being."[127] The dream's validity, therefore, is in inverse proportion to its raison d'être; the very impoverishment of objectivity is what endows the dream with meaning. It is at this juncture that Foucault invokes Spinoza's discussion of the dream and prophecy, above all noting that his account of the prophetic dream illustrates the tendency of the imagination to extend beyond the content of experience to access a truth that surpasses the human mind, but that nonetheless communicates to it in concrete images. It is in this sense that the dream, the "sign of transcendence" experienced under the "sign of the imaginary,"[128] engenders human freedom "in its most original form."[129]

Viewing the dream through the lens of the anthropological approach to the imagination highlights this sense of freedom in the plurivocality of symbolic significations and semiotic possibilities that any given oneiric drama might yield.[130] Only thence can one "bring into full light the constituting feature of dream subjectivity." Again, contrasting his view (informed by the work of Binswanger, who is indebted predominantly to Husserl and Heidegger)[131] with Freud's, Foucault remarks that the "subject is not characterized as one of the possible meanings of one of the personages of the dream, but as the foundation of all its eventual meanings." The dream subject, consequently, is not simply a later adaptation of a "previous form" or an "archaic stage of personality." It is rather that which "manifests itself as the coming-to-be and the totality of existence itself."[132]

The shift in orientation also summons a change in understanding the temporal component of the dream: "But the essential point of the dream lies not so much in what it revives of the past as in what it declares about the future.... The dream anticipates the moment of liberation. It is a prefiguring of history even more than an obligatory repetition of the traumatic past." The subject of the dream cannot be limited to a past history, for its "constituting moment" is an "existence which makes itself through time," a "movement toward the future."[133] Foucault does not completely deny the recurrence of the past in the psychodynamics of the dream; he does, however, maintain that "repetition is precisely the experience of a temporality which opens upon the future and constitutes itself as freedom."[134] In this conception of authentic time, there is no binary opposition—significantly, Foucault speaks of Binswanger setting forth a "Hegelian dialectic of a dream"[135]—reliving the past induces the unprecedented future. In the constitution of time as freedom is the anchoring of destiny as the recurrence of what is yet to come in the expectation of what has always been.

In addition to these "temporal pulsations," the existential meaning of the dream—the dream as the expression of the ontological ground of existence (*Existenz*) in and through which the modalities of the being-there (*Dasein*) of the human condition are defined—is uncovered as well from its spatial coordinates. Through the lived experience of the dream, one can retrieve the primordial sense of space before it is demarcated geometrically or geographically, the spatiality that "presents itself first and foremost as scene or landscape." Just as in the case of the dreamtime, the replication of the past constitutes the innovation of the future, so we can say of the dreamspace that it is "paradoxically closed by the infinite openness of the horizon." In the geographic space of waking reality, "motion is nothing but displacement: a concerted change of position from one point to another according to a previously established trajectory." In the lived space of the dreamscape,

> the displacement preserves an original spatial character; it does not cross, it travels along; until the very moment it stops, it remains a proffered trajectory of which only its point of departure is known for certain; its future is not prearranged by the geography of the setting, but is awaited in its authentic historicity.... The dream deploys itself in this original spatiality of the scene and finds there its principal affective meanings.[136]

Both the temporal and spatial dimensions of the dream call attention to indeterminacy as the salient feature of the oneiric. Indeed, in spite of the wide-ranging nature of Foucault's analysis, the common thread that ties together his disparate thoughts is his insistence on this quality of the dream. This is most conspicuous in his claim that "every act of imagination points implicitly to the dream. The dream is not a modality of the imagination, the dream is the first condition of its possibility."[137] The dream is the first condition of the possibility of the imagination because with respect to the dream, the image is not defined eidetically by reference to the real, whether in the positivistic sense of the image as a residue of perception or in the negativistic sense (advanced phenomenologically by Sartre) of the imaging consciousness that posits its object as irreal. The imaginary is transcendent, not in the sense of objective transcendence, but as the "movement of freedom which makes itself world and finally anchors itself in this world as its destiny. Through what it imagines, therefore, consciousness aims at the original movement which discloses itself in dreams." Dreaming, therefore, "is not a singularly powerful and vivid way of imagining," but rather "imagining is to take aim at oneself in the moment of dreaming; it is to dream oneself dreaming."[138]

The imagination is marked by the reflexivity expressed most perfectly in the prospect of dreaming that one is dreaming. The dream of death is thus assigned paradigmatic status insofar as it discloses the "ultimate meaning of the dream" linked to the "movement of the imagination" whereby the self is *derealized* as a presence to the very world penetrated by the presence of that self. Again, we confront the paradox of the "cosmogony" of the dream state: what is experienced in the dream belongs entirely to the dreamer, but only to the extent that the dreamer is absent from the dream. Through the freedom of this derealization one can fathom and totalize the curve of destiny.[139] Ironically, suicide is upheld as the "absolute of imaginary behaviors":

> every suicidal desire is filled by that world in which I would no longer be present here, or there, but everywhere, in every sector: a world transparent to me and signifying its indebtedness to my absolute presence. Suicide is not a way of cancelling the world or myself, or the two together, but a way of rediscovering the original moment in which I make myself world, in which space is still no more than directedness of existence, and time the movement of its history.

There is a homology between the dream and suicide: the former is the genesis, the "absolute origin," of the imagination and the latter the "ultimate myth," the "Last Judgment."[140]

The imaginary thus is not false or illusory, not a "mode of unreality," but a "mode of actuality," "a way of approaching presence obliquely to bring out its primordial dimensions." Appropriating the language of Bachelard, Foucault speaks of the *realism of unreality* that holds sway through the imagination. The dream, in particular, can be profitably described in these terms, for, strictly speaking, it is the image one has after the cessation of imagining, the image that partakes of the order of "as if" par excellence.[141] And in this regard, the dream imagination may be compared to the proliferation of metaphors on the part of the poet that are meant to lead back to a presence, the "depth of immediacy," that is beyond metaphor.[142] "The imagination, in its true poetic function, meditates on identity. If it is true that the imagination circulates through a universe of images, it does not move to the extent that it promotes or reunites images, but to the extent that it destroys and consumes them. The imagination is in essence iconoclastic." The freedom of imagination thus imposes itself on the poet as the refusal of the imagination, "the inner destructive power of the image."[143] Similarly, we imagine that "the image makes up the weave of the dream," but this is only from the viewpoint of waking consciousness, which seeks to recoup something of the dream imagination. From the vantage point of the dream, "the movement of the imagination is directed toward the primary moment of existence where the original constitution of the world is achieved." Freud is to be given credit for discerning that the meaning of the dream is not to be sought at the level of the image content, because the phantasmagoria of the dream hide more than they reveal. The tension, however, is not between repressed impulses and overt routines. It is

> between the authentic movement of the imaginative and its adulteration in the image. If the meaning of the dream is always beyond the images gleaned upon waking, this is not because they veil hidden forces, but because wakefulness can reach the dream only mediately, and because between waking image and dream imagination, the distance is as great as between quasi-presence in a constituted world and original presence to a world being constituted.

Dream analysis, therefore, effects the "transcendental reduction of the imaginary" to the extent that it has the "goal of bridging the distance between image and imagination."[144] The dream itself "breaks away from images" and thereby "restores the imagination to its truth and gives it back the absolute meaning of its freedom. All imagination, to be authentic, must once more learn to dream, and '*ars poetica*' has no meaning unless it teaches us to break with the fascination of images and to reopen, for imagination, its path of freedom toward the dream that offers it, as its absolute truth, the 'unshatterable kernel of night.'"[145] Contrary to conventional wisdom, the dream is the "alienation of the imaginative," and thus it serves as the fire in which the flame of the images is purified. "The image is no longer image *of* something, totally projected toward an absence which it replaces; rather, it is gathered into itself and is given as the fullness of a presence."[146] Foucault utilized the reflections of Binswanger to argue, in agreement with Maimonides, that human imagination is directed to the fullness of a presence that is beyond images, a fullness that can be ascertained only through the attenuation of its own abundance. The dream thus signifies the movement of the imagination to the center that is the absolute limit where the imagination dissolves in the collapse of its own power to sustain anything but the imagining of images that cannot be imagined.

CHAPTER THREE

A Letter Over/written: Hermeneutics and the Textuality of the Dreamscape

My friend, that is the poet's art,
His dreams to cherish and impart.
Trust me, the best ideas of men
In dreams are opened to their ken:
All book-craft and all poetry
Are naught but dreams made verity.
—Richard Wagner, *The Mastersingers of Nuremberg*

In this chapter, I will investigate in greater detail the view that the dream phenomenon should be treated principally as a text and the corollary proposition that dream interpretation is a form of exegesis. The portrayal of oneiric images as nocturnal ciphers is to be found as far back as the literary reports of enigmatic dreams in Mesopotamian and Israelite divination practices;[1] the roots for this orientation may also be uncovered in the Greek mythological notion that Hermes, the chthonic god of revelation, is responsible for bringing dreams to mortals.[2] In particular, as Jung and analysts who have followed his path have well understood, underlying the ascription of this role to Hermes (or Mecurius) is the presumption that dreams are to be viewed as omens that exact interpretation.[3] The further depiction of this god as androgynous, typified, for example, in his being described in the *Papyri Graecae Magicae* as "spherical and square,"[4] resounds as well with the delineation of the dream as the *coincidentia oppositorum*, a theme that will be analyzed more expansively in the next chapter.

Oral Affixation: All Dreams Follow the Mouth

According to one trajectory within the rabbinic corpora, which reflects an older mantic convention, the dream is compared more specifically to a scriptural text.[5] This comparison was expressed chiefly in one of two ways, either as the importation of exegetical techniques from the oneirocritica familiar to the rabbis into their own midrashic practices[6] or in the application of the canons of scriptural interpretation developed by the rabbis to the analysis of dreams.[7] An oft-cited tradition preserved in a section of the Babylonian Talmud that has been characterized as the centerpiece and fulcrum of the rabbinic dreambook, a supposedly independent literary unit that was affixed to the ninth chapter of the tractate Berakhot,[8] relates that Bar Hedya, an interpreter of dreams (*mefashshar ḥelmei*),[9] would offer felicitous interpretations to those who paid him a fee and ill-fated ones to those who would not pay. The tradition is supported by an account concerning Abbaye and Rava, two celebrated fourth-century *amoraim*: the former was willing to compensate Bar Hedya, and thus he received favorable interpretations, whereas the latter was not willing to do so, and thus the interpretations he received were unfavorable. In the end, Rava mended his ways, and by offering to pay Bar Hedya, the fate of the interpretations of his dreams was modified accordingly. The change of fortune is encapsulated in Bar Hedya's assurance that miracles would happen to Rava.

At this juncture of the talmudic tale, the redactor includes a narrative that substantiates, but also in some sense subverts its didactic point: Bar Hedya was once traveling with Rava in a boat, and he calculated that since he had predicted that miracles would occur to this sage, if the boat would sink, the latter would be the one to be saved. Bar Hedya decided, therefore, to disembark, and as he did so, a book fell from him. Rava is said to have found the book and to have discovered written therein "all dreams are consequent to [literally, follow after] the mouth" (*kol ha-ḥalomot holkhin aḥar ha-peh*), which led him to exclaim: "Wicked one! It all depended on you, and you caused me all this suffering."[10] The reader is told, moreover, that Rava was willing to forgive Bar Hedya for everything he foretold with the exception of the death of his wife. For this reason, he placed a curse on the dream interpreter's head, "May it be the will [of God] to give this man over to the [foreign] government, which should have no mercy upon him!" In an effort to circumvent the curse, Bar Hedya exiled himself and fled to the Romans, ending up sitting at the door of the keeper of the king's wardrobe, who enunciated his dreams to him, but, as was his custom, he demanded payment before he would interpret them. When Bar Hedya heard that the man dreamt that worms filled the whole of his hand, he gave in and interpreted it (pro bono) as a sign that all the royal silk garments would be spoiled by worms. The story concludes with the keeper of the king's wardrobe pleading for his life by laying the blame on Bar Hedya, since he refused to interpret the prior dreams in a timely fashion, and had he done so, the damage may have been averted.

There is surely much to discuss in this passage. What seems especially noteworthy to my ear is the confluence of economic and hermeneutic concerns. Reflecting a common attitude of the ancient world, the predictive value of dreams to foretell the future (either directly or allegorically) is of major interest.[11] In this regard, not only is the meaning of the dream thought to be determined by its interpretation, but the latter transforms that meaning into reality.[12] The worth of the interpretation, however, is contingent upon whether or not the interpreter is reimbursed for his services. Is delimiting the effectiveness of the interpreter to his request for payment some kind of joke, a mocking caricature of expert dream interpreters, who may have exacted payment dishonestly for false explanations?[13] Might the rabbinic disquiet be comparable to the institution of expert witnesses in the American legal system, specialists who come to court to offer purportedly impartial testimony, but who are usually compensated for their assistance and therefore subject to the suspicion that their opinions are tainted? Is the rabbinic tale polemically charged, intended to put the (evidently nonrabbinic) dream interpreters[14] on notice that oneirocriticism is a practice that is best executed by the sages, for not only do they possess the skill necessary to crack the encoded symbolism of dreams effectively, but they have the moral fortitude not to be swayed by mercenary objectives?[15]

Curiously, the rabbinic story echoes the method of dream interpretation proffered by Artemidorus, which, as noted already by Freud, takes into account "not only the content of the dream but also the personality and circumstances of the dreamer . . . so that the same element in the dream has a different meaning for the rich man, the married man, or the orator from the meaning it has for the poor man, the unmarried man, or, say, a merchant."[16] Looking more closely at the talmudic text, one discerns that the commodity of exchange is implicitly criticized by both the response of Rava and the story of the king's wardrobe keeper. The oneirocritical capacity should not be made dependent on a financial arrangement, even if it is accepted that the interpretation of dreams is a professional calling, maybe a dubious one, subject, as it is, to attract charlatans, though clearly not disregarded completely by rabbinic authorities, as the vocational identity of Bar Hedya itself indicates.[17] Prima facie, it would seem that the narrative sponsors a structural homology between economic and semantic systems of exchange,[18] but in fact, the intertwining of these two thematic vectors achieves the opposite result. Culturally speaking, from the standpoint of this text, the linguistic sign, and not the monetary object, is determinative of meaning; even though currency and language are both modes of emblematic representation, they are not manifestations of the same epistemic configuration. The rabbinic sages seem to be resisting the commoditization of the discursive practice of dream interpretation—just as they might be suspicious of the hired gun who serves as an expert witness. Nevertheless, their convergence is understandable; the dream proffers an omen of what will transpire socioeconomically, and thus it is reasonable to expect that a dream interpreter would demand capital for his or her services.[19] Without denying the ability of professional dream interpreters to decode the premonitional dimension of dreams, the rabbis seek to uphold a greater force that allays the potential of oneiric determinism. A similar implication may be elicited from another dictum that affirms the power of prayer to overturn a fate forecast in a dream, "R. Ḥanan said: Even if the master of dreams [*ba'al ha-ḥalomot*] says to a person that on the morrow he will die, he should not desist from [beseeching divine] mercy, for it says 'Since much dreaming leads to futility and to superfluous talk, one should fear God' (Ecclesiastes 5:6)."[20]

In a somewhat ironic turn, Rava discovers that the maxim "all dreams follow the mouth" was written in Bar Hedya's book, most likely a manual of oneirocritica. This statement may be viewed as the most important comment in the talmudic dreambook, since it encapsulates formulaically the quintessential aspect of the rabbinic hermeneutic related to deciphering dream symbols. If the point of the story, as I suggested before, was to portray the dream interpreters negatively, the discovery of what was written in Bar Hedya's book complicates the picture and leaves the criticism somewhat more ambiguous. The tactic employed by Bar Hedya is precisely the one promulgated by the sages, and if this is so, then we must further assume a shared hermeneutic. The insinuation of this adage is not only that every dream demands an interpretation, for a dream that is not interpreted, in the language of another proclamation recorded in the name of R. Ḥisda, is like a letter that has not been read,[21] but that the upshot of the dream is determined by its interpretation.[22] Dream interpretation is a mode of performative speech that has the potential to change the course of events,[23] just as the practice of certain ritual actions (for example, the dream fast, *taʿanit ḥalom*, which, as one rabbinic authority argued, was even allowed on the Sabbath)[24] can offset the impending doom foreseen oneirically. To say that dreams depend on interpretation does not mean simply that the interpretation retroactively bestows sense on the dream, but that the interpretation protentitively confers reality upon the dream and, as a consequence, the dream shapes reality.[25] The circularity of my reasoning here illumines the reversibility of cause and effect that we may infer from the case of the dream and its interpretation—the cause occasions the effect that is its cause. The saying in the Babylonian Talmud "all dreams follow the mouth" is thus parallel to R. Yoḥanan's statement in the Palestinian Talmud that "all dreams follow their interpretations [*kol ha-ḥalomot holkhin aḥar pitroneihen*] except for wine; there is one who drinks wine and it is good for him (the scholar) but there is another who drinks wine and it is bad for him (the ignoramus)."[26] The stuff of the dream is determined by its interpretability, though the latter is determined by the stuff of the dream.

We are reminded of this wisdom in the seemingly innocuous statement passed on in the name of Bar Qappara, "There is no dream that does not have an interpretation" (*leit ḥalom she-ein lo pitron*).[27] The crux of this maxim is not the trivial fact that every dream has an interpretation, but that the latter is constitutive of the former; to speak of a dream without interpretation, therefore, is as meaningless as speaking of a text without a reader. The suchness of the text, textuality as such, must be considered from the angle of an ostensibly banal correlative logic: there is no text without reader and no reader without text. Interpretation fulfils the same purpose vis-à-vis the dream: there is no dream without an interpreter and no interpreter without a dream. The same mind-set undoubtedly underlies the counsel (recorded in *Sefer Ḥasidim*, the compilation of exempla attributed for the most part to Judah ben Samuel he-Ḥasid, one of the central figures of the Rhineland Jewish pietists, who were active in the twelfth and thirteenth centuries, and in *Sefer ha-Zohar*, the anthology of kabbalistic lore and practice that began to circulate in the thirteenth and fourteenth centuries in fragmentary units, whence, through an extensive process of scribal transmission whose contours may not be entirely available to scholarly discernment, the manuscript witnesses were redacted into the printed versions of the Mantua and Cremona editions, the prototypes for all subsequent editions)[28] that one should disclose one's dream only to a friend:[29] what actualizes the dream is its interpretation, the tenor of which will reflect the way the interpreter feels about the dreamer. A positively disposed comrade will be inclined to explicate the matter compassionately and, as a consequence, constructively affect the reality wrought by the dream.

In this regard, it is of interest to ponder that in his collection of halakhic responsa received from heavenly revelations, *She'elot u-Teshuvot min ha-Shamayim*, composed in the early part of the thirteenth century, Jacob of Marvège dedicates a whole section to inquire precisely about this matter. After recounting the depiction of Bar Hedya's modifying his interpretation in accord with the payment he received as well as the general dictate that "all dreams follow the mouth," Jacob poses the following query to his celestial interlocutors:

> Concerning this we are perplexed and we ask, is it possible that the decrees of the Creator will be altered on account of the interpretation of the interpreter? And is the statement that dreams follow the mouth, whether for good or evil, to be taken literally, or is it not to be taken literally, since the decrees of the Creator are not changeable? Bar Hedya was naught but an interpreter, and if so, why was it written in his book "all dreams follow the mouth"? They responded: It is a decree, examine it and you will find [that it

is so]. I inquired a second time, and they responded as they did at first, and I was distressed by this and I asked again as I did the first time. They responded: You know and you have heard that there are some people whose destiny is that their eyes and their tongues will be evil, and their feet, too, are evil . . . and there are those whose feet are for good. . . . So do not wonder about those whose destiny it is to be interpreters of dreams, which will be fulfilled, whether for good or evil, as long as it is in accord with the matter, and Bar Hedya was among them. The interpretations were not established on account of his merit but rather on account of his fortune, and thus Rava got angry at him and cursed him. And what was written in his book—"all dreams follow the mouth"—was not said except about those people whose destiny is such. All this they responded to me. Again I asked: If so, why must one say one's dream to one who has compassion for him? They responded: One must never open one's mouth to the adversary.[30] The one who has compassion for him must interpret [the dream] favorably because the angel that stands to his right takes the word from the mouth of the interpreter, snatches it, and says "Amen, so must it be." And if one hates him, he opens his mouth for evil, and the angel that stands to his left snatches the word and says "Amen." For this reason what is done is done, whether for good or evil. After an hour they answered a third time: Do not think about our words, for in truth we have informed you, and the secret is deep.[31]

Despite his persistent probing, Jacob of Marvège does not receive a satisfactory answer to his query concerning the rabbinic principle that the outcome of the dream is dependent on the hermeneutical stance of the interpreter, a principle encapsulated in the passage allegedly written in the book of Bar Hedya, "all dreams follow the mouth." For the medieval sage, this idea clashes with the theological credo that events unfold providentially in accord with the necessity of the divine directive. The angelic voices assure the inquiring rabbinic scholar that it is the destiny of some people, including the aforementioned Bar Hedya, to be dream interpreters, which implies that the interpretation of specific dreams offered by such people are to be considered expressions of God's volition. Jacob of Marvège pushes forward and asks about another talmudic proverb that one should convey one's dream only to one who has compassion. If everything about a dream is determined by God, why should it matter to whom I recount my dream? After two attempts to explain this, the angels advise Jacob that he should not dwell on their words, since the "secret is deep." The matter of how interpretation actually affects the realization of the dream is thus left to stand as an irresolvable mystery.

Arguably, the most important precept of rabbinic oneirology, surely the one that had the most significant reverberations in subsequent homiletical, commentarial, philosophical, and mystical literature, is thus considered inherently enigmatic; indeed, the more light that is shed on it, the obscurer it becomes. From this we can adduce a valuable insight about the apophatic element in dream analysis, a theme we explored in detail in the preceding chapter. In a spirit reminiscent of current deconstructionist and/or postmodernist hermeneutics, the rabbinic assumption is that the substance of the dream is molded by interpretation; since the latter is inscrutable, however, the finale of the dream must necessarily remain a pure contingency. Translating this thought philosophically, I would say the underlying issue concerns the relation of the openness of the future and the determination of the past, or perhaps it is the openness of the past and the determination of the future.

A Dream Interpreted within a Dream

Phenomenologically, dreaming entails double vision, or better, a vision folding in on itself, a seeing of the seen that is seen only in the seeing that lacks any seen apart from the seeing. I surmise this idea is implied in R. Yoḥanan's formula "a dream interpreted within a dream" (*ḥalom she-niftar be-tokh ḥalom*).[32] What is a dream interpreted within a dream?[33] Like the dream of Penelope reported in the *Odyssey*,[34] the remark of R. Yoḥanan suggests that the content of the dream contains its own interpretation. As I noted in the previous chapter, Maimonides proffered an explanation of the talmudic dictum according to which the one who dreams the interpretation of one's dream while dreaming is compared to the prophet who receives the parable and its explanation in the vision.[35] The iteration implied in the phenomenon of the dream interpreted within a dream—to dream that one has awakened from the dream, situated in the interstice between wakefulness and dream that is delineated rabbinically by the phrase *nim we-lo nim tir we-lo tir*, "asleep but not asleep, awake but not awake,"[36] the space where it is not possible to distinguish the two, since to be awake, one must be dreaming, but to be dreaming, one must be awake—sheds further light on the meaning of dreams more generally in the rabbinic mentality: the dream can never be detached from its interpretation. We may assume that the imaginal topography, the "hyperspace" of the dream, changes with each effort to interpret it, whether to oneself or to another—in line with the part accorded in quantum physics to the observer in determining the properties of an observable object, which I discussed briefly in Chapter 1—but in keeping with the dynamic of a dream interpreted within a dream, the very supposition that the dream can be separated, ideationally or experientially, from its interpretation must be jettisoned. Recounting the dream is akin to explaining a text that is, textually speaking, already an interpretation of a text; the dream is itself a narrative retelling that is on a par with dreaming a dream that one is dreaming a dream or dreaming a dream that one is not dreaming—in either case, the dreamer awakens into another dream, an endless flight from any fleeing that is not an eternal fall into the lattice of dreaming.[37]

It seems to me dubious, therefore, to contrast dream interpretation with the technique of rabbinic midrash on the basis that the "essential thrust" of the latter is to find "multiple interpretations of Scripture," whereas the former harbors the "singleminded desire to unravel the one and only meaning of the dream."[38] Closer to the mark is the description of rabbinic hermeneutical practice offered by Levinas:

> the intention of the signified by the signifier is not the only way of indicating significance. In its other modes, the significance of the signifier responds only to the mind that seeks it, thus becoming part of the process of signification; interpretation necessarily includes that seeking without which the non-said, inherent in the texture of what is declared, would be extinguished by the weight of the texts and sink into their letters.[39]

Just as the reader actively participates in the creation of the meaning of the text—indeed, in a profound sense, interpretation is part of the constitution of the text, including the manner in which a particular verse may be vocalized[40]—that gives shape to the identity of the reader, so the dreamer weaves the dream through which the dreamer is woven. To be sure, there are passages in rabbinic literature and other documents of the ancient world that posit a one-to-one correspondence between dream images and symbols, but this by no means intimates that the dream yields only one meaning.

Quite the contrary, some rabbis entertained the notion that the dream has multiple meanings. Consider the following comment that is attached to a tradition transmitted in a chain of several sages, culminating with the elder R. Bena'ah:

> There were twenty-four interpreters of dreams [*potrei ḥalomot*] in Jerusalem. One time I dreamt a dream and I went to all of them, and what one interpreted for me was not what the other interpreted—yet all of them were fulfilled in me, to substantiate what is said, "all dreams follow the mouth." Is the statement that "all dreams follow the mouth" scriptural? Yes, as stated by R. Eleazar, for R. Eleazar said: Whence do we know that all dreams follow the mouth? As it says, "as he [Joseph] interpreted to us, so it was" (Genesis 41:13). Rava said: This is only if he interpreted it in accord with one's dream, as it says, "according to each man's dream did he interpret" (*ibid.*, 12).[41]

The teaching that all dreams follow the mouth is offered as the rationale to legitimate the multivalency of the dream, which, in the talmudic context, means not only that manifold interpretations of a dream are possible, but that they all will be fulfilled, a harder thing for the human mind to comprehend.[42] The example of Joseph, the paradigmatic explicator of dreams in Jewish lore, is cited as the biblical basis for the oneirocritic principle, the wide-ranging repercussions of which may be adduced by the qualifying remark ascribed to Rava: it is valid to say that the meaning of the dream is made real by the interpretation only in the case that the interpretation corresponds to the content of the dream. Rava's caveat notwithstanding, the rabbinic idea bespeaks a radical hermeneutic that would endow the interpreter with the power to make the images of the dream come true, which, in my understanding, conveys the notion that the reality presumed to be true consists of the images that are so interpreted. Veracity and duplicity are not inherent properties of the phenomenon that is dreamt, but they are relative to the expository condition of the dreamer.

The polysemic underpinnings of the claim that all dreams follow the mouth derive precisely from the view that Rava seems to have challenged.[43] As Alexander has expressed it, "the outcome of a dream is determined by the interpretation that is put upon it: its fulfillment—whether for good or for ill—is somehow activated by interpretation."[44] The capability of interpretation to actualize the dream, and in so doing to shape reality, is not limited to a situation where there is ostensible accord between the interpretation and the dream content. To insist on this qualification is to miss the significance of the rabbinic approach entirely. That the various interpretations are all valid implies that the dream, when divested of any interpretative cloak, is hermeneutically neutral. This neutrality is well captured in the teaching—attributed alternatively to R. Meir, R. Abbahu, or the Rabbis—that the words of dreams are inconsequential, *divrei ḥalomot lo maʿalin we-lo moridin*, literally, they "do not raise up or bring down." In several talmudic passages, the statement is cited to underline that one cannot rely on information divulged in dreams to settle legal or ritual matters.[45] But in other midrashic contexts,[46] the intention is not so restricted, and the point is, rather, that the content of dreams in general has no ultimate consequence or meaning apart from what is imparted by the act of interpretation that makes intelligible the ascription of the properties "true" and "false" to images that are intrinsically neither true nor false because they are concurrently true and false, that is, true precisely because false, false precisely because true. The interpretative token, as it were, transmutes the mimetic relationship of representation and represented and, in the process, upends the conventional hierarchy of appearance and reality; the latter is as much shaped by the former as the former is by the latter. There is no way to fathom the text of the dream but through the veil of interpretation and no way to unveil the veil of the dream but through the text of interpretation.[47] Following Nietzsche's surmise regarding the poetic symbol, we can say of the dream that it signifies the "nature of being as interpreted being," that is, that there is no being of which to speak discriminately that is not already a being of which one has spoken indiscriminately, no sense of the real that is not real because it appears to some observer as real. Hence, interpreting a dream, like reading a text, requires the "rigorous philology" of a "genealogical decipherment."[48]

Dream Exegesis and the Hermeneutic Circuit

Dream interpretation and textual study share an elemental hermeneutical postulate. The point has been well expressed by James Kugel with reference specifically to the emphasis in the book of Daniel on the need to retell the dream and then to interpret it: "Both features represent the same basic idea: interpretation begins by the interpreter reproducing the text itself, for the latter, whether dream or scribbling, is itself a gift from God granted afresh to the interpreter; proper understanding is inseparable from prophecy itself."[49] One may apply this insight to the rabbinic sensibility: interpretation requires translocating a text, to use Celan's locution[50]—either a dream writ on the palimpsest of the imagination or an actual inscription etched on a material surface—that is given anew to the interpreter in each moment of reading; the exegetical and visionary dimensions are interwoven.[51] The point is epitomized in a midrashic text from an anonymous fourteenth-century compilation appended to the list of thirty-three[52] rules by which the aggadah—the rabbinic term for nonhalakhic material, which encompasses folkloristic, mythical, theological, cosmological, and anthropological insights—is interpreted:

> There are the rules by which the aggadah is interpreted, and the multifaceted explanations of Scripture emerge from them. And thus it says "Behold, my word is like fire—declares the Lord—and like a hammer that shatters rock!" (Jeremiah 23:29). The house of R. Ishmael taught: just as this hammer divides into several sparks, so one verse can yield several explanations, but one explanation is not derived from two verses. Hence it says "Just as a dream comes with much brooding" (Ecclesiastes 5:2), and the matter [can be explained by the method of] *a minori ad maius*: If with respect to the words of dreams that have no effect, one dream can yield several explanations, how much more so with respect to the words of Torah, which are more significant, that one verse will yield several explanations. And

> thus it says "For this is not a trifling thing for you" (Deuteronomy 32:47). There is no letter in the Torah, and all the more so no word, and all the more so no verse, and all the more so no chapter that does not yield several meanings and that is interpreted in several ways.[53]

One would obviously expect that a higher status be conferred on the Torah than the dream, but it is significant that the polychromatic nature of the former is derived from the latter through the deductive rule of *a minori ad maius*, that is, if the dream yields multiple explanations, we may infer that this is the case with scriptural verses. Although not stated explicitly, the selection of the dream to make this argument rests on the conjecture that the dream may be compared to a text, and hence, the manner of interpreting it proceeds in line with the regulations of textual analysis.

The rabbinic wisdom is reinscribed in the following passage in *Sefer Ḥasidim*:

> Why does a dream come "with much brooding" (Ecclesiastes 5:2) and when it is interpreted in accordance with its matter it goes after the mouth? Nothing comes to a man, whether good or evil, if he does not first see in the dream some simulacrum [*me'ein dugma*]. But no man is worthy to see in a dream a simulacrum of [things] in the future as they will be without any doubt or hesitation, for thoughts are not reliable, and when a person sleeps [they are] mixed with the words of the angel, and therefore they "follow the mouth"[54] when they are interpreted in accordance with their matter. They said that "a dream is one-sixtieth of prophecy,"[55] and it is written "in the hands of the prophets I was imaged" (Hosea 12:11), and it is written "I see a branch of an almond tree [*maqqel shaqed*].... For I am watchful [*shoqed*] to bring my word to pass" (Jeremiah 1:11–12)—by means of a parable [*mashal*] the heart of man will comprehend. Thus "and taking up his parable he said" (Numbers 24:3), and it is written "to comprehend the parable and the epigram" (Proverbs 1:6). With respect to the dream of the prophets, their thoughts were not intermingled nor [were they] the words of the demon, but in the [ordinary] dreams of people the words of the demon are intermingled.... All of these dreams and others akin to them are not dreams told by the angel, but rather through [one's] thoughts one sees in one's dream their simulacra, and concerning them it

> says "they spoke false dreams" (Zechariah 10:2).... All of these dreams are on account of the demon, and concerning them it says "how can straw be compared to grain?" (Jeremiah 23:28), for there is no substance in them.... Concerning the dreams of an angel it is said "through a dream I will speak to him" (Numbers 12:6), for the angel speaks through the thoughts of a man like one who leads the blind... since at times he thinks truth and at times deceit, and so it is in a dream.... Therefore the knowledge of a man during a dream is like a blind man or a child. Sometimes he thinks truth and sometimes deceit, and most thoughts are not intended.[56]

In this passage, many of the older talmudic dicta about dreams are reworked in light of some of the predominant anthropological and cosmological assumptions of Ḥasidei Ashkenaz. Based on a rabbinic text in which a distinction is made between a dream that comes through an angel and a dream that comes through a demon,[57] Judah he-Ḥasid distinguishes between prophetic and ordinary dreams: the agent of the former is always an angel, and that of the latter is occasionally an angel (in which case the dream partakes of prophecy to a degree) and occasionally a demon. Translated psychologically, when the dream derives solely from the repository of one's own thoughts, an idea that is averred explicitly in another rabbinic teaching,[58] it is deemed the work of the demon and therefore false.[59] When, however, the source is an angel, then a distinction is drawn between commonplace dreaming, which is a hybrid of truth and falsehood, and prophecy as such, which is unfailingly trustworthy, an imagistic representation without any taint of pretense.

The link between prophetic vision and the angelic presence is highlighted in other works of the Rhineland Jewish pietists, including Eleazar ben Judah of Worms (ca. 1176–1238),[60] on occasion in such a manner that would not corroborate the effort in the above passage to distinguish the source of the vision as either the storehouse of one's thoughts or an angel. That is, there is sufficient textual evidence to demonstrate that some of the pietist masters also understood the angel to be a theophanic form that takes shape within, but exists in a universe parallel to an individual's mind, the mirror reflection, the image of the image. In addition to envisioning the glory prophetically, this idea is deployed to explain several crucial spiritual phenomena, particularly the proper intentionality in prayer. The angels are imaginal forms (*dimyonot* or *demuyot*) that the divine places in the mind/heart of the prophet and/or worshipper and by which the nonphenomenalizable is encountered phenomenally. The imagination (*dimyon*) is the faculty that mediates between the corporeal and spiritual, and thus the ocular forms (*maḥazot* or *mar'ot*) it produces are visible representations of the invisible.

Clearly, these images do not objectively correspond to the truth, but neither are they entirely subjective. The imaginary is both real and illusory. The paradox is pithily expressed in the assertion preserved in several sources that God is both outside and within the image.[61] The glory can be imagined in concrete forms, including most importantly that of an *anthropos*, but God, the transcendent One, is not the image; yet one can worship that very image because God is present therein. The positive value accorded to the imagination is also underscored by the theological claim that it is the will of God itself that is responsible for placing these thoughts (*da'atanot*) within the prophet's visual mind (*maḥashevet ha-re'iyyah*).[62] The same explanation is applied to the phenomenon of the dream: God's volition is communicated through an angelic presence that corresponds to a person's inner thought and its corresponding celestial angel (*sar mazzal*), which assumes the image of that person upon descending to the world.[63] Moreover, this is how the pietists explained the biblical idea that Adam was created in the divine likeness, that is, the human being is fashioned in the likeness of the angelic form that is one's own image.[64] The depiction of the imagination as the locus of the corporalization of the incorporeal implied in this angelophany puts into sharp relief the inadequacy of distinguishing between the prophetic and dream visions on the grounds that the former are perfectly true and the latter are a blend of truth and untruth.

Beyond this distinction, two more points are made with respect to the dream phenomenon. The dream is understood mainly as a form of prognostication. Indeed, the matter is presented as a general principle that does not appear verbatim in earlier sources: A portent of everything that will occur in a person's life first appears in a dream. However, since no human is capable of foretelling perfectly what will transpire in the future, there is the necessity for interpretation. Without the hermeneutical clarification, the dream is muddled, or, in the scriptural idiom, "the dream comes with much brooding" (Ecclesiastes 5:2). The dream is thus a textual artifact, a point reinforced by the paraphrase of the statement that Rava reportedly discovered in the book of Bar Hedya, "all dreams follow the mouth." The maxim is treated at length in another passage from *Sefer Ḥasidim*.[65] The relevant discussion occurs after it has been established that it is efficacious to fast in order to deter the dire consequences foretold in a dream, such as the passing of an individual with a name similar to the person who dies in the dream. It is impossible for the dream not to come about at all, but it is possible "to transpose the image of the constellations" (*lehithappekh dugmat ha-mazzalot*) so that the fate below will be altered.[66] At this point, the author comes to the decisive part of his discussion:

> Why does the dream follow the mouth? For if the dreams did not follow the mouth, we would say that dreams are not from the blessed holy One, for the Torah is from him, and it follows the mouth and the interpretation. Now it is not possible to know the dream, but concerning everything that is from the blessed holy One, he gives one a heart to know and a mouth to explicate. If not, why is there a dream? It is to tell us that it is from the blessed holy One, to inform us that he knows all of the future and he notifies human beings about what will come to pass in the future, so that one will repent, pray, and not transgress. Moreover, they said there were twenty-four dream interpreters in Jerusalem, and what one interpreted the other did not interpret, but all of them were fulfilled.[67] Just as one verse can yield several explanations, and the interpretation of the verse should be in accord with its literal sense, so the [interpretation of the dream] should be comparable to the dream. Then it is possible for one to intend the interpretation.... Another reason why the dream follows the mouth is because it is hidden. If it did not follow the mouth, it would not be possible to repent on account of it. Since it is possible to know, one can comprehend what it is.[68]

The principal objective of the dream is to inform one about the future, but in this extract, the matter is contextualized more specifically as part of the divine plan to afford one an opportunity to repent and to change one's ways. Indeed, it is this need that assures us that dreams derive ultimately from a godly source, the rationale invoked to explain the rabbinic sentiment that dreams follow the mouth, that is, their intent and realization are both dependent on an act of interpretation. The dream in itself is unknowable, and yet we are given the aptitude to decipher it, for if that were not the case, we could not say that the dream was from God, since God allegedly would not bequeath a message utterly beyond our ability to comprehend. The analogy to the scriptural text is drawn overtly: just as the Torah, which is from the divine, is made known through interpretation, so too the dream. The textual comportment of the latter is made even more explicit in the analysis of the talmudic tradition that there were twenty-four dream interpreters in Jerusalem. Judah he-Ḥasid expounds this tradition by combining two hermeneutical principles culled from rabbinic literature, the notion that one verse engenders multiple interpretations (*miqra eḥad yoṣe le-khammah ṭe'amim*)[69] and the idea that no verse can be completely removed from its literal or contextual sense (*ein miqra yoṣe midei peshuṭo*).[70] The combination of these two tenets—obviously explicated in a manner distinctive to the historical moment of the pietists and not reflecting the meaning of the dicta in their original context—forges a rather sophisticated hermeneutics that bears resemblance to at least one trend in postmodern critical theory: meaning is polyvalent, but there must always be allegiance to the text. Multivocality does not discredit philological attunement; on the contrary, the latter is precisely what facilitates the former. The same may be applied to the dream: there are multiple interpretations, and each is correct as long as it is tied to the intent of the dream, even though that intent is exposed only through the weft and warp of exegesis that unravels in time. The conclusion offers another explanation for the rabbinic assertion that the dream follows the mouth. Since the meaning is hidden, the latent must be made manifest through the interpretative gesture, and in the process, knowledge assumes a transformative goal.

The rabbinic declaration "all dreams follow the mouth" is elucidated as well in a passage in *Sheva Netivot ha-Torah*, a treatise on the seven exegetical paths composed by Abraham Abulafia:

> What is written of necessity requires two primary matters even according to the mind of the populace: One of them is the need to know the script [*ha-mikhtav*], that is, its simple reading [*ha-qeri'ah*

> *ha-peshuṭah*], and the second is the need to know the explanation [*ha-perush*], for this is similar to the matter of the dream itself, for a dream needs an interpretation [*pitron*], and every dream that is not interpreted is comparable to a parable and an allegory that are written, but not expounded, because these exist entirely for the sake of their interpretation and explanation.[71]

The dream is compared to Scripture, which has an external and an internal meaning, the contextual sense (*peshaṭ*) and its explanation (*perush*), a notion that Abulafia would have culled from both classical rabbinic authorities and Maimonides. Appropriating the axiom of the Maimonidean hermeneutic, Abulafia insists that if the literal does not contradict reason, then there is no justification for ignoring it. If, however, there is such a contradiction, both the revealed and the hidden meanings are to be approved, even as it is understood that the literal in this case is not to be explained literally, since the contextual sense overlaps with the figurative. To frame the matter in terms of an opinion preserved in one talmudic passage in the name of R. Judah, the story about the resurrection of the dead in the vision of the dry bones (Ezekiel 37:1–14) "in truth was a parable" (*emet mashal hayah*). R. Neḥemiah objects to R. Judah's comment, "If it is true, why is it a parable, and if it is a parable, why is it true?" The view of R. Neḥemiah, which presumes that the parable and truth are mutually exclusive opposites, is undermined by R. Judah's insight that the truth of the parable consists precisely of its being parabolically true.[72]

The seemingly negligible pairing of the words "truth" and "parable" brings to the fore the far-reaching theoretical consequence of the comparison of the scriptural text to the dream. At first glance. we might be tempted, like R. Neḥemiah, to say that if something is parabolic, it cannot be historically factual, and, alternatively, if something is historically factual, it cannot be parabolic; upon closer inspection, however, we appreciate that the dream destabilizes the certitude of this binary insofar as there is no criterion of referentiality apart from what is fabricated—the images of the dream alone constitute the reality of what is dreamt, and thus their truth is determined by what is imagined to be true. Analogously, in the mind of the enlightened reader, there is no external meaning in the text to be distinguished from the internal. At best, the literal serves politically as a partition to shield the metaphorical truth from the unworthy.[73] The whole of the revealed word is likened therefore to a dream, exemplifying the paradoxical notion of fictional truth, the truth that is true because it is fiction. Abulafia, it seems to me, is drawing out the full inference of Maimonides' own insistence on the inherently parabolic nature of the Torah.[74] It is in this sense, moreover, that we can apply to the Torah his characterization of divine actions as the work of "wily graciousness and wisdom"[75] or in the frequently utilized locution of the rabbis to articulate the principle of accommodation, "the Torah speaks in human language,"[76] that is, the utterance of truth in the form of true figures that are literally untrue.[77]

Let us consider the following extraordinary passage in *Sefer ha-Edut*, a composition in which Abulafia's visionary experiences are presented under the pseudonym Raziel, the angel of divine mysteries, chosen because its numerology (200 + 7 +10 + 1 + 30) is the same as his first name, Avraham (1 + 2 + 200 + 5 + 40):[78]

> Raziel said in the fifth month, which is the month of Av, on the first and second days of the month, the Lord showed me two visions in one form. Know that concerning what the prophet gives testimony about, which is a vision, a dream, or a parable, and the like, there is no need for any person to raise difficulties about his words, for the mouth of a person is like one hundred witnesses.[79] All of the dispute is only in places where it appears that his words are entirely in accord with their literal sense, and therefore it is possible to explain them according to their literal sense and through their mysteries. And even though they are in accord with their literal sense, and all of these matters transpired, there is nothing preventing them from being explained in their mysteries, for every literal sense bears the concealed, but not every concealed sense bears the literal. Know that at times I will explain many issues in these books, which happened verily according to their literal sense, by way of the concealed.[80]

In the purview of the dream, what is revealed of the concealed conceals the revealed of the concealed. The exposure of the exposure perforce is a double concealment, a withholding of withholding, and hence, just as one cannot expect to understand the scriptural text without recourse to interpretation, one cannot expect to do so with respect to eliciting meaning from the dream. But as we have already seen, this is not simply to say (in a commonsensical and even pedestrian way) that interpretation makes explicit the implicit import of the dream. After all, interpretation is as much a covering up as it is an uncovering. The point, then, is that elucidation itself is a form of obfuscation. Comprehending the parabolic status of the dream leads to a recognition of the dreamlike character of the parable. The inner exposes the outer as the outer that conceals the inner.

A similar revisioning of the rabbinic posture can be elicited from a passage in *Sefer ha-Zohar*:

> It has been said, "All dreams of the world follow the interpretation of the mouth," and it has been established, as it written "As he explained it to us, so it was" (Genesis 41:13). What is the reason? Because there is deception and truth in the dream, and the word rules over everything, and hence the dream requires a good interpretation. Rabbi Judah said: Because every dream is from a lower gradation and the word rules over it, every dream follows its interpretation.... R. Ḥiyya and R. Yose were in the presence of R. Simeon. R. Ḥiyya said: We have learned that a dream that is not interpreted is like a letter that is not read.[81] Is this because it exists and he did not know it, or did it not exist at all? He said to him: It exists, but it was not known, for the power exists over that dream, but it is not known, and he does not know if it exists or not. There is no matter in the world that is not dependent on the dream or on the messenger before it comes into this world, as it is said that prior to each and every matter that comes into the world there is a decree about it from heaven, and from there it disseminates into the world and it is given by the messenger. And all of this because it is written "the Lord God does not do anything if he does not disclose his secret to his servants the prophets" (Amos 3:7)—this is when prophets are found in the world, and if not, even though prophecy no longer resides, the sages are preferable to the prophets,[82] and if not, it is given in a dream, and if not, the matter is found with the birds of the sky.[83]

As we find often in zoharic homilies, the above passage is a tapestry woven from the threads of various rabbinic dicta. The cord that weaves the disparate sources together is the belief that nothing in the terrestrial world materializes except through a divine decree that can be delivered in the form of prophecy, a dream, or the chirping of the birds (the art of augury inspired in the history of Jewish exegesis by Ecclesiastes 10:20. "For a bird of the air may carry the utterance, and a winged creature may report the word"). What is of particular importance to mark is that the talmudic maxim that all dreams follow the mouth is explained by reference to the view (also expressed in rabbinic literature) that the dream comprises both truth and deception, that the truth of the dream relies on the untruth by which it is imaginally enframed. Interpretive prowess, therefore, is required to separate the wheat from the chaff, to extract the diamond from the ore. I will return to this idea in the next chapter, but suffice it here to note how the different motifs combine to accentuate the point that precisely because there is this admixture, the dream can portend good or evil, and thus its result will be dependent on how it is interpreted. Interpretation is an apparatus through which events in time can be molded. This creative ("demiurgical" might be the more suitable adjective) potency is related to the larger metaphysical premise that the word rules over everything. One can take this remark at face value as a verification of the primacy accorded to language, an essential postulate of Jewish esotericism through the ages; insofar as the word is the instrument of creation, it continues to demonstrate control over the things that were created through it, in this case, through the hermeneutic dexterity of the human being applied specifically to dreams.

To grasp the intent of this remark, however, we need to take stock of the sefirotic symbolism encrypted therein: the word (*millah*) corresponds to the last of the ten divine emanations, *Shekhinah* or *Malkhut*. In the exact language of this text, the meaning of the dream is determined by the interpretation of the mouth (*pishra de-fuma*)—an amalgamation of the dicta that appear respectively in the Palestinian and Babylonian Talmuds—for the words that issue from the mouth correspond to the divine word, which is superior to the level of the dream. Put more technically, the "word" is a symbolic allusion to *Shekhinah*, the divine gradation that is also referred to as the "vision" (*mar'eh*) of prophecy,[84] the "speculum that does not shine" (*aspaqlaryah she-einah me'irah*),[85] the prism (*ḥeizu*) through which all the colors are seen, whereas the dream (*ḥalom*) is one-sixtieth of prophecy, according to another rabbinic dictum,[86] that is, "the sixth gradation from that gradation of prophecy, and this is the gradation of Gabriel, who is appointed over dreams."[87] The depiction of Gabriel is predicated on the fact that there are six rungs separating the source of prophecy in the divine pleroma from the source of dreams in the angelic world (*olam ha-mal'akhim* or, in the original Arabic whence the Hebrew phrase probably derived, *'ālam al-malā'ika*, which is closely linked to the invisible, spiritual domain known as *'ālam al-malakūt*, the "world of sovereignty"), that is, the four lower sefirotic emanations, *Neṣaḥ*, *Hod*, *Yesod*, *Malkhut*, and the two archangels, Michael and Gabriel.[88] Confirmation of this explanation is found in several other zoharic passages, as well as in the writings of Moses de León,[89] although another possibility, attested in Joseph Angeleṭ's *Livnat ha-Sappir*,[90] is that the order of the six angels in the camp beneath the divine presence consists of Metatron, Sandalfon, Uriel, Rafael, Michael, and Gabriel.[91] It is likely, moreover, that the specification of Gabriel as the locus of dreams is related to the association of this archangel and prophecy that some Jewish thinkers took over from Islamic philosophers, who assigned this role to Gabriel based on his identification with the Active Intellect.[92] In the zoharic passage, the emphasis is placed on Gabriel's being appointed over dreams, but the connection to prophecy is obviously kept intact.[93] The contrast between the two is specified in sharper terms in the following comment:

> What is the difference between prophecy and the dream? Prophecy is in the world of the masculine, the dream in the world of the feminine, and from one to the other there is a descent of six gradations. Prophecy is on the right and the left, the dream on the left.[94] The dream is divided[95] into several gradations below, and therefore the dream is in the whole world, even though one sees in accord with one's gradation, one's gradation is in accord with the person. Prophecy does not spread forth except in its place.[96]

The prophetic vision belongs properly to the sefirotic pleroma, *alma di-dekhura*, the "world of the masculine," a term that usually refers either to *Binah* or to the sefirotic potencies from *Binah* to *Yesod*, whereas the dream vision is assigned to *alma de-nuqba*, the "world of the feminine," a technical designation of *Shekhinah* or the angelic potencies beneath it.[97] The two types of vision are further contrasted in the zoharic homily on the grounds that prophecy is on the right and left, perhaps alluding respectively to the seventh and eighth emanations, *Neṣaḥ* and *Hod*, while the dream is aligned exclusively on the left, which is linked to Gabriel, the angel whose power derives from the aspect of strength (*gevurah*) on the left side.[98] Finally, a topographical distinction is made: prophecy is said to be limited to its place—just as the rabbinic teaching restricted prophecy (with a few notable exceptions) to the land of Israel, so the kabbalists confined the prophetic influx to the divine realm, and especially *Shekhinah*, the theosophic correlate to the geographic space—and the dream, by contrast, is dispersed over the world. Given the ubiquity of the dream, it is emphasized that each person sees the nocturnal vision in conformity with his or her level of attainment.

The implications of the zoharic symbolism can be discerned by considering passages in several of de León's works, especially *Shushan Edut* (1286). Before engaging this passage, let me state candidly that I am not concerned if this Spanish kabbalist had the precise zoharic texts, or even versions of them, before him when he worked on his own compositions, an issue that is still debated by scholars of the field; far more significant, in my estimation, is whether he articulates a view that is consistent or inconsistent with what we may elicit from those texts. In this case, we can assent to the former option. Turning to the passage from *Shushan Edut*, de León explicates the rabbinic teaching[99] that the dream is the unripe fruit of prophecy: "Contemplate that the fruit of prophecy is the dream, everything is hewn from one place, but since it is unripe, the maturation[100] is not as it matures in its place."[101] De León goes on to juxtapose this dictum with the characterization of the dream as one-sixtieth of prophecy:

> As you already know, the gradations whence prophecy issues are the pillars of Torah, "disciples of the Lord" (Isaiah 54:13), "the precious children of Zion, once valued as gold" (Lamentations 4:2). The prophets drew from there the sustenance of prophecy. Know that what falls from there descends from gradation to gradation until six gradations below whence the dream spreads forth. The gradation of the dream falls and descends from the gradation of prophecy.[102]

Prophecy is from the seventh and eighth sefirot, *Neṣaḥ* and *Hod*, labeled variously as the "pillars of Torah," "disciples of the Lord,"[103] and "precious children of Zion." From these attributes, the efflux of prophecy overflows until the sixth gradation beneath them, the source of the dissemination of dreams. Daniel is upheld by de León as someone who was not a prophet, but who was nevertheless granted dream visions that are correlated with, or better, replicate, the supernal emanations. Similarly, we read in a zoharic homily:

> What is written of Daniel? "The mystery was revealed to Daniel in a night vision" (Daniel 2:19)—in a night vision. What is "in the night vision?" This is Gabriel, for he is a vision [*ḥezwa*], a prism from a prism [*ḥeizu min ḥeizu*]. Come and see what is written: "And there, coming from the east with a roar like the roar of mighty waters, was the glory of the God of Israel, and the earth was lit up by his glory" (Ezekiel 43:2). And what is written after it? "The vision was like the vision I had seen when I came to destroy the city, the very same vision that I had seen by the Chebar Canal, and I fell on my face" (*ibid.*, 3). All of these visions added up to six,[104] for they are the visions [*mar'ot*] and the prism of vision [*ḥeizu de-ḥezwa*], the prism through which the colors above are seen, and they are seen in that prism, and there is a prism of the prism [*ḥeizu le-ḥeizu*]—a prism of the prism, one above the other! All them exist in gradations that are known, and they reign, and they are called the "prism of the night" (*ḥeizu de-leilya*), and through them all the dreams of the world disseminate,[105] and these are in the pattern of those above them.[106]

The role of Gabriel as interpreter of dreams is affirmed in the book of Daniel itself (8:16, 9:22), but for the author of the zoharic passage, this angel does not just fulfill this task; he is the agency that brings about the appearance of dreams, and thus he is referred to as the vision (*ḥezwa*)—it is likely this identification reflects the fact that *gavri'el* and *mar'ah* (or *mar'eh*) both equal 246[107]—or more specifically, in the language of the verse, the "night vision" (*ḥezwa di-leilya*), and demarcated as the "prism from a prism" (*ḥeizu min ḥeizu*). Through this vision/prism the mystery was revealed to Daniel. The nature of the mystery, the mystery of the mystery, can be ascertained by attending to the dual connotation of the term *ḥeizu* in the zoharic lexicon as "vision" and "prism" and its symbolic application to *Shekhinah*, since this divine potency is both the speculum through which the upper sefirotic potencies become visibly accessible to the human imagination and the psychic faculty by means of which the visualization is achieved.[108] To speak of Gabriel as the "prism from the prism" (*ḥeizu min ḥeizu*) or, alternately, as the "prism of the prism" (*ḥeizu le-ḥeizu*), signifies that dreams are visions by which one can glimpse the sefirotic images as reflected in *Shekhinah*,[109] the "prism of vision" (*ḥeizu de-ḥezwa*), the prism through which the invisible supernal colors are seen.[110] Dreaming, on this score, is a triple mirroring, beholding the forms in the mirror of the mind that mirrors the angelic mirror of the divine mirror.

Further support for this hypothesis may be adduced from another text that appears as part of the zoharic stratum known as *Sitrei Torah*. Commenting on the verse describing the vision of Jacob on his journey from Beer-sheba to Haran, "He had a dream, a stairway was set on the ground and its top reached the sky" (Genesis 28:12), the anonymous exegete wrote: "The dream is from the sixth gradation from the two gradations of prophecy, from that gradation there are six gradations, and hence the dream is one-sixtieth of prophecy."[111] Even more pertinent is the following remark in a homily on the same verse from what is commonly referred to as the main body of the *Zohar*:

> Come and see: The dream [*ḥelma*] is through Gabriel, for he is below in the sixth gradation from prophecy. The vision [*mar'eh*] is through that gradation that is the celestial beast [*ḥayyah*] ruling at night. And if you say, it is written "Gabriel, make that man understand the vision" (Daniel 8:16), so it most certainly is, for the matters of the vision are more concealed, and in the dream they are better explicated, and it explains the secrets of the vision. And thus Gabriel was appointed to interpret the matters of the vision, which is more concealed.[112]

Gabriel is the angel assigned to the dream, which is contrasted with the prophetic vision associated with the celestial beast that rules at night, a symbolic reference to *Shekhinah*.[113] The aim of the dream is to illuminate the concealed matters of the vision. The text ratifies the rabbinic conviction that after the demise of the institution of prophecy, the matter of prophetic inspiration is the patrimony of the sages, although it is found as well in dreams and in the speech of birds. What all of these divinatory phenomena share is the need for interpretation, which is connected to the last of the sefirotic potencies. To cite one final zoharic passage that drives the point home:

> Why is it written "So Joseph said to them, 'Do not interpretations belong to God [*le'lohim pitronim*]? Tell me, please!'"(Genesis 40:8). What is the reason? Because this is how the one who interprets dreams should allocate the interpretation to the blessed holy One, since the foundation of everything is there, and the interpretation subsists there. Come and see: It has been said that the gradation of the dream is below, and it is the sixth gradation, for from the place where prophecy abides until the gradation of the dream there are six gradations. The interpretation ascends from the gradation of the dream to another gradation. The dream is the gradation below, and the interpretation stands above it, the interpretation exists in the word, and hence the matter is established by the word [*be-dibbur qayyema millah*], as it is written "Do not interpretations belong to God?"—to God [*le'lohim*] certainly![114]

The interpretation rises from the dream, which is six degrees below in the angelic realm, to its source in the aspect of the divine marked as the word (*dibbur*), a term that is associated in many zoharic passages (as well as other kabbalistic sources) with *Shekhinah*, the speech that makes audible the as of yet inaudible voice (*Tif'eret*), which emerges from an even more inaudible voice (*Binah*), everything ultimately murmuring forth from infinite silence. This is the esoteric import of Joseph's retort to Pharaoh's cupbearer and baker, *le'lohim pitronim*: explication of dreams draws its efficacy from the gradation to which the name *elohim* is assigned, that is, the tenth emanation. Joseph's relation to this dimension is tied to his symbolic association with *Yesod*, the phallic potency that showers light upon *Shekhinah*. Zoharically, this place, referred to as the "foundation of everything" (*qiyyuma de-khola*), is the source whence interpretation of the dreams comes forth. Joseph incarnates that potency, and thus, while he can proceed to interpret dreams only once he is confident that he has imparted to those who have sought his services the wisdom that the facility to explicate issues from *Shekhinah*, in fact, his hermeneutic agility is sustained primarily by *Yesod*.

The phallomorphic character of dream interpretation is attested in a plethora of kabbalistic texts. Here I will illustrate the point with two examples. The first is a passage from Ḥayyim ben Joseph Viṭal (1543–1620), one of the foremost disciples of Isaac Luria (1534–1572):

> Know that the secret of the dream [*sod ha-ḥalom*] is the secret of the three [states] of expanded consciousness [*moḥin de-gadlut*], which are the three [permutations of] YHWH [10 + 5 + 6 +5 = 26 x 3 = 78], and they are numerically equivalent to [the letters that spell the word for dream] *ḥlm* [8 + 30 + 40 = 78].... And you already know that the entire reality of sleep is in [the condition of] diminution [*qaṭnut*], and thus the dream is from the aspect of expansion that persists within the diminution, and it is concealed there, and thus the dream is hidden and it is not explicated except by the interpreter, who is Joseph, the foundation [*yesod*] of *Ze'eir Anpin*, and all the supernal lights are gathered there.... And this is the secret of "Joseph is a fruitful bough" [*ben porat yosef*] (Genesis 49:22), for in *Yesod*, which is Joseph, all the consciousness gathers, and as a consequence, he is called *ben porat yosef*, and he becomes an interpreter of dreams [*poter ḥalomot*]. Therefore, the level of the interpretation is greater than the dream, for the dream is the secret of the [states of] consciousness alone when they are concealed in the throat, and the interpreter is the secret of the [states of] consciousness when they are revealed below in *Yesod*, for then the hidden reality of the dream is disclosed as it is above.[115]

There are many fascinating elements in this passage, but for our immediate purposes, I will stress again that the capacity to interpret dreams is allocated specifically to Joseph, the biblical figure who corresponds symbolically to the divine phallus (designated by the technical parlance *yesod di-ze'eir anpin*). Curiously, the dream is tagged as being "from the aspect of expansion that persists within the diminution" (*mi-beḥinat ha-gadlut she-nish'ar tokh ha-qaṭnut*), that is, the dream ensues from an amplification of the three states of consciousness, which are marked previously in the text as wisdom (*ḥokhmah*), understanding (*binah*), and knowledge (*da'at*), but since this occurs during sleep, a state of decreased mindfulness, the interpretation is indispensable in exposing what was hidden, and hence it is said to be greater than the dream. That the act of interpreting has been apportioned to Joseph is insinuated in the scriptural blessing associated with his name, *ben porat yosef*; the letters in the word *porat* can be rearranged to spell *poter*, the "one who interprets." Building on this passage from Viṭal,[116] the ḥasidic master, Ṣadoq ha-Kohen of Lublin (1823–1900) commented:

> The vain imaginings [*dimyonot shel hevel*] are the diminished consciousness [*moḥin de-qaṭnut*], but in the case of Israel, since each one has a root in the Torah in which is written truth and not an image, the expanded consciousness [*moḥin de-gadlut*] is concealed in the diminished consciousness, but nevertheless on account of the diminution that encompasses it, it is impossible that there will not be something nonsensical [*davar baṭel*], even though there is also within it wheat. The one who comprehends this matter of the inner content of the imaginings is one who is untainted from desires like Joseph with respect to lust for women and Daniel with respect to craving for food. They were interpreters of dreams, for the root of all the idle thoughts [*hirhurei beṭelah*] is in the desires. The heart yearns to contemplate, but the one submerged in the imagination cannot exchange and bring out the true matter that is garbed in the imaginings. Only one who is not submerged can remove the good from the bad, and this is the secret of the elevation of alien thoughts in prayer.... Of necessity this is similar to prophecy, that is, a thing that one cannot understand based on the faculty of wisdom [*koaḥ ha-ḥokhmah*], which is in the faculty of the intellect [*koaḥ ha-sekhel*] in the brain, but rather through the imaginative faculty [*koaḥ ha-medammeh*] through which one understands the word of Torah.[117]

This text is embellished in language that is reflective of several doctrines that shaped the ideas and practices of modern East-European Ḥasidism, especially the notion of alien thoughts (*maḥashavot zarot*), the carnal temptations that arise unexpectedly in the mind of the worshipper.[118] These "vain imaginings" are wayward thoughts—from the ḥasidic perspective, the ontic reality of something is determined by the nature of one's thought in relation to that entity—that fall from their supernal source into a state of diminished consciousness. For Jews, whose souls are enrooted in the Torah, the mystical essence of the Tetragrammaton, the expanded consciousness is garbed within the diminished consciousness, a process that is common to prophecy and to dreams. Because of the diminution, the truth is conveyed through images that are outwardly preposterous. Only one who is abstemious and pure of carnal desire is capable of interpreting the visions to separate the wheat from the chaff. The core idea can be traced back to zoharic symbolism: Joseph epitomizes the interpreter of dreams because he represents the mundane embodiment of the phallic energy. The explanatory suppleness is linked to the latter, but invertedly. That is, the hermeneutic empowerment of Joseph (and presumably this could be extended potentially to anyone that attains his symbolic status) is augmented not through satisfaction of the libidinal passion, but through its renunciation, exemplified in his withstanding the temptation and advance of the wife of Potiphar. The example of Daniel's overcoming of gluttony validates the claim, since, in consonance with many traditions, the hunger for food is posed as a counterpart to the appetite for sex. Only the mind that executes ascetic control can separate the truth of the dream from the false images within which it is enclothed.

Sacred Dream Text and the Psychoanalytic Narrative

In contemporary terms, the insight that retelling the dream is an integral part of the exegesis of the dreamwork is associated especially with the psychoanalytic approach of Freud.[119] As he put it in a memorable passage from *The Interpretation of Dreams*, "In interpreting dreams, we paid equal attention to every nuance of the verbal form in which the dream before us was expressed." Contrasting his own approach with other forms of analysis, Freud maintained that nothing in the dream should be ignored, no image should be viewed as arbitrary or inconsequential. Indeed, the dream is to be scrutinized "like a sacred text" (*wie einen heiligen Text*).[120] Surely, this language is summoned by Freud to convey the idea that just as the traditional believer does not think there is an extraneous word in holy Scripture, so the individual dreamer (through the help of the analyst) must be careful to heed and interpret every facet of a dream. Here it is also important to remember Freud's notion of the condensation of visual images and the composite makeup of the dream content.[121] Although

Freud explicitly uses the example of the drawing to elucidate the manner in which disparate images are fused together into a new unity in the dream, I would propose that these characteristics aid us in understanding his comparison of the dream to a holy text, as well, for a text similarly is a complex aggregation of divergent elements that cohere in an integrated, but not necessarily harmonious way.

On occasion, Jung was critical of viewing the dream as a text, which may have been a tacit condemnation of Freud. For instance, in one context, he wrote: "Dreams have no general meaning, one cannot translate them as one can a text. They are compensatory to a particular conscious and unconscious situation in a particular individual."[122] Elsewhere, however, he embraced the textual nature of the dream, even if he still felt the need to mark his disagreement with Freud. One passage, in particular, is worthy of mentioning. In a lecture delivered in April 1931, "The Practical Use of Dream-Analysis," Jung insisted that the analyst must be vigilant to dissuade patients, who seek to resemble their doctors in displaying an "insuperable desire to understand and to interpret offhand, especially when they have been primed by ill-digested reading or by a previous analysis that went wrong." Such an impulse betrays an aspiration "to get behind the dream at once in the false belief that the dream is a mere façade concealing the true meaning. But the so-called façade of most houses is by no means a fake or a deceptive distortion; on the contrary, it follows the plan of the building and often betrays the interior arrangement." Just as in the architectural model the distinction between external and internal is not cast in iron, so in the case of dreams, there is no need to distinguish the overt and the covert inflexibly:

> The "manifest" dream-picture is the dream itself and contains the whole meaning of the dream.... What Freud calls the "dream-façade" is the dream's obscurity, and this is really only a projection of our own lack of understanding. We say that the dream has a false front only because we fail to see into it. We would do better to say that we are dealing with something like a text that is unintelligible not because it has a façade—a text has no façade—but simply because we cannot read it. We do not have to get behind such a text, but must first learn to read it.[123]

Leaving aside the accuracy and fairness of Jung's rendering of Freud, he here challenges the latter's claim that understanding the dream requires taking hold of the latent aspects that both hide and reveal the manifest. The dream is like a text, which, for Jung, does not display the duality of exteriority and interiority. To comprehend the dream, one "must stick as close as possible to the dream images."[124] In the lecture "Psychology and Religion," delivered at Yale University in 1937, Jung corroborated his view that the gist of the dream is not supplemental to its images by referring to the talmudic notion (mentioned above) that "all dreams follow their interpretations," which he transmits as "The dream is its own interpretation."[125] With respect to these images, Jung appropriates a critical dimension of Freud's insight, translating it into a rudimentary principle of analytic psychology: "the dream images are to be understood symbolically; that is to say, that they are not to be taken literally just as they are presented in sleep, but that behind them a hidden meaning has to be surmised."[126] However, rejecting "Freud's dogmatic rigidity,"[127] Jung insists that dream symbols are not merely expressions of an individual's neuroses, which could be tracked more specifically to the trauma of primal incest, but are archetypal or primordial images, and thus they should not be regarded "semiotically, i.e., as signs or symptoms of a fixed character, but as true symbols, i.e., as expressions of a content not yet consciously recognized or conceptually formulated.... Instead of yielding to a dogmatic conviction based on the illusion that we know something because we have a familiar word for it, I prefer to regard the symbol as an unknown quantity, hard to recognize and, in the last resort, never quite determinable."[128] Or, as he puts it elsewhere: "Just as dreams do not conceal something already known, or express it under a disguise, but try rather to formulate an as yet unconscious fact as clearly as possible, so myths and alchemical symbols are not euhemeristic allegories that hide artificial secrets. On the contrary, they seek to translate natural secrets into the language of consciousness and to declare the truth that is the common property of mankind."[129]

It is of interest to recall here the observation of Tomoko Masuzawa that "the contrast between Jung's outlook on religion and Freud's probe into its origin shows up in the constitutional difference between their objects of attention: on the one hand, universal archetypes and the mythic structure of the unconscious, and on the other, traces (*Spuren*) of what once took place. One calls for the contemplative gaze, the other, for reading."[130] Magnifying this insight, I would say that the variance between the Freudian and Jungian approaches with respect to the nature of the symbolic can be sketched in terms of the distinction between the archetype of the trace and the trace of the archetype. Notwithstanding this disparity, the hermeneutic of the unconscious implied by the process of decoding, whether through the Freudian technique of free association or through Jung's notion of establishing the "whole context" of the dream image,[131] may be profitably likened to the midrashic manner of exegesis as a "stringing together" of words from the Torah, Prophets, and Writings,[132] which is based on the assumption that the scriptural text is one interconnected whole, a presupposition that has been adroitly designated the "enchainment (*ḥarizah*) of possibilities."[133] In Kristevan terms, the same intertextual approach may be applied to dream interpretation: the parts of a dream can be explained atomistically, but this is possible only because of the confederation of each of the components in what we could call the body of the text that constitutes the text of the body of the dreamer embedded in the narrative language of the dream.[134] The interconnectivity is not an essential quality abstracted from the plethora of particulars, but is rather an expression of those very particulars, the cluster of which is constantly coming to fruition from the proliferation of fragments. The textual connectedness is infinite in potential, even as it must already be presupposed in order to discern that it cannot yet be discerned. To think otherwise would implicate one in what Alfred North Whitehead (1861–1947) called the fallacy of misplaced concreteness, that is, the tendency to disregard the relationality of actual entities (or occurrences), which results in the error of mistaking a general abstraction for the totality of the concrete reality.[135]

Additionally, it must be borne in mind that the textual approaches of the rabbinic sage and the psychoanalyst do not reduce the nature of what is real to the point of asserting (as Derrida notoriously did) that there is nothing outside the text. The point rather is to comprehend, as Ricoeur noted with respect to psychoanalysis, that "symbolic activity lacks autonomy," for it is "bound activity," which is to say, the "symbolic function" is always attached "to this or that non-symbolic or pre-linguistic activity." The symbolic activity is a "boundary phenomenon linked to the boundary between desire and culture, which is itself a boundary between impulses and their delegated or affective representatives." The former is a "primary repression" and the latter a "secondary repression," which occasions the appearance of "derivative offshoots" or "indefinite substitute signs." The psychoanalytic sign, which is technically a sign of a sign, arises "on the boundary between a conflict of impulses and an interplay of signifiers." Psychoanalysis, accordingly, "must develop a mixed language, which connects the vocabulary of the dynamics or energetics . . . of impulses with that of a textual exegesis." Ricoeur illustrates the point by referring to the concept of censorship that Freud introduced in *The Interpretation of Dreams*, "which expresses the repressive action of a force at the level of the production of a text, albeit a text which is first revealed as erased or disfigured." Jung eclipsed, even ignored, this important insight regarding Freud. The text of the dream is a text that is initially revealed as erased or disfigured. Only by taking this into account can we understand the psychoanalytic dream work, which operates "mechanically as displacements, condensation, decomposition . . . procedures that Freud sums up under the general heading *Entstellung*. . . . At the same time, however, this interplay of forces can be read in the text of the dream account understood as a kind of palimpsest, riddle, or hieroglyph. Psychoanalysis must therefore assume the mixed epistemological status which these hybrid concepts impose upon it insofar as these deep conflicts resist any reduction to linguistic processes, yet cannot be read anywhere else than in the dream or symbolic text." The place where psychoanalytic discourse occurs, therefore, is "in the intermingling of force and meaning, impulse and discourse, energetics and semantics."[136]

On the basis of this analysis, Ricoeur finds support for the distinction between symbol and metaphor: the latter "occurs in the already purified universe of the *logos*," and thus, one word can substitute for another word, whereas the former "hesitates on the dividing line between *bios* and *logos*. It testifies to the primordial rootedness of Discourse in Life."[137] The ramification of Ricoeur's remarks bring us back to the discussion of Foucault in the previous chapter. The symbolic nature of the dream is expressive of an inherent tension between word and life, image and imagined, the force of being and the form we seek to impose thereto; to heed the language of the dream—and hence to comprehend the nature of its textuality—is to be guided to the borderline of the linguistic sign, where the spoken conveys what cannot be spoken, for whatever is spoken cannot but be what is never spoken. Bearing this in mind, we can better understand how the textualization of the dream, and by extension of the dreamer, sanctioned by Freud and Jung (whatever the discrepancies between them) resonates with the oneiric perspective that has similarly informed rabbinic sages through the generations.[138]

To thwart potential misunderstanding and what strikes me as an altogether anachronistic charge of anachronism, I state unequivocally that I am not suggesting that the traditional Jewish material anticipated modern and postmodern theories of dream interpretation. I would not be so bold as to say, together with David Bakan,[139] that "Freud, when interpreting dreams, follows the pattern of the *Zohar*"[140] or that "the fundamental principles of dream interpretation used by Freud are already present in the Talmud,"[141] but I do find the drift of the argument instructive and provocative. In a far more temperate tone, Fromm observed that the talmudic interpretation of dreams "follows Freudian lines," because it is "apparently based on the idea that a symbol always stands for something else."[142] Within the textual parameters of the dream, each image is an encoded reference to another reality that is both manifest and occluded by the dream. In this respect, there is a connection between the ancient art of divination and the contemporary practice of diagnosis.[143] The Freudian orientation is predicated on a way of viewing the dream and dreamer that exhibits affinity with ideas expressed in classical rabbinic and medieval kabbalistic sources, especially regarding the symbolic deportment of the dream and the primacy accorded interpretation as a mechanism to decode, and thereby differentiate, the latent meaning from its patent covering.[144] But at an even deeper register, the distinction between the clandestine and blatant is not sustainable if viewed as antinomical. Jewish and psychoanalytic textual practices persistently resist dichotomizing the symbolic and the real. The mythopoeic nature of the dream, which was discussed in Chapter 1, rests on the dehiscence of the signified and the porosity of the signifier. What allows us to think of the poet as dreamer and the dreamer as poet is the presumption, as Ricoeur put it,[145] that "the manifest meaning refers endlessly to hidden meaning"—to refer endlessly suggests that there is no closure, no final determination, no resolution that would preclude the possibility of reiteration of the future in the past. Set within a larger hermeneutical framework, these novel ideas are not so much extreme breaks with perspectives remembered from the presumably immemorial past, but rather subtle reinscriptions of them. Primary and secondary sources, therefore, can and perhaps should be positioned as mirrors facing one another, yielding an inversion of the presumed linear causality of time—what comes before may be construed as the effect of what comes after, and what comes after as the cause of what comes before.[146] This reversal presages the machination of time that one may elicit from the narrative sequence of dreams and their emblematic imagery, a theme that will be expanded in the final chapter.

CHAPTER FOUR

Coincidentia Oppositorum and the Mythologic of the Dream

So lived I and lived not, so wrought I and wrought not,
with creatures of dreams,
In a long iron sleep, as a fish in the water goes dumb as a stone.
—William Butler Yeats, *The Wanderings of Oisin*

The dream incarnates human imagination in a distinctively excessive way. As the phenomenologist Edward S. Casey expressed the matter:

> in dreaming, as in free-associating, there is a proliferation of types and modes of content—often to the point of surfeit and even of absurdity. In each case the imagery is of many different sorts, and what is conveyed to the mind seems kaleidoscopic in its diversity: we are as surprised at the multitude of things that show up in free-associating as we are at what appears in our nocturnal dreams.[1]

Of the many ways that the imaginal superfluity can be detected, I will here mention two: first, a dream may embody competing sensibilities, defying the commonsense assumption that a thing cannot be the same as its opposite; second, the *omnia* of dreams may augur the reverse of what we regularly expect of them.[2] Both of these possibilities are attested in the rabbinic dreambook to which I referred in Chapter 3. The former is the underlying intent of the tradition attributed to R. Josiah ben Levi that if one dreams of any of the following items—river, bird, pot, grapes, mountain, ram's horn, dog, lion, razor, well, reed, or ox—one should rise early and utter a particular verse where the relevant image is used positively before another verse where that same image has a negative connotation.[3] The image itself, accordingly, is not intrinsically abhorrent or appealing; it can be one or the other, its outcome left in the hands of the dreamer. The same assumption is at work in the anonymous rabbinic statement that the intent of seeing a cat in one's dream depends on if the word used for cat is *shunara* or *shinra*; the former is a sign that a "beautiful song" (*shirah na'ah*) will be composed for the dreamer, the latter, that the dreamer will undergo a change for the worse (*shinnuy ra*).[4] That paronomasia—the playing with homonyms based on local linguistic practice[5]—assists in determining the meaning of the dream object indicates the extent to which the reality within the dream is semantically determined. Looking at the matter from a broader vantage point, we can say that implicit here is the supposition that human, world, and language are three rings fastened in what Husserl referred to as the "inseparable relational unity" that constitutes the "linguistic embodiment" (*sprachliche Verleiblichung*) or the "linguistic living body" (*Sprachleib*) of the "intrasubjective structure" (*innersubjektiven Gebilde*).[6] The world's objective being (*objektives Sein*) presupposes human beings with a "common language" (*allgemeinen Sprache*). This does not imply that there could ideally be one language out of which all dialects spoken by humans emerge, an *Ursprache*, but rather that to presume external objectivity presupposes an ideality of meaning, which, in turn, rests on a shared "world-horizon" within which "everything has its name" and is therefore "linguistically expressible," albeit in a potentially indefinite number of cultural-historical forms. "Language, for its part," wrote Husserl,

> as function and exercised capacity, is related correlatively to the world, the universe of objects which is linguistically expressible in its being and its being-such. Thus men as men, fellow men, world—the world of which men, of which we, always talk and can talk—and, on the other hand, language, are inseparably intertwined; and one is always certain of their inseparable relational unity, though usually only implicitly, in the manner of a horizon.[7]

Despite the vast cultural and historical distance that separates the world of rabbinic piety and Husserlian phenomenology, I think the hermeneutic temperament of the latter easily maps onto the former (and, by extension, to the kabbalistic *imaginaire*), especially as it relates to the dream. That is, the ontological is determined from the perspective of the linguistic: what is given to human consciousness is what is named; any and every activity, even if it cannot be marked linguistically, is a matter of naming—ineffability itself is a semantic construct. A noticeable divergence is that rabbis and kabbalists hyperliteralized the principle of the linguisticality of all being by identifying Hebrew as the matrix language. The limitation of this specification (which has and can continue to have grave ethical and political consequences) should not prevent us from seeing the potential it contains to overflow its own boundaries and thereby liberate the tradition from the clutch of its obdurate confinement. The cosmological hypothesis that all things are created by divine fiat—when stripped of its theistic embellishment—implies that every being is what it is in virtue of its nameability, not by a particular name rooted in a specific cultural environment, but instead as a result of the potential for being named, the meaningfulness of all things experienced within the lifeworld of human subjects is due to their linguistic enframing, even acts that are either before or after language. This phenomenological seeing undergirds the talmudic tradition that the manner in which the dream images are verbally expressed reflects and informs the nature of the reality to which they refer.

An interesting example of the possibility that the *omnia* of dreams signal the opposite of their conventional signification may be culled from the story about Bar Qappara approaching Judah the Prince to obtain an explanation of the four images that he has dreamt. His nose falling off in the dream is interpreted as a sign that intense anger has been removed from him; his hands cut off that he will no longer require manual labor; his legs cut off that he will ride on horseback; and the premonition that he would die in the month of Adar, and thus be prevented from seeing the month of Nisan, is decoded as a sign that he would die in honor (*adruta*) and not be brought into temptation (*nisayon*).[8] The curiousness of this exchange is highlighted by comparing it with the narrative that immediately succeeds it: a "certain heretic" relates some of his dreams to R. Ishmael, but in this case, there is the more predictable correlation of the image and interpretation, for example, pouring oil on olives is decoded as an indication that one has outraged one's mother or the plucking of a star that one has stolen an Israelite. R. Judah's explanations, by contrast, render the meaning of the various images contrary to what one might suppose.

It is reasonable to assume something similar underlies the following rabbinic tradition: If a man dreams that he has intercourse with his mother, he may expect to obtain understanding; if he dreams that he has intercourse with a betrothed maiden, he may expect to obtain knowledge of the Torah; if he dreams that he has intercourse with his sister, he may expect to obtain wisdom; and if he dreams that he has intercourse with a married woman whom he did not know beforehand, he can be certain that he has earned a share in the world to come.[9] Prima facie, one is struck by the audacity of this dictum and the moral depravity—an assessment based on the mores of the rabbinic ethos—it promotes; one would not expect illicit behavior to be a harbinger of such profitable consequences. On the contrary, the more predictable response to incestuous dreams would have been reserve and even embarrassment, as we find in other cultural contexts.[10] And yet the opposite reaction is sanctioned by the text. From his analysis of this passage, Alexander adduces that there is a crucial discrepancy between the Freudian and rabbinic approaches to interpreting dream symbols. He readily admits that both acknowledge a rift between manifest and latent meaning, but, unlike Freud, the rabbis "use the distinction at times to diffuse the disquieting implications of dreams." Citing the specific case of a man dreaming about having sex with his mother, Alexander asserts that "mother" does not literally mean the biological parent, but metaphorically, "wisdom," and that "sexual intercourse" does not literally mean carnal relations, but metaphorically, "gaining understanding." Whereas psychoanalysis would be inclined to correlate the evident very directly with the nascent, the rabbinic orientation allegedly turns the "apparent urge to commit incest into something benign." Since the dream is symbolic, the image of the mother should not be taken any more literally than any other potential image, for example, a monkey or turnip.[11]

In my judgment, the connection between the dual layers of meaning on the part of the rabbinic sages is closer in spirit to what is here purported to be the Freudian hermeneutic. To be clear, let me repeat that I am not advocating that a psychoanalytic reductionism be applied to the rabbinic dicta, nor am I affirming that the latter anticipated Freud in some simplistic sense.

Nonetheless, it does seem that the figurative rendering of dream symbols on the part of some of the rabbis rests on grasping a more intricate correlation between revealed and concealed as it is enunciated explicitly by Freud. To dream of having intercourse with one's mother is not irrelevant to deciphering the hidden intent implied by this image, and it will not do to substitute that image arbitrarily. Something intrinsic is to be inferred from the coupling of the image of an actual mother and the allegorical topos of understanding; acquiring the metaphoric import of the latter bears something of the actual experience of the former. Indeed, we might go further and aver that metaphoricity is precisely what accords veracity to what we consider to be genuine. From this standpoint, the divide between reality and dream, what is and what appears, is tenuous at best: the image is as real as it seems to be.

It is important to note that in all but the last example, a scriptural verse is cited as a proof text. Intercourse with one's mother, the sign of understanding, is tied exegetically to Proverbs 2:3; intercourse with a betrothed maiden, the sign of knowledge, to Deuteronomy 33:4; and intercourse with one's sister, the sign of wisdom, to Proverbs 7:4. I would conjecture that the "original" version of this tradition included only these three examples, the triad of wisdom, understanding, and knowledge, which is of biblical origin.[12] Be that as it may, the use of scriptural verses should not obscure the radical implication of what is being asserted; the very citation may suggest that the strangeness of the claims required textual support. The timespace of the dream is an inversion of our world; what is deemed reprehensible from the naturalistic perspective functions in the dream as a sign of moral and spiritual perfection. As Judah he-Ḥasid later expressed the matter, wakefulness vis-à-vis sleep is like the relation of this world to the world to come, and just as the wicked feel no remorse for their transgressions, so in a dream, one experiences no sense of shame.[13] The dream is the antithesis of our wakeful state—an *olam hafukh*, a "topsy-turvy world," appropriating the depiction of the world to come, according to one rabbinic narrative[14]—and hence its images indicate the opposite of what we habitually experience.[15] Perhaps this is the intent of the epigram recorded in the name of R. Huna, "A good dream is not shown to a good man and an evil dream is not shown to an evil man."[16] Since the dream heralds the converse of what will transpire, the worthy person does not experience fortuitous dreams, and the unworthy person does not experience ill-fated dreams. Along similar lines, a tannaitic sage reportedly said in the presence of R. Sheshet that if one sees a serpent in a dream, it foretells that his livelihood is assured, and if it bites him, his life will be doubled, but if he kills it, he will lose his livelihood.[17] Even R. Sheshet is surprised at the counterintuitive nature of this claim. Common sense would dictate that if one kills a serpent, one's life should be doubled, rather than curtailed! The redactor of the passage insists, however, that it is not as R. Sheshet (and we) might expect. The dream is a mirror image of our empirical expectations—to kill the serpent, therefore, foreshadows loss of life.

To be sure, the imaginal scope of the dreamscape can have its own idiosyncrasies, and the contours thereof are often determined by the dreamer's own wishes and desires, which, we can reasonably assume, are informed by the memories of past experiences. This insight, accentuated by the psychoanalytic approach, is expressed in the aphorism attributed to R. Yonatan and transmitted by R. Samuel ben Naḥman, "A man is shown [in a dream] only what is suggested by the thoughts of his own heart" (*ein mar'in lo le-adam ella me-hirhurei libbo*). Rava glosses this by noting that it is proved "by the fact that a man is never shown in a dream a date palm of gold or an elephant going through the eye of a needle."[18] It is not clear to me that this was the intent of the original teaching or that this view is consistently ascribed to Rava in the extant rabbinic literature.[19] A person's dreams may betray the tenor of his or her lived experience, a point underscored by a second gloss on this dictum ascribed to R. Joshua ben Ḥaninah,[20] but this does not preclude the possibility of combining sensory images in new and unpredictable patterns. The dream imagination is not restricted by the catalog of past experience, and thus, the yoking together of dispersed images may present itself in the manner I have described; one may indeed behold a date palm of gold! We might even say that the dream has the potential to subvert the past that it upholds by unbolting the future of the present from the present of the future.[21]

In Chapter 1, I noted the observation of Freud in *The Interpre-*

tation of Dreams that dreams license the coexistence of incompatible sensibilities, even to the point of generating monstrous combinations, an idea that can be traced to ancient theories regarding the role of the dream imagination to create fantastic images by combining sense data that are ordinarily unrelated. Significantly, as I also remarked, Freud linked this insight exegetically to Virgil's statement in the *Aeneid* (vii.313), "If Heaven I cannot bend, then Hell I will arouse." In assessing the meaning of this quote, we should remember that it served as the epigraph of Freud's book. Surely, then, we are justified to presume that the poet's oration holds a key for apprehending Freud's understanding of the unconscious as a psychic domain wherein "instinctual impulses are co-ordinate with one another, exist side by side without being influenced by one another, and are exempt from mutual contradiction."[22] Within the dream, therefore, opposites and contradictions are disregarded, or they are drawn together into a unity in which they are represented as one.[23] In the brief treatise *On Dreams*, written in 1901, one year after the publication of the first edition of his magnum opus, Freud turns this principle into a rule for dream interpretation:

> In analyzing a dream, if an uncertainty can be resolved into an "either-or," we must replace it for purposes of interpretation by an "and," and take each of the apparent alternatives as an independent starting point for a series of associations. If a common element of this kind between the dream thoughts is not present, the dream work sets about *creating* one, so that it may be possible for the thoughts to be given a common representation in the dream.[24]

In the continuation, Freud notes that one of the "most convenient ways" to bring together two supposedly disconnected dream thoughts is "to alter the verbal form of one of them, and thus bring it halfway to meet the other, which may be similarly clothed in a new form of words. A parallel process is involved in hammering out a rhyme, where a similar sound has to be sought for in the same way as a common element is in our present case."[25] It is significant that Freud draws an analogy between poetic composition and dream work in an effort to elucidate the psychological leaning to loop together incongruent images in a logic of unifying contradiction. In a second passage, Freud elaborates:

> The alternative "*either-or*" is never expressed in dreams, both of the alternatives being inserted in the text of the dream as though they were equally valid. I have already mentioned that an "either-or" used in *recording* a dream is to be translated by "and." Ideas which are contraries are by preference expressed in dreams by one and the same element. . . . Opposition between two thoughts, the relation of *reversal*, may be represented in dreams in a most remarkable way. It may be represented by some other piece of the dream content being turned into its opposite—as it were by an afterthought. We shall hear presently of a further method of expressing contradiction. . . . The dream work makes use of such cases as a foundation for dream condensation, by bringing together everything that shows an agreement of this kind into a *new unity*.[26]

Doubtlessly influenced by Freud, Fromm commented: "Most of our dreams have one characteristic in common: they do not follow the laws of logic that govern our waking thought."[27] Fromm's language will surely strike postmodern ears as a bit overreaching in its essentializing tone. But let us forgive him his rhetorical hyperbole and concentrate instead on the chief point behind his words: A recurrent component of dreaming is a loosening of the knot of reason that dominates what could still be considered the commonsensical attitude to the natural world. There is another logic, however, or, to be more precise, mythologic, to which we have access in alternate ways, the dream being perhaps the most ubiquitous. I assent, therefore, to the assessment that in the setting of the dream, "the unreal and the imaginative, because they are possible, cannot be judged by the standards of waking reality. It is a device to lend credence to the marvelous."[28] The way to a deeper cognizance of world and self and of the reciprocal relation that binds them in their difference is through the imaginal corridor of the dream. Hobbes, it will be recalled, observed, "In sum, our dreams are the reverse of our waking imaginations; the motion when we are awake, beginning at one end; and when we dream, at another."[29] I am not inclined to accept that all dreams fit neatly into this Procrustean bed, but it would be foolhardy to deny the fact that many of our dreams demonstrate a (non)sense that stands in inverse relationship to what we assume are the cogent patterns that shape and are shaped by waking reality. This inversion has been emphasized, more recently, by John

R. Wiksein: "Dreams speak the language of imagination. They do so through images that do not obey the laws of noncontradiction, through metaphors which bring together and focus our emotional ambivalences."[30] Norman Malcolm made a similar point when he observed, "In a dream I can do the impossible in every sense of the word. I can climb Everest without oxygen and I can square the circle."[31] Events in the dream are not bound by what reason typically determines to be logically impossible.[32]

This insight also calls to mind the reflection of Bachelard that the value of the imagination lies in its polyvalence, which elicits a "psychological ambivalence," since every image is a "*poetic double* which allows endless transpositions." The imagination, therefore, displays a "manichaeism of reverie," an inherent twofoldness that calls for a "*dual participation* of desire and fear, a participation of good and evil, a peaceful participation of black and white."[33] Hillman has reminded us that Bachelard's phrase "black and white" can be traced to Philostratus, who depicted the god of dreams as "wearing a white garment over a black one,"[34] an image that intimates that "the dream presents in the robes of duplicity, stating simply that an ambiguity of significance is its habitual presentation. If dreams are the teachers of the waking-ego, this *duplicity is the essential instruction they impart*."[35] Bachelard himself expressed the matter elsewhere by noting that the dream exemplifies an "active participation in two opposite characteristics," a "double participation in one act" that "corresponds to a true Manicheism of motion.... This metallic realism of good and evil provides a way of measuring the universality of images."[36] The reference to Manichaeism in this passage and the aforecited one is understandable, but it does not well serve Bachelard's true intention. The "dual destiny" of the dreams does not imply an unmitigated dualism, as the Manichaean reference might suggest. On the contrary, the poiesis of the dream imagination is better characterized by the paradoxical identity of opposites, the *coincidentia oppositorum*, which Jung exploits when exploring the self in relation to the collective unconscious and the alchemical nature of dream symbolism.[37] This quality, moreover, undergirds the property of the dream image to conceal what it reveals by revealing what it conceals, a dynamic I discussed in my exposition of the oneiric mask in Chapter 1. The "dreamer truly contemplates what is hidden," writes Bachelard, "making use of reality, he manufactures mystery."[38] Duplicity invariably occasions elusiveness, and the latter is a measure of mystery, the inscrutable allusion, evocative of eluding evocation, prompting the production of secrecy by withdrawing in expanding and expanding in withdrawing.

The deportment of dreaming presents a striking affinity with the mystical sensibility. For those who identify the latter as a nondual state, characterized, as well, as pure or empty mindfulness, it goes without saying that a claim regarding the identity of opposites would be appropriate, since there is no longer any epistemic basis, let alone ontic ground, for discrimination or differentiation. But even in a state of visionary consciousness still beholden to a structure of intentionality, it is possible for clashing images to coalesce. This hybridization might be viewed as a form of *phenomenological disorientation*,[39] seeing the world invertedly, a destabilization of the temporal and spatial coordinates of the mundane apperception by deepening the temporal and spatial coordinates of the imaginal, a realm of virtuality retrieved as real through the imagination of the dreamer. The words of Patricia Cox Miller, interpreting the dream of Alcyone, wife of King Ceyx, in book 11 of Ovid's *Metamorphoses*, are especially fitting: "What is unreal is real—the unsubstantial figment of the imagination (the 'phantasm') conveys the essential message. What is counterfeit is true, what is alive is dead, what is divine is human—and also the reverse." By affording one the possibility of traversing the chasm that superficially severs candor and pretense, death and life, mortal and immortal, the figural bricolage of the dreamworld "does not dissolve reality but rather crystallizes it."[40]

Dreaming (Non)Sense

Even those of us who scarcely recollect our dreams will readily admit that this type of mental activity is distinguished by the proclivity of the brain to combine images we ordinarily deem to be true with others that strike us as evidently false. What in the dreamscape is real conforms to our shared sense experience—a term that has no evaluative function, but simply denotes the range of intersubjective experiences that, as we can conventionally concur, constitute our common cultural lot—and what is fictitious contradicts our expectations. The judgment "true" or "false," therefore, does not reflect an absolute standard of either an epistemological or an ontological nature; it simply expresses the credibility and incredibility that we are likely to accord respectively to images in dreams that correspond to our everyday lived experience and those that do not. Even so, ancient thinkers such as Artemidorus already discerned that the dream illustrates the adage that there is truth in lying, and hence, the line separating "creative imagination" and "willful mendacity" could easily be blurred.[41]

The rabbinic oneiric tradition, too, has given voice to this insight. According to a dictum attributed to Simeon ben Yoḥai and transmitted in the name of R. Yoḥanan, "Just as wheat cannot be without straw, so there can be no dream without nonsense [*devarim beṭelim*]."[42] This maxim is presented in the Babylonian Talmud as an exegetical explication of the verse "Let the prophet who has a dream tell the dream; and let him who has received my word report my word faithfully! How can straw be compared to wheat?—says the Lord" (Jeremiah 23:28). These words occasion a query on the part of the redactor, "What is the connection of wheat and straw in relation to the dream?" If we attend carefully to Simeon ben Yoḥai's response, we notice that the rabbinic interpreter inverted the scriptural intent. The prophetic utterance seeks to establish a clear boundary between the true reception of the divine decree and the false dream, the former compared to wheat and the latter to straw.

An adaptation of the talmudic dictum is found in several zoharic passages.[43] Here I will translate and analyze two examples.

> "[When a prophet of the Lord arises among you, I make myself known to him in a vision] I will speak with him in a dream" (Numbers 12:6). This is one-sixtieth of prophecy, as it has been established,[44] and this is the sixth gradation from that gradation of prophecy, and this is the gradation of Gabriel, who was appointed over the dream, as it has been said.[45] Come and see: every dream that is appropriate issues from that gradation, and thus, there is no dream that is not mixed with false matters, as we have established, and hence some of them are true and some of them are false, and there is no dream that is not both from this side and from that side. Since everything is in the dream, as we said, all dreams of the world follow the interpretation of the mouth, as it has been established with respect to

what is written "as he interpreted to us, so it was" (Genesis 41:13). Why? Because in the dream, there is deception and truth, but the word rules over everything, and therefore the dream needs a good interpretation.[46]

R. Yose began to expound and said "Just as a dream comes with much brooding, the voice of the fool comes with many words" (Ecclesiastes 5:2). "Just as a dream comes with much brooding," it has been established that the dream has various powers and agents, gradations upon gradations, so that some dreams are entirely true and some in which there is truth and falsehood. But to the truly righteous, fabricated matters are not revealed, only that which is entirely true. Come and see what is written of Daniel, "The mystery was revealed to Daniel in a night vision" (Daniel 2:19), and it is written "Daniel saw a dream and a vision of his mind in bed; afterward he wrote down the dream" (*ibid.*, 7:1). If there were false matters in it, why was it inscribed among the Writings? However, when the souls of the truly righteous ascend, only holy words are conjoined to them, to instruct them about true words, enduring words that are never uprooted.... Come and see: when a person is asleep on his bed, his soul departs and wanders in the world above, and it enters the place that it enters. Several troops of alluring [demons][47] come forth and go about in the world, and they strike that soul. If it is virtuous, it ascends above and it sees what it sees. If not, it cleaves to that side and they inform it of false matters or of things that are about to happen soon. When he awakens, the soul that is within him informs him about what it has seen. Therefore, a person who is not worthy is shown a good dream that is not true, all in order to lead him astray from the path of truth. Since he has swayed from his path, the path of truth, they defile him. For whoever comes to purify himself, they purify him, and whoever comes to defile himself, they defile him.[48]

One can detect two principal interpretations in the zoharic milieu of the rabbinic maxim that there can be no dream without nonsense, either that some dreams are true and others are false[49] or that there is no dream that is not a concoction of truth and falsity, "from this side and from that side."[50] In the aforecited extracts, there is an echo of both explanations, but the predominant drift seems to be to stress that every dream is a confluence of the veridical and the specious, which may indeed have been the intent of the original dictum. In the first passage, the admixture is related to the idea that dreams are consequent to the interpretation of the mouth. Since the dream contains both guile and truth, it can be either true or false based on its interpretation. In the second, a distinction is made between worthy and unworthy souls. The dreams of the former (personified by Daniel) are exclusively truthful, whereas the dreams of the latter comprise both true matters, limited to what will take place in the proximate future,[51] and false matters imparted by demonic forces that seek to tempt the soul with their illusive shimmer, so that it will swerve from the way of truth.

A similar sentiment is articulated in another passage where it is argued that the dream is a form of revelation that replaced both prophecy (*nevu'ah*) and the disclosure of the divine voice (*bat qol*):

> Come and see: the dream is seen by everyone because the dream comes from the left side, and it descends in several gradations. The dream is seen even by the wicked and even by the idolatrous nations, for sometimes the evil types seize the dream, hear it, and inform human beings. Some of whom mock human beings and inform them of false matters [*millin kedivin*] and sometimes of true matters [*millin di-qeshoṭ*] that they have heard, and sometimes they are sent to the wicked and they inform them of supernal matters [*millin illa'in*].[52]

Of the three kinds of communication, the dream is the most egalitarian, since it is seen by everyone, even the wicked and non-Jews. To deny that non-Jews dream would, of course, be ludicrous. This is, however, an extraordinary assertion in light of the fact that the dream is labeled an inferior prophecy, which is consistently understood as an idiosyncratic heritage of the Jewish people.[53] To be sure, in the above passage, the dreams seen by the idolatrous nations are said to be brought about by evil forces. This proviso notwithstanding, the barrier that characteristically separates the holy seed of Israel and the demonic seed of the Gentiles is effaced to some degree. More expectedly, in another zoharic context, the reader is told about the Jewish soul (specifically the *nefesh*, which is the lowest of the five levels demarcated in rabbinic parlance in ascending order as *nefesh*, *ruaḥ*, *neshamah*, *ḥayyah*, and *yeḥidah*) that cleaves to the unholy forces and is notified by them of worldly events in truthful and false images; the idolatrous nations are similarly described as dreaming of truthful things that will come about in the future on account of the fact that they are conjoined to the side of impurity.[54] Kabbalistically, the dream derives from the left side, a symbolism that also underlies the identification of Gabriel as the angelic prince of dreams, since he, too, as his name indicates, draws his power from the attribute of strength (*gevurah*) on the left, as I noted in the preceding chapter.[55] Thus, the sinister forces occasionally take hold of the dream and toy with human beings by alternately conjuring images that are false and images that are true. The complexity and perhaps imprecision of the zoharic view is amplified by the remark that at times, the oneiric spectacle is the tool by which these forces inform the wicked of what takes place above.

An even more arresting formulation is found in another zoharic passage, where the evil spirit Sarṭiya and the myriad beings beneath him in the second of the seven palaces of the demonic other side—the shadowy counterparts to the seven palaces of the side of holiness, the seven compartments of the supernal Garden of Eden, one of the standard symbolic prisms for *Shekhinah*, which correspond to the seven palaces of the Garden of Eden below and to the seven sefirotic emanations above[56]—are said to communicate to the soul through a dream in which deceptive words (*millin kedivin*) are mixed with veritable words (*mit'arvei be-millei qeshoṭ*), since a lie can be sustained only if it is expressed truthfully.[57] From this, one may adduce that the dream issuing from the satanic powers dissembles its truth in the guise of the deceitful; the blending of the two blurs the boundary between divine and demonic. By contrast, consider the unequivocally negative assessment in the following passage from the *Ra'aya Meheimna* stratum of zoharic literature:

> Sleep is one-sixtieth of prophecy, and therefore the rabbis, masters of the academy, established "And dreamers speak lies" (Zechariah 10:2), but is it not written "I speak with him in a dream" (Numbers 12:6)? There is no difficulty, for here it is by means of a demon and there by means of an angel; the dream by means of an angel is one-sixtieth of prophecy, the dream by means of a demon is a lie, from the side of death, and it is straw, as it has been established, just as it

is impossible for there to be wheat without straw, it is impossible for there to be a dream without false matters.[58]

The last line might suggest an encroachment of the border between the two, but a closer look at the full context indicates that the author, likely reinterpreting an earlier zoharic microform, is making a more rigid differentiation between the angelic dream and the demonic dream: the former is wheat, and the latter straw. The presumption that the two kinds of dream can be kept apart is to be distinguished from the view that truth and treachery will always be jumbled together.

In his exposé of the second palace of impurity, which is called *shaḥat*, based on one of the metaphorical designations for death in some parts of Hebrew Scripture (Psalms 30:10, 55:24, 94:13; Job 33:18, 24, 30), the Safedian kabbalist Moses Cordovero (1522–1570) elaborated the zoharic perspective:

> In this palace, there is another impure force, and his name is Sarṭiya, and there are a myriad of destructive angels beneath him, and they are summoned when the dream descends into the world from the side of holiness. This spirit and all the destructive angels who are with him descend with this dream and are mixed in with it, and they inform this man of fraudulent words, mischievous words, together with the honorable dream. Thus, the rabbis, blessed be their memory, said that just as wheat cannot be without straw, so there can be no dream without nonsense.[59]

Cordovero's reading is that the dream occasioned by demonic forces is a mishmash of honesty and mendacity. In its descent from the divine realm, the dream can be entwined with the spirits of unholiness, and this results in the synthesis of the real and fantastic images. Moses Ḥayyim Luzzatto (1707–1746) also attempted to harmonize the divergent views that can be culled from zoharic literature:

> Hence the principle of dreams—forms of the imagination [*ṣiyyurei ha-dimyon*], whether from itself or from what arouses the soul according to what it comprehends, but what is activated in all of these is one of the spiritual powers, which informs the soul, and the soul extends to the imagination ... and if that power is from the holy servants, the matter will be true, and if from one of the adversative

> powers, the matter will be false, and this is what the sages, blessed be their memory, said,[60] "here by means of an angel and there by means of a demon." But in all of them there are mixtures of wayward images of the imagination, and this is what the sages, blessed be their memory, said,[61] "it is not possible for there to be a dream without idle things."[62]

Similarly, the Iraqi kabbalist Yehudah Pedaya (1859–1942) distinguished sharply between angelic and demonic dreams. The dream brought about by an angel is well ordered and not a mixture of miscellaneous things, and hence the dreamer does not feel any anxiety or fear in the moment of dreaming, whereas the dream caused by a demon is a compound of unrelated matters that confound and startle the dreamer.[63] Utilizing an idiom that is implied in a few zoharic passages,[64] but that is made explicit in Lurianic sources,[65] Pedaya makes a further distinction between dreams that are caused by "Gentile demons" (*shedin nukhra'in*) and those caused by "Jewish demons" (*shedin yehuda'in*), for in the case of the latter, there is the additional element that they assume the veneer of the patriarchs, prophets, rabbinic sages, or judges, and instead of bewildering the dreamer, they manifest an image of heaven or an image of the throne and the attending angels. They also instruct him to study the *Zohar* or the book of Psalms each day, to rise every night to perform the midnight vigils (*tiqqun haṣot*), and to implement ascetic practices such as ritual immersion, exchanging garments, refraining from touching a woman, and fasting. One must be especially vigilant with respect to the Jewish demons, therefore, since their mode of appearance and manner of operating (in a nocturnal dream or when one is awake) could more readily dupe the person to the point of madness.[66] Most of the dreams that come through the medium of an angel are to be explained according to the secret (*al pi ha-sod*), for the angel is a spiritual being (*ruḥani*), and thus they produce the allusion (*remez*) in accord with their way; the dreams that come through the medium of the demons, whether Jewish or Gentile, are not to be explained in this manner because they are inherently bogus and muddled.[67]

This perspective should be contrasted with the explanation offered centuries before by Joseph Gikatilla (c. 1248–1305), another Spanish kabbalist with close ideational ties to the zoharic compilation and possibly an active member of one of the circles responsible for a part of its literary invention.

> Know that if not for the fact that combined together with dreams is a mixture of the corporeal residue, how great would they be for human beings, for the name *ḥalom* ["dream"] intimates that a human being comprehends more than what matter comprehends, and this is the subject of dreams. One can mentally concentrate [*mitboded*] in concurrence with the dream of prophecy, even though there are some parables [*meshalim*] in it, but with respect to the rest of the dreams, if not for the straw and the refuse mixed in with them, they would be a great thing. And this is what the rabbis, blessed be their memory, said, "Just as there is no wheat without straw, so there is no dream without false matters." They informed us that if not for the false matters compounded with the dream, even the dream of a commoner would be one-sixtieth of prophecy. The person who comprehends more than what the body comprehends is called *ḥolem* ["dreamer"].... You will find that the name *ḥolem* alludes to the comprehension of people in the lower world when they ascend to comprehend a level superior to what the bodies comprehend. If the dreams are not perfect, their deficiency is due only to the abundance of the mixture.... It is impossible for a dream to be entirely true, as we have explained, but part of it of necessity will be true.... From all of these words we can learn that when an ordinary human comprehends more than his matter comprehends, that comprehension is called *ḥalom*, from the language of *ḥolem*, for from the vowel of the *ḥolem* thousands of myriads of lights burst forth, and the [dreamer] merits that some of the lights that burst forth from the vowel of the *ḥolem* will be revealed. Therefore, according to the power of the light that bursts forth in the one who sees the dream from the emanation of the vowel of the *ḥolem*, so will his dream be true; if it bursts forth minimally, a small part of his dream will come to be, and if maximally, the dream will be fulfilled to the end of its matter. According to the bursting forth, so shall the measure of the dream be realized. The one who knows the secrets of these mysteries hidden in the matter of the *ḥolem* will know the secret of the comprehension of the dreams [*sod hassagat ha-ḥalomot*].... Now contemplate well and you will see the secret of the rank of the *ḥolem* over the rest of the vowels,[68] and you will already know in these places the secret of the dreams, and how they are dependent on the *ḥolem*, which is

> the secret of the supernal vowel, and according to the efflux that descends from it, the comprehensions will come following their types, whether of prophecy or of the rest of the matters.[69]

Every dream is a fusion of vain matters and truth—even the dream of prophecy, which is distinguished from commonplace dreams insofar as it is completely truthful, employs figurative language that is literally false (with the exception of the prophecy of Moses)[70]—because of the inherent limitations of the material body, but the knowledge that we access through dreams transcends those very limitations. The artifice of the dream is a means to reach a higher level of gnosis that is connected to the *ḥolem*, the vowel that theosophically symbolizes the emanation of *Keter*, since, orthographically, it is the highest of the vowels, positioned on the top of the consonants. I will return to this symbolism in the next chapter, but suffice it here to underline that dreams are explained by Gikatilla as the outcome of the stream of light that issues from the first of the sefirotic gradations, an efflux that facilitates the mental ascent of the soul of the dreamer separated from corporeal embodiment and the succeeding state of contemplation (*hitbodedut*), a depiction of the dream alluded to in the following zoharic homily interpreting the verses "In a dream, a night vision, when deep sleep falls on men, when they slumber on their beds. Then he opens men's ears, and by disciplining them leaves his signature" (Job 33:15–16) in light of the well-attested motif of the nocturnal separation of the soul from the body and its ensuing ascent:

> What is written? "In a dream, a night vision." When people lie asleep in their beds, and the soul leaves them, as it is written "when they slumber on their beds. Then he opens men's ears." Then, through the gradation presiding over the dream, the blessed holy One informs the soul of the matters that will come upon the world or of things that concur with the imaginings of one's heart,[71] so that one will take a path of admonition in the world. For one is not informed when one is still existing in the strength of the body, as we have said. Rather, an angel informs the soul, and the soul, the person, and that dream is from above, when souls leave their bodies and ascend, each one in accord with its own way.[72]

The mechanics of the dream as a mental ascent dependent on separation of mind from body—in part resonant with an idea expressed in older sources (traceable to Aristotle) that explains the prophetic propensity of the dream to see the future as a consequence of the soul no longer being preoccupied with bodily needs during sleep[73]—is developed by later kabbalists, for example, Meir Ibn Gabbai,[74] Ḥayyim Viṭal,[75] Moses Ḥayyim Luzzatto,[76] and Menasseh ben Israel.[77] Even so, the rabbinic idea that just as there is no wheat without straw, so the dream comprises truth and falsity imposed itself on subsequent interpretations of the oneiric phenomenon. For Gikatilla, the gist of this dictum is that the source of the dream is the infinite will,[78] the "world of mercy" (*olam ha-raḥamim*),[79] where opposites coincide, and hence, there is no truth that is not also untrue and no untruth that is not also true.[80] That dreams are a mix of the truthful and disingenuous signifies that they issue from the aspect of infinity wherein it is no longer possible to differentiate antinomies. The rabbinic insight, consequently, insinuates that the dream is a superior, indeed the supreme, mode of knowledge, which is the absence of knowledge, an unknowing that destabilizes the distinction between sense and nonsense.

Exile, Dream, and the Night of Annihilation

This apophatic subversion can be discerned in the characterization of the dream as the *coniunctio oppositorum* of truth and deception, a theme that has come to the fore on a number of occasions in this analysis. The soundness of the dream cannot be severed from its spuriousness, inasmuch as what is factual in this arena is the fictitious. In the remainder of this chapter, I will examine this motif in the mystical ruminations of Shneur Zalman of Liadi (1745–1812), one of the prominent disciples of Dov Baer, the Maggid of Międzyrzecz (1704–1772), himself a follower of Israel ben Eliezer (1698–1760), the Ba'al Shem Ṭov, "master of a good name," better known by the acronym of this title, the Beshṭ, the man to whom credit is given for spearheading and inspiring a revivalist pietism (Ḥasidism) that flowered in the late eighteenth and early nineteenth centuries into a vibrant social phenomenon throughout East European Jewish communities.[81] Shneur Zalman is notorious for being the progenitor of the ḥasidic dynasty known as Ḥabad or Lubavitch. The former name is an acronym for *ḥokhmah*, *binah*, and *da'at*, "wisdom," "understanding," and "knowledge," a reference to the three upper aspects of the ten enumerated divine emanations[82] and their corresponding psychic faculties, *nefesh*, *ruaḥ*, and *neshamah*, which constitute the triadic nature of intellect (*sekhel*);[83] the latter is the Yiddish version of Lyubavichi, the town in Russia where the headquarters of the movement were established by Dov Baer Schneersohn (1773–1827), son of and successor to Shneur Zalman.

Before discussing this motif in Ḥabad sources, I will note a striking parallel in the Spanish Ṣūfi Muḥyīddīn Ibn al-ʿArabī (1165–1240). Let me remark briefly that Ibn al-ʿArabī—in some respects continuing the orientation of al-Ghazālī[84]—accords a special status to the imagination, the faculty that gives one entrée to the intermediary realm (*barzakh*) of soul situated between the invisible and visible,[85] what Corbin called the imaginal world (*mundus imaginalis*, *ʿālam al-mithāl*), the universe of symbol or archetypal images "in which spirits are corporealized and bodies spiritualized."[86] By the metrics of reason, the divine, or the spiritual domain, more exclusively, is not phenomenologically available, since hiddenness and manifestation are antinomical, but the imagination opens the way to the dialectic whereby the antinomies are synchronized in their difference, and "God is manifest through self-disclosure when He is hidden, but He is hidden through the forms that appear when He is manifest."[87] Insofar as the dream is viewed as the most pervasive inculcation of this active imagination, it is considered, in the words of William C. Chittick, a "key to unlock the mystery of cosmic ambiguity and the constant transmutation of existence."[88] The dream is an instrument by which the incorporeal is corporealized and the invisible visualized, and thus it typifies the role of the imaginative faculty of the mystical visionary to emulate the divine by effectuating the coincidence of opposites (a conception often linked exegetically to qur'ānic description of Allāh in *surā* 57:3, "He is the first and the last, the manifest and the nonmanifest," which is itself partially based on Isaiah 44:6).[89] Accordingly, the dream is designated the "homestead (*mawṭin*) of the imagination," for through it, one can have a vision of the formless Real (*ḥaqq*) in "corporeous form,"[90] a process that is compared to the unveiling (*kashf*) of the self-disclosing veil (*ḥijāb*) of the divine that the prophets and the gnostic elite, the "friends of God" (*awliyā'*), visually experience when awake.[91]

I have explored a similar phenomenon in medieval kabbalistic theosophy, the anthropomorphic construction of the sefirotic emanations in the imagination. Thinking in Corbin's footsteps,[92] I have characterized the suprasensible knowledge (*hierognosis*) propagated by kabbalists in a comparable way as being the imaginal intermediary that facilitates the disclosure of the concealed in the concealment of the disclosed, a conversion of contraries that destabilizes the opposition between concealment and disclosure.[93] A number of kabbalists spoke of the nocturnal dream as the medium by which secrets of Torah are revealed,[94] but, to the best of my knowledge, they fall short of depicting the speculative vision of the divine as a dream in the manner of Ibn al-ʿArabī. Precisely such a position, however, is attested in a passage from the *Qelaḥ Pitḥei Ḥokhmah*, a treatise traditionally attributed to Moses Ḥayyim Luzzatto: "The *sefirot* can be seen in images that even conflict with one another [*yekholot ha-sefirot lera'ot badimyonot afillu hafkiyyim zeh la-zeh*], just as one verily sees in a dream that subjects change before him in one moment [*kemo mammash ha-ro'eh ba-ḥalom she-mitḥallefim ha-nos'im lefanaw berega eḥad*]." In contrast to the waking sensation, the dream imagination demonstrates the capacity to portray a matter in varying and conflicting images in tandem, a characteristic of prophetic visions, as well. Since the sefirotic emanations are also configured concurrently in contradictory terms, for example, as circular and linear, as above and below, the oneiropoetic imagination is the most apposite epistemic modality to comprehend the imaginal nature of the divine.[95]

We find a similar view in the work of Yosef Ḥayyim of Baghdad (1832–1909), known honorifically as the Ben Ish Ḥai. After citing several prominent kabbalists, including Isaac Luria, Ḥayyim Viṭal, and Shalom Sharabi, who affirmed emphatically that the divine secrets should not be taken literally, since this would lead inevitably to the erroneous conception of a corporeal God, the Ben Ish Ḥai comments, "We cannot comprehend the truth of the matter, as it is impossible for us to configure this matter in our intellect, but rather we learn these matters as a dream."[96] The point here is not simply that mysteries are disclosed in a dream, a phenomenon discussed in Chapter 2, but that their comprehension itself assumes the form of a dream. It is of interest to mention here the remark of Rosenzweig in his commentary to Judah Halevi's poem *liqra't meqor ḥayyei emet aruṣah*, which he translates as *Sehnsucht*:[97] "For this poet, the forerunner of the great Kabbalistic movements for whom the vision of God served as Israel's topical heritage and always to be newly actualized on the holy ground, sleep and dream are the legitimate ways to the goal."[98] This is a remarkable passage that both demonstrates a subtle grasp of Halevi's protokabbalistic sensibilities and offers an incisive understanding of the centrality of the visionary dimension in the kabbalistic worldview.[99] Rosenzweig's recognition of the ocularcentric nature of kabbalistic gnosis is impressive, but even more so is his insistence that the nocturnal dream is the most appropriate means to attain that vision. In consonance with this view, I propose that, in the mind of kabbalists, what makes the oneiric condition commensurate with esoteric knowledge is that the formless object of the contemplative vision can be seen only in the imaginal forms in which it (dis)appears, the sefirotic potencies configured in the heart, and hence, there is no substantial difference between appearance and reality.

The dream, as metaphor, is a transference that presupposes a gap continuously crossed but never collapsed, an opening that begets the merger of dissimilar entities without resolution of their difference.[100] Rendered metaphorically, the metaphor is the bridge that spans the breach between literal and figurative, truth and fiction, the verbal leap that propels one across the space of an irreducible reducibility. Metaphor, on this score, is a form of language that materializes in the fissure that connects by keeping apart. The understanding of metaphor—both a movement of thought as well as an analogue for existence[101]—as bridging, rather than obliterating distance reflects a peculiarly Heideggerian reading of Nietzsche's characterization of metaphor as displacement and dissimulation.[102] In *On Truth and Lying in a Non-Moral Sense* (1873), Nietzsche writes:

> We believe we speak of trees, colours, snow, and flowers, we have knowledge of the things themselves, and yet we possess only metaphors of things which in no way correspond to the original entities.... What, then, is truth? A mobile army of metaphors, metonymies, anthropomorphisms, in short a sum of human relations which have been subjected to poetic and rhetorical intensification,

> translation, and decoration, and which, after they have been in use for a long time, strike a people as firmly established, canonical, and binding; *truths are illusions of which we have forgotten that they are illusions*, metaphors which have become worn by frequent use and have lost all sensuous vigour, coins which, having lost their stamp, are now regarded as metal and no longer as coins.[103]

Metaphors, as Nietzsche put it in a fragment from one of his unpublished notebooks (summer 1872–early 1873), produce the "inclination of truth" (*Hang zur Wahrheit*), but the truthfulness (*Wahrhaftigkeit*) that comes to light through the veil of metaphor necessarily consists of illusion. That is, inasmuch as metaphorical truth is truth revealed through the guise of an image, it is laid bare to the degree that it is cloaked. The human being, in Nietzsche's judgment, "senses stimuli rather than truths. He dreams, he imagines divine human beings as nature." The "pathos of truth" (*Pathos der Wahrheit*) and the "genesis of knowledge" (*Entstehen des Erkennens*) proceed from the "mendacity and illusion in which human beings live. Lies and speaking the truth—myth, poetry."[104] Speaking truth and lying are not antithetical; to speak truth is necessarily to camouflage the truth, because there is no word that is not a mask hiding some other word[105]—this is the essence of the mythopoeic enterprise and hence the place where the vectors of the oneiric and the aesthetic intersect: the task of the artist is not simply to preserve the vision that has come in the dream, but to mimic the dream by maintaining the illusion of truth in the truth of the illusion. Following Heidegger's appropriation of Nietzsche, I would speak of metaphor as *a covering of truth by the facade of truth*. The following account by Janet Love seems especially suitable:

> In a different context, Heidegger speaks of the between as that which, reaching from the earth to the sky, is measured out for the dwelling of man. Perhaps the function of metaphor can be thought of in the same way, as a spanning of the "between" that rests within the poles of, or the movement from, literal to metaphorical. For Heidegger, the possibility of measuring lies with the disclosure of the unknown, insofar as it remains unknown and against which man's familiarity shines forth. Something similar happens within a metaphor, although reversed: as meaning is carried across the span,

> the meaning itself, like man in his measuring, shines forth. But what shines forth is what is known; the familiarity of meaning is what allows the metaphor, and the discretion of metaphor protects this familiarity. And yet behind this shining forth stands, obscured, the between itself, which is unknown as long as the metaphor goes unquestioned. Once questioned, however, metaphor reveals an innocent literalism at its core. Difference is always assumed in the metaphorical leap, difference that the leap proposes to bridge.[106]

The dream may present us with one of the more viable ways to bridge the difference in the metaphorical leap, for the dream seems inaccessible except through the portal of discerning that there is *no truth that is not also a lie*, since every lie must be true to itself, and hence no face escapes the fate of being but another disguise that covers up the face. Even more germane to my understanding is the insight of Derrida that metaphor entails a withdrawal (*re-trait*) of "truth as non-truth," a withdrawal that "is no more proper or literal than figurative," "neither thing, nor being, nor meaning," inasmuch as it "withdraws itself both from the Being of being as such and from language, without being or being said elsewhere; it *incises* ontological difference itself."[107] What is implied in this *re-trait*, this withdrawal of truth as nontruth? How can we juxtapose truth and nontruth such that the truth withdrawn as nontruth lingers as the truth that is withdrawn? For truth to be withdrawn as nontruth, it must persist as the truth of nontruth, which can only be as the nontruth of truth, but a truth that is true as nontruth can be neither literally nor figuratively so. Alternatively expressed, it can be literal only as figurative and figurative only as literal, literally figurative because figuratively literal.[108] Kabbalistic knowledge of the divine realm, as the Ben Ish Ḥai perceptively intuited, is similarly entangled in the web of metaphoricity, a mode of knowing predicated on a conflation of opposites by which the incorporeal is rendered corporeal and the invisible visible. Reversing the Platonic hierarchy to which I referred in Chapter 1, the dream is not a spurious and deficient reason concerned with the image of what is real—that which is false made to seem true—but rather a superior cognition through which one envisions the image that is real. Esoteric wisdom, accordingly, is likened to a dream, and as a consequence, a profound affinity between the two is established as a focus of meditation.

Let me turn at this juncture to a passage from *Torah Or*, the anthology of Shneur Zalman of Liadi's homilies on Genesis and Exodus compiled by his grandson, Menaḥem Mendel (1789–1866), the third leader of the Ḥabad-Lubavitch sect and the namesake for the seventh and presumably last rebbe of the movement.[109] It is characteristic of the rhetorical style of the Ḥabad masters that any cross section of their dense and sweeping oral sermons and/or written treatises can serve as a window through which to view the philosophical perspective they promulgated. Their own texts hermeneutically endorse the meontological premise that one can see in every particularity a manifestation of the hidden essence, the mystery of the infinite nothing revealed through being concealed in the veil of nature.[110] This is surely the case in the following passage, whence we will elicit the complex nexus between imagination, dream vision, nocturnality, exile, redemption, and mystical annihilation.

The pertinent text appears in the context of Shneur Zalman's attempt to explicate the celebrated dreams of Joseph:

> "A song of ascents. When the Lord restores [the fortunes of Zion], we will be as dreamers" (Psalms 126:1). The dream joins two opposites in one subject, and it combines two contradictory matters as if they were one, for during sleep, the brain of the intellect that makes distinctions [*moaḥ ha-sekhel ha-mavḥin*] is removed, and all that remains is the imaginative faculty [*koaḥ ha-medammeh*], and the imaginative faculty can combine two contradictory matters [*yakhol leharkiv shenei inyanim hafkiyyim*]...but when one is awake, the intellectual faculty is aroused, and it rules over the imaginative faculty, and it does not permit it to combine, since one sees with the eye of one's intellect that these are separate things and they are not at all unified. Similarly, in the matter of the exile, the divine spark that is in the human soul is in the aspect of sleep and the removal of consciousness [*bi-veḥinat sheinah we-histallequt ha-moḥin*], so it can combine two opposite things.[111]

The opening verse from Psalm 126 forges a connection between the hope for redemption, the restoration of Zion, and the act of dreaming. But as we are quick to learn, the dream is also aligned with exile, since the latter is depicted metaphorically as sleep, and the dream occurs during sleep, when the intellectual faculty, which is marked by the facility to distinguish one thing from its opposite, retreats, and the imagination, which is characterized by the tendency to combine one thing and its opposite, dominates. Sleep, therefore, should be understood metaphorically as a topos for exilic dormancy, submergence of the soul in the darkness of matter.[112]

In the continuation of the passage, Shneur Zalman offers further clarification of the incongruous images combined in the dreamscape. Utilizing the symbolism of Lurianic kabbalah, the nature of exile, the proverbial night in which all cows are black, is described as the enclothing of the pneumatic spark in the garment of the body,[113] a union that impels the soul to carry on the gnostic drama of liberating through the act of purification (*berur*)[114] the light that is entrapped in the physical world.[115] The overcoming of body, however, is achieved through transformation rather than obliteration of the somatic. This basic tenet of Ḥabad—a specific application of the doctrine of *avodah be-gashmiyyut*, "corporeal worship," often singled out as a distinguishing element of the East European pietism traced back to the Besht[116]—is expressed by Shneur Zalman in his insistence that even when one is enwrapped in liturgical worship, love of God[117] of necessity is realized through the love that one enacts with and in the body.[118] To appreciate this point, it should be borne in mind that Shneur Zalman distinguishes two kinds of worship. The first is the form of ecstasy (*hitpa'alut*), the "great love" (*ahavah rabbah*), which is so intense (*aṣumah*) that the heart cannot contain it, and hence the soul yearns to leave the body; the second is a form of ecstasy that can be contained by the vessel of the heart, and its primary purpose is to draw down the divine surplus from above into the material world.[119] The intent of this passage, as may be gathered from other texts that preserve Shneur Zalman's teaching,[120] is that worship consists of two phases, the self-annihilation that results from the conjunction (*devequt*) of the soul in the infinite light (*or ein sof*),[121] on the one hand, and the drawing down of that light through the fulfillment of Torah and ritual commandments to sustain the cosmos, on the other. From a chronological perspective, the latter is consequent to the former, as Shneur Zalman himself put the matter: "It is precisely the nullification of something into nothing that causes the drawing down of nothing into something" (*u-viṭṭul ha-yesh le-ayin dawqa gorem hamshakhat ayin le-yesh*).[122] However, from the perspective of the incorporation (*hitkallelut*) of all things in the infinite essence,[123] and the corollary principle of the *complexio oppositorum*,[124] the two must be viewed as expressions of a single phenomenon.[125] In metaphoric terms, the dual movement of worship may be depicted as the ascent and descent (*aliyyah wi-yeridah*) of the angels on the ladder envisaged by Jacob in his dream at Bethel (Genesis 28:12) or as the running to and fro (*raṣo wa-shov*) of the creatures seen by Ezekiel in his vision of the chariot by the Chebar Canal in Babylonia (Ezekiel 1:14). The ascent must be followed by descent, the running out by return, but one conjoined to the essence reaches the place of indifference where the opposites are viewed as identical in virtue of their opposition.[126] On this account, the going up and coming down, the running hither and thither, are the same other and consequently other to the same. Worship may be compared to the dream, for it, too, partakes of the paradoxical collusion of polarities: only the one divested of corporeality is in the position to sustain the corporeal. I will cite an extensive portion of Shneur Zalman's articulation of this point:

> But, in truth, the root of the aspect of the dream is above, and its foundation is in the mountains of the supernal holiness.... Exile is the aspect of sleep and the removal of consciousness [*histallequt ha-moḥin*]...and then his soul draws life from above, and there it is in the aspect of circles, which have no above or below, but rather everything is in one equanimity [*ha-kol be-hashwwa'ah aḥat*], the containment [*hitkallelut*] and unification [*hitaḥadut*] of all the matters without any separation or division, as the dictum of the rabbis, blessed be their memory,[127] "these and those are the words of the living God," is known. When it is drawn forth by way of the lines, then there is division...which is not the case with the aspect of the circles, wherein there is no division at all, and there all the things that are separated below are joined and comprised together and there does not appear to be any separation or division amongst them. However, for this aspect to be revealed below, it is only by means of the aspect of sleep and the removal of consciousness in exile. Concerning this it says "I will clothe the heavens in blackness" (Isaiah 50:3). The heavens are the aspect of the circles, and they are arrayed in the aspect of blackness and darkness, which is the concealment

> and hiddenness [*he'lem we-hester*], for then it shines and radiates from the supernal world above, which is the aspect of the circles in the aspect of the dream, the faculty of the imagination to combine two opposites in one subject [*leḥabber shenei hafakhim be-nose eḥad*] as if they were actually one, since in truth they are conjoined and unified in their source in the supernal world, for there is the aspect of circles, as was mentioned above. Only below is there a division of the lines [*hitḥallequt ha-qawin*] by means of *Ḥokhmah* and *Da'at*, so that one line will be like this and the other like that, and then will the opposite be seen and be revealed, for the one is the opposite of the other, and consequently they are separate and distant from one another. Therefore it is impossible for there to be a revelation of the aspect of integration [*gilluy beḥinat ha-hitkallelut*] in the aspect of the disclosure of *Ḥokhmah*, which is the beginning of the division of the lines, but in the aspect of sleep and the removal of consciousness in exile, then the supernal light shines and radiates. It is hidden and concealed in the aspect of blackness and darkness, that is, in the aspect of the investiture of the concealment [*hitlabbeshut ha-he'lem*] and not in the aspect of disclosure, for the disclosure is the aspect of *Ḥokhmah* and *Da'at*, which is according to the lines.[128]

A positive valence is accorded exile and sleep, because it is only through the removal of consciousness (*histallequt ha-moḥin*) associated with them that the mind can reach the level beyond duality.[129] The root of the dream, therefore, is in the "mountains of the supernal holiness," that is, the aspect of the light of infinity positioned in the interiority of *Keter*,[130] the "incomposite will that is above intellect and comprehension" (*raṣon pashuṭ she-lema'lah me-ha-sekhel we-hassagah*),[131] the "essential concealment" (*he'lem aṣmi*)[132] that is the "actual nothing" (*ayin mammash*).[133] The matter is expressed as well in the portrayal of the source of the dream as a circle (*iggul*), the geometric figure that symbolizes the property of equanimity (*hashwwa'ah*),[134] the integration (*hitkallelut*) and unification (*hitaḥadut*) of all things in a nondifferentiated unity. By contrast, the line (*qaw*), which begins with the attributes of *Ḥokhmah* and *Da'at*, demarcates the division of the divine pleroma into right, left, and center columns.[135] In the circle, opposites converge, and there is thus no way to distinguish beginning from end, and the dream, which arises as a result of the imagination's ability to combine disparate images, is assigned supreme value as the channel through which one can reach the light beyond discrimination, the supernal light (*or ha-elyon*) so luminous that it is described as "blackness" (*qadrut*) and "darkness" (*ḥoshekh*),[136] the luminescence that is the arrayment of concealment, the hiding of hiddenness,[137] a double occlusion whose disclosure can be gauged from the circular indifference of the infinite essence, as opposed to its linear division into dichotomies in the constellation of the sefirotic potencies in all of their permutations.[138] By means of the dream, therefore, one can attain the mystical state of (dis)integration (*hitkallelut*)[139] in which all disparity is overcome, and the semblance of existence independent of the essence—the nothing that is everything in virtue of being nothing—is annihilated. The propensity of the dreaming imagination to combine opposites is the psychological analogue to the ontological *coincidentia oppositorum*, the "great mystery" that is encapsulated in the cliché often reiterated in Ḥabad teaching, "two opposites in one subject" (*shenei hafakhim be-nose eḥad*).[140] To cite Shneur Zalman again:

> For the one who sees in a dream it is possible that two opposites will be in one subject actually.... By way of comparison, the community of Israel in the time of exile are called "dreamers," because it appears that opposite things in contrast to one another in the extreme are united, and the one is not a contradiction to its opposite, like all the effort of Israel in commerce and matters of this mundane world, which is the opposite and conflicting greatly in relation to the aspect of the nullification of holiness that is found in Israel during the time of prayer, when the saying of the Shema is recited with intention, "Hear O Israel [the Lord, our God] the Lord is one" (Deuteronomy 6:4), and "there is no other apart from him" (*ibid.*, 4:35). Since there is none apart from him, how is it possible afterward to be involved in mundane matters, in the needs of this world, issues of material sustenance with which one toils greatly in heart and soul? And if it is said that since one's engagement is with matters of this world all day, it is necessary that one does not pray with intention, and one should not direct one's heart in truth, this, too, is not the truth, for even so, one must direct one's heart in truth through prayer, and this is not contradictory, for even though this is a matter and its opposite in actuality, it is like the dream in which one dreams of a thing and its opposite in one substance.... The root of the dream is in the aspect of the supernal perimeter [*ha-maqqif elyon*] that comprises all the

opposites in one union [*ha-kolel kol hafakhim be-ḥibbur eḥad*], for it encompasses from every side in an equanimity without a linear division at all [*she-maqqif mi-kol ṣad be-hashwwa'ah aḥat beli hitḥallequt qawin kelal*]. Before him, the darkness and light are equal, everything is considered as equal, and he renders equal the small and the big, all things are esteemed as one in the aspect of nullification before him...he surrounds and encompasses all the worlds equally, and he is entirely removed from the category of division. Therefore, he comprises all the opposites together in one unity.[141]

The dream is enrooted in the "supernal perimeter" (*maqqif elyon*), the aspect of the Godhead that precedes division into binaries, the place of equanimity where opposites coincide. As Shneur Zalman puts it in another context, "the root of the dream is from the world of chaos" (*olam ha-tohu*),[142] that is, the amorphous plenum before there is a separation into discrete beings. In the Lurianic lexicon, whence this terminology is derived, the world of chaos (based exegetically on the description of the earth as *tohu wa-vohu* in Genesis 1:2) has a decidedly negative connotation as it came to be applied to the world of punctiform lights (referred to both as *olam ha-nequddot* and *olam ha-niqqudim*) in the divine economy wherein the breaking of the vessels (*shevirat ha-kelim*) occurred, a cataclysmic event (also designated on the basis of the scriptural language as the death of the Edomite kings or in accord with the rabbinic legend as the destruction of the primordial worlds)[143] that brought about disorder that had to be ameliorated by a rebalancing of the forces in the "world of rectification" (*olam ha-tiqqun*).[144]

Needless to say, it lies beyond the purview of this chapter to enter into the details of this cosmological myth. What I have noted, however, is sufficient to make the main point. Ḥabad sources retain this older conception, but there is also a positive tint accredited to the world of chaos, insofar as the light contained there was in abundance and therefore above the delimitation associated with the emanation of the *sefirot* through the agency of the line of measure (*qaw ha-middah*), a zoharic elocution that denotes the attribute of judgment by means of which the limitless light is delimited in the configuration of the divine gradations.[145] By locating the source of the dream in the world of chaos, Shneur Zalman is implying that the imagination during sleep draws from this excess of light—it is even too constricting to speak of this light as light, since in the world of chaos, dark and light are not yet distinguished—that is above comprehensible knowledge (*da'at ha-mussag*).[146]

I surmise that the description of the dream as combining opposites is inspired by the view proffered in several zoharic texts discussed above. In at least some of those passages, as we have seen, the dream is characterized as a mélange of what is true and what is untrue. This, I suppose, is the kabbalistic underpinning of the emphasis given by Shneur Zalman to the confabulatory power of the dream to combine discordant images. Support for my conjecture may be elicited from the following comment of the sixth Lubavitcher rebbe, Yosef Yiṣḥaq Schneersohn (1880–1950):

> In the time of sleep, one dreams a dream, for in the dream, two opposites come together in one subject in actuality to the point that it is possible that the foundation of the matter or of the edifice that he sees is a true foundation, and upon it the matter is constructed or the opposite matter entirely, for this is the substance of the dream, the combining of two opposite matters, one truth and the other falsehood, and both of them appear as one, and from this example, worship at the time of prayer can be comprehended.[147]

Prima facie, the final assertion is startling, since it implies that prayer, like the dream, is a compound of truth and perfidy. But how can this be? In what manner is subterfuge a legitimate part of liturgical observance? To grasp the secret implied here, we must recall, as I noted above, that for Ḥabad masters, the highest rank of worship is the complete eradication that ensues from the worshipper being bound to the infinite light, a nullification so absolute that not only worshipper, but worship and worshipped, too, are annihilated in the total (dis)integration of all being and nonbeing into the void that is the essence. Yet even this form of veneration requires verbal gesticulations and bodily gestures of an incarnate nature. From the ritual obligation to recite the words of the statutory prayers, the contemplative, who has been absorbed in the radiance that is beyond linguistic and/or conceptual demarcation, is compelled to bear in mind that the multiple worlds in the ontic chain come to be through the agency of the supernal word (*hithawwut ha-olamot hu al yedei dibbur ha-elyon*), and thus, "the entire concatenation is merely an illumination" (*kelalut ha-hishtalshelut he'arah bilevad*) of this word, which is the ineffable name YHWH.[148] Just as the truthful elements of the dream are enmeshed in what is patently false, so, too, in the matter of worship in the exilic state, one's continued sense of autonomy as an embodied being in a finite universe thought to be independent of the infinite divinity is the dissimilitude—the dream is the deceit that dissimulates as truth (*sheqer nidmeh la-emet*), as opposed to the deceit that covers truth (*sheqer mekhasseh al ha-emet*)[149]—that is necessary for one to see through the veil of concealment (*he'lem*) that is the world (*ha-olam*), according to the wordplay that appears repeatedly in Ḥabad teaching,[150] and in so doing, one can discard the concealment of the veil by carrying out the purification of the light in all worldly matters.[151] "This is [the intent of] 'we will be as dreamers,' to combine two opposites as one, for if his worship in prayer was authentic, then all day long [he will fulfill] 'In all your ways know him' (Proverbs 3:6), for the trace of the prayer will remain with him, and he will be mindful of divinity constantly in all affairs and activities."[152] Beyond this insight, the very prospect of the pietistic ideal of annihilation is inconceivable but from the perspective of the imagination, because the possibility of something becoming nothing rests on the comingling of ostensibly divergent matters in a fashion that defies the law of noncontradiction. The imaginative faculty is integral to the act of nullification, since to become nothing, one must imagine that one is something, that the nothing is shrouded in the affectation of something that must be incorporated into the nothing to which something cannot be attributed, the nothing that is so utterly nothing that to say it is nothing is already to ascribe too much something to it.

An astute articulation of this point is found in an extraordinary passage by one of Shneur Zalman's pupils, Aaron Halevi Horowitz of Staroselye (1766–1828). This text has been discussed in previous scholarship as evidence for a pluralistic approach to religious fervor that challenged the more exclusionary and elitist stance of Dov Baer Schneersohn.[153] By emphasizing this indisputable difference, the affinity between the two disciples of Shneur Zalman of Liadi with respect to the central role of the imagination in the abolition of individuated ego consciousness (*biṭṭul ha-yesh*) has been obfuscated to some extent. Expounding the credo of his teacher that the objective of worship (*avodah*) and realization (*hitpa'alut*) is to "remove the awareness of oneself" (*lehasir hargashat aṣmo*), Aaron Halevi notes that "this victory [*niṣṣuaḥ*] is achieved by each person according to his merit, for there are innumerable levels, and what appears to the imagination of the worshipper as his removing the awareness of self is vis-à-vis the level above him a complete awareness of self." This is the esoteric import of the divine proclamation "and through the prophets I was imaged," *u-ve-yad ha-nevi'im adammeh* (Hosea 12:11); the transcendent essence takes on form in accord with each person's imaginative capacity, and in that sense, "the imagination is the aspect of awareness [*ha-dimyon hu ha-beḥinat hargashah*], for his being has not yet been abrogated completely, and his nullification is only in accord with his imagination [*raq biṭṭulo hu lefi dimyono*]." Moses alone attained the level of complete annihilation, and thus he saw through a translucent speculum, that is, an imageless vision, whereas all the other prophets saw through an opaque speculum—"their comprehension was through the garbing in the aspect of something [*hassagatam hayah be-hitlabbeshut beḥinat yesh*], and they would nullify only in accord with their imagination." If this was the case for the prophets, it is surely so with respect to all other Jews:

> for each and every one, the truth is in accord with his imagination [*lefi dimyono hu emet*], because the purpose of creation is that his divinity [*elohuto*], blessed be he, will be revealed precisely from the perspective of the imagination [*mi-ṣad ha-dimyon*]. The purpose of all of creation is to reveal his divinity, blessed be he, even from the perspective of something [*afillu mi-ṣad ha-yesh*], and from the perspective of something, there are incalculable gradations, but from the true perspective [*mi-ṣad amittit*], everything is true [*ha-kol hu emet*], for the imagination is also his power, blessed be he, which descends to the imaginative faculty of each and every person.[154]

There is one reality, the formless and incorporeal essence, but the only way to access it (for all human beings with the exception of Moses) is through the multiplicity of forms that cohere in the sensible world. Prayer, Torah study, and performance of the precepts, mystically conceived, provide the lens by which one can peer through the charade of there being something ontically distinct from the indistinct nothing outside of which there is nothing that is not assimilable into the nothing. The unveiling of the acosmic secret—the disclosure of the disclosure as concealment in the concealing of the concealment as disclosure—could not be accomplished, however, unless one were to imagine the seemingly autonomous cosmos as the raiment that shelters the essence in the propinquity of what is withdrawn. In Aaron Halevi's own words:

> This is the worship of each and every one from Israel, to ponder with his mind in what manner to abrogate his soul [*levaṭṭel nafsho*], even with the aspect of the imagination [*afillu bi-veḥinat dimyon*], for the imagination, too, is true from the perspective of the root [*mi-ṣad ha-shoresh*], since from the perspective of the essence [*mi-ṣad ha-eṣem*], in truth "there is none beside him" (Deuteronomy 4:35)...and, consequently, the imagination is also true.[155]

From the vantage point of the inessential essence, the essence whose essence it is to resist essentialization, opposites coincide, and therefore what appears to be false is true, just as what appears to be true is false. In uncovering the truth of the ruse that is the corporeal world, the dissonance between real and make-believe is effectively undermined.[156] The essential truth of (non)being, consequently, is neither true nor untrue, for to say that it is either true or untrue would be too limited for the limitless truth of the essence. As I have suggested elsewhere,[157] to comprehend this meontological perspective, it is beneficial to adopt a logic akin to the *madhyamaka*, the middle way, in the Mahāyāna tradition, a logic that posits the identity of opposites in the opposition of their identity, a reclaiming of the middle excluded by the law of the excluded middle. Betraying an affinity to the Buddhist wisdom, Ḥabad speculation on the nature of being and nonbeing posits an emptiness—the void (*efes*) that is above the nothing (*ayin*)—in which all things become empty, even or especially of their own emptiness. The comportment of the dream to combine conflictual images provides a mechanism by which one can reach the abyssal indifference of the essence of infinity (*aṣmut ein sof*). The imagination, accordingly, is allocated a prominent role on the pietistic path as the means by which the visible cosmos is exposed as the epiphany of the invisible and the mask of truth is unmasked as the only truth that cannot be (un)masked.

The implications of Shneur Zalman's text are made explicit by his son, Dov Baer, who thus commented that the root of dreams

> is extremely high in the aspect of the circles and the perimeters of the aspect of the chaos [*bi-veḥinat iggulim u-maqqifin di-veḥinat ha-tohu*]...for in the dream, there are two opposites, as when he dreams that he is very uplifted and then he immediately dreams that he is greatly downtrodden, a thing and its opposite are as one, like life and death are as one. Analogously, with regard to the disclosure of divinity in the soul of Israel in exile, which is called "sleep," there are two opposites, the submission of self [*mesirat nefesh*] in reciting the Shema and then, immediately, one is engaged [in loving God] with all one's heart, through commerce [*be-massa u-mattan*], but this is not a thing and its opposite at all, as in the dream, for each is a true matter unto itself, and their coming together as one is from the aspect of dreams that join together two opposites. That they come as two opposites, mercy, which is a true matter unto itself, and judgment, which is a true matter unto itself, instructs about the aspect of chaos. In the aspect of the circles of chaos [*ha-iggulim de-tohu*], everything comes together as one without any division at all [*ba'im ha-kol ke-eḥad beli hitḥallequt kelal*], and it is comparable to the time of sleep, when all the faculties of the intellect [*koḥot ha-sekhel*] and the properties of the essence of the soul [*middot be-eṣem ha-nefesh*] in the aspect of *yeḥidah* withdraw in elevation after elevation, and there remains only the aspect of the faculty of the imagination in the mind. Even though the aspect of the imagination of dreams is very low, its source is in the supernal perimeter [*be-maqqif ha-elyon*] of *yeḥidah* to which all the intelligibles [*sikhliyyim*] and desires [*reṣonot*] ascend, the source of all the intelligible desires in the supreme elevation of the integration as one precisely [*meqor kol ha-reṣonot sikhliyyim be-illuy muflag be-hitkallelut ke-eḥad dawqa*].... Thus the potency of dreaming that is in the imagination is in *yeḥidah*, for there, everything comes as one without division of the will and intellect...like a circle in which there is no division at all.[158]

Although the withdrawal of intellect during sleep and the exclusive role accorded the imagination places the dream at the lowest end of the gnoseological spectrum, its root is implanted in the highest level, which has both a theosophical and a pneumatic correlate,[159] the encompassing circle (*maqqif*) of the world of chaos that precedes the dichotomization of the indivisible essence[160] and the dimension of the human soul that is called *yeḥidah*, because it denotes its indissoluble unity and consubstantiality with God.[161] Given the status of the source of the dream, we can well understand the contention that it exhibits the quality of combining contrasting images.[162] Worship may be compared profitably to the dream, since it, too, revolves about this paradox.[163] The paradigmatic illustration of the point is the recitation of the Shema, the traditional confession of Israel's monotheistic faith. Transposed esoterically, the avowal of God's oneness is an expression of the mystical truth that the divine essence is the sole reality. For the enlightened adept, then, to proclaim that God is one means to give witness to the insight that all existence, including one's own self, is rendered as nothing in relation to the light of infinity. The nullification is so thorough that one has no feeling of oneself at all, not even the sense of being nullified—the ultimate annihilation, perforce, is the annihilation of the annihilation.[164] And yet the mandate of the Shema is to express the love of God with one's full embodied presence in the world, a point epitomized by reference to the business transactions with which one must be engaged to fulfill the needs of the physical body.[165]

Menaḥem Mendel Schneerson (1902–1994), the seventh and hitherto last rebbe of Lubavitch, remarked that the "totality of worship" (*kelalut ha-avodah*) involves the descent of the soul and its "engagement with the external in the manner of adornment" (*hit'assequt im ha-ḥuṣah be-ofen shel hitlabbeshut*), the technical term used by Ḥabad masters to denote the incarnation of the spiritual in the physical, the "matter of the amalgamation of two opposites" (*inyan shel ḥibbur shenei hafakhim*). The sensory example (*dugma muḥashit*) that illumines this truth is the dream, which comes about as a result of the imagination's ability to combine opposites,[166] "the enclothing of the expansive consciousness in the diminished consciousness" (*hitlabbeshut moḥin de-gadlut be-moḥin de-qaṭnut*),[167] that is, the pairing of mercy and judgment, the power to expand, which is engendered as male, and the capacity to restrict, which is engendered as female. By this account, divine worship is manifest in this world in the form of dissimilitude, an idea conveyed by the outwardly bizarre expression, *biṭṭul idyoṭ* (ביטול אידיאט). To comprehend this diction, we must recount the story that is the original setting in which it appears.[168] A group of ḥasidim were engaged in a discussion on the matter of nullification, and as they were walking home late at night, still preoccupied with the topic, a Russian officer called out to them *kto idyot* (кто идёт), "Who goes?" and one of the ḥasidim responded *biṭṭul idyoṭ*.[169] A double entendre is thus implied by the expression *idyoṭ*, the Russian идёт conveying the sense of "going" and the Yiddish homonym אידיאט, as its English equivalent, "idiot." The intent of the story, then, is that the ḥasid responded to the guard in a way that was outwardly respectful, but actually derogatory. Speaking out of both sides of his mouth, as it were, the ḥasid was saying "Idiot, no one is going about," that is, the one who has become nothing through *biṭṭul* is the one you have addressed. The response *biṭṭul idyoṭ*, accordingly, is duplicitous, communicating truth through the artifice of untruth. According to Schneerson's interpretation, this jarring wording calls attention to the fact that annihilation is a matter that must be manifest in the phenomenal realm—the one who goes about in the world is precisely the one who experiences somatically[170] the utter extermination of existence (*biṭṭul bi-meṣi'ut*)[171] to the point of not feeling any ontological separation from God[172]—so that the divinity will be fully revealed in every corner of the universe,[173] even the place most remote from holiness, a harnessing of the sacred and profane that is signified by the combination of Russian and Hebrew in the phrase *biṭṭul idyoṭ*.[174] The nullification that is attained through devotion and sacrifice is not a disincarnate state; the stripping away of physicality is itself an incarnality of being, an embodiment that is realized through the idiocy of the unfettered imagination, the psychic faculty that juxtaposes what apparently does not belong together, that is, the material something rendered as nothing essential through its integration into the essential nothing that is the immaterial something, the ultimate concealment that must be concealed from being what it is concealed not to be. It is in this sense that the quietistic ideal of abnegation, which is the most perfect implementation of the pietistic virtue of love, betrays "the image of the dream that blends two opposites."

In combining opposites, the dream instantiates that which must be judged by reason as "most impossible" (literally, the "impossible of the impossible," *nimna ha-nimna'ot*),[175] the manifestation of the essence (*gilluy ha-aṣmut*) that is essentially beyond manifestation, the intermingling of corporeality and spirituality (*ḥibbur bein gashmiyyut we-ruḥaniyyut*),[176] and hence it anticipates the messianic future[177] in which there will be a disclosure of the divine quiddity (signified linguistically in Ḥabad thought by the terms *aṣmut*, "essence," and *mahut*, "substance") without any obstacle, an idea that is anchored exegetically in the eschatological predictions "and your master will no longer be covered and your eyes will see your master" (Isaiah 30:20) and "for every eye shall behold the Lord's return to Zion" (*ibid.*, 52:8). The seeing without a garment is the mystical import, as well, of the verse "on that day the Lord shall be one and his name shall be one" (Zechariah 14:9), the prophetic promise that "he will not be attired and covered in an encasement, and he will be called as he is written,"[178] that is, the name YHWH will no longer be pronounced through the epithet Adonai, but it will be vocalized as it is inscripted. This, too, is the meaning of the opening verse of Shneur Zalman's discourse, "When the Lord restores the fortunes of Zion, we will be as dreamers" (Psalms 126:1): "this gradation and aspect of the dream will be revealed to the point that everyone will fathom, know, and comprehend the vitality [*ḥiyyut*] that emanates upon them in the time of exile, which is the aspect of the dream. Therefore, it says 'we will be as dreamers.'"[179]

The dream is a prolepsis of redemption, which is depicted as a seeing of the essence without any garment (*beli levush*),[180] beholding the real, one might say, beyond the veil of metaphor. But Shneur Zalman and those who followed his path appropriated and elaborated the dialectic of disclosure and concealment enunciated by previous kabbalists, a dialectic especially conspicuous in the sixteenth century, and thus they discerned that there can be no disclosure of the divine that is not concomitantly a concealment.[181] What is revealed is the infinite essence, but the infinite essence cannot be essentialized and remain the essence that is infinite; hence, what is revealed must always remain concealed, and the seeing without a garment amounts to seeing that there can be no seeing without a garment.[182] Utilizing apophatic modes of speech, it can be said of this essence that there "is no comprehension with respect to it" (*ki ein bo shum tefisah*),[183] that it is the "negation of thought" (*afisat ha-ra'yon*),[184] the silence that is the "complete nullification of essence" (*biṭṭul ha-aṣmut mi-kol we-khol*),[185] the void (*efes*) that is "more than nothing" (*mer eyder nisht*),[186] the "essential concealment that is not in existence at all, as it is also concealed to itself" (*he'lem ha-aṣmi she-eino bi-meṣi'ut kelal we-hu he'lem gam le-aṣmo*).[187] We can speak of the essence, so to speak, only to the extent that it is unspoken. The oneiric imagination is privileged, because the way to reach the unknowable and unnamable is through the mental faculty that combines opposites and thus points to the mystery of equanimity, the state of indifference wherein opposites are identical in their opposition.[188] Restoration to infinity—the mystical nuance of the traditional notion of repentance, *teshuvah*, which is etymologically from a root (*shin waw beit*) that means to return—is predicated on the removal of consciousness, which is indicative of exile, but also on the illumination of the supernal light, the vestment of concealment, since it is only by being concealed that the concealment can be revealed as concealed. Through the dream, therefore, the schism between sleep and wakefulness, exile and redemption, is itself transcended in the luminal darkness where the difference between dark and light is no longer operative. Esoterically rendered, one will awaken to the dream no longer dreamt as a dream, the vision of truth imagined to be true.

CHAPTER FIVE

Undoing Time and the Syntax of the Dream Interlude

> The language of love is only present; dream and reality, sleep of the limbs and wakefulness of the heart are inextricably woven one into the other, everything is equally present, equally fleeting and equally alive.
>
> —Franz Rosenzweig, *The Star of Redemption*

In pondering temporality and the phenomenon of dreaming, a prudent place to begin would be to acknowledge that the time of the dream must be thought from the time of the dream, that the duration of the dream can be measured only from the duration of the dream. The reversal of the time line, such that one can progress to the past and regress to the future, and the consequent assumption that the effect may, in effect, be the cause of the effect—characteristics of the dreamtime that I discussed briefly in the section on quantum physics in Chapter 1—are sufficient to account for the circular reasoning of these tautologies. The matter, however, should also be considered in light of the Husserlian notion of the *temporal field* wherein the objects of experience both fabricate and are fabricated by the unity of time intuition.[1] Herein lies the fundamental paradox of what Husserl construed to be the uniqueness of the human condition in the world. Despite his best efforts, Husserl was finally not able to flee from the intractable grip of this paradox. Rather than being a shortcoming, the self-contradictory nature of Husserl's cogitation on internal time-consciousness provides a useful lens through which to speculate on the temporal curvature of the dream. If an object is constituted by the mental intuition that is itself constituted by the object, then the sense of time—or what might amount to nonsense—conveyed by this circularity puts into question the strictly linear conception of a sequence commencing at a certain point and culminating at another, the egological inscripting of the tale we routinely identify as the story of our lives. The larger problem looming here concerns the hermeneutical role of imagination and the temporal concocting of the imagined objects that cohere in the myriad lifeworlds of our experience. This is obviously not the context to do justice to this topic, but it is requisite to ask if there is something eccentric about the dream image in this regard. Many philosophers, especially those who adopt phenomenological psychology, have engaged the matter of time and dreaming. I initiate my reflections by turning to the view tendered by Sartre.

In exploring the claim that "the time of the object as imaged is an irreality," Sartre provides the example of dream images as "irreal objects that appear to consciousness without any temporal determination."[2] Elaborating the point, he writes:

> It is well known that most of our dreams are extremely short. Nevertheless the dreamed drama can occupy several hours, several days. It is impossible to make this drama that is spread through a whole day coincide with the rapid flow of the consciousness that dreams it. One will perhaps attempt to reduce the duration of the dream to that of the dream consciousness, to make of the dreamed *story* a rapid procession of images. But this explanation is very ambiguous. What should we understand here by image? Will one speak of the imaging consciousness or of the imaged object? If it is a case of the imaging consciousness, it is evident that it can flow neither faster nor slower than it does flow: all that one can say is that it absolutely fills (*remplit*) its duration and that it is this very fullness (*plénitude*) that measures the duration. In what concerns the imaged object, can one truly speak of a more rapid succession?... It is necessary therefore to admit here a phenomenon of *belief*; a positional act. The duration of irreal objects is the strict correlate of this act of belief: I *believe* that these truncated scenes are welded one to another in a coherent whole, which is to say I join the present scenes with past scenes by means of the empty intentions accompanying positional acts. Moreover, I *believe* that these scenes together occupy a duration of several hours. Thus the duration of the object as imaged is the transcendent correlate of a special positional act and consequently participates in the irreality of the object.[3]

Building upon the groundwork laid by Sartre, we may say that the temporality of the dream is to be discerned from the confluence of the irreal duration of the object and the real duration of the flow of consciousness parallel to it. It is exactly this convergence that both facilitates and helps us comprehend the commonly attested phenomenon that a brief span of time in a dream can be experienced as if it were long, sometimes interminably so, or that an expansive span of time can be experienced as if it were short, a flash of light in the dark, as it were. It is even possible that a whole lifetime may pass in a dream that in actual time–which is not to say that I think there can be any time that is actualized outside the mind that is not itself a product of mentation[4]—is naught but a moment,[5] the "trifle that holds a lot,"[6] indeed a moment, we are inclined to say, that vanishes like a dream.

The matter of dreamtime problematizes the prevailing computation of time in wakeful states, a temporal register determined by an objectifying intentionality that is shaped principally by the structures of presentation and judgment. The dream, by contrast, embodies a nonobjectifiable intentionality that presumes an ideality wherein the kinesthesic-noematic sense is not regulated or restricted by logical coherence or linguistic meaning.[7] The destabilizing of the chronoscopic offers an alternate perspective on human temporality as it relates to memory in its dual deportment as retention and protention. In Chapter 2, I noted that Foucault challenged the dominant Freudian conception by arguing that the dream is not primarily about reliving a past trauma, but is the "future making itself, the first moment of freedom freeing itself."[8] The psychoanalytic perspective on the regressive component of the dream is a consequence of Freud's more general allegation that processes of the unconscious "are *timeless*, i.e. they are not ordered temporally, are not altered by the passage of time; they have no reference to time."[9] Since the past is not subject to time, it is simultaneous with events of the present and thus can be replayed at any time with the prodding of the proper therapeutic intervention. The sense of biographical time, therefore, is irrelevant to the dream; all experiences within the oneiric landscape coexist on a "timeless plane of psychical interaction."[10] For Foucault, by contrast, the dream, which is the future repeatedly making itself, is not timeless, but rather the fullest endowment of time. One does not simply revive an experience that is decisively terminated; one refashions it as a memory that is steadfastly underway to becoming once more what it always never was. More recently, Kelly Bulkeley has emphasized that dreaming can be described as a means to expand the range of our temporal perceptions. This expansion can extend in either direction, stretching back or extending forward, but more weight appears to be placed on the latter, particularly as this relates to the predictive nature of the dream or its prophetic potential. Bulkeley recommends that we view the premonitional aspect of dream phenomenology against the backdrop of the human mind's enriched aptitude to think ahead and to plan for the future, which he further claims is ingrained in the complex physiological development of our brain, specifically its larger and more densely interconnected cerebral cortex.[11]

In spite of or perhaps due to the soundness of this contention, it is incumbent upon us to shake loose of the temptation to view the temporal sway of our experience as insufferably auspicious—even finding hope in hopelessness may be too hopeful[12]—stimulated by our experience of the "rhythmic time marked by oscillations, a seasonal time where absence is always a pledge of return, and death, the pledge of resurrection."[13] Near the conclusion of the Preface, I spoke of the hope imparted by the dream renewing itself sporadically as the hope deferred perpetually. Neither pessimism nor optimism seems apposite to categorize the surpassing of hope to which I allude in professing the bequeathing of hope in the dream through its adjournment, a sentiment that circumvents the adjudication of an axiological appraisal basic to our navigating the currents of the world—as Heraclitus reportedly mused, "He who does not expect will not find the unexpected, for it is trackless and unexplored."[14] Perhaps it is hopeless to imagine letting go of the inclination to hope, but then, we would do better to think of hope, phenomenologically, as the unremitting projection of an elementally calibrated retrospection, to foretell what has been in the recollection of what is to come. Every undertaking, on this score, would be a return of what can never be but what can never be, the loop of the double negative that yields the positivity of our becoming the being we are not, a penchant well understood through time by mystic visionaries and contemplative masters.

Commemorating the Future/Awaiting the Past

The promise we customarily associate with the dream, an association that doubtless underlies the archaic alliance of dream and prognostication, is veritably a call to reminiscence, or what may be termed *prospective memory*. In this regard, the retroactive and imminent are not to be positioned dyadically. The example of ancient Israelite prophecy is instructive: the prophet is so certain of the truth of the vision that the forecast of what is to come seems to him as if it has already taken place, and thus the future prediction is expressed in the past tense.[15] Thinking beyond the theological parameters of prophecy, we can apply this bending of time's arrow to dreams more generally. Furthermore, with respect to this constituent of consciousness, the dream state and waking reality are on an equal phenomenal footing, since there is no compelling reason to ascribe more credibility to what is recollected in the latter than to what is recollected in the former, a point confirmed by experimental data that indicates the susceptibility of the reality-monitoring function of the brain to misattribute memories of imagined experiences to actual experiences.[16] Not only is there no deficiency of memory with respect to the dream, but there seems to be an intricate connection between the facility to remember and the propensity to dream—not necessarily the ability to evoke the dream, but the very activity of dreaming; the fiber of the dream, as it were, is woven from memory threads encoded in and thus retrievable from various regions of the brain,[17] especially the hippocampus and prefrontal cortex, an internal stream of imagery that one researcher has called the "autonomous imagination," in contrast to the emotionally coded memory register of outside consciousness.[18] To translate the neurobiological datum mythopoeically: in the truth of its appearance, the dream is an interior state of anticipatory remembering. Even if we propose a scenario in which one dreams that one has forgotten one's dream, this is still a manner of recollecting, and as such, it provides the prospect for anticipation. Viewing time from within the dreamscape, we can ascertain that expectation, in its deepest modulation, is a form of commemoration.

In this spirit, let us consider the following passage in a zoharic homily in which an anonymous Jew, who is described as having carried a wineskin (*qapṭira de-ḥamra*) while escorting R. Yeisa and R. Ḥizqiyah on their sojourn from Cappadocia to Lyda,[19] expounded a number of esoteric matters, including the mystery of the dream (*raza de-ḥelma*), anchored exegetically in the verse "And Joseph recalled the dreams that he had dreamed about them" (Genesis 42:9):

> He remembered them because there is no forgetfulness before the blessed holy One.[20] A person should remember a good dream, so that it will not be forgotten, and then it will be fulfilled, for just as it is forgotten before a person, so it will be forgotten above him. Come and see: A dream that is not interpreted is a like a letter that has not been read[21] . . . because it is not remembered, it is as if no one knows it. Accordingly, the one who forgets the dream and does not know it, it is not primed above him to be fulfilled. Therefore, Joseph remembered his dream, so that it would be fulfilled, and so that the dream would never be forgotten by him, and he waited for it constantly.[22]

On the face of it, the main point pronounced in this passage is obvious enough, indeed even somewhat trite: to know a dream, it must be remembered, and only then will it be implemented. It seems to me, however, that a more sublime meaning may be elicited from the text. Utilizing the dream, the author of this zoharic segment instructs us about lingering in the interval of the present lodged between past and future, the time lag that propels the temporal obstinacy of human destiny to keep moving, to get on with life, as we are wont to say. The dream informs us, therefore, about the most salient feature of memory alluded to in the comment at the end of the citation: by remembering his dream, Joseph *waited for it constantly*.

Common sense would dictate that the quality of human remembrance that is most characteristic is not anticipation, but retrospection. Nevertheless, since the dream both happened and did not yet happen, to remember it is to anticipate it. Hence, the zoharic passage reminds us that from recalling our dreams, we learn about the nature of waiting and the incongruity it entails. We cannot wait for something about which we have no knowledge, but not to know is integral to waiting; the capriciousness of what may be or not be endows the waiting with its tensiveness—I may think I am confident about the time of an incident for which I am waiting, however, if there is no possibility that it will not take place, if I can prognosticate with certainty that it will occur at the time of my expectancy, then the waiting is depleted of the temporal tension that confers upon it existential gravitas. The dream affords the dreamer the possibility to envision an experience that in some sense transpired beforehand, but in the interlude of the dream, there is no beforehand that is not also afterward, and thus, we do not merely foresee what is still to come, we recollect, and thereby await, what is no more because it is what has already been what has always never been. The oneiric mystery lurks in the chasm that opens the past to the presentness of its future in revisioning the future of its present as the originary advent. In the intensity of the dream, as refracted through the prism of the Foucauldian notion of pure difference of which I spoke at the very beginning of the Preface to this book, the difference that disrupts and thereby duplicates itself, what was and what will be are not turned into what is; the absolute now that is the dream is the moment that, like a sword, cuts the triple chord of time.[23]

Joseph, in particular, typifies the paradox. It is not immaterial that in the kabbalistic symbolism, especially prominent in the zoharic anthology, this biblical figure incarnates the phallic potency of the divine, the covenantal sign, the locus of memory, the primal act of re/membering,[24] a truth implied in the rabbinic dictum that there is no forgetfulness before God.[25] However, there is something puzzling about the opening statement that Joseph remembered his dreams because there is no forgetfulness before God. If the cause of Joseph's recollection is the constitutional inability of the divine to forget, then how do we explain the subsequent maxim that a person must remember a good dream so that it will not be forgotten? If in the case of Joseph the matter is dependent on there being no lapse of memory in God, then this would imply that the dream would be recalled irrespective of any human effort. It seems to me that the commencement of the passage is meant to underscore that just as Joseph remembered his dreams because he embodied the attribute of the Godhead that corresponds to memory, so it is incumbent on each person to remember one's dreams in the manner that God remembers, that is, a memory that is free of the constraints and vagaries of time, a memory that is completely guarded from the corrosive effect of forgetfulness and the inevitable disintegration of the self. Precisely the dream, which epitomizes the evanescence and contingency of existence, becomes the locus of this deeper sense of temporality in which the vestiges of memory are no longer erased by the ravages of amnesia. That this kind of recollection and the responsibility for the dream analysis that ensues therefrom should be tied to Joseph—positioned according to the end of this homily in the world of the masculine (*alma di-dekhura*), in contrast to the other tribes, who were in the world of the feminine (*alma de-nuqba*)[26]—follows from the (conspicuously androcentric) correlation of the phallus and interpretation attested in kabbalistic literature and even more particularly from the dialectical disclosure and concealment of the secret, a dialectic that is fixed symbolically in this divine gradation and its corresponding location in the human anatomy.[27]

Interpretation issues from the very place of memory.[28] To know one's dream, but not its interpretation, thus gives rise to some degree of agitation; the distress, however, is doubled when one forgets both the dream and its interpretation.[29] Joseph is extolled for recalling the dream, because the fulfillment, based on its explication, cannot be actualized if the dream is submerged in the waters of oblivion. But to recall the dream is to await its coming to pass. The past is anticipated in the future that is recollected. In the preceding chapter, I invoked the observation of Fromm that dreams do not follow the laws of logic that govern our wakeful consciousness. Expanding the point, he wrote:

> The categories of space and time are neglected. People who are dead, we see alive; events which we watch in the present, occurred many years ago. We dream of two events as occurring simultaneously when in reality they could not possibly occur at the same time. We pay just as little attention to the laws of space. It is simple for us to move to a distant place in an instant, to be in two places at once, to fuse two persons into one, or to have one person suddenly be changed into another. Indeed, in our dreams we are the creators of a world where time and space, which limit all the activities of our body, have no power.[30]

While I would agree that dream consciousness demonstrates the quality of interrupting the temporal and spatial suppositions that fashion our habitual way of being in the world, I would not go so far as to say that time and space have no power in the dream. I would counter that the dream discloses a different inkling of time and space. Turning the focus specifically on the temporal vector, we note again the striking inversion of the chronological, the inability to differentiate definitively between before and after, a disorientation that renders problematic the commonsensical presumption that one unvaryingly progresses linearly or even cyclically. With respect to this characteristic, moreover, the isomorphism between the dream and the scriptural text according to the rabbinic hermeneutical principle "There is no before or after with respect to the Torah" (*ein muqdam u-me'uḥar ba-torah*) should be mentioned.[31]

The view I am expressing has a close parallel in the following passage from the *Genjōkōan* (*Manifesting Suchness*), one of the oldest texts included in the *Shōbōgenzō* compilation of the teachings of Eihei Dōgen (1200–1253), the celebrated Japanese monk and founder of the Sōtō branch of Zen:

> Once firewood turns to ash, the ash cannot revert to being firewood. But you should not take the view that it is ashes afterward and firewood before. You should realize that although firewood is at the dharma-stage of firewood, and that this is possessed of before and after, the firewood is at the same time independent, completely cut off from before, completely cut off from after. Ashes are in the dharma-stage of ashes, which also has a before and after.[32]

The asymmetrical irreversibility implied by the normal sequence of our experience—the firewood that is burnt turns into ash, but we do not imagine that the ash reverts back to being firewood—can be attributed to both terms of the corollary, "it is ashes afterward and firewood before." However, it is also possible to consider each of these terms independently of this temporal demarcation. In the continuation, Dōgen draws the larger implication of this line of thinking for the question of birth and death. We can view these serially, the one ensuing from the other, but, as in the example of the firewood and ash, we should not presume that there will be life that follows the dissolution of the body. Birth and death are stages of a continuum of what Dōgen called in another fascicle from his anthology "being-time" (*uji*)[33]—the transition from living to dying is designated as being "unborn" or as "undying"—and just as the enlightened "do not suppose that winter passes into spring or speak of spring passing into summer," there is no need to align the two restrictedly in a succession of causal contiguity.[34] The example of the seasons verifies the belief that time does not proceed straightforwardly from what came previously to what will come subsequently; the temporal comportment of our destiny might seem "irreversible and iron-clad," in the language of Borges, but in each moment of time's being the being-time, this directionality is undermined by the intransience of the transient, the permanent impermanence that casts everything as concomitantly the same because intermittently different. Borges himself instantaneously tempered his observation, "Time is the substance I am made of. Time is a river that sweeps me along, but I am the river; it is a tiger which destroys me, but I am the tiger; it is a fire which consumes me, but I am the fire."[35]

This characteristic of time and the self in dreams, or the nature of the unconscious more generally, was noted by Jung—reflecting the view of Freud mentioned above—in his comments on the "timelessness of mind" in which "past, present, and future are blended together." Referring to the example of John William Dunne's *An Experiment with Time* (1927), Jung observed that it is viable to dream the night before what one ought logically to have dreamt the night after.[36] The temporal simultaneity experienced in the dream—a sensibility that undergirds Jung's conception of synchronicity as the acausal connecting principle, that is, the rupture in time that induces the meaningful coincident occurrences of events that are apparently disconnected[37]—does not fit neatly into either the mold of the punctiform or the extended. The tenor of temporality in the dream state must be imagined from the paradoxical stance of the linear circle or the circular line in which nothing changes because everything changes insofar as there is no thing to change. The memory that coheres in the crease of the dream partakes of the fabric of time stitched through this undoing of time. The activity of dreaming reminds us—if we care not to forget the remembering that can be remembered only through forgetting the need to remember—that the moment comes to be periodically in its passing away incessantly, that the durability of the temporal consists precisely in its ephemerality.[38]

In the dream sequence, as in the design of a story, the antecedent may appear consequent to the consequent and the consequent antecedent to the antecedent, since neither one nor the other comes before without also being after, that is, the meaning of before and after is dependent on what is before or after. It is thus possible to reverse the timeline without affecting the mythologic of the narrative: one can follow the plot whether told from beginning to end or from end to beginning.[39] Predictably, this perception has an ancient precedent. In the second century, Artemidorus commented in his *Oneirocritica* (1.11), "When judging dreams, the dream interpreter must regard some of them from the beginning to the end . . . some, from the end to the beginning. For sometimes the beginning indicates the end, which is obscure and not to be grasped as a whole; sometimes, however, the end shows the beginning."[40] We may be accustomed to view the trajectory of life as a unilateral progression from beginning to end, and on occasion dreams, too, follow that predictable pattern, but at other times they invert the order, thereby reminding us of the shortsightedness of the one-sided way of seeing time's ebb and flow. Eschewing the monochromatic temporality bolstered by the perspective of the ego that initiates the measure of time's duration at birth and terminates it at death, the dream illustrates that the inception of a yarn may portend its conclusion, and the conclusion its inception. Hermeneutically, therefore, the dream is like a text, which, as Rosenzweig reminded us, may be read either from start to finish or from finish to start.[41] Within the swerve of this linear circularity, we must seek an opening to what has been called the "hyperdimension of the dream . . . in which life and mind seem to be embedded."[42]

Fore/giving Time and the Dream of Prayer

In kabbalistic literature, the imaginary intentionality has sometimes been exhibited through the correlation of time, dream, and the first of the ten emanations, *Keter*, the "crown," which is also designated as nothing (*ayin*), the infinite void of being that is the plenum of all becoming. The lingering impact of this nexus of symbols can be seen in a brief section with the title "Way of the Dream" (*derekh ha-ḥalom*) in the anonymously published contemporary kabbalistic work, *Yam ha-Ḥokhmah* (*Sea of Wisdom*), which records the teachings of Isaac Meir Morgenstern. As an entry into our deliberations on the dream of prayer and the forgiving of time, I will explicate this text.

The expression "way of the dream" communicates the notion of a path in the mystical-pietistic sense, much like *ṭarīqah* in the Ṣūfi tradition, where the "way" connotes a method and practice to attain the end marked as "truth" (*ḥaqīqah*). The goal set forth in the teaching of Morgenstern is "to unify with the light of pleasure" (*lehityaḥed im or ha-ta'anug*). Drawing upon a long history regarding each of these terms,[43] he identifies the "light of pleasure" as the "light of *Keter*." The way of the dream, therefore, is "one of the ways to reach the light of *Keter*," a motif that we have already encountered in the explication of the Ḥabad material in the previous chapter. Perhaps influenced by these sources,[44] Morgenstern establishes a connection between dreams and prayer: "However, by means of the power of prayer, that is, when one prays in the aspect of 'I am prayer' [*wa-ani tefillah*] (Psalms 109:4), can one also merit the light of *Keter*, which is the aspect of unification and fusion with the actual light [*hitaḥadut we-ḥibbur im ha-or mammash*], for *Keter* is the power that unifies [*koaḥ ha-me'aḥed*], that is, it is in its power to unify the emanated and the emanator [*asher be-khoḥo le'aḥed et ha-ne'eṣal im ha-ma'aṣil*]."[45] The way of the dream leads notionally to the summit of the *scala contemplativa*, the place of the *coincidentia oppositorum* in the Godhead, where limitlessness and limitedness intersect and collude in the identity of their (in)difference, where nothing becomes something and something nothing. To aid in the acquisition of this ultimate mystery, Morgenstern provides instruction from a lower station on the way, one that involves the union of the tenth and ninth emanations, *Nuqba* and *Yesod*, the feminine countenance and the (phallic) foundation:

> You must know that when *Nuqba* prays and beseeches, she begs from *Yesod*, which is the gradation above her, for he bestows and overflows. When *Yesod* is implored and overflows, then the unity between the emanation and emanated is achieved. Then the person[46] who is directed can reach the gradation of *Yesod*, and since *Yesod* has the potency to rise in one moment to *Keter*, from there, the light of knowledge opens up and illumines the person, for it is the six

> extremities of *Keter*, and thus one feels an actual light inside, which is the light of *Keter*.[47]

The task is to ascend to the point where emanator and emanated are conjoined. From this point, which is no point at all, the nonlocality of the pointless, one is absorbed in the infinite. Epistemically, being attached to this spot propagates the awareness that unification is discriminated through division, that identity is envisaged against the foreground of heterogeneity. The dream guides one contemplatively on the path that peaks with being bound to the light of *Keter*, the dark luminescence, where opposites converge in their opposition. The dream is thus compared to prayer, another motif we have discussed, but it is a special type of prayer,[48] one that is encoded in the psalmist's words *wa-ani tefillah*. Prima facie, two seemingly simplistic words are here juxtaposed, "I" (*ani*) and "prayer" (*tefillah*), and yet attunement to their juxtaposition is the key to open the door of gnosis that leads to vision and union.

At the base level, the words *wa-ani tefillah* allude to the entreaty of God on behalf of one's own needs, which, Morgenstern notes, is performed ceremonially in the eighteen benedictions, the central part of the rabbinic liturgy. The lowest rung of prayer, accordingly, involves the worshipper imagining a reciprocal relation to a transcendent other. As one mystically illumined comes to understand, however, both the self of the former and the icon of the latter are products of an egocentric consciousness programmed instinctually to perceive reality from the standpoint of individual needs (at its best coalescing in the altruistic obligation to maximize the good for the greatest number). The psychological inclination translates theologically into the inexorable need to render the divine in human terms. When conjured theistically, prayer ensnares one inescapably in a trap of metaphoricity, and hence, the face of the other, presumed to be incapable of representation, is shrouded anthropomorphically and anthropopathically. Even if the image of the face is meant to intimate an alterity that cannot be known or named, the "trace of illeity," in Levinas's telling terminology mentioned in the Introduction,[49] the mind is still coerced to construct an image of the imageless. In examining Ḥabad teachings on dream and prayer, I reached a similar conclusion:

> Worship is thus compared to the faculty of the dream imagination; just as the dreamer demonstrates the ability "to combine two opposites in one subject"... since the "root of the dream" is from the aspect of the supernal perimeter... wherein opposites are no longer distinguishable, so only the worshipper, completely divested of corporeality, is in the position to maintain the corporeal. As if in a dream, we must take hold here of the convergence of opposites: the world is constituted as virtually something by the one who has become nothing actually. Embedded deeper in the comparison of worship to the dream is the discernment that pious life, at least as it is construed (mono)theistically, entails a form of dissimilitude, perpetuating the charade of a dialogic encounter between a personal deity and a personal self. Truth appears, finally, through the mask of this untruth, the mask unmasked as the face that is the mask through which one can see the face.[50]

The aim is to decipher that the true purpose of prayer is not to request of a supposedly willful God to fulfill one's needs, but "to arrive at the complete unity of the emanated and its emanator" (*lehagi'a le-iḥud gamur shel ha-ne'eṣal im ma'aṣilo*).[51] In obtaining this higher realization, the enlightened soul overcomes the allure of theopoesis to project the human ego into a conception of a personal deity that exercises providential care and governance over history and the natural world. The acme of the ascent is the atheological showing, an apophatic venturing beyond the anthropomorphic need to configure the transcendent. But the route to this disfiguration, the facing of the face that necessarily cannot be faced, the contemplation of the meta/figure, the inessential essence that is (non)human,[52] is through the veil of the divine anthropos/human imagination.[53] Morgenstern insists, therefore, that the superior rationale for prayer is to be appraised by considering the relation of *Shekhinah* (or *Nuqba*) to *Yesod*, the dynamic of the feminine imploring the masculine, or, specifically, the phallic potency. When the latter overflows, there is heteroerotic union. From this conjugation, we comprehend the point of intersection of emanator and emanated, the pleromatic crevice—the crack before the egg[54]—where identity of difference is both identical to and different from difference of identity. Moreover, the one conjoined to *Yesod* can ascend "in one moment" (*be-rega eḥad*)—time in its fullest sense, the (non)event that cannot occur in the temporal flow, but that nonetheless is the very condition that incites that flow, the continuity of time's discontinuity that is the perdurance of the world[55]—to *Keter*, whence the light of knowledge (*or ha-da'at*), an "actual light" (*or mammash*) felt inside, illumines the worshipper. Since this is the "unifying light" (*or ha-me'aḥed*), one can detect from it the "complete fusion of the emanated and the emanator" (*ḥibbur gamur shel ha-ne'eṣal im ha-ma'aṣil*). The one who fathoms that unity, moreover, is incorporated within it; indeed, only one incorporated in the incomposite unity of the nothing can be cognizant of it, but the one so incorporated is nothing and therefore no longer the one who may be cognizant of anything, including the unity wherein all things are no thing.

The language of Morgenstern is unequivocal and quite bold: "It must be known that this aspect of complete union [*ha-yiḥud ha-gamur*] is what the soul in truth needs and desires, and this is the whole matter of prayer, to yearn to be in complete oneness [*aḥdut gemurah*] with the creator." The form of rhetorical delivery remains theistic, but this should not obfuscate the radical implications of the claim that the purpose of prayer is for the worshipper to be in *total union* with the divine,[56] a unity so inclusive that there is nothing outside it, *ein ḥus mimmenu*, in the language Azriel of Gerona used to describe *Keter*, the nothing of infinity, no other that is excluded by this inclusivity.[57] To contemplate this point is to concede that the ontic distinction between creator and creation is not sustainable and that the dialogical underpinning of the petitionary aspect of worship is severely compromised. As a consequence of attaining this state of mindfulness, the "light of the pleasure of *Keter* enters into and encompasses" the person until the attribute of *Yesod* "emanates and pours out ideas and holy thoughts, and this is the gradation of the dream." The dream, then, is understood as the overflowing of *Yesod* set off by the light of knowledge or the light of the pleasure of *Keter*. The issue of gender is utilized again to account for the difference between the wherewithal to feel the light of pleasure, which is aligned with the feminine (*Malkhut*), and the "power of the formation of the dream" (*koaḥ ha-ṣiyyur de-ḥalom*), which comes from the phallic potency (*Yesod*).[58] The privileging of the masculine is explained by referring to the fact that in the physical dream (*ḥalom de-gashmiyyut*), the imagination dominates over other cognitive faculties, and therefore truth is mixed with deception; the imaginative faculty during sleep is on a lower level than the imagination when one is awake, and it is associated with the shell of *nogah*—the innermost of the four husks surrounding *Malkhut*, whose denomination together with the other three, *ruaḥ se'arah*, *anan gadol*, and *esh mitlaqqaḥat*, are derived from Ezekiel 1:4—which is portrayed as a mixture of good and evil.[59] Pinpointing both the origin of the dream and the power to interpret in the divine phallus is meant to provide a mechanism by which veracity can be separated from duplicity and the precarious danger of the dream averted:

> Thus the aspect of the dream is made from the power of *Yesod*, and not from the power of *Malkhut*, for *Yesod* is the one that bestows and overflows, and it makes the dream interesting, for if not, the thought of the person would not be conjoined to it. When one wants to comprehend the dream and to find the truth in it, one needs an interpreter of dreams, in the aspect of Joseph the righteous, for he is in the aspect of *Yesod*, and by means of the power of his holiness, he elevates the holy spark in the dream from the refuse, and then the holy thought is purified, and it is possible to comprehend it.... And in greater depth it can be explained that, in fact, the gradation of the dream is bound to the emanations of *Yesod* and *Keter*.... In truth, the secret of the dream is, in fact, the liturgical worship, for the entire matter of prayer is the joining of creation to the infinite light, and this is essentially the matter of the dream, for it purifies all the imaginings [*dimyonot*], which are the aspect of this corporeal world, and it elevates them to the aspect of truth, which is the light of the Lord, blessed be his name.[60]

Prayer with the proper intention brings about attachment of the mind to *Malkhut*, but from there, it ascends to *Keter*. *Malkhut* is the personification of prayer, or, in her guise as *keneset yisra'el*, the "community of Israel," she gathers the multiple prayers of the Jewish people. The elevation of *Malkhut* to *Keter* can be viewed as a theosophic reworking of the ancient motif concerning the hoisting of the prayers of Israel by an archangel (Sandalfon or Metatron) as a crown placed on the head of the glory.[61] Kabbalists have understood this elevation as a form of psychic transport, recognizing thereby, like masters of esoteric lore in other traditions, that the going up is in truth a delving within. Following the phallocentric arc of the tradition, Morgenstern emphasizes that the ascent to *Keter* occurs through the agency of *Yesod*. We can say, therefore, that from the standpoint of the kabbalistic symbolism affirmed by this teacher in consonance with many that came before him, the dream is the vision that eventuates from the phallic escalation that climaxes in the dreamer's being conjoined to and integrated within the infinite nothing and the consequent flowering of the light of knowledge in the heart.[62] This is the meaning of Morgenstern's statement that the "secret of the dream [*sod ha-ḥalom*] is, in fact, the liturgical worship [*avodat ha-tefillah*]." The goal of the latter is the "joining of creation to the infinite light [*ḥibbur ha-beri'ah le-or ein sof*]," the quintessential (im)materialization of the *coincidentia oppositorum*, the cosmological principle of apophatic embodiment that complements the pneumatic paradigm of *unio mystica*. Only the psyche in the dream state is capable of imaginally instigating the amalgamation of finitude and infinity.[63] Contemporary physics may have led us to this very place, but this would not weaken the kabbalistic perspective. That is, if we have the scientific technology to survey the paradox of a finite universe being the substratum of the infinite light, then this technology itself is buttressed by a theoretical mind-set imbued with the dream mythologic, for which such a coincidence of opposites is not implausible.

Left unspoken in Morgenstern's words is another, much older kabbalistic motif, the representation of *Keter* (or, more accurately, an aspect of *Keter* referred to in some zoharic passages as *boṣina de-qardinuta*, the "hardened spark") as the upper phallus that corresponds to *Yesod*, the lower phallus.[64] Given the structural affinity between the divine and human bodies, we can presume that there is an equivalent correlation between the crowning region of the head and the male organ in the fleshly anatomy (ideally incarnate in the ethnos of Israel). Countless texts could be cited to substantiate this claim—the cacophony of voices critical of my interpretation of the kabbalistic symbolism as phallomorphic notwithstanding[65]—but I will mention one passage from the circle of Moses Ḥayyim Luzzatto, the notorious eighteenth-century man of letters. While there is some question about the authorship of the work I will cite, there is no doubt that it does preserve

Luzzatto's teaching.[66] The perfection of the phallus (*tiqqun ha-yesod*), we are told, comes about exclusively through the disclosure of *Arikh Anpin*, the title of the divine countenance (*parṣuf*) that overlaps, more or less, with the sefirotic configuration of *Keter*. Elevating the phallus to the crown is both the trigger and upshot of the process of redemption; exile, inversely, is portrayed as phallic flaccidity or, in the scriptural elocution, as the downfall of the righteous man (Proverbs 24:16)—a truism that is mined eisegetically from God's directive to Moses "And you lift up your rod and hold out your arm over the sea and split it, so that the Israelites may march into the sea on dry ground" (Exodus 14:16).[67] Poetically, the image of Moses raising the rod signifies phallic empowerment through ascetic withholding and psychic rechanneling. This conforms to my argument in an earlier work that the symbolic homology between *Yesod* and *Keter* is the conceptual underpinning of the erotic ascesis embraced by kabbalists, the tantric-like lifting of the libidinal energy from the genital region to the skull, a climb of the mind, as it were, that results in the mindless cleaving to the infinite and the consequent profusion of light seed in the expanse of distended consciousness.[68] I suggest that the quietistic ideal of self-abnegation is intimated by the expression *wa-ani tefillah*, read appositively, "I am payer," that is, *ani*, the I, is humbled and transformed into the nothing of *ayin*. In that nothing is the crossing of infinity, the space where emanator and emanated are joined as one, where cause and effect merge in the circuitry of the moment, where the eternal is temporalized and the temporal eternalized, the site of the incipient redundancy, the beginning that must have already begun to be the beginning before the beginning had begun.

The textual roots for the correlation of the dream and *Keter* seem to lie in the following passage preserved in *Sefer ha-Bahir*, which began to circulate in the twelfth and thirteenth centuries. The difficulties related to the composition and redaction of this collection are, in my judgment, beyond the ability of scholars to settle, given the nature of the material artifacts with which we must work,[69] but it can still be asserted confidently that this aggregate preserves the mythologoumena whence many of the basic tenets of medieval kabbalah evolved. According to the pertinent text, the disciples inquired of their master,

R. Amora, regarding the inner import of the Hebrew vowel *ḥolem*. He responded that it relates to the soul (*neshamah*),

> for if you heed it, you will cause your body to be vigorous [*taḥalim*][70] in the future to come, and if you rebel against it, illnesses [*ḥolim*] will fall upon its head, and the malady [*ḥolyah*] will be on its head.[71] Moreover, he said that every dream [*ḥalom*] is in the *ḥolem*, and every white pearl is in the *ḥolem*, as it is written "and an amethyst [*we-aḥlamah*]" (Exodus 28:19).[72]

By a play of words, the vowel *ḥolem* is linked to the dream (*ḥalom*), which is further associated with the amethyst (*aḥlamah*), the jewel that has the apotropaic potency to protect one from infirmities. The bahiric exegesis is based on the presumed folkloristic notion that the amethyst has the property of facilitating the perspicuity of mind and the concentration of imagination related to nocturnal dreaming. A possible literary conduit of this idea, as Gershom Scholem conjectured,[73] may have been the remark of the twelfth-century Spanish exegete, philosopher, and poet Abraham Ibn Ezra that the term *aḥlamah* is related to Arabic *al-ḥilma*, for by wearing this stone on one's finger, one can visualize one's dreams.[74]

Unsurprisingly, the bahiric text is laconic and hence somewhat murky. A reworking of the passage appears in the seventieth section of *Tiqqunei Zohar*, dedicated to a symbolic elucidation of the application of the different vowels to *Shekhinah*, "And she is called *ḥolem* [when she is in] in the likeness of the side of the central pillar [*Tif'eret*], 'from there the shepherd, the rock of Israel' (Genesis 49:24), 'the stone that the builders rejected has become the chief cornerstone' (Psalms 118:22). Every precious stone is in the *ḥolem*, as it is written 'a jacinth, an agate, and an amethyst' [*leshem shevo we-aḥlamah*]' (Exodus 28:19), and through it 'we had dreams' [*wa-naḥlemah ḥalom*] (Genesis 41:11)."[75] The implications of this text are made explicit in the following comment by Cordovero:

> *Ḥolem* is from the side of the central pillar. It has already been explained that at times *Malkhut* is a diadem [*aṭarah*] on the head of *Tif'eret*, and then she is called the "glorious diadem" [*aṭeret tif'eret*], and then she is a *ḥolem* on the top of the *waw*, and then it says concerning her "the stone that the builders rejected has become the chief cornerstone." When she is a diadem on his head, "from there the shepherd, the rock of Israel," that is, the patriarchs and the

> edifice are sustained, for even Jacob is nourished by her . . . and then she is a precious gem. A proof is brought from the verse "a jacinth, an agate, and an amethyst." . . . Another proof is brought from "we had dreams," and the dream is from the side of *Malkhut*.[76]

In Chapter 3, we educed from a zoharic homily the distinction between the prophetic vision and the dream vision: the former is allied with *Shekhinah* and the latter with Gabriel, the sixth gradation in the angelic sphere beneath the divine. At times, prophecy can occur in a night vision, *mar'ot ha-laylah*, in the biblical vernacular (Genesis 46:2), which, rendered kabbalistically, is an allusion to *Shekhinah*,[77] but even this is to be distinguished from an ordinary dream. By contrast, in the aforecited text from the *Tiqqunim*, the last of the sefirotic emanations is branded as the locality of dreams in the imaginal realm. I hasten to add that this role is related, more specifically, to the positioning of the feminine as a diadem on the head of the masculine, for which reason she is called *aṭeret tif'eret*. The anonymous Spanish kabbalist responsible for this text was likely influenced by a second passage in the bahiric compilation in which the image of the diadem (*aṭarah*) on the head of the king appears;[78] the deployment of the word "head" (*ro'sh*) in both passages presumably suggested a pairing of the crown and the *ḥolem*.[79] I have engaged the gender implications of this symbolism extensively in prior writings, and thus I will refrain from reiterating the details of my argument.[80] Nevertheless, it behooves me to mention that the repercussions of the transposition of gender implied in the text from the *Tiqqunim* are critical to our assessment of the way that kabbalists viewed the phallic intimation of the nocturnal vision.

The source of the dream (*ḥalom*) is to be located in *Malkhut*, but only when the precious stone is elevated like a crown on the male, for in that posture, she corresponds to the *ḥolem*, the vowel point that is calligraphically marked above the letter, as Cordovero made clear in his explication. In assuming this position, the feminine presence is restored to the masculine, or, in the exact language of the text, she is in "the likeness of the side of the central pillar," which is another name for *Tif'eret*, the sixth emanation, and hence the stone that was rejected by the builders (also referred to as the stone of Israel, based on Genesis 49:24) becomes the cornerstone, *ro'sh pinnah* (Psalms 118:22), literally, the "head of the corner," a turn of phrase whose Hebrew cadence (when intoned kabbalistically) likely has a phallic connotation.[81] Support for this suggestion is found in other passages in this zoharic stratum where the orthographic form of the *ḥolem*, a dot atop the *waw*, is said to take the shape of the *zayin*,[82] the letter that symbolically stands for *zakhar*, the male, or its weaponry (*zayin*) and adornment (*ziyyun*). This would be consistent with the identification of *Yesod* as the source of the prowess to interpret dreams, a view explored in Chapter 3. I cite here one interesting example from Moses David Valle, a member of Luzzatto's circle:[83] "Thus it was decreed by the supernal governance that everything would come to Joseph through a dream, in the secret of the providence of *Tif'eret* over *Yesod*, which is the Tetragrammaton in the vocalization of the *ḥolem*, as these are the letters of *ḥalom*."[84] The phallic intent of the correlation of the dream (*ḥalom*) and the *ḥolem* made explicit by Valle validates the reading I have proffered. Many more texts could be cited as support, but this one will be sufficient.

I surmise, moreover, that behind this symbolism is the association of *ḥolem* and *Keter*,[85] because the central pillar in the sefirotic edifice (*Tif'eret* and *Yesod* are the key nodal points) extends to infinity at the apex, the quarry, as it were, whence the dream stone is hewn.[86] In the preceding chapter, we discussed a passage from Gikatilla according to which the source of the dream is situated in *Keter*, the world of pure mercy, the simple unity that precedes the severance into the right side of extension (benevolence) and the left side of constriction (judgment), portrayed respectively as masculine and feminine. The dream mimics the coincidence of opposites allied with *Keter*, and this is so mainly in its being a blending of truth and untruth. The dream, as I have noted at several junctures in this book, is true only inasmuch as it is untrue, and hence untruth is the metric that measures the truth. In the ecology of the dream, the surface is the depth.[87]

A similar portrayal is put forward in the anonymous fifteenth-century Byzantine treatise *Sefer ha-Peli'ah*:

> Why is it called *ḥolem*? He responded that the *ḥolem* is from the word *ḥalom*, a matter that is not comprehended, but rather this vowel is compassionate [*ḥomel*] and forgives. It is also from the word *melekh*, to teach you that just as salt [*melekh*] is a matter that preserves and

sustains, so the vowel that is called *ḥolem* is the bread [*leḥem*] that nourishes the upper and lower beings. Thus you see with your eyes all the good things produced by the vowel called *ḥolem*. But you see as well that in the future to come it will battle [*loḥem*] against the enemies. And all of this because it is white as snow and ashen as the wool and it is merciful forever.[88]

In the first instance, the bond between *ḥolem* and *ḥalom* is related to the matter of incomprehensibility. This reflects the long-standing depiction of *Keter*, in the language used by Gikatilla at the end of the thirteenth century, as the "utter nothing" (*afisah muḥleṭet*) beyond apprehension and linguistification, the inaccessible and boundless will that wills nothing but the nothingness of its will,[89] the "place of negation" (*meqom ha-shelilah*) about which, technically speaking, one can converse only through apophatic formulae (*ledabber mi-derekh ha-shelilah*), expressions of inexpressibility.[90] Additionally, it is highlighted that the dream, like the sefirotic gradation to which it is correlated, comports with the qualities of forgiveness and compassion, a point ratified by juxtaposing the words *ḥalom* and *ḥomel*, since they (like the word *ḥolem*) are composed of the same consonants, *ḥeit*, *lamed*, and *mem*. The *ḥolem* is also referred as the king, *melekh* (*mem lamed kaf*), which is homonymous with the word *melekh*[91] (constituted by the same consonants as the words *ḥalom*, *ḥolem*, and *ḥomel*, but in the order *mem*, *lamed*, *ḥeit*), for, like salt, it has the capability of preserving and sustaining, and therefore it is also designated *leḥem* (*lamed*, *ḥeit*, *mem*), the bread that nourishes the beings in the supernal and terrestrial worlds. Finally, we are told, somewhat startlingly, that in the future, the attribute of mercy will do battle, *loḥem* (*lamed*, *ḥeit*, *mem*), against the enemies, referring, in all probability, to the adversaries of Israel. This, too, is an expression of the *coincidentia oppositorum*, since it is the divine mercy that will enact punishment through the exercise of judgment. Be that as it may, the various permutations of the three letters forge a nexus between the vowel (*ḥolem*), dream (*ḥalom*), compassion (*ḥomel*), salt (*melekh*), bread (*leḥem*), and combat (*loḥem*).

For the purposes of this chapter, I will focus on the third ring in the chain, the correlation of the dream (*ḥalom*) and the act of clemency (*ḥomel*), which rests on the theosophic assumption that mercy is the quality affixed to *Keter*, the sefirotic attribute associated grammatically with the *ḥolem*. Since there is no element of judgment in this mercifulness, all transgressions are eliminated. In the concise formulation of Gikatilla: "Know that this *sefirah* is the place of pure mercy, and it transforms sinners, for even though people are worthy of obliteration, by means of this *sefirah*, he atones for them and has mercy and pity over them, as the matter of 'and the grace that I grant and the compassion that I show' (Exodus 33:19)."[92] In the secret of forgiveness, guilt is transmuted to innocence, and the stain of sinfulness is absolved in the whiteness of pure mercy, the divine indifference that effaces all difference, even the difference between right and wrong. The kabbalistic doctrine, far-reaching in its hypernomian potential,[93] is an elaboration of the rabbinic idea that God pardons human indiscretion by annulling the standard of rectitude mandated by the Torah. Simply put, in the act of forbearing, the criterion of reward and punishment sanctioned by the strict canon of law would have to be overturned.[94]

From this perspective, we can enlist the Derridean idea and speak of the nonjuridical dimension of forgiveness—the unconditional as opposed to the conditional notion of forgiveness that eludes any sense of economic exchange and therefore can function without any apology, remorse, or hope of reconciliation—and the implied suspension of the order of lawfulness,[95] a state that parallels the juridical concept of imprescriptibility insofar as both lead to "a sort of eternity or transcendence, the apocalyptic horizon of a final judgement in the law beyond the law, in history beyond history."[96] To cross that horizon—a crossing that continually consists of not being able to cross that which is to be crossed—one must appropriate the paradox that there can be forgiveness only in relation to the unforgivable, for in the absence of the unforgivable, there would be no need for forgiveness. In Derrida's own aporetic formulation: "Thus forgiveness, if it is possible, if there is such a thing, is not possible, it does not exist as possible, it only exists by exempting itself from the law of the possible, by impossibilizing itself, so to speak, and in the infinite endurance of the im-possible as impossible."[97] In the last analysis, Derrida acknowledges that his idea of the purity of forgiveness, a state that is *unconditional, but without sovereignty*, is an impossible task that endures as a "dream of thought."[98]

Analogously, in the halakhic mind-set, which informed rabbinic sages and kabbalists alike, the interruption of law entailed in the impossibility of the possibility of forgiveness is at the very foundation of the law. Ostensibly, the full accomplishment of this infringement is for all time postponed until the end-time, but it is proleptically accessible at any time as a retrieval of the origin that precedes the beginning, the attribute of *Keter*, the nihility of the divine plentitude, the absolute necessity that is pure contingency, the locus of forgiveness and of the dream. The act of human repentance, in particular, occasions the divine forgiveness, for this is the gesture, according to a talmudic tradition,[99] that is invested with the capacity to turn intentional wrongdoing (*shegagot*) into merit (*zedonot*), to convert one thing into its opposite such that the opposition that informs the nomian axiology is surmounted. That the dream exemplifies a similar potency was expressed in the following comment on a passage from *Tiqqunei Zohar*[100] transmitted in the name of Phineḥas ben Abraham Abba Shapiro of Korzec (d. 1790/91),[101] one of the Ukrainian ḥasidic masters and a close companion of the Beshṭ:

> All of the dreams [*ḥalomot*] come from the vowel *ḥolem*, and from this vowel they can do what they want to do, and they can overturn [*lehithappekh*], and this is like the hylic matter [*ha-hiyyuli*], through which they can do what they want, and hence the righteous can transform the attribute of judgment to the attribute of mercy, and this is the meaning of "tear up our evil decree,"[102] and this is the essence of repentance [*iqqar ha-teshuvah*], for repentance transforms the attribute of judgment to the attribute of mercy.[103]

Given its origin in the vowel *ḥolem*, which corresponds to *Keter*, the place where opposites coincide, the dream imbues one with the capacity to turn something into its opposite, judgment into mercy, which is the quality of forgiveness on the part of the divine and repentance on the part of the human.

The use of the philosophical notion of hylic matter is meant to underscore that the dream, or better, the locus of the dream in the Godhead, signifies the actuality that is circumscribed as pure potentiality—what it is to become is the essence of what it is. As I have argued elsewhere,[104] the connection between *Keter* and forgiveness signifies that the latter bears within itself the limitlessness of its own delimitation, the laying at hand of what is remembered, that which proceeds (or slips) from the past into the present and thereby is anticipated in the future, the retrieval of the irretrievable.[105] Here again, it is beneficial to invoke Derrida. Noting that forgiveness is dependent on taking to heart the "im-passbleness" and "impassivity" of the past, one might be led to conclude that forgiveness is "the being of time insofar as it involves the indisputable and the unmodifiable past."[106] Yet as Derrida cautions the reader, the "pastness of an eventness" (*passéité d'une événementialité*), the certitude that something has happened, is not sufficient to serve as a foundation for the concept of forgiveness.[107] The past event must continue to echo unremittingly, albeit intermittently, in the present, and in this respect, forgiveness, like the dream, is a "ghostly disturbance," an "interruption of onto-temporal identity."[108]

On this point, kabbalistic sources are instructive, insofar as they convey the notion that forgiveness wells from the mediated sense of time's immediacy, indeed, from the experience of time as the irreducible possibility of there being something, even if that something is nothing. Forgiveness is the fore/giving, the giving before, that grounds the fecundity of temporality in the *nunc stans*. By this term, I intend the *tempus discretum*, the cut that binds one synchronically to the diachronic opening of time, the discontinuity of the continuous present, the noncoincidental coincidence, the blink of the eye that is concurrently repetitive and diremptive. Not only is repetition not adverse to difference, but the possibility of the latter is actualized by the former. Thus, we can apply the following words of Deleuze to the kabbalistic notion of the time swerve that emerges from the conception of forgiveness as the giving before:

> The order of time has broken the circle of the Same and arranged time in a series only to re-form a circle of the Other at the end of the series.... The form of time is there only for the revelation of the formless in the eternal return.... In this manner, the ground has been superseded by a groundlessness, a universal ungrounding which turns upon itself and causes only the yet-to-come to return.[109]

Anthropologically, to forgive must always be an unprecedented recurrence, a renewal of covenant between two parties, the aggrieved and the perpetrator. Theosophically, as well, in the moment of fore/giving, no more turns into not yet, and time endures in its transience. The correlation of *Keter* and the dream—the *ḥolem* that is the *ḥalom*—signals that the dreamtime similarly partakes of the infinite kenosis of what has always been what is to come.

One of the main vehicles by which kabbalists have expressed their conception of time as the genuine repetition of an inceptual replication, the intermingling of the novel and erstwhile in the letting go of what is held in reserve, is the attribution of the term *ehyeh* to *Keter*, which stems from the name revealed by God to Moses in the theophany at the burning bush, *ehyeh asher ehyeh*, "I will be as I will be" (Exodus 3:14). There are, of course, a multiplicity of readings of this scriptural verse that may be excavated from kabbalistic texts.[110] The interpretation I will advance, however, relates to the predominant nuance of *ehyeh* as it pertains especially to the eternality of time and the temporality of eternity. Read hyperliterally, *ehyeh* denotes that in each instant, nothing becomes something that forever is not what it has become—it will be what it will be, but what it will be must always not be what it is. This is the esoteric significance of the dogma of the creation of something from nothing (*yesh me-ayin*): the something contained in the nothing whence it came (not) to be. In other technical kabbalistic parlance, the something (*yesh*) is *Ḥokhmah*, the second gradation, the divine thought (*maḥashavah*), which comprises the other gradations within itself indivisibly,[111] and thus it is symbolized by the letter *yod*, the first letter of the Tetragrammaton and the numerical equivalence of ten, and the nothing (*ayin*) is the first gradation (for some kabbalists identical with the infinite and for some divergent) that both is what it is not and is not what it is. The *nihil* is the divine abundance, and not the privation of being, as the conventional understanding of the creed would necessitate.[112] As I noted above, this conception of *creatio ex nihilo* renders suspect the ontic distinction between creator and creation that is endemic to a theistic portrait of God. What I did not emphasize is the implication of this shift for the understanding of time. The temporal consequences of this obfuscation were considered by Scholem in his presentation of the kabbalistic symbol.[113] This aspect of Scholem's thought has been discussed by many scholars,[114] but to the best of my knowledge, the element to which I have called attention has been neglected. In Scholem's own words: "The symbol in which the life of the Creator and that of creation become one, is—to use Creuzer's words—'a beam of light which, from the dark and abysmal depths of existence and cognition, falls into our eye and penetrates our whole being.' It is a 'momentary totality' which is perceived intuitively in a mystical *now*—the dimension of time proper to the symbol."[115]

The alteration from nothing that is something to something that is nothing opens the gate to the esoteric implications of kabbalistic esotericism, the laying bare of the secret of the secret. Just as, hermeneutically, we are compelled to uncover the mystery by discovering rather than discarding the cover, so the process of emanation, meontologically, is a recovery, an unveiling of the veiled in a manner that the unveiled is veiled, otherwise it would not be the veiled that is unveiled. *Keter* is the excessive lack that contains the totality (*kelal*) of particulars (*peraṭim*) in the simplicity of its (non)being, and thus it is marked by the first-person singular imperfect, *ehyeh*, which connotes, in the language of one zoharic passage, the impetus of the infinite will "summoned to extend and to produce everything" (*zammin le'amshekha wi-le'olada khola*).[116] From here, we retrieve the axiom that the essence of time (*zeman*) may be deduced from the gesture of beckoning (*zammin*), the calling into the open of what was concealed as what was to become, but what was to become is enclosed in the (non)being that is from eternity—hence the meaning of the titles *Attiq Yomin*, the "ancient of days," *Attiqa*, the "ancient one," and *Attiqa Qaddisha*, the "holy ancient one," applied to *Keter* in some strata of zoharic literature—the pledge of the eternal now, resolutely stipulated by the indeterminacy of its primeval futurity, the hiddenness that is unwaveringly the not yet manifest one.[117]

In a second zoharic text, we find a comparable portrayal of *Keter*, although in that context, the image of the continual dispersal of the unlimited nothing more overtly undercuts a substantialist metaphysics: "The primordial one is *ehyeh*, this is the supernal concealed one [*setima illa'ah*], as it is said 'I am what I am' [*ana ma'n da-ana*],[118] but it is not known what it is [*we-lo ityyeda ma'n hu*]. Subsequently, *asher ehyeh*, I am that which is summoned to be revealed [*ana de-zammin le'itgalyya*]."[119] *Ehyeh* denotes the insubstantiality intrinsic to *Keter*, "I am what I am" (*ana ma'n da-ana*); the nature of that "I," however, is not known apart from what is unfurled in the disclosure of this concealment, which perforce must be a concealment of disclosure; the impending I that will be exposed (*ana de-zammin le'itgalyya*) is the I that has always been, the primordial one (*qadma'ah*) that is innately inscrutable. *Ehyeh*, therefore, is a peculiar name insofar as it names the withheld that is perpetually forthcoming, the same that is always newly constellated. The description of *Keter* yields the ideational structure that underlies the kabbalistic conception of time as a circular linearity—a present determined contemporaneously by the past of the future that is yet to come as what has already been and by the future of the past that has already been what is yet to come. Language here falters, and the notion of temporality can be properly enunciated only through the renunciation of speech, a silence that bespeaks the purging of thought at the point of its fullest fruition.[120] The same point in all of its opaqueness was articulated cogently by Moses de León:

> The first name, *ehyeh*, is the secret of the unique name [*shem ha-meyuḥad*], and this is the name of the unity that is unified [*ha-shem ha-aḥdut ha-meyuḥad*] in the totality of his names. However, as we have already noted,[121] the secret of the subtle ether that is not comprehended has no known name or a delimited boundary or anything by which one might comprehend it.[122] The first being [*hawayah ha-ri'shonah*] that comes to be from its secret is the totality of all the unity [*kelal kol ha-aḥdut*] in the secret of the point of thought [*ha-nequddah ha-maḥashavit*][123] about which no one knows anything of its secret until the wellspring issues forth to be built. Thus, the secret of its unified name is *ehyeh* (Exodus 3:14), that is, "I still will be and I will emanate the secret of being in the secret of my existence," that is, "I will be and I will construct my existence, and I will emanate the emanation of being so that it will exist." Indeed, this is the secret of the first name that was communicated to Moses in the bush, in the secret of the beginning of the prophecy of Moses, peace be upon him. . . . The secret of the first name is concealed and elevated without any disclosure, and thus it is the secret of *ehyeh*, this is the name that stands in its being in the secret of the hidden depth, until the secret of *Ḥokhmah* comes forth, whence there is the

> dissemination of everything. Thus it says subsequently *asher ehyeh*, that which is summoned to be revealed [*ha-mezumman lehitgalot*].[124]

Time is the unraveling of the (k)not of eternity, a metaphysical disentanglement captured semantically in the expression *ehyeh asher ehyeh*, "I will be what I will be." The first *ehyeh* is decoded as a reference to *Keter*, the abyss that is at once pure actuality and pure potentiality—in the nothingness empty of everything, even its own nothingness, there is no point to position actual and possible as antinomical. From a kabbalist's perspective, therefore, we would be wise not to speak of the possible as either becoming or not becoming actual, since everything possible is actual, because what is actual is nothing but the possible. As I pointed out in an earlier publication, the nothing (*efes*) of the infinite is the potency of all that was, is, or will be in the panoply of possible beings, and thus it is itself the im/possible that is both and therefore neither possible nor impossible. Nothing is the potentiality that is fully actual as the actuality that is fully potential in being nothing. I also compared the kabbalistic view (extrapolated from Azriel of Gerona in the thirteenth century) to Nicholas of Cusa's identification of God as the "potency as such," the precondition for conditionality, the "possibility-to-be" (*posse esse*) of what may come to be as the actualized possibility (*possest*). In this negative infinity, there is no distinction between potentiality (*posse*) and actuality (*esse*).[125]

This is the sense insinuated by the esoteric reading of *ehyeh asher ehyeh* we have come across in the zoharic corpus and in de León, the convening of that nothing to become all that exists in the concatenation of being. Time (*zeman*), we might say, is the concealment summoned to be revealed (*ha-mezumman lehitgalot*), a revelation, to repeat, that must be a concealment, if it is the concealment—the "hidden matter" (*davar ne'lam*) that is "neither something nor nothing" (*lo yesh we-lo ayin*)[126]—that is revealed. The interpretation of the verse effectively undermines any ontology of substance or metaphysics of presence with regard to the nothing in which everything is incorporated, a conception that I have dubbed *meontology*. I avail myself of this idiom to mark the inability to separate being and nonbeing in the recognition that in the infinite, which is nothing, being is what it is to be and thus it cannot be but as nonbeing. The "I" of the Godhead is *what will be*, but what will be, *ex definitio*, can be only what will be, not anything that is; the letters of *ani* (*alef, nun, yod*) are transposed into *ayin* (*alef, yod, nun*). The equation of these words has often been noted; what is worthy of emphasis is that this signifies not only that the first and last of the emanations, the commencement and termination of the circle, *Keter and Malkhut*, are identical, but in the more baffling sense, the identity of opposites within *Keter* itself. Mystically speaking, in its profoundest individuation, the I is nothing other than the nothing it relentlessly is by not being.

The name *ehyeh*, therefore, can be said to denote the future that is rejuvenated recurringly in the breach of the beginning within the origin whence time is engendered from the past of the infinite eternality (*niṣḥiyyut*) constantly renewed in the present. The moment, in the language of Blanchot, displays the quality of noncontemporaneity, insofar as it "is a passage always passed over," the "passive" that, "outside time, disarranges time as pure and empty form.... Time that is deranged and off its hinges still lets itself be drawn—if only through the experience of the crack—into a coherence which unifies and universalizes itself.... The crack: a fissure which would be constitutive of the self, or would reconstitute itself as the self, but not as a cracked self."[127] These words nicely capture the kabbalistic notion of the evolution of the divine persona (in the form of the *sefirot*) from the abyss of Ein Sof whence the eternal coil unwinds—through the fracture that is the core of its being, the opening that comprises the possibility of all possibilities, including the possibility of the impossible contained in the impossibility of the possible—as the endless chain of temporal becoming. Time, then, is conceived to be a gift in the most exacting sense, an unreserved graciousness that withholds nothing but the grace of reciprocity, the impossible possible, possible because of the impossibility of every possibility,[128] a quality that is uniquely matched to the dream phenomenon in which nothing seems impossible. Appropriating Hölderlin's diction, we might say that in the dream, we are suspended in a "state between being and non-being" where "the possible becomes real everywhere, and the real becomes ideal."[129] Gikatilla expressed it as follows:

> *Ehyeh*, this is a name that ascends to the head of *Keter*, concerning which there is no knowledge except for it. This is the name hidden

in the concealment of its abode, and it is the one appointed over the world of mercy [*olam ha-raḥamim*]. . . . Know that the function of the supernal name, which is *ehyeh*, is the activity of the complete mercy [*ha-raḥamim ha-gemurim*], and this is the name that is beneficent; it bestows a free gift [*matnat ḥinnam*] and it is compassionate, not from the perspective of judgment, but from the perspective of complete mercy, as it is said "I will proclaim before you the name YHWH, and the grace that I grant and the compassion that I show" (Exodus 33:19).[130]

The medieval kabbalist characterizes the benevolence of *Keter* as the conferral of a "free gift" (*matnat ḥinnam*),[131] a rabbinic coinage used to label the gifting of divine grace (*ḥinnun*)[132] and especially in some passages as a response to the act of human prayer (often tied exegetically to the words allegedly spoken by Moses *wa-etḥannan el yhwh*, "I pleaded with the Lord," in Deuteronomy 3:23).[133] For Gikatilla and other kabbalists, such as David ben Yehudah he-Ḥasid,[134] the gift—the meontology presupposed by kabbalists justifies the use of the term in the manner that I criticized in the Introduction, namely, ascribing agency to the event of giving, such that we think and speak of it as a gift of being—is located in *Keter*, about which we can say nothing, since it is unknowable to all but itself. Thus, it is also signified by the third person pronoun *hu*, which may be translated as "he" or "it."[135] I prefer the neutrality of the latter as a safeguard against eliding into theopoetic personifications, even though this seems inevitable, if one is to think at all, surely if one is to commit one's thoughts to verbal or written communication. Not only is *Keter* beyond knowledge, but even to speak of its being is problematic, except as "it is vis-à-vis the essence of its truth and not to any other" (*she-hu le-eṣem amittato we-lo lezulato*), an explanation that Gikatilla submits for the name *ehyeh*.[136] From this unmitigated mercy, the source of being beyond being, the no-thing, one may discern the nature of time as the overflow that springs ceaselessly from the "essence of the primordial existence [*iqqar meṣi'ut qadmon*], from whose truth the *sefirot* were revealed."[137]

Time, so conceived, is treated by Gikatilla as a "deep matter" (*davar amoq*), and the term *qadmon*, the "primordial," reveals "several mysteries." The impersonal pronoun *hu* is used to name the connection of *Keter* to the other sefirotic emanations, for "this matter is very deep, and a person must transmit it in an oral tradition, so that one will know the way in which to go to comprehend how the *sefirah* of mercy is revealed by means of the rest of the *sefirot*, and how it transforms the attribute of judgment into the attribute of mercy."[138] An appeal to oral tradition (*qabbalah peh el peh*) is significant for Gikatilla, a kabbalist whose written treatises, especially *Sha'arei Orah*, are expansive in their diffusion of esoteric wisdom.[139] In another work, the exposition of the thirteen attributes that come forth from *Keter*, Gikatilla repeats this view, underlining that the containment of all the emanations in *Keter* in an indivisible unity is something that can be transmitted as a matter of faith (*emunah*) and is not subject to comprehension (*hassagah*). *Keter* itself is denominated as the "essence of all faith and the root of trust," and "whoever believes in the existence of *Keter* is called a 'faithful spirit,'[140] but whoever does not believe is uprooted from the plants that emanate from *Keter*."[141] We must take special notice, therefore, of the requirement to transmit this notion orally. From both contexts it is clear that this caution relates to the impenetrability of the topic to be divulged. Secrecy is demanded, in the first instance, by the complexity of the relationship of *Keter*, which for Gikatilla is identical with the infinite (*ein sof*), to the lower nine emanations—other kabbalists, who distinguished the infinite more sharply from *Keter*, would transfer the dilemma addressed by Gikatilla to the emergence of *Keter* from its source—and second, by considering the apparent absurdity of judgment being transformed into mercy, one thing becoming its opposite. What Gikatilla is alluding to is the speculative conundrum of the beginning, mentioned above, a puzzle that still challenges scientists and philosophers: can the beginning begin without us assuming that it has already begun, for had it not begun, how could it begin? The beginning, as kabbalists were given to say, is the *beit*, the opening letter of the Torah, the first that is second, the initial iteration, the stammer of the naming of the nameless as the inexpressible name, the concealment of *alef*, the origin before beginning, the hiddenness hidden by being revealed.[142]

The two aspects of the arcane assist us in the effort to attend the pulse of temporal eternity from the timbre of eternal temporality, the coming to be of the delimited something (whatever it will be) from the limitless nothing (never what it has been).

In that transition, the moment of creative tension, the schism between old and new cannot be upheld. The point is underscored by the simultaneous attribution of the terms *qadmon* (or *qedem*) and *ehyeh* to *Keter*, the former denoting primordiality and the latter posteriority. The combination of these two names relays the paradox that what was is what will be. Extrapolating the intent of applying *qedem* to *Keter*, Gikatilla wrote:

> Since the *sefirah* of *Keter*, which is called *ehyeh*, precedes all [*qadmah la-kol*], and all the *sefirot* were contained and hidden in it prior to the world's having been created, and when it arose in thought to create the world, the *sefirot* were revealed from the mystery of *Keter*—therefore, it is called *qedem*, for it preceded everything [*qodemet la-kol*], because it is the *sefirah* whence the secret of the *sefirot* was revealed.[143]

The rabbinic designation for God, the "primordial one of the world" (*qadmono shel olam*), is applied to *Keter* because all the *sefirot* "emanate and proceed infinitely and boundlessly" from it.[144] The meontological mystery—the nothing temporally becoming the something it eternally is not—is elucidated by the verse "The Lord God planted a garden in Eden from old,"[145] *wa-yiṭṭa yhwh elohim gan be-eden mi-qedem* (Genesis 2:8):

> The secret of the plants of the Garden were arranged in Eden and planted in the Garden. That is, the plants were planted in the Garden and the Garden was planted in Eden, and this is the secret of the true perfect unity [*sod ha-yiḥud ha-shalem ha-amitti*]. Whence were the Garden and Eden revealed? "From old" [*mi-qedem*], from the supernal Crown [*keter elyon*]. "The Lord God planted a garden in Eden"—whence were they planted? "From old." It is all explained, and thus I will hint at [in the verse] "And his goings forth were from old, from ancient times" (Micah 5:1)—"and his goings forth" certainly were "from old," for from the ancient one the emanation of thought emerges and the secret of the disclosure of the *sefirot*.[146]

Gikatilla's exegesis of the verse provides a succinct sketch of the unity of the sefirotic pleroma: all the forces are comprised in the garden (*Malkhut*), which is comprised in Eden (*Ḥokhmah*), and this, in turn, is comprised in the ancient one (*qedem*) that is the crown (*Keter*). What unfolds differentially was enfolded indifferently within the incomprehensible nothing in which "there is no face or back, and no matter of opposition at all."[147] In the absence of opposition, there is no need to espouse belief in the one in contradistinction to another (even if the other is deemed to be false), because there is nothing but the nothing that egresses endlessly into the nothing of its nothingness. Needless to say, the credo of Jewish monotheism regarding the unconditional dissimilarity between God and world is subverted in the kabbalistic theosophy and displaced by a meontological monism. The wellspring of light that overflows the primeval font is renewed each moment as that which has formerly been, the absolute potential of all that actually exists. The time/summoning (*zeman/zimmun*) that ensues from the interminable largesse, the world of unqualified purity without any admixture of impurity—indeed, a purity beyond the polarity of pure and impure—surpasses the discrepancy between guilt and innocence, merit and blame. This unadulterated white (*loven*)—whence *Keter* assumes the appellation "white head" (*ro'sh lavan*)[148]—is the achromatic peak of the color spectrum, the translucent invisibility that occasions the showing of all visions through the black opacity of *Malkhut*, the prismatic periphery at the other end of the spectrum, although, as I have already duly noted, the first and last of the sefirotic gradations are as much a circle as a line, and thus the absolute fullness of light in the whiteness of *Keter* and the absolute emptiness of light in the blackness of *Malkhut* are identically different in virtue of being differently identical.[149] What we see in the dream, therefore, is an archetypal image cast from and upon the screen of the blank space of infinity mirrored in the infinity of the blank space that is deflected in the imagination of each individual.

The pulsation of time that permeates the whole of reality is this "gratuitous gift,"[150] the rhythmic throb that exceeds the dyad of the (masculine) compulsion to give and the (feminine) aspiration to take. Within the domain of infinite compassion, bestowing is a form of receiving, and receiving a form of bestowing. Transposing this mutuality in temporal terms, we can speak of *Keter* as the timeless time, the time beyond the disjunction of night and day, the time in which day is night and night day. In Gikatilla's own words:

> From *Keter* there flow the wellsprings of everlasting mercy, goodness, and pleasure that do not change and are not altered . . . and this place is called neither day nor night, for there is no day without night and no night without day, and this is the secret of all the nine emanations beneath *Keter*, but *Keter* is called neither day nor night. In the time that it will appear, then there will be a perfect redemption [*ge'ullah sheleimah*], after which there will be no misfortune or sorrow. This is the secret of "But there shall be a continuous day—only the Lord knows when—of neither day nor night" (Zechariah 14:7), and this is the secret of "and there shall be light at eventide" (*ibid.*), for in the rest of the days [it is said] "and this was morning." And this is the secret of "in that day the Lord shall be one and his name shall be one" (*ibid.*, 9).[151]

There is neither day nor night in *Keter*, not because there is both day and night (a difference of identity), but because the darkness of night has been converted into the light of day (an identity of difference).[152] Interestingly, the time of the "continuous day" (*yom eḥad*),[153] which transcends the oscillation of the dimorphic rhythm, characterizes both creation and redemption. The latter, moreover, is presented as the "day" in which God and his name are one. A thematic connection is thus forged between the spontaneous diremption/recurrent irruption and the Tetragrammaton. Similarly, in a passage from the *Tiqqunim*, the name *ehyeh* and the traditional notion of the compresence of the three temporal modes in the Tetragrammaton is accentuated:

> *Ehyeh* is above being [*al hawayah*], and this breath of the heart [*hevel de-libba*] governs[154] the voice of YHWH [*Tif'eret*]; it is the cause of all causes [*illat al kol ha-illot*], hidden and concealed, and it is not revealed, and it governs and rules over everything. *Ehyeh* indicates that the cause of causes [*illat ha-illot*] was, is, and shall be [*hayah howeh we-yihyeh*], and it is the breath that rises to infinity [*ein sof*] by means of which the causes of all causes governs.[155]

Ehyeh is described as "above being" (*al hawayah*); the term *hawayah* has a twofold signification in this context: first, as a generic noun, it signifies the composite of being as such, that is, the being that comprises all beings, and, second, as a proper name, it is assigned to that which can have no proper name, the ineffable name (*shem ha-meforash*), the Tetragrammaton (the letters *yhwh* are a variant permutation of *hwyh*), but, in this case, as in numerous other sources, it is attributed to *Tif'eret*. Confirmation of this interpretation may be adduced from the continuation, where we are apprised of the symbolic depiction of *Keter* as the "breath of the heart," *hevel de-libba*, which governs the "voice of the Tetragrammaton," *qol yhwh*, another reference to *Tif'eret*. Moreover, *ehyeh* is the supernal cause that executes providence (literally, "rides upon") all that exists, the supreme concealment that shows the way to the infinite, the "cause of causes" (*illat ha-illot*), the ontic foundation distinguished from *Keter*, the "cause of all causes" (*illat kol ha-illot*). The paramount emanation divulges the paradoxical compresence of the three tenses comprised in the name; that is, the unutterable name, whether vocalized as *ehyeh* or as *yhwh*, alludes symbolically to the fact that, in the infinite, was, is, and, will be (*hayah howeh we-yihyeh*), past, present, and future, are unified—the mystery of the threefold unity that is a unified trinity, a mystery apprehended as mystery by the spirit carried on the wings of the upward breath, the breath of the heart, that ascends to and evaporates in the impenetrable infinity.[156]

The secret of time is exemplified by *ehyeh*, the name that demarcates the junction of eternality and temporality instantiated in the moment wherein past, present, and future cease to be distinct. Astonishingly, the kabbalistic understanding of temporality as the an-archical infinity actualized, time after time, in the *purely present future*, the future that is already present as the present that is always future—a chiastic paradox that is at the heart of Jewish messianism[157]—is well suited to the remark of Levinas concerning "the zero point in the scale of time: the point where what is comes to be—or is the point of being produced. The present is the future making itself present."[158] *Keter* can suitably be marked as this zero point, where "what is" can be only what "comes to be," the future making itself present as the presence that persists as presently absent.

From the experience of dreaming, episodic as it might be, we can access this point of zero, the negative infinity, in the scale of time, because the dream informs us about the past through a future that is present as the future that is past. Mathematically, the superfluidity of the incursion of the dreamtime is constricted to a triadic point that potentially can expand infinitely. I suspect that such a model inspired Merleau-Ponty's observation that eternity is the "time that belongs to dreaming, and the dream refers back to waking life, from which it borrows all its structures.... It is the field of presence in the wide sense, with its double horizon or primary past and future, and the infinite openness of those fields of presence that have slid by, or are still possible."[159] In Chapter 1, I had the opportunity to engage Merleau-Ponty's reinscription of the Husserlian notion of the field of presence at some length. Suffice it here to underline the aspect of his thinking that bears upon the matter of the temporality of the dream. Eternity and time are not posed oppositionally; on the contrary, the former belongs to dreaming as a mode of the latter. The time of the dream—and I would further presume the dream of time—is described as the *infinite openness* of the field of presence in its double horizon as past and future. Eternity is the circle of time squarely open at the always-ending beginning that is the always-beginning ending.

Waking to a Dream Waking from a Dream

I conclude with an extraordinary passage from Moses de León's *Mishkan ha-Edut* (1293). Introducing the first part of his treatise, a clarification of mundane matters, the author notes that "some of the sages" (*ḥakhamim*)—by which he means philosophers—have comprehended that "the foundation of this world corresponds to the way of nature, where all things decay and perish, and that this world vis-à-vis the supernal world is like the dream vis-à-vis prophecy." De León goes on to contrast the two on the grounds that the dream is pointless and transitory, whereas prophecy is an "enduring matter" (*davar qayyam*) that is "in the divine secret and essentially true " (*be-sod elohi we-iqqar emet*), for when the

> prophet is unified in the level of his wisdom to be conjoined in his form in proximity to the supernal form [*behityaḥed ha-navi be-ma'alat ḥokhmato ledabbeq be-ṣurato eṣel ha-ṣurah ha-elyonit*], he divests himself of all corporeal matters and from all elements of this world [*mishtolel mi-kol ha-devarim ha-gufaniyyim u-mi-kol yesodei ha-olam ha-zeh*], and when through the thought of his form [*be-maḥashevet ṣurato*] he is divested from all corporeal matters, he is conjoined to the supernal forms [*mitdabbeq ba-ṣurot elyonot*].[160]

This concise presentation undoubtedly reflects the Aristotelian-Neoplatonic view (widespread among intellectual elites in the late Middle Ages, but likely known to de León primarily from Maimonides)[161] that prophecy is the conjunction of the human intellect with the supernal form, a disembodied mental state, or at least as far as is humanly possible.[162] Against this backdrop, a stark contrast is made between prophecy and the dream. The former deals with the veritable and the abiding, the latter with the fictitious and the evanescent. Echoing this much older perspective, de León draws the conclusion: "And thus, one should not believe in this world at all, because it is undeniably a dream, as it says, 'Like one who is hungry and dreams he is eating, but wakes to find himself empty' (Isaiah 29:8)."[163] Upon waking, one appreciates that the satiation of hunger was a dream, and this stands metonymically for the whole of our experience in the world of coming to be and passing away. A close parallel to de León's aside is found in Abraham Ibn Ḥasdai's *Ben ha-Melekh we-ha-Nazir* (*The Prince and the Ascetic*), a thirteenth-century Hebraic adaptation of the Barlaam and Josaphat tale, which in all likelihood derived from an Arabic rendering (perhaps based on an earlier Persian version) of the ancient Sanskrit story of the young Buddha: our wakeful state is, in truth, sleep, and hence what we consider to be actual experience with a correspondence to external nature is merely the internal topography of a dream; in death alone is one aroused from the repose of one's wakefulness.[164]

De León is quick to point out the biblical verses where prophecy and dreaming are juxtaposed (Numbers 12:6, Deuteronomy 13:2, Jeremiah 23:28), some of them validating an essential difference and others problematizing it. The difference is epitomized by the prophecy of Moses, which is described (following Maimonides)[165] as most perfect, since it was a vision denuded of all corporeality, seeing through the transparent speculum, the "true splendor, pure and clear" (*zohar amitti zakhah u-varah*), which "does not materialize in a physical vision at all" (*einah nigshemet bi-rei'yyat gufani kelal*). All other prophets see through the opaque speculum, and thus the epiphany does "materialize in accord with their vision" (*nigshemet kefi re'iyyatam*); hence they see only a "bodily image" (*demut guf*). When a dream vision is attributed to a prophet, the verse is speaking about the phenomenon of non-

Mosaic prophecy, but this only fortifies de León's assertion that the world is like a dream.[166] The philosophical point is illustrated by the story he recounts (in the name of the rabbis) of one of the ancient Indian sages (*ḥakhmei hoddu ha-qadmonim*) who came before some other wise men to inquire into the nature of the world; not having received an adequate response, he decided to go to Egypt to ask again about this matter, and there he was instructed about a great king who ruled for more than forty years while holding a cup of wine in hand from which to drink. The sage inferred from what he was told that the "the world is a dream and futile [*ha-olam hu ḥalom we-hevel*], and it has nothing advantageous."[167]

It is hardly coincidental that de León uses a tale about an Indian sage as a didactic point of emphasis. The portrayal of India as a repository of mysterious and remote wisdom, sometimes classified negatively as pagan or barbaric superstition, is well documented in medieval Jewish authors (Saadya Gaon, Judah Halevi, Maimonides, Moses Ibn Ezra, and Shem Ṭov Ibn Falaquera). This Orientalizing myth, originating in the Hellenistic accounts of Indian antiquity, was enhanced by the augmented circulation of oral traditions and written texts amongst Jewish scholars, whence it permeated to more popular forms of cultural transmission, such as the Hebrew versions of the Alexander Romance, the tenth-century chronicle *Sefer Yossipon*, and the especially germane collection of fables *Kalilah and Dimnah*, rendered into Hebrew in the thirteenth century by the Spanish poet Jacob ben Eleazar.[168] De León utilized this topos to chronicle the truth that the world is a dream,[169] a reverberation of the well-known Hindu doctrine of *māyā* (especially as it was elaborated by proponents of the nonduality of the Advaita Vedānta school), the conviction that the sensible world of differentiation obscures the nondifferentiated oneness of ultimate reality.[170]

It lies beyond the scope of this chapter to enter into a lengthy discussion of the philosophical intricacies of this topic—rooted in the older mythological conception of the world arising from the dream of the creator-god Viṣṇu[171]—but I will present a brief reckoning to orient the reader toward my main objective, which is to shed light on de León's cursory comment. I am mindful of the peril of offering a generalization culled from such an intricate and multifaceted complex of traditions; we are today more sensitive to the fact that any ideational-cultural phenomenon exceeds both our taxonomic classifications and our attempts at historiographical reconstruction, which for the most part are retrospective inventions that enable us to group together differing and perhaps even conflicting factors under the rubric of a distinct entity. Nonetheless, in my judgment, it is still theoretically warranted and heuristically viable to account for the variant expressions in different historical periods by identifying patterns of thought and unified systems. Moving beyond the postmodern critique of essence and the deconstructionist appeal to *différance*, both of which preserve the dichotomous reasoning they seek to undermine, we are justified in adopting a hermeneutical method that may be labeled *polychromatic essentialism* or *essentialist polychromatism*, that is, an essentialism that presumes that sameness is precisely what generates difference, that the discontinuity of the continuous prompts the continuity of the discontinuous, that polysemy is fostered by resemblance and diversification by integration.[172]

With regard to the particular topic at hand, we can say that the core belief is that the cosmos in all its corporal vivacity is a delusion, which implies that everything is either a mental projection of individual consciousness[173] or a magical chimera brought about by the sportive power (*śakti*) of Brahman personified in the form of Īśvara, the Lord of the world, the Self of the universe.[174] Both interpretations, however, yield the same insight: whether we imagine that the human mind is duped by the transcendental mirage that is God's ploy or by the empirical hallucination that is the collective cognitive error we suffer as sentient beings,[175] the objects we experience are construed as real, but in the truth of their untruth, they are apparitions to which neither reality nor unreality can be justly ascribed. The enlightened mind, which attains release (*mokṣa*) from the cycle of death and rebirth (*saṃsāra*), comprehends that the universe is like a dream,[176] which, in the words of the *Brahma-sūtra*, "is only an illusion, for its nature is not completely manifest."[177] To be more precise, in terms of the Advaitic epistemological hierarchy, based on the four states of consciousness delineated in the *Chāndogya* and *Māṇḍūkya Upaniṣads*—waking, dreaming, deep sleep, and a state that encompasses, but supersedes all three—just as dreaming exhibits radical discontinuity vis-à-vis waking, so the world of conditionality is radically discontinuous with nondual consciousness (*Brahma-caitanya*). Wakefulness is a sublation of dreamful sleep, and dreamful sleep a sublation of the slumber in which there is no consciousness, but in comparison with the ultimate attainment, wakefulness is itself a dream state, and the objects that one perceives in the former are as illusory as the entities that one imagines in the latter; in perceiving this, one awakes from the dream of wakefulness in the wakefulness of the dream.[178] In the language of the *Āgama-prakaraṇa*, the first section of the *Āgama Śāstra*, the earliest known treatise of the Śaṅkara school of Advaita Vedānta, which is attributed to the eighth-century guru Gauḍapāda, the four states of self—waking (*viśva*), dreaming (*taijasa*), sleeping (*prājña*), and the fourth (*turya*) beyond the threefold—are described as follows:

> The first two (i.e. waking and dreaming) are joined with dream and sleep; *prājña*, on the other hand, is bound with sleep but not with dream. Those with firm conviction see neither sleep nor even dream in *turya*. Dream is for one comprehending otherwise (i.e. falsely); sleep is for one who does not know reality (*tattva*). When these two errors are destroyed, one attains *turīya*. When the individual who is asleep owing to the beginningless illusion awakens, then he awakens to the birthless, sleepless, dreamless nonduality.[179]

In another part of the *Āgama Śāstra*, the *Vaitathya-prakaraṇa*, less likely to have been written by Gauḍapāda, the illusionistic (*māyā-vāda*) interpretation of the Vedānta is more pronounced; the distinction between dream and reality dissolves inasmuch as the entities perceived in both are ascertained to be unreal:

> Verily, the wise say that dream and waking states are one, on the basis of the well-established reasoning concerning the sameness of the entities in the two states.... Though on a par with things unreal, things are seen as if they were not unreal.... Even in the dream state, again, what is imagined by the mind within verily does not exist; what is apprehended by the mind outside does exist. The unreality of both these is seen. Even in the waking state, again, what is imagined by the mind within verily does not exist; what is apprehended by the mind outside does exist. The unreality of both

> these is reasonable.... As dream and magic (*svapna-māyā*) are seen, and as an illusory city in the sky, so is this universe seen by those who are well-versed in the Vedānta.... This world is not manifold at all, either by the nature of the Self or by its own nature. Nothing whatever is different or non-different. The knowers of the truth (*tattva*) know this.[180]

As Gauḍapāda's successor and disciple, the Indian philosopher Śaṅkara (788–820), remarked:

> the entire complex of phenomenal existence is considered as true as long as the knowledge of Brahman being the Self of all has not arisen; just as the phantoms of a dream are considered to be true until the sleeper wakes. For as long as a person has not reached the true knowledge of the unity of Self, so long it does not enter his mind that the world of effects with its means and objects of right knowledge and its results of actions is untrue; he rather, in consequence of his ignorance, looks on mere effects... as forming part of and belonging to his Self, forgetful of Brahman being in reality the Self of all.... The case is analogous to that of a dreaming man who in his dream sees manifold things, and, up to the moment of waking, is convinced that his ideas are produced by real perception without suspecting the perception to be a merely apparent one.[181]

Śaṅkara is adamant that while we may label the effects of a dream as "unreal," this is not true of the consciousness that the dreaming person has of them. "This consciousness is a real result; for it is not sublated by the waking consciousness. The man who has risen from sleep does indeed consider the effects perceived by him in his dream such as being bitten by a snake, bathing in a river, &c. to be unreal, but he does not on that account consider the consciousness he had of them to be unreal likewise."[182] In a manner reminiscent of the blurring of the distinction between dream and wakefulness that emerges from the phenomenologies of Husserl and Merleau-Ponty discussed in Chapter 1,[183] Śaṅkara subtly distinguished the content and the event of dreaming. Just as one does not comprehend the unreality of the former until one awakens from the latter, so, too, waking consciousness is prone to judge its objects real until it awakens to nondual awareness and perceives the spectral nature of everything experienced.[184] Paul Deussen, the noted Sanskritologist, summarized the "higher doctrine" (*parā vidyā* or *samyagdarçanam*) of Śaṅkara's Vedānta philosophy:

> In the department of Theology it teaches that the Brahman is not thus or thus, but altogether without attributes (*guṇa*), distinctions (*viçesha*) and limitations (*upâdhi*), and therefore in no way capable of being defined or conceived. And this Brahman, devoid of all limitation, is the only being, outside which nothing is; therefore, in the department of Cosmology, there can be as little question of the origin of the world as of its existence, but only of there being neither anything different (*nânâ*) from the Brahman, nor any plurality of things (*prapañca*), and that the world extended in names and forms is non-existent (*avastu*), is only a glamour (*mâyâ*) which Brahman, as master-magician (*mâyâvin*), projects (*prasârayati*), as the dreamer projects dream forms.[185]

The Vedāntic principle of *māyā*, according to Walter Y. Evans-Wentz, was adapted in the various schools of Buddhism, which affirmed that "the whole world and cosmic creation, subjective and objective, is illusory, and that mind is the sole reality.... *Māyā* is the Magic Veil, ever worn by Nature, the Great Mother Isis, which veils Reality. It is by *yoga* alone that the Veil can be rent asunder and man led to self-knowledge and self-conquest, whereby Illusion is transcended."[186] Substances within the universe, therefore, are "mind-made; they are of the marrow of which dreams are shaped. It is their illusiveness which is *māyā*.... Through innumerable myriads of forms, through innumerable myriads of eyes and sense-organs of creatures, through innumerable myriads of microcosms, Mind knows Itself to be the Dreamer of *Māyā*'s Kingdom. But until the Mirage of Being is scattered by Bodhic-Enlightenment, the many know not the One."[187] The dream "shows that even as all sensuous experiences of the waking state are illusory, equally illusory are all sensuous experiences of the dream state; these two states forming the two poles of human consciousness. In other words, nature as a whole is the Dream of One Mind; and until man conquers nature, and thereby transcends *māyā*, he will remain asleep, dreaming the Dream of ignorance."[188] The meditational praxis provokes "the *yogin* to arise from the Sleep of Delusion, from the Nightmare of Existence, to break the shackles in which *māyā* thus held him prisoner throughout the aeons, and so attain spiritual peace and joy of Freedom, even as did the Fully Awakened One, Gautama the Buddha."[189]

Grasping the dreamlike nature of experience, the mind, emancipated from nescience (*avidyā*),[190] attains the *samādhi* of the "sphere of neither-ideation nor-nonideation," the "all-knowing awareness" in which saṃsāric existence is severed,[191] and the disparity between actual and apparent dissipates, a hyperrealism—what is most real is the unreal—that resonates with what some have marked as a distinguishing trait of certain strands of modern-day physics.[192] The Upaniṣadic-Vedāntic hypothesis that reality is a dream culminated in the Buddhist teaching—encapsulated in the Mādhyamika precepts of emptiness (*śūnyatā*) and dependent origination (*pratītyasamutpāda*)—that all phenomena are empty, devoid of inherent existence, phantasms like the echo in the cave or the moonlight on the water. In the poetic rendering of the hymn to the Buddha Śākyamuni, *In Praise of the Incomparable*, transmitted in the name of Nāgārjuna, the renowned Indian philosopher of the first two centuries, who purportedly established the Madhyamaka school of Mahāyāna Buddhism:

> O blameless One, you have realized
> That the world of beings, just like an echo,
> Is free from unity and multiplicity
> And lacks transmigration and destruction.
>
> Lord, you have realized that cyclic existence
> Is free from permanence and extinction
> And lacks characteristics and what is to be characterized,
> Just like a dream or an illusion.[193]

The wheel has turned full circle with the explicit delineation of awakened mindfulness as perceiving the image as image, seeing through rather than disposing of the veil of visuality.[194] Enlightenment is beholding the emptiness that cannot be held, envisioning the reality of the dream from the dream that is reality, a cognizance that is central to the Yogācāra school, as well.[195] In the forty-fifth verse of *Yuktiṣaṣṭikā*, Nāgārjuna wrote:

> Those who accept dependent things
> As being like the moon in water,

> Neither [intrinsically] real nor unreal,
> Are not deprived by addictive views.[196]

In the continuation of the poem (53–56), the second Buddha, as Nāgārjuna is nicknamed, compares the unenlightened, the "worldly people," to a child who falls in love with a mirror image and mistakes it for truth, and hence they "are trapped in a thicket of objects." The enlightened, by contrast, are the "great souls," who see with the "eye of intuitive wisdom" that "things" are actually "like mirror images," that is, they pierce through the image of the image through the image. Understanding the formless nature of forms, they are not stuck in the "quicksand of objects." Being neither attached to nor detached from the beauty of those objects, they perceive it as empty, like an illusory person, and thus they reach nirvāṇa.[197] Following the logic of this argument, which carries us beyond the binary of subject and object, the dreamer would be no more real than what is dreamt; the irreality of the one is inconceivable without the irreality of the other, and thus, neither should be privileged. Indeed, as the Third Karmapa of the Tibetan Karma Kagyü sect, Rangjung Dorje (1284–1339), commented on the thought of nonduality in the *Zabmo Nangdon* (*The Profound Inner Reality*):

> But the thought, "There is no duality of apprehender and apprehended, and they are empty" is not real or ultimate either. For, just as you may think, "[My] son is no more" after you have dreamt that he died, though there is no son who could [really] die in a dream, this consciousness about the lack of thought that thinks, "Apprehender and apprehended are not established as two" [just] turns into a great thought, with which you boast to yourself. Śāntideva['s *Bodhicaryāvatāra*] says:
>
> > Therefore, the lack of a delusive entity
> > Is clearly delusive [too].
> > Thus, when one's son dies in a dream,
> > The conception "He does not exist"
> > Removes the thought that he does not exist,
> > But it is also delusive.[198]

The dream is a "double delusion," the verity of which is apprehended when one comes to know one is dreaming while one is dreaming, and in so doing, one sees the cloud through the transparency that is the cloud.[199]

From the nondualist vantage point, illusion is truth, and hence the dream is accorded the liberative capacity of awakening—one awakens not from, but into the dream.[200] This is the crux of the remarks of Dōgen in the fascicle of the *Shōbōgenzō* (*The True Dharma-Eye Treasury*) entitled *Muchū Setsumu* (*Disclosing a Dream within a Dream*):

> The domain and association of the Buddhas, and the Way and cushion of the patriarchs, is realization beyond realization . . . and disclosing a dream within a dream. . . . This is the way the Buddhas turn the Dharma-wheel. . . . Each and every manifestation of the entire universe is a dream . . . you must understand that the path to attaining the Way is realized through illusion surpassing illusion. . . . Because supreme enlightenment is supreme enlightenment, a dream is called a dream. It is a dream disclosing a dream within . . . or, within a dream disclosing a dream. . . . If there is no within a dream, there is no disclosing a dream. If there is no disclosing a dream, there is no within a dream. If there is no disclosing a dream, there are no Buddhas. If there is no within a dream, the Buddhas do not appear to turn the wondrous Dharma. The Dharma-wheel is [transmitted] only between a Buddha and a Buddha; that is disclosing a dream within a dream. Indeed, the supreme enlightenment of all Buddhas and all patriarchs only appears in disclosing a dream within a dream. . . . Just as emptiness pervades itself, disclosing a dream within a dream grasps objects while allowing them to play in emptiness. This is the manifest body of balance in emptiness, for balance is the great Way of the scales. . . . A dream is the entire world, and the entire world is balance.[201]

For Dōgen, to disclose the dream within the dream, that is, to comprehend that the world is a dream, brings one to the supreme truth of the nonduality of mind and matter, the realization that the phenomenal is the absolute, that the contingent is necessary because only the necessary is contingent, that the sentient universe of conditioned beings is the unconditional, insentient Buddha nature, that even the distinction between nirvāṇa and saṃsāra is overcome (as Nāgārjuna had already taught) in the truth-body (*dharmakāya*) that appears as everything possible because it is nothing actual, the emptiness that is the true nature of things.[202] Recapitulating the point in the *Busshō* (*Buddha-nature*) fascicle of the *Shōbōgenzō*, Dōgen renders the statement from the twenty-seventh chapter of the *Mahāparinirvāṇa Sūtra*, "All sentient beings without exception have the Buddha-nature," as "*entire being* is the Buddha-nature" or "*entire being* is in itself completely and totally emancipated suchness. "[203] From the vantage point of this meontology, there is no basis to discriminate dream and reality: what is seems to be what seems to be what is. The comprehension of this (un)truth leads to a reversal specified by Dōgen in the *Genjōkōan*: buddhas "greatly enlighten illusion," as opposed to sentient beings, who are "greatly deluded amid enlightenment." The latter seek enlightenment—the letting go that cannot be seized but by the self that realizes there is no self to be realized that is neither self nor not-self[204]—and thus they "proceed amid their illusion deeper into further delusion," whereas the former "go on realizing Buddhahood continuously," without the need to perceive that they are buddhas, attaining the state of enlightenment in which "all trace of enlightenment disappears."[205] To be of bodhi mind, then, is to apperceive that even the "supreme and perfect awakening" (*anuttara-samtak-sambodhi*) is fleeting and flimsy like a dream.

Remarkably, de León seems not only to have approved of this worldview, but to have considered it conceptually on a par with Jewish esotericism, even though he does not contend that the Indian wisdom originated with the secret teaching of the Jews, an idea reinforced by the phonetic association of the name "Abraham" and the term "Brahmin."[206] This dimension of kabbalistic gnosis is corroborated in an especially poignant way by a number of leading masters of East-European Ḥasidism. In the previous chapter, I delved into some Ḥabad sources that articulate this perspective. I will here provide a modest sampling of a few more examples. Jacob Joseph of Polonnoye (d. 1782), one of the most important disciples of the Besht, thus commented on Jacob's nocturnal vision at Bethel: "'He had a dream' (Genesis 28:12), that is, he saw that this entire world is like a dream, as it is written 'we will be as dreamers' (Psalms 126:1). He saw that the only benefit of this world is that it will be for a person 'like a ladder set on the ground' (Genesis 28:12), so that one can do preparation in this world by means of which one ascends, 'and its top reached to the sky' (*ibid.*)."[207] From the fuller context, we learn that the pneumatic ascent comes about through the noetic elevation of the Hebrew letters by means of one being conjoined to the "inwardness of the spirituality of the light of the infinite" (*penimiyyut ruḥaniyyut or ein sof*) contained therein. The escalation of mind is predicated on discerning the linguistic essence of material substances, a rudimentary precept affirmed uniformly by practitioners of the various trends of Jewish mysticism/esotericism through the ages.[208] When Jacob was passionately conjoined to the letters of the Torah, he was divested of corporeality (*nitpashet me-ha-gashmiyyut*), and he dreamt the dream that educates us more generally about the dreamlike nature of the universe, that the materiality that appears to be real is in fact nothing but the facade that the luminosity of the letters assumes in the guise of an ontically autonomous world vis-á-vis the divine. In truth, the sole substance that is real is the light of infinity, the nameless essence that is arrayed in the letters of the Tetragrammaton, or the Torah, which comprises all of the Hebrew alphabet. We can speak of the corporeal world manifesting the divine presence, therefore, only if we apprehend that the manifestation is an occlusion—precisely by hiding the light beyond space and time does nature expose it through the guise of spatiotemporal coordinates. Conjunction of human thought with divine thought, the pinnacle of the contemplative ladder, is predicated on discerning this ontological truism, which is the conceptual basis for the pietistic mandate to transfigure the somatic semiotically, to transform the carnal body into the linguistic body.[209] Jacob's perceiving that the universe is a dream signifies his awakening from the dream within the contours of the dream. It is in this sense that the oneiric accords one the possibility to see the veil of truth through the truth of the veil.

In a compilation of dicta ascribed to Dov Baer, the Maggid of Międzyrzecz, a distinction is made between our sense of sight in the day and the ability to dream at night: in our wakefulness, we see the material reality and contemplate that the spiritual is garbed therein, whereas in sleep, we are capable of seeing the "spiritual naked without any garment" (*ha-ruḥani arum beli levush*). The Hebrew term for dream, *ḥalom*, conveys this notion inasmuch as it is connected to the expression "moments of lucidity" (*ittim ḥalim*),[210] that is, when the soul is divested of the body, the person can envision the vitality of being without any investiture, imagining the form that is without form, the form of the formless. The capacity to dream bestows on everyone the opportunity to attain the gradation of prophecy (with the exception of Moses, who was capable of seeing the vitality within the material while awake).[211] But how can there be a vision of denuded truth when the truth is a matter of spirit that cannot be seen? The task of contemplation is to see through—rather than to eliminate—the shroud, to comprehend that concealment is what makes disclosure possible, since what is disclosed can be disclosed only to the extent that it is concealed. The dream is upheld as the locus of enlightened consciousness; it is the speculum through which we grasp that the world is like a dream, that there is no way to access truth in this world except through the dissimilitude of the image. The dream is likened to the world to come, for just as the latter is thought to be above time, so while dreaming, one can traverse a long distance in a single moment; in the dream, time is undone (*ha-zeman baṭṭel mi-meṣi'ut*).[212] In the final analysis, what the dream divulges is that the phenomenal world is the dream from which one must awaken by waking to the dream that one is merely dreaming that one is awake. The oneiric, therefore, symbolizes not only exile, but redemption; indeed, one might say the dream signifies both at once to the degree that through the dream, one ascertains the wakeful character of the dream and the dreamful character of wakefulness.

According to a tradition transmitted in the name of Phineḥas of Korzec, but perhaps preserving the teaching of another disciple of the Besht, Shmeril of Virchivkeh:[213] "For the *ḥolem* is above the letters, and the world was created by means of the twenty-two letters, and this is [the meaning of] 'When the Lord restores the fortunes of Zion, we will be as dreamers' (Psalm 126:1), we will be above the way of nature [*lema'lah mi-derekh ha-ṭeva*] just as the *ḥolem* is above the letters."[214] The *ḥolem* is located on top of the letters, but is still one of the ways that the letters are vocalized, so the dream lifts one above nature, but in the manner of remaining as part of nature. To be above nature, therefore, is not to inhabit a supernatural realm; it is to perceive nature for what it is, the metaphysical within the physical, the transcendent within the immanent. According to another exegesis attributed to Phineḥas of Korzec: "All of the sciences [*ḥokhmot*] are the refuse of Torah [*pesolet ha-torah*], for by means of them, the Torah is purified [*nitbarer*], and this is 'When the Lord restores the fortunes of Zion, we will be as dreamers,' for then it will be revealed to everyone that all the sciences and the whole exile were for the sake of purifying consciousness [*levarer moḥin*], like the aspect of the dream."[215] The purifying capacity of exile is explained by the comparison of the secular sciences and the wisdom of Torah. In the period of darkness, the former serve the role of cleansing human consciousness so that it can eventually receive the true light of the latter, and in that sense, the sciences are called the refuse of Torah. Correspondingly, the dream is labeled the "refuse of consciousness" (*pesolet ha-moaḥ*), because consciousness is purified by means of the dream,[216] that is, sleep is the apparatus by which the heart—the "point in the dream"[217]—can form images of that which is beyond all images. If we follow the logic of the argument, then liberation from exile consists not of departing therefrom, but rather of becoming more deeply enrooted therein until one apprehends that there is nothing from which to be delivered but the expectation that one will be delivered.

That the dream is singled out as the most fitting metaphor to convey the ideal of deliverance from the need to be delivered is commensurate with the fact that it is by nature a virtual reality. The point is made even more explicit in an interpretation of the verse "He had a dream, a stairway was set on the ground and its top reached the sky, and angels of God were going up and down on it" (Genesis 28:12) transmitted in the name of Phineḥas of Korzec:

> The dream is the refuse of thought [*pesolet ha-maḥashavah*], and as the thought is more subtle, so the dream is superlative. And [in the case of] the magnanimous righteous men, the dream is through an angel [created from] his own thought... therefore it is written by Jacob, "He had a dream, a stairway was set on the ground etc. and angels of God were going up and down on it," [and it is mentioned that] they ascended first, for those angels were from his very thought; thus, they ascended initially and afterward they descended to him in his dream. From the exceptional thought of the magnanimous righteous

> men an angel is produced, and that angel comes to him in a dream, for there are ten gradations of angels, *er'elim*, *ishim* etc.[218] They are called *ishim*, for they are created from human beings, and thus sleep comes to draw down the refuse from thought below.[219]

At first blush, the classification of the dream as the "refuse of thought" would seem to imply an inferior epistemic level. In fact, however, it indicates the opposite, for it is only through the refuse of thought that thought can be purged. To ascertain that the angels that came to Jacob—and, by extension, to any righteous being—were produced by his thoughts is the crucial step on the path to the purification of thought, which is the spiritual meaning of redemption. The dream instrumentally brings one to apprehending that the reality that is thought to be external to the mind is confabulated mentally. This explains the inherently figurative nature of the dream. Thus, commenting on the verse "When a prophet of the Lord arises among you, I make myself known to him in a vision, I will speak to him in a dream" (Numbers 12:6), Phineḥas of Korzec taught:

> For in a dream, that matter is garbed in allusion [*remez*] and this is like the content of a matter that is comprehended through a parable [*mashal*], for without the parable, we could not comprehend the content of the matter, which is sublime. Through this you can understand the prophecy [related in the words] "I will speak to him in a dream"; it is for him only a dream, but he comprehends from it the truth of the very sublime matter. Your prophecy in relation to him is merely a garment to comprehend more from it.[220]

Parabolic images, the material of the dream, are the apparel by which one journeys to the shore without images, the place beyond place, the time beyond time. From the voyage, the dreamer gathers that the escape from bondage consists of discerning that there is no bondage from which to escape but the bondage of thinking that there is something from which to escape. To know that the universe is a dream is to be privy to the truth that untruth lies coiled like a serpent in the heart of truth. The wise comprehend that there is no way for truth to be manifest but through the concealment of truth.

Moses Ḥayyim Ephraim of Sudlykow, the grandson of the Beshṭ, notes in his exposition of Psalms 126:1 that the comparison of exile to a dream is based on the fact that the dreamer imagines false things to be true. Redemption, by contrast, will consist of seeing the "complete truth" as it is, without any semblance of deceit.[221] It is interesting to note that there is a written record of some of the oneiric revelations that this master experienced, including visitations of his illustrious grandfather.[222] We can safely assume that the dream was considered by him and his followers to be an important source of knowledge. That the dream vision is comparable to exile does not denote an inferior state; on the contrary, the metaphor signifies the dream's superiority, since to be redeemed is to wake from the dream that we call life. Emancipation from exile, accordingly, consists first and foremost of knowing that one is exiled. In this vein, Ṣadoq ha-Kohen of Lublin remarked: "Thus, this entire world is called a 'world of deceit and imagination' [*alma de-shiqra we-dimyon*] as it written 'When [the Lord restores the fortunes of Zion], we will be as dreamers' (Psalms 126:1). But in this world, it appears as truth [*nidmeh la-emet*]."[223] In another context, he wrote: "It is known that this world is called the 'world of deceit,' that is, in truth, all that is seen by the eye is deceitful and imaginary, for what is momentary is called 'deceit,' but in the future there will be the resurrection of the dead, and it will become clear that death is imaginary,[224] as it is written 'we will be as dreamers,' and what is in a dream is not true at all."[225]

Oddly, this facet of Jewish esotericism (admittedly incubated in the world-denying cosmology that was rife in medieval Europe) has been largely neglected by academic exponents and traditional practitioners. To be enlightened means to peer through—and not to abolish—the veneer of nature by perceiving that all that exists is naught but a veil by which the enframing light beyond the veil is manifestly hidden in the hidden manifestation of that veil. We can speak of the sensual world disclosing the essence (within, but outside that world) if we comprehend that disclosing here means hiding; what worldliness reveals is the concealment of nothing that is concealment and hence concealed only when revealed with the lifting of the curtain to expose, as Shakespeare famously put it, that "nothing is but what is not" (*Macbeth* 1.iii). By means of this vision, as dim as it might seem, one may be roused to awaken from the dream that one is not dreaming the dream that one is not dreaming. To take in that we are indeed "such stuff as dreams are made on" (*The Tempest* IV.i) is to be stirred from the dream of life into the truer reality that is the life of dream.

Let me conclude by noting that the appropriation of the Indian wisdom on the part of masters of Jewish esotericism has an analogue in Islamic mystical sources. To illustrate the point, I mention two examples. The first is from the interpretation of the *ḥadīth* "Men sleep, and when they die, they shall awake" in the section on Joseph's dreams and visions in Ibn al-'Arabī's *Fuṣūṣ al-ḥikam*:

> all that is seen in sleep being of a similar nature . . . his whole earthly life was after this fashion, [earthly existence] being a dream within a dream. All things of this kind come within the realm of the Imagination, because of which they are interpreted. That means that something that of itself has a certain form appears in another form, so that the interpreter proceeds from the form seen by the dreamer to the form of the thing in itself. . . . If what we say is true, the Cosmos is but a fantasy without any real existence, which is another meaning of the Imagination. That is to say, you imagine that it [the Cosmos] is something separate and self-sufficient, outside the Reality, while in truth it is not so. . . . If things are as we have decided, know that you are an imagination, as is all that you regard as other than yourself an imagination. All [relative] existence is an imagination within an imagination.[226]

From the viewpoint of the illuminated wisdom (*al-ḥikmat an-nūrīyah*) of the Ṣūfi, to say that the world is imagination combines the Indian tradition of the illusory character of the world with the notion that all that exists in the sensible world is an analogical image of the spiritual realities that assume form only in the human imagination. The universe can be called, therefore, the "world of imagination" (*'ālam al-khayāl*), as well as the "world of analogies" (*'ālam al-mithāl*). In the same text, Ibn al-'Arabī depicts the cosmos as the "shadow" of God.[227] The affinity between this language and the Vedāntic notion of the world as Māyā has been duly noted.[228]

The second illustration of the utilization of this theme in Islamic esotericism is found in the following verses from the majestic narrative poem *Mathnawī*, composed by the Persian mystic R mī (1207–1273), who was more or less contemporary with de León:

> This world is a dream—do not rest in (false) opinion.... The Prophet said of this world, which is substantial in appearance, that it is the sleeper's dream.
>
> You have accepted this (statement) conventionally, (but) the travellers (on the mystic Way) have beheld this (truth) clairvoyantly, without (relation from) the Prophet.
>
> You are asleep in the daytime: do not say that this is not sleep. The shadow (reflexion) is derivative, the origin (of it) is naught but the moonlight.
>
> Know, O comrade, that your sleep and waking (your life in this world) is as though a sleeper should dream that he has gone to sleep.
>
> He thinks, "Now I am asleep," (and is) unaware that he is (really) in the second sleep.[229]

The perspicacity by which one apprehends that the world is "substantial in appearance" (*bi-ṣūrat*), and hence akin to a "sleeper's dream" (*ḥulm-i nāyim*), is attributed to Muḥammad. Reynold A. Nicholson, the editor and translator of Rūmī's text, records that in the *Fātiḥu 'l-abyāt*, a Turkish commentary on the *Mathnawī*, Ismā'īl Anqirawī cites a *ḥadīth* on the authority of Jābir ibn 'Abdallāh al-Anṣārī "to the effect that a fair-complexioned man, who really was the Archangel Gabriel, came to the Prophet and asked, 'What is this world?' The prophet replied, '*Ḥulmu 'l-ná'im*.'"[230] The poet, too, cites the tradition that the world is a dream of one asleep; however, he points out that those who traverse the mystical path (*sālikān*) behold that truth by themselves, without any recourse to the words of the prophet that most people accept as a matter of convention (*taqlīd*). Just as the shadow is a reflection of the moonlight, so everyday consciousness is in truth a state of ignorance in which the sensible world seems to be real. The alternation of sleep and wakefulness is compared, therefore, to a sleeper who dreams that he has gone to sleep. Thinking in the dream that he is now asleep, he is not aware that he had to have already been in a somnambulant condition in order to dream that he is going to sleep. The objects perceived in waking hours are themselves material images of the dream world (*'ālamu 'l-mithāl*); passing from being awake to sleep, consequently, is not crossing a radical disjuncture, but rather swinging like a pendulum from one chimerical realm to another.[231] From the perspective of one who is enlightened, wakefulness is itself a state of somnolence—or, as Rūmī puts it in the tale of the Sūfī engaged in meditation in the garden, the "heedless sleep" (*khvāb-i ghaflat*)[232]—and what is deemed to be sleep is in fact a "second sleep." The universe, as 'Abdu 'l-Karmīn ibn Ibrāhīm al-Jīlī wrote in his *Insānu 'l-kāmil* (*Perfect Man*), exists as a dream in the perception of the dreamer, and thus it is nothing but "a thought within a thought within a thought" (*khayālun fī khayālin fī khayāl*).[233]

Many more examples from various other religio-cultural contexts could have been adduced to lend credence to what Foucault spoke of as the "last stage" of the "great mythology of the dream, the fantastic cosmogony of the dream where the whole universe seems to conspire at a momentary and vacillating image," an idea he supports by citing the following passage from Schelling: "The world becomes dream, the dream becomes world, and the outcome in which one believes can be seen coming from afar."[234] I will conclude this chapter with a glimmer of this vision that may be gleaned from a stanza in Allen Ginsberg's poem "The Change: *Kyoto-Tokyo Express*," written on July 18, 1963:

> In this dream I am the dreamer
> and the Dreamed I am
> that I Am Ah but I have
> always known[235]

Noteworthy is that the American bard verbalized the collapse of the partition of subject and object in the spacetime of the dream by invoking the name that God revealed to Moses. To be sure, for Ginsberg, the unity of dreamer and dreamed within the confines of the dream is illumined by a decidedly nontheistic (perhaps "a/theistic" would be more suitable) application of the biblical slogan (rendered in accord with the King James version). Just as self-autonomy breaks down in the appreciation that in the dream, there is no difference between the one who dreams and what is dreamt, so in the case of the nothing, there is no substance of being that can be distinguished from the process of becoming. Ironically, through a Buddhist-inflected exegesis—that the poem was written in Japan is hardly inconsequential—Ginsberg was able to recover the zoharic understanding implied in translating *ehyeh asher ehyeh* as *ana ma'n da-ana*, "I am what I am," that is to say, there is no ego (divine or human) that can be severed from the eternal oscillation of temporal fluctuation. This is something the "I" has always known, as long as the I realizes that there is no I to realize that there is no I to realize. In attaining the self that is to be eradicated, the self of no-self[236]—negating the affirmation of negation by affirming the negation of affirmation[237]—one is liberated from the need to posit a personal deity, even if presumed to be invisible.[238] Deliverance from the impulse for theolatry, a quagmire into which theism seems always susceptible of falling,[239] comes by surrendering to the awareness that what we think of as reality in contrast to the dream is naught but a dream of there being reality apart from the dream.

The trail of philosophical inquiry we have embarked upon thus leads back to the poetic word declaimed at a previous moment as the disclosive withdrawal of what is always belatedly still to come:

> there is a dream
> that dreams itself
> before the dream begins—
> a dream dreamt
> in the dreamless dream
> of a dream that no longer dreams
> the dream dreamt in the dream[240]

In the dreamless dream, the dream before the dream, one dreams the dream that is dreamt as the dream one no longer dreams. By interpreting that dream, the dream within the dream, we edge ever closer to waking from the dream that we are dreaming that we are waking from the dream.

Notes

PREFACE

1. Peter Struck, *Birth of the Symbol: Ancient Readers at the Limits of Their Texts* (Princeton: Princeton University Press, 2004), p. 177. See also Eva T. H. Brann, *The World of the Imagination: Sum and Substance* (Lanham: Rowman & Littlefield, 1991), pp. 335–36: "Dreams are of all representational events the most imaginal in two senses: They are imagistic insofar as they consist largely of mental imagery, and they are imaginative insofar as they contain the most abandoned fancies. Dreaming is also, to tell the long and the short of it, a mystery. . . . if by a mystery is meant a phenomenon that conceals itself in the very act of revealing itself, dreams may be called mysteries."

2. David Foulkes, *Dreaming: A Cognitive-Psychological Analysis* (Hillsdale: Lawrence Erlbaum Associates, 1985), pp. 32–37.

3. The term "mythopoetic function" was coined in the nineteenth century by Frederic W. H. Myers to name the tendency in people to weave fantasies when in a trance or reverie. See Henri Ellenberger, *The Discovery of the Unconscious: The History and Evolution of Dynamic Psychiatry* (New York: Basic Books, 1970), p. 314, cited in Douglass Price-Williams, "The Waking Dream in Ethnographic Perspective," in *Dreaming: Anthropological and Psychological Interpretations*, edited by Barbara Tedlock (Cambridge: Cambridge University Press, 1987), p. 246. See also Rollo May, "Introduction," in Leopold Caligor and Rollo May, *Dreams and Symbols: Man's Unconscious Language* (New York: Basic Books, 1968), pp. 4–5: "We need to remind ourselves that dreams are *trans*logical as well as *pre*logical. They are a form of communication with ourselves and our world which includes many dimensions at once, and therefore it is entirely understandable that they should, as Jung and Fromm (in his early work) have argued, include insight and reveal not only greater error and evil but also greater wisdom and ethical sensitivity than the person was aware he possessed in his conscious life." And see *ibid.*, pp. 8–9: "Unconscious experience does

have its own *form*.... This form has more in common with art than with logical forms. The language which is unique to unconscious experience is the symbol and myth. Here symbol and myth come into their own, not as rationalized explanations but as their own language.... The symbol and myth present a totality of meaning which 'grasps' us, a meaning which contains a union of feeling, willing, and thinking. It seems to me we lose the power of a dream and other unconscious experience when we reduce them to rationalized words, for they then become 'signs' rather than 'symbols'" (emphasis in the original). For May, the sign is "arbitrary," whereas the symbol is "an organic expression of the meaning of the total living experience of the person" (p. 16). For a still helpful discussion of the relationship between dreams and myths, the former presumed to be private and the latter public, see Wendy Doniger, "When a Lingam is Just a Good Cigar: Psychoanalysis and Hindu Sexual Fantasies," in *Vishnu on Freud's Desk: A Reader in Psychoanalysis and Hinduism*, edited by T. G. Vaidyanathan and Jeffrey J. Kripal (Delhi: Oxford University Press, 1999), pp. 279–82.

4. Michel Foucault, "Theatrum Philosophicum," in *The Essential Works of Foucault, 1954–1984*, vol. 2, *Aesthetics, Method, and Epistemology*, edited by James D. Faubion (New York: New Press, 1998), p. 357. Foucault's view was anticipated in different terminology in a 1908 essay by Henri Bergson, included in *Mind-Energy*, translated by H. Wildon Carr, edited by Keith Ansell Pearson and Michael Kolkman, with an introduction by Keith Ansell Pearson (New York: Palgrave Macmillan, 2007), pp. 123–24: "The dream is not something fantastic hovering above and additional to the reality of being awake; on the contrary, that reality of the waking state is gained by limitation, by concentration and by tension of a diffuse psychical life, which is the dream-life. In a sense, the perception and memory we exercise in the dream-state are more natural than those in the waking state: there does consciousness disport itself, perceiving just to perceive, remembering just to remember, with no care for life, that is, for the action to be accomplished.... To be awake means to will. Cease to will, detach yourself from life, disinterest yourself, and by that mere abstention you pass from the awake-self to the dream-self—less *tense* but more *extended*" (emphasis in the original).

5. Michel Henry, *Philosophy and Phenomenology of the Body*, translated by Girard Etzkorn (The Hague: Martinus Nijhoff, 1975), p. 61.

6. Jorge Luis Borges, *Labyrinths: Selected Stories and Other Writings*, edited by Donald A. Yates and James E. Irby, preface by André Maurois (New York: New Directions, 1964), p. 221. The context in which Borges uses this expression is a deliberation on the "unstable world of the mind" affirmed by philosophical idealists: "A world of evanescent impressions; a world without matter

or spirit, neither objective or subjective; a world without the ideal architecture of space; a world made of time, of the absolute uniform time of the *Principia*; a tireless labyrinth, a chaos, a dream."

7. Gaston Bachelard, *The Poetics of Reverie: Childhood, Language, and the Cosmos*, translated by Daniel Russell (Boston: Beacon Press, 1971), p. 17.

8. See, for example, Bronislaw Malinowski, *The Sexual Life of Savages*, with a new introduction by Annette B. Weiner (Boston: Beacon Press, 1987), p. 327. Speaking about the vision of departed spirits in the "standardized dreams" of the Trobrianders, Malinowski notes that not all such dreams are considered true, for the appearance of a dead person may be either an illusion (*sasopa*) or a real spirit (*baloma*). See *ibid.*, pp. 332–33, where the more general distinction is made between "spontaneous" dreams and "stereotyped" dreams: the former are a lie or illusion, and the latter, which are induced by magic or spirits, are true and prophetic.

9. The language here reflects the influence of Michael Riffaterre, *Fictional Truth* (Baltimore: Johns Hopkins University Press, 1990).

10. My formulation is indebted to the analysis of Deleuze's "reversed Platonism" offered by Foucault, "Theatrum Philosophicum," pp. 344–45.

11. See Sue Savage-Rumbaugh and Kevin McDonald, "Deception and Social Manipulation in Symbol-Using Apes," in *Machiavellian Intelligence: Social Expertise and the Evolution of Intellect in Monkeys, Apes and Humans*, edited by Richard W. Byrne and Andrew Whitten (Oxford: Oxford University Press, 1988), pp. 224–37; Richard W. Byrne and Andrew Whiten, "The Manipulation of Attention in Primate Tactical Deception," in *Machiavellian Intelligence: Social Expertise*, pp. 211–23; Marc D. Hauser, "Minding the Behaviour of Deception," in *Machiavellian Intelligence II: Extensions and Evaluations*, edited by Andrew Whiten and Richard W. Byrne (Cambridge: Cambridge University Press, 1997), pp. 112–43. Many of the other relevant studies on tactical deception in primates by Richard W. Byrne and Andrew Whiten are listed in the bibliography to the introduction in *Machiavellian Intelligence II*, pp. 18 and 23.

12. Maurice Blanchot, "Literature and the Right to Death," in *The Gaze of Orpheus*, translated by Lydia Davis (Barrytown: Station Hill Press, 1981), p. 30.

13. Rodolphe Gasché, "The Felicities of Paradox: Blanchot on the Null-Space of Literature," in *Maurice Blanchot: The Demand of Writing*, edited by Carolyn Bailey Gill (London: Routledge, 1996), pp. 43–44.

14. Maurice Blanchot, *Friendship*, translated by Elizabeth Rottenberg (Stanford: Stanford University Press, 1997), pp. 142–43. On this dimension of Blanchot's thought, see Herschel Farbman, "Blanchot on Dreams and Writing," *SubStance* 34 (2005): 118–40.

15. Maurice Blanchot, *The Infinite Conversation*, translated and foreword by Susan Hanson (Minneapolis: University of Minnesota Press, 1993), p. 38.

16. See Gerald L. Bruns, *Maurice Blanchot: The Refusal of Philosophy* (Baltimore: Johns Hopkins University Press, 1997), pp. 188–90 193–94; *idem*, "Anarchic Temporality: Writing, Friendship, and the Ontology of the Work of Art in Maurice Blanchot's Poetics," in *The Power of Contestation: Perspectives on Maurice Blanchot*, edited by Kevin Hart and Geoffrey H. Hartman (Baltimore: Johns Hopkins University Press, 2004), pp. 121–40, esp. pp. 126–33; Zoltán Popovics, "'Counter-time: A Non-dialectical Temporality in the Works of Maurice Blanchot," *Colloquy: Text Theory Critique* 10 (2005): 42–56.

17. Blanchot, *Friendship*, p. 145.

18. *Ibid.*, p. 147. Blanchot considers this aspect of the dream to be parallel to the condition of insomnia, which many writers have marked as the catalyst that inspires their creativity.

19. *Ibid.*, p. 146.

20. On the eccentricity of the dream, see Blanchot, *Friendship*, pp. 144–45.

21. Artemidorus, *The Interpretation of Dreams: Oneirocritica*, translated and commentary by Robert J. White, 2nd edition, revised and enlarged (Torrance: Original Books, 1990), p. 183. For select references to studies on Artemidorus, see Chapter 3 n. 16.

22. See Roger Caillois, *L'incertitude qui vient des rêves* (Paris: Gallimard, 1956).

23. Thus, for example, I am not ignorant of anthropological studies of the dream phenomenon in what are currently called "indigenous" or "aboriginal" peoples, even though these will not figure in my own analyses. The privileging of the philosophical over the ethnographic should not be construed as an intellectual judgment on my part regarding the relative merits of each methodological orientation.

24. Robert Moss, *The Secret History of Dreaming* (Novato: New World Library, 2009), pp. xii–xiii (emphasis in the original).

25. Alain Badiou and Slavoj Žižek, *Philosophy in the Present*, edited by Peter Engelmann, translated by Peter Thomas and Alberto Toscano (Cambridge: Polity Press, 2010), pp. 26–48.

26. Alondra Yvette Oubré, *Instinct and Revelation: Reflections on the Origins of Numinous Perception* (Amsterdam: Gordon and Breach, 1997), p. 113. On symbolic thought, the unconscious and dreaming, see *ibid.*, pp. 154–60.

27. *Ibid.*, p. 158. The author relies primarily on the works of Jonathan Winson, *Brain and Psyche: The Biology of the Unconscious* (Garden City: Anchor Press, 1985) and "The Meaning of Dreams," *Scientific American* 243 (1990): 86–96.

28. See David Tacey, "Imagining Transcendence at the End of Modernity: Jung and Derrida," in *Dreaming the Myth Onwards: New Directions in Jungian Therapy and Thought*, edited by Lucy Huskinson (London: Routledge, 2008), pp. 58–68.

29. The reader interested in exploring in greater detail this dimension of my thinking should consult Elliot R. Wolfson, *Open Secret: Postmessianic Messianism and the Mystical Revision of Menaḥem Mendel Schneerson* (New York: Columbia University Press, 2009), pp. 265–300.

30. It is of interest to recall the popular legend that the poem *u-netanneh toqef* was dictated by Amnon of Mainz to his teacher, Qalonymus ben Meshullam, in a dream on the third night after he had been killed. See Joshua Trachtenberg, *Jewish Magic and Superstition: A Study in Folk Religion* (New York: Behrman's Jewish Book House, 1939), p. 234.

31. *Maḥazor la-Yamim ha-Nora'im*, edited and annotated by Ernst Daniel Goldschmidt, vol. 1: *Rosh ha-Shanah* (Jerusalem: Qoren, 1970), p. 171. The English translation is my own. In homage to my father, I note that during my childhood, he would often repeat this refrain to me on the walk back from synagogue on the night of Yom Kippur.

INTRODUCTION

1. Paul Ricoeur, *Freud and Philosophy: An Essay on Interpretation*, translated by Denis Savage (New Haven: Yale University Press, 1970), p. 162.

2. Eric R. Dodds, *The Greeks and the Irrational* (Berkeley: University of California Press, 1951), pp. 103–104, argues persuasively that conformity to a particular cultural pattern not only affects the interpretation of a dream, but also has a hand in shaping its structural content.

3. Harvie Ferguson, *The Lure of Dreams: Sigmund Freud and the Construction of Modernity* (London: Routledge, 1996), p. 3: "The history of dreams, and the history of the interpretation and explanation of dreams is, then, more than a scale of changing values. The reality which constitutes the dream and dreaming itself changes."

4. *Traum und Existenz* was first published in *Neue Schweizer Rundschau* 9 (1930): 673–85, 766–79, and was then reprinted in Ludwig Binswanger, *Augewähtle Vorträge und Aufsätze*, vol. 1 (Bern: A. Francke, 1947), pp. 74–97.

5. Ludwig Binswanger, *Le rêve et l'existence*, translated by J. Verdeaux (Paris: Desclée de Brouwer, 1954). Foucault's introduction appeared on pp. 9–128, and it was reprinted in Michel Foucault, *Dits et ècrits 1954–1988*, edited by Daniel Defert and François Ewald, with the collaboration of Jacques Lagrange, vol. 1:

1954–1969 (Paris: Gallimard, 1994), pp. 65–119. An English translation by Forest Williams, entitled "Dream, Imagination and Existence," appeared in Ludwig Binswanger, *Dream and Existence*, translated by Jacob Needleman, edited by Keith Hoeller (Atlantic Highlands: Humanities Press, 1993), pp. 29–78 (first published in 1985 as vol. 19 of the *Review of Existential Psychology and Psychiatry*). I have consulted the French text of Foucault, but for citational purposes, I have availed myself of the English translation.

6. Foucault, "Dream, Imagination and Existence," p. 45. In his challenge to Freud's conception of the dream as wish fulfillment, a similar sentiment was expressed by Wilhelm Stekel, *Sex and Dreams: The Language of Dreams*, translated by James S. Van Teslaar (Boston: Gorham Press, 1922), p. 24: "The dream seeks solutions for unsolvable problems.... Its realm is inexhaustible and it is not to be encased within the narrow limits of a formula. The dream is in fact as inexhaustible as the riddle of man and yet as transparent as man, provided one does not start out with any preconceived notions.... The dream is the stream of our mental life as it flows out of the unexplored depths through the filter of conscience and up to the level of awareness."

7. Foucault, "Dream, Imagination and Existence," p. 49.

8. *Ibid.*, p. 51.

9. Alain Badiou, *Saint Paul: The Foundation of Universalism*, translated by Ray Brassier (Stanford: Stanford University Press, 2003), pp. 41–42, considers this facet to be a distinctive cultural marking of Judaism: "What is Jewish discourse? The subjective figure constituted by it is that of the prophet. But the prophet is one who abides in the requisition of signs, one who signals, testifying to transcendence by exposing the obscure to its deciphering. Thus, Jewish discourse will be held to be, above all, the discourse of the sign.... Jewish discourse is a discourse of exception, because the prophetic sign, the miracle, election, designate transcendence as that which lies beyond the natural totality.... Greek discourse bases itself on the cosmic order so as to adjust itself to it, while Jewish discourse bases itself on the exception to this order so as to turn divine transcendence into a sign." My own thinking, informed by a particular reading of kabbalistic sources, resists this Jewish-Greek dichotomy, and hence the transcendence denoted by the prophetic sign is not necessarily positioned beyond nature. For discussions of Badiou's interpretation of Pauline theology, see Stephen Fowl, "A Very Particular Universalism: Badiou and Paul," in *Paul, Philosophy, and the Theopolitical Vision*, edited by Douglas Harink (Eugene: Cascade Books, 2010), pp. 119–34, and in the same volume, the essays by Neil Elliott, "Ideological Closure in the Christ-Event: A Marxist Response to Alain Badiou's Paul," pp. 135–54, and Geoffrey Holsclaw, "Subjects between

Death and Resurrection: Badiou, Žižek, and St. Paul," pp. 155–76.

10. This stance was famously taken by Carl G. Jung. Of the many passages in which Jung's idea is expressed, I cite from his *Mysterium Coniunctionis: An Inquiry into the Separation and Synthesis of Psychic Opposites in Alchemy*, translated by R.F.C. Hull (Princeton: Princeton University Press, 1970), p. 390. Jung insists that by treating dream-symbols "as psychic phenomena, we remove them from the inaccessible realm of metaphysics, about which nothing verifiable can be said, and this disposes of the impossible question as to whether they are 'true' or not. We take our stand simply and solely on the facts, recognizing that the archetypal structure of the unconscious will produce, over and over again and irrespective of tradition, those figures which reappear in the history of all epochs and all peoples, and will endow them with the same significance and numinosity that have been theirs from the beginning." See, however, the remark of Jung cited in Chapter 1 n. 306, where in the context of denying intentionality to the act of dreaming, he characterized the dream as a *natural phenomenon*.

11. Edith Wyschogrod, "The Civilizational Perspective in Comparative Studies of Transcendence," in *Transcendence and the Sacred*, edited by Alan M. Olson and Leroy S. Rouner (Notre Dame: University of Notre Dame Press, 1981), pp. 59–60. A useful account of the connotation of the term and the philosophical issues related to it can be found in Marvin Farber, "Experience and Transcendence," *Philosophy and Phenomenological Research* 12 (1951): 1–23.

12. Gilles Deleuze, *Expressionism in Philosophy: Spinoza*, translated by Martin Joughin (New York: Zone Books, 1992), p. 109: "Spinoza's doctrine is rightly called 'parallelism,' but this because it excludes any analogy, any eminence, any transcendence. Parallelism, strictly speaking, is to be understood neither from the viewpoint of occasional causes, or from the viewpoint of ideal causality, but only from the viewpoint of an immanent God and immanent causality." See *ibid.*, pp. 180–81, 256, 269.

13. Gilles Deleuze, *Pure Immanence: Essays on A Life*, with an introduction by John Rajchman, translated by Anne Boyman (New York: Zone Books, 2001), pp. 26–27. Compare the discussions of the Deleuzian sense of immanence in Giorgio Agamben, *Potentialities: Collected Essays in Philosophy*, edited and translated, with an introduction, by Daniel Heller-Roazen (Stanford: Stanford University Press, 1999), pp. 220–39, and Daniel W. Smith, "Deleuze and Derrida, Immanence and Transcendence: Two Directions in Recent French Thought," in *Between Deleuze and Derrida*, edited by Paul Patton and John Protevi (New York: Continuum, 2003), pp. 46–66, esp. 51–52 and 62–63. In a manner similar to my own thinking, Smith concludes that the philosophy of the future "needs

to move in the direction of immanence" by accepting its "demystificatory role" in exposing the "fictional" or "illusory" status of the idea of transcendence (p. 61). For discussion of immanence as the thread that connects the various stages of Deleuzian thought and as that which distinguishes philosophy from religion and ontotheology, see Miguel de Beistegui, "The Vertigo of Immanence: Deleuze's Spinozism," *Research in Phenomenology* 35 (2005): 77–100.

14. Gilles Deleuze and Felix Guattari, *What is Philosophy?* translated by Janis Tomlinson and Graham Burchell (New York: Columbia University Press, 1994), p. 47. See also Chin-Tai Kim, "Transcendence and Immanence," *Journal of the American Academy of Religion* 55 (1987): 537–49; Ignace Verhack, "Immanent Transcendence as Way to 'God': Between Heidegger and Marion," in *Religious Experience and the End of Metaphysics*, edited by Jeffrey Bloechl (Bloomington: Indiana University Press, 2003), pp. 106–18, esp. 112–16; and the innovative approach of Sami Pihlström, *Naturalizing the Transcendental: A Pragmatic View* (Amherst: Humanity Books, 2003). Finally, mention should be made of Jürgen Habermas, "Transcendence from Within, Transcendence in this World," in *Religion and Rationality: Essays on Reason, God and Modernity*, edited by Eduardo Mendieta (Cambridge, MA: The MIT Press, 2002), pp. 67–94. Habermas affirms a postmetaphysical sense of transcendence that does not posit anything external to the world, but is immanent in the world and grounded in human language and a communicative rationality that secures ideally social tolerance and pluralism. That is, our attempt to assert truth claims presupposes a community of communication that transcends personal interest and regional communication. As is to be expected, many have written about this notion of this-worldly as opposed to other-worldly transcendence. For representative studies, see the informative comments by Eric Bain-Selbo, "A Review of Jürgen Habermas, *Religion and Rationality: Essays on Reason, God, and Modernity*," *Journal for Cultural and Religious Theory* 5 (2003): 139–43, and Ali Muhammed Rizvi, "Habermas' Conception of 'Transcendence from Within': An Interpretation," Ph.D. dissertation, La Trobe University, Melbourne, 2007. See also Robert Erlewine, *Monotheism and Tolerance: Recovering a Religion of Reason* (Bloomington: Indiana University Press, 2010), pp. 21–25.

15. Tim Maudlin, *The Metaphysics within Physics* (Oxford: Oxford University Press, 2007). Maudlin's orientation is summarized in the following paragraph: "Metaphysics is ontology. Ontology is the most generic study of what exists. Evidence for what exists, at least in the physical world, is provided solely by empirical research. Hence the proper object of most metaphysics is the careful analysis of our best scientific theories (and especially of fundamental physical theories) with the goal of determining what they imply about the constitution

of the physical world" (p. 104). Historically, this conception of metaphysics can be traced to Aristotle, who offered three different perspectives: the science that investigates the being that is eternal, immovable, and separable from matter (*Metaphysics* 1026a 10); the science that investigates the first principles and causes of all that exists (982b 9, 1003a 26); and ontology, or the science that investigates being as being (1003a 21). The second definition relates, more specifically, to the four causes that apply to nature, and hence metaphysics is an integral dimension of physics. Moreover, if the only knowledge we can have of God is derived from the cosmos—not about God's essence as such, but about the existence and governance of a divine principle—it follows that metaphysics is not about describing nature pneumatically, as Nietzsche put it (*Human All Too Human*, sec. 8), but rather it is itself part of the naturalistic explanation of what exists. Something similar is in play in medieval Aristotelian-Neoplatonic cosmologies, which struggled to balance two divergent views, one that maintained that we can infer the being of the First Cause from the universe and the other that upheld that the universe may point to the First Cause, but there is absolutely no resemblance between the two. For a concise discussion of the tension in Islamic and Jewish thinkers, see Shlomo Pines, "Translator's Introduction," in Moses Maimonides, *The Guide of the Perplexed*, translated with an introduction and notes by Shlomo Pines, with an introductory essay by Leo Strauss, 2 vols. (Chicago: University of Chicago Press, 1963), pp. xciv, cxii–cxiii, cxiv–cxv.

16. Edmund Husserl, *The Basic Problems of Phenomenology From the Lectures, Winter Semester, 1910–1911*, translated by Ingo Farin and James G. Hart (Dordrecht: Springer, 2006), sec. 28, pp. 59–60. See also Edmund Husserl, *Ideas Pertaining to a Pure Phenomenology and to a Phenomenological Philosophy. First Book: General Introduction to Pure Phenomenology*, translated by F. Kersten (Dordrecht: Kluwer, 1983), secs. 42–44, pp. 89–98; *idem*, *Cartesian Meditations: An Introduction to Phenomenology*, translated by Dorion Cairns (The Hague: Martinus Nijhoff, 1977), sec. 47, pp. 103–105; John D. Caputo, "Transcendence and the Transcendental in Husserl's Phenomenology," *Philosophy Today* 23 (1979): 205–16; Michael Theunissen, *The Other: Studies in the Social Ontology of Husserl, Heidegger, Sartre, and Buber*, translated by Christopher Macann with an introduction by Fred R. Dallmayr (Cambridge, MA: The MIT Press, 1984), pp. 50–51.

17. Compare Michel Henry, *The Essence of Manifestation*, translated by Girard Etzkorn (The Hague: Martinus Nijhoff, 1973), p. 238: "*Exteriority designates precisely the ontological character of this belonging, namely, the mode according to which the reception by the essence of this pure content which it itself is takes*

place. To give a rigorous ontological meaning to the concept of an exterior content is to extend it to all represented reality in general, and primordially to the ontological reality of the essence itself insofar as it projects itself under the form of a horizon into the pure milieu of exteriority. Precisely because it is constituted by this horizon, namely, by a milieu of pure exteriority, the ontological content, which the essence represents to itself in the act whereby it objectifies itself in it, is an exterior content, *and this in a radical sense in conformity to which exteriority, which qualifies such a content, is not a property added-on, but rather determined this content itself in its own ontological reality*" (emphasis in the original).

18. *Ibid.*, p. 240: "That which manifests itself in the form of the transcendental horizon of Being is the phenomenological form of this horizon itself, it is not the essence. Or else, if the horizon manifests the essence, it is in an altogether different meaning, namely in the sense in which 'to manifest' means 'to be the appearance of something,' nevertheless, in such a way that that which manifests itself in this appearance is not the thing of which it is the appearance, but merely refers to this thing as to that which does not show itself in the effective phenomenological content of the appearance itself. In this sense 'to manifest' signifies 'to hide' as well, or more precisely, to indicate something as differing in itself from appearance which indicates it."

19. For a fuller discussion of incarnation and phenomenological sensibility, see Michel Henry, *Incarnation: Une philosophie de la chair* (Paris: Éditions du Seuil, 2000), and the analyses in Michael O'Sullivan, *Michel Henry: Incarnation, Barbarism, and Belief* (Oxford: Peter Lang, 2006), pp. 84–96, and *idem*, *The Incarnation of Language: Joyce, Proust, and a Philosophy of the Flesh* (New York: Continuum, 2008), pp. 30–41.

20. Henry, *The Essence of Manifestation*, p. 385.

21. Compare the assessment of May, "Introduction," in *Dreams and Symbols*, p. 4: "I believe also that dreaming has some connection with man's distinctive capacity for transcendence, i.e., his capacity to break through the immediate objective limits of existence and bring together into one dramatic union diverse dimensions of experience."

22. See Kierkegaard's description of the infinite in the entry "To Be Nothing" in *Søren Kierkegaard's Journals and Papers*, vol. 2, F–K, edited and translated by Howard V. Hong and Edna H. Hong (Bloomington: Indiana University Press, 1970), sec. 2089, p. 449: "The infinite in the guise of being nothing, purely and simply 'man' (somewhat like the lily and the bird, which indeed are not something), is in the world the point outside of the world which can move all existence. If the infinite is something, it can move only relatively." For the

intellectual background of the point made by Kierkegaard, see Karl Menges, "Romantic Anti-Foundationalism and the Theory of Chaos," in *Romanticism and Beyond: A Festschrift for John F. Fetzer*, edited by Clifford A. Bernd, Ingeborg Henderson, and Winder McConnell (New York: Peter Lang, 1996), pp. 33–56, esp. 48: "according to Romantic thought... all theoretical foundationalism is stuck in the performative contradiction of trying to formulate an Absolute in a relativistic way."

23. Jean-Luc Marion, "The Saturated Phenomenon," *Philosophy Today* 40 (1996): 103–24, reprinted in *idem*, *The Visible and the Revealed*, translated by Christina M. Gschwandtner and others (New York: Fordham University Press, 2008), pp. 18–48; *idem*, "In the Name: How to Avoid Speaking of 'Negative Theology'," in *God, the Gift, and Postmodernism*, edited by John D. Caputo and Michael J. Scanlon (Bloomington: Indiana University Press, 1999), pp. 39–42, reprinted in Jean-Luc Marion, *In Excess: Studies in Saturated Phenomena*, translated by Robyn Horner and Vincent Berraud (New York: Fordham University Press, 2002), pp. 158–62; *idem*, *Being Given: Toward a Phenomenology of Givenness*, translated by Jeffrey L. Kosky (Stanford: Stanford University Press, 2002), pp. 199–221; *idem*, *The Visible and the Revealed*, pp. 119–44; and the critical evaluations by Robyn Horner, "The Betrayal of Transcendence," in *Transcendence: Philosophy, Literature, and Theology Approach the Beyond*, edited by Regina Schwartz (New York: Routledge, 2004), pp. 61–79, esp. 70–76; Christina M. Gschwandtner, *Reading Jean-Luc Marion: Exceeding Metaphysics* (Bloomington: Indiana University Press, 2007), pp. 59–86, 150–55, 233–42; Shane Mackinlay, "Exceeding Truth: Jean-Luc Marion's Saturated Phenomena," *Pacifica* 20 (2007): 40–51, and the fuller treatment in *idem*, *Interpreting Excess: Jean-Luc Marion, Saturated Phenomenon, and Hermeneutics* (New York: Fordham University Press, 2009). See below, n. 57.

24. Jean-Luc Marion, *God without Being: Hors-Texte*, translated by Thomas A. Carlson, with a foreword by David Tracy (Chicago: University of Chicago Press, 1991), pp. 25–52. See the analysis in Bruce Ellis Benson, *Graven Ideologies: Nietzsche, Derrida, and Marion on Modern Idolatry* (Downers Grove: InterVarsity Press, 2002), pp. 188–223. I concur with Benson's conclusion: "Instead of facing the excruciating demands of an orthodox Christology that attempts to navigate between the Scylla of transcendence and the Charybdis of immanence, Marion denies the true iconic nature of Christ and so succumbs to the idolatry of transcendence." See also Felix Ó Murchadha, "Glory, Idolatry, Kairos: Revelation and the Ontological Difference in Marion," in *Givenness and God: Questions of Jean-Luc Marion*, edited by Ian Leask and Eoin Cassidy (New York: Fordham University Press, 2005), pp. 69–86, and Mark Dooley,

"Marion's Ambition of Transcendence," in *ibid.*, pp. 190–98.

25. Calvin O. Schrag, *God as Otherwise Than Being: Toward a Semantics of the Gift* (Evanston: Northwestern University Press, 2002), p. 64.

26. Compare Schrag, *God as Otherwise*, p. 72: "We are thus invited... to examine the possibility of a robust and hyperbolic transcendence that would at once proceed beyond the concept of God fettered by the categories of metaphysics, the concept of God as framed by a fundamental ontology, and the role of deities in poetic thinking and dwelling.... If the conversation about God as truly otherwise than a grammar of beings and Being, outside the economy not only of metaphysical and ontological reflection but also that of the poetic imagination, is to continue, we will need to maneuver a semantic shift in our discourse about the Deity." On the terms "theopoetic" or "theopoiesis," see Amos N. Wilder, *Theopoetic: Theology and the Religious Imagination* (Philadelphia: Fortress Press, 1976), p. iv; David L. Miller, "Theopoiesis," in Stanley R. Hopper, *Why Permissions and Other Poems: Transformations of Theology in Poetry* (Atlanta: Scholars Press, 1987), pp. 1–12; *idem*, *Hells and Holy Ghosts: A Theopoetics of Christian Belief* (Nashville: Abingdon Press, 1989); *idem*, *Christs: Meditations on Archetypal Images in Christian Theology* (New Orleans: Spring Journal Books, 2005), p. xviii; Stanley R. Hopper, "Introduction," in *Interpretation: The Poetry of Meanings*, edited by Stanley R. Hopper and David L. Miller (New York: Harcourt, Brace and World, 1967), pp. ix–xxii, esp. xix; Catherine Keller, *God and Power: Counter-Apocalyptic Journeys* (Minneapolis: Fortress Press, 2005), pp. 140, 145–46, 149–52.

27. This insight has been essential to my thinking, already attested in my first major monograph *Through a Speculum That Shines: Vision and Imagination in Medieval Jewish Mysticism* (Princeton: Princeton University Press, 1994), but unfortunately, the larger implications of my scholarship for the study of the phenomenology of religious experience have been largely ignored. Similar conclusions have been reached by other scholars whose work has commanded more attention in the marketplace of ideas. See the analysis of this dimension of Richard Kearney's thought in B. Keith Putt, "Theopoetics of the Possible," in *After God: Richard Kearney and the Religious Turn in Continental Philosophy*, edited by John Panteleimon Manoussakis (New York: Fordham University Press, 2006), pp. 241–69, esp. 242–50. See also the dialogical exchange on the "theological character of the saturated phenomenon" in Jean-Luc Marion and Richard Kearney, "Hermeneutics of Revelation," in *After God*, pp. 320–24. The concern I raise can also be framed in terms of the matter of divine concealment, that is, rather than appealing to the aspect of hiddenness as an integral proof of theism and a defense of supernaturalism, I would contend,

such an approach engenders a concealing of the concealing and thus leads to an obfuscation of the phenomenon of concealment. For a relatively recent articulation of the view that I am opposing, see Robert Oakes, "Life, Death, and the Hiddenness of God," *International Journal for Philosophy of Religion* 64 (2008): 155–60.

28. Graham Ward, "Transcendence and Representation," in *Transcendence: Philosophy, Literature, and Theology*, p. 135: "That which lies beyond can be either theistically or atheistically interpreted; it can either be plenitude or void." Ward relies on the remark of Steven T. Katz, "Language, Epistemology, and Mysticism," in *Mysticism and Philosophical Analysis*, edited by Steven T. Katz (Oxford: Oxford University Press, 1978), p. 48.

29. Regarding this turn of phrase, see John D. Caputo and Michael J. Scanlon, "Do We Need to Transcend Transcendence?" in *Transcendence and Beyond: A Postmodern Inquiry*, edited by John D. Caputo and Michael J. Scanlon (Bloomington: Indiana University Press, 2007), pp. 2–5.

30. My own thinking here, as in other crucial contexts, is reflective of the logic of the middle way (*madhyamaka*) of the Mahāyāna tradition, a logic based on the tetralemmic scheme: S is P; ~P; both P and ~P; neither P nor ~P. I will refrain from citing relevant bibliography on this topic because I have done so elsewhere, but I will note the study of Robert A. E. Thurman, "Transcendence and the Sacred in the Mahāyāna Middle Way," in *Transcendence and the Sacred*, pp. 100–14, which analyzes the matter of transcendence, or what is called "the utter transcendentality of ultimate reality" (p. 107), in the Buddhist teaching of nonduality and the indiscriminate emptiness (*śūnyatā*) that is the discriminated thusness (*tathātā*) of all that exists. Perhaps even more pertinent to the drift of my thinking is the study by Sara L. McClintock, "The Role of the 'Given' in the Classification of Śaṅkarakṣita and Kamalaśīla as Svātantrika-Mādhyamikas," in *The Svātantrika-Prāsaṅgika Distinction: What Difference a Difference Makes?* edited by George B. J. Dreyfus and Sara L. McClintock (Boston: Wisdom Publications, 2003), pp. 125–71. There is also affinity to the characterization of the void in quantum physics as the empty space that is nonetheless seething subatomically with the creation and destruction of protons and neutrons. For a lucid account, see Henning Genz, *Nothingness: The Science of Empty Space* (Cambridge, MA: Perseus Publishing, 1999), and the summation on p. 305: "the line that separates *something* from *nothing*, matter from empty space is blurred—just as we are accustomed in our daily lives to an indistinct separation of subject from object. The universe is but one immense unit; it cannot be separated into spatial domains that are totally empty and others that are completely filled with matter. Matter and space can be distinguished from each other,

but where we draw the blurred line between them is largely a matter of taste" (emphasis in the original). See also Richard H. Jones, *Science and Mysticism: A Comparative Study of Western Natural Science, Theravāda Buddhism, and Advaita Vedānta* (Lewisburg: Bucknell University Press, 1986), pp. 186–91; William L. Ames, "Emptiness and Quantum Theory," in *Buddhism and Science: Breaking New Ground*, edited by B. Alan Wallace (New York: Columbia University Press, 2003), pp. 285–302. See below, n. 112.

31. Catherine Keller, "The Flesh of God: A Metaphor in the Wild," in *Theology That Matters: Ecology, Economy, and God*, edited by Darby Kathleen Ray (Minneapolis: Fortress Press, 2006), pp. 101–102 (emphasis in the original). My gratitude to Virginia Burrus for drawing my attention to this essay.

32. *Ibid.*, p. 102.

33. Elliot R. Wolfson, "Negative Theology and Positive Assertion in the Early Kabbalah," *Da'at* 32–33 (1994): v–xxii; *idem*, *Language, Eros, Being: Kabbalistic Hermeneutics and Poetic Imagination* (New York: Fordham University Press, 2005), pp. 22–23, 219–20, 343.

34. For a sensitive, but, in my judgment, not persuasive grappling with this problem from the perspective of the liturgical practice of Judaism, see Elliot N. Dorff, *Knowing God: Jewish Journeys to the Unknowable* (Northvale: Jason Aronson, 1992). I thank the author for gifting me a copy of his book. Dorff offers a judicious account of the dissonance between the abstract and personal depictions of God that have shaped the Jewish religious sensibility. He argues that this tension is best resolved through an integrative approach that recognizes variegated contexts shaped by different human needs. The God of the philosophers is not identical with the God of biblical-rabbinic faith, but both are "legitimate and complementary conceptions of God, and we need both to be true to the totality of our experience as human beings and as Jews" (pp. 206–207). Dorff is correct to mark prayer as the critical source of interaction with the personal God of the Jewish tradition (pp. 207–208), and he is aware of the potential idolatry of the anthropomorphic representation of the divine (pp. 209–16), but he still wishes to assign a cognitive status to images in worship to the extent that those images speak to the devotional needs of the religious individual and the community (pp. 223–40). Much like Keller, albeit from a somewhat varied philosophical perspective, Dorff distinguishes between good and bad images: "Ultimately, we have no recourse but to think of God in images. The only real question is how we choose the images we use. In that process we would reject images that are ineffective because they do not touch us; those which distort or falsify our experience; and those which undermine the community's cohesiveness. On the other hand, we must seek images that

have the immediacy of meaning that we seek in images as against creeds and symbols; those that evoke the emotions and actions that powerful images should; those that are true to our experience, even if they cannot be totally so; and those that enjoy the community's validation in thought and action. Above all, we must make sure that our images are not idolatrous, that they do not pretend that the part is the whole, for that would be to deny the truth and to give up our special mandate to be a people true to God" (pp. 247–48). There are various aspects of Dorf's argument that I cannot accept, for instance, what seems to me to be an a priori commitment to community and the assumption that the ideals of that community are inherently laudable, and perhaps more importantly, the circularity of his reasoning: a personal imaging of the divine is said to be necessitated by the experience of prayer, but that experience is the main vehicle through which we access this knowledge of a personal God. In the final analysis, what is demanded by prayer is used to substantiate what is elicited from prayer. For a recent attempt that has an affinity with the approach of Dorff, albeit drawing directly on kabbalistic and ḥasidic sources, as opposed to Maimonides, see Arthur Green, *Radical Judaism: Rethinking God and Tradition* (New Haven: Yale University Press, 2010). In contrasting his own "mystical-panentheist" theology with the "personalist" theology of his teacher, Abraham Joshua Heschel, Green acknowledges that for him, "the personal God is a bridge between soul and mystery, a personification of the unknown, a set of projected images that we need and use, rather than an ultimate reality" (p. 158). The metaphorical understanding of the theistic representation of God does not, however, lead to discarding the traditional liturgical idiom. In Green's own words: "Yet I still affirm there is God who seeks us out. The inner One, Y-H-W-H inseparable from existence itself, still wants to know where I am. It needs me . . . as its embodiment . . . called upon to do its work, to move the process of evolution ever forward, and, in our age as in none other, to help our planet to survive. I still hear the One ask me 'Where are you?' I respond to that question as a Jew, from within my people's covenant. This means *mitzvah*, an act in which I intend to be aware of God's presence. . . . In doing this, I retain a sense of partnership with the divine One, a conviction that the human deed makes a difference" (p. 159). Green goes on to describe this mystery, signified by the Tetragrammaton, as the "Source and Giver of all life," which "calls upon us to become givers, our own lives being the gift." Philosophically speaking, if the images of the divine personhood are merely metaphors (pp. 44–58, 73), I do not see any reason to affirm the covenantal language of divine commandment as a response to a call (see Green's own reservation on p. 108) or as a justification to attribute a standard of ethical behavior and intent to this "ultimate Oneness," which is the "single universal Mind and Heart" (p. 180 n. 34), let alone to continue to use the dialogical language of "partnership" between human and God organized around the image of the gift. In spite of marking the difference between himself and Heschel, Green succumbs to language that is very similar to the latter's when he notes that "all God can do is call out to us, now as always. All we can do is respond—or not.... God is indeed in need of humans; and we humans are in need of guidance, seeking out the hand of a divine Partner, one who 'speaks' from deep within the heart, but also from deep within our tradition and its wisdom" (p. 166). Even when acknowledging that the "personalist theism" of Judaism will have to be transformed by the nondualism of Buddhist and Vedāntic teachings, Green cannot avoid lapsing into theistic language: "The Judaism emerging from such a process would clearly assert the holiness of all life, seeing the face of God both in the uniqueness of each individual creature and in the underlying and mysterious unity of all. The worship of the personified 'God' needs to be clearly described as a symbolic way to express this truth and to deepen its expression through the rich echo chambers of a traditional religious language" (p. 73). If the worship of a personified God needs to be understood as merely symbolic, then why translate the monist conception of an underlying unity into the theistic language of the face of God? In my own thinking, which is indebted to a sustained study of Hindu, Taoist, and Buddhist sources for over three decades (see above, n. 30, and below, n. 54), we need to advance to the notion of giving that does away with both giver and gift, to see the veil of nature as a veil without presuming there is a face of God behind or even within it. I note, finally, another relatively recent work, Michael Fishbane, *Sacred Attunement: A Jewish Theology* (Chicago: University of Chicago Press, 2008), which is similarly attentive to grounding the theological orientation in the phenomena of the world of sense experience. Unlike Green, however, Fishbane's worldview is not pantheistic or panentheistic; on the contrary, even though he emphatically denies the possibility of contemporary theologians reverting to some form of otherworldliness, whether the Platonic ideal forms or the Kantian noumena, he is not willing to concede that "all that remains is some mode of natural piety" (p. 12). Borrowing the locution of Jean Wahl (see below, n. 100), Fishbane marks the difference between the "immanent transcendence" (*l'immanence transcendante*) of ordinary perception and the "transcendent immanence" (*le transcendance immanente*) of the "unsayable ground," the "radically Other" that cannot be "delimited by human language and consciousness" (pp. x–xi). One entrusted to the divine covenant must "actualize the principles of Sinai," the historical locus of revelation, which symbolizes the "junction of heaven and earth" (p.

109; see pp. 128–29, where Jacob's ladder is also interpreted as symbolic of the conjunction of immanence and transcendence). Through religious commitment, therefore, "we may live at the intersection of transcendence and immanence—the transcendent immanence of world-being perceived as (actualities of) immanent transcendence" (pp. 109–10). Theology is meaningful only if it is "grounded in earthly experience and understood from within its forms," but, in a manner akin to, although surpassing, the aesthetic sensibility, it also must point to infinities that are "intuited as more than a trace of the elusiveness of experience ... the given (or 'shadow') of an unsayable, and insensate, and utterly transcendent Giving, to which we can only orient ourselves in silence." The transcendence that Fishbane affirms is to be sought in the "unfolding of the Godhead into world-being" (p. 14), so that the person of faith intuits "God's informing presence in all the realities of existence, the infinite modalities of divine effectivity" (p. 35). Religious imagination, accordingly, is a "bimodal consciousness" (p. x) encompassing the fullness that is the "illimitable transcendence of Divinity, the Life of all life, ever exceeding human knowledge and grasp" and the "experience of God's immanent actuality as the Life of the life we find in the world" (p. 123). It is in this sense that Fishbane situates theology "at the border of the known and unknown, of the manifest and the concealed. It is at this nexus that the self seeks God." The excess of all that transpires in space and time extends to the "utmost depths of Being and beyond," for "all our worldly experiences are prismatic revelations of a deeper elementariness," and hence, "through a wholly natural attitude toward the world a deeper phenomenality is disclosed." The ideal of theology is essentially the attunement of the heart to the "ultimate Source of all things," the "most primal Depth (beyond the Beyond of all conception)." Indeed, the word *God* is the "thought-image of a supernal Font of Being" (p. 34), the transpersonal infinity that surpasses any imaginary construct of the divine person (pp. 158–59). In the final analysis, Fishbane's theology embraces the paradox well-rooted in the Jewish mystical cosmology of kabbalists and ḥasidic masters: "if all existence is not God as such, it is also not other than God, Life of all life" (p. 34). Understandably, Fishbane utilizes the figurative trope of the gift to depict the mystery of God's effectivity (pp. 38, 42, 123, 131–33, 136, 166, 204), an act of bestowing that is related mythopoeically to the giving of the Torah, which is rendered metaphorically as "God's absolute gift and giving of world-reality," the "sacred gift of freedom, grounded in God's goodness, allowing all things to be and to happen" (pp. 158–59). Technically speaking, the anthropomorphization of the generative force of divine transcendence along these lines has the potential of becoming a "verbal idol" (p. 86). Fishbane is well aware that theology is, first and foremost, a "construct of thought and imagination" (p. 32). Needless to say, this is not meant to suggest that the divine is nothing more than a projection of the human psyche. What is intended is that theology is a "symbolic form which takes our experiences in the natural world and reshapes them" such that we may cross over "to the numinous qualities of the unsayable origin inhering in every moment of existence" (pp. 33–34). It remains unclear to me, however, why the particularities of the phenomenal realm, the "specific concrescences of existence," are to be "experienced as the gift of God's all-unnamable 'Shall-Be" (p. 124), an abbreviated form of the name revealed to Moses at the epiphany of the burning bush, *ehyeh asher ehyeh*, "I shall be as I shall be" (Exodus 3:14). From my perspective, the task is to get beyond the double bind of the anthropomorphic configuration of the divine and the theomorphic configuration of the human.

35. Catherine Keller, *On the Mystery: Discerning Divinity in Process* (Minneapolis: Fortress Press, 2008), p.18 (emphasis in the original). For a more technical discussion of the *via negativa* and the *docta ignorantia*, see Catherine Keller, *The Face of the Deep: A Theology of Becoming* (London: Routledge, 2003), pp. 200–12. Keller is one of a number of thinkers who have looked to the apophatic tradition to articulate a constructive theological response, often utilizing Derridean thought, in particular. See Toby Foshay, "Introduction: Denegation and Resentment," in *Derrida and Negative Theology*, edited by Howard Coward and Toby Foshay (Albany: State University of New York Press, 1992), pp. 1–24; David E. Klemm, "Open Secrets: Derrida and Negative Theology," in *Negation and Theology*, edited by Robert P. Scharlemann (Charlottesville: University Press of Virginia, 1992), pp. 8–24; Mark C. Taylor, *Nots* (Chicago: University of Chicago Press, 1993), pp. 33–39 and 46–50; Martin C. Srajek, *In the Margins of Deconstruction: Jewish Conceptions of Ethics in Emmanuel Levinas and Jacques Derrida* (Dordrecht: Kluwer, 1997), pp. 214–33 and 255–57; Shira Wolosky, "An 'Other' Negative Theology: On Derrida's 'How To Avoid Speaking: Denials'," *Poetics Today* 19 (1998): 261–80; Marion, "In the Name," pp. 20–53; Hent de Vries, *Philosophy and the Turn to Religion* (Baltimore: John Hopkins University Press, 1999), pp. 305–58; *idem*, "The Theology of the Sign and the Sign of Theology: The Apophatics of Deconstruction," in *Flight of the Gods: Philosophical Perspectives on Negative Theology*, edited by Ilse N. Bulhof and Laurens ten Kate (New York: Fordham University Press, 2000), pp. 166–94; Ilse N. Bulhof, "Being Open as a Form of Negative Theology: On Nominalism, Negative Theology, and Derrida's Performative Interpretation of Khôra," in *Flight of the Gods*, pp. 195–22; John D. Caputo, *The Prayers and Tears of Jacques Derrida: Religion without Religion* (Bloomington: Indiana University Press, 1997), pp.

1–68; *idem*, "Shedding Tears Beyond Being: Derrida's Experience of Prayer," in *Théologie Négative*, edited by Marco M. Olivetti (Milan: CEDAM, 2002), pp. 861–80; Mary-Jane Rubenstein, "Unknow Thyself: Apophaticism, Deconstruction, and Theology after Ontotheology," *Modern Theology* 19 (2003): 387–417; Dirk Westerkamp, *Via Negativa: Sprache und Methode der negativen Theologie* (Munich: Wilhelm Fink Verlag, 2006), pp. 200–209; Anslem K. Min, "Naming the Unnameable God: Levinas, Derrida, and Marion," *International Journal for Philosophy of Religion* 60 (2006): 99–116; William Franke, "Apophasis and the Turn of Philosophy to Religion: From Negative Theology to Postmodern Negation of Theology," *International Journal for Philosophy of Religion* 60 (2006): 61–76. For critical assessments of the endeavor to construct a negative atheology on the basis of Derridean deconstruction, see Robert S. Gall, "Of/From Theology and Deconstruction," *Journal of the American Academy of Religion* 58 (1990): 413–37; Clayton Crockett, "Post-Modernism and Its Secrets: Religion without Religion," *Cross Currents* 52 (2003): 499–515; Siebren Miedema and Gert J. J. Biesta, "Jacque Derrida's Religion without Religion and the Im/Possibility of Religious Education," *Religious Education* 99 (2004): 23–37; Martin Hägglund, *Radical Atheism: Derrida and the Time of Life* (Stanford: Stanford University Press, 2008), pp. 144–45.

36. Miller, *Hells and Holy Ghosts*, p. 153.

37. See references cited above, n. 26, to which may now be added David L. Miller, "The Body Is No Body," in *Apophatic Bodies: Infinity, Ethics, and Incarnation*, edited by Christopher Boesel and Catherine Keller (New York: Fordham University Press, 2009), pp. 143–45.

38. Jean-Luc Nancy, "A Deconstruction of Monotheism," in *Religion: Beyond a Concept*, edited by Hent de Vries (New York: Fordham University Press, 2008), p. 383.

39. *Ibid.*, p. 386. For a critique of the theistic conception, see H. J. Adriannse, "After Theism," in *Religion: Beyond a Concept*, pp. 392–412.

40. Jean-Luc Nancy, *Dis-Enclosure: The Deconstruction of Christianity*, translated by Bettina Bego, Gabriel Malenfant, and Michael B. Smith (New York: Fordham University Press, 2008), p. 15.

41. David L. Miller, "The Brokenness of Beauty and the 'Beauty' of Brokenness: Toward a Postmodern Theopoetics," Drew Tripple-Vosburgh Lecture, October 2009. I am indebted to Virginia Burrus for sending me a copy of the lecture.

42. See Catherine Keller, "Rumors of Transcendence: The Movement, State, and Sex of 'Beyond,'" in *Transcendence and Beyond*, pp. 129–50; *idem*, "The Apophasis of Gender: A Fourfold Unsaying of Feminist Theology," *Journal of*

the American Academy of Religion 76 (2008): 905–33.

43. Henry Corbin, *Creative Imagination in the Ṣūfism of Ibn ʿArabī*, translated by Ralph Manheim (Princeton: Princeton University Press, 1969), pp. 268–69. See also *idem*, *Le paradoxe du monothéisme* (Paris: Éditions de L'Herne, 2003), pp. 24–27, and the analysis in Christian Jambet, *Le caché et l'apparent* (Paris: L'Herne, 2003), pp. 64–65.

44. See B. Alan Wallace, *Contemplative Science: Where Buddhism and Neuroscience Converge* (New York: Columbia University Press, 2007), pp. 149–69.

45. Here, too, my thinking has affinity with Schrag, *God as Otherwise*, pp. 34–73. See as well references to the work of Mark C. Taylor cited below, n. 109.

46. Jean-Paul Sartre, *Being and Nothingness: An Essay on Phenomenological Ontology*, translated and with an introduction by Hazel E. Barnes (New York: Philosophical Library, 1956), p. 198. For Sartre, as is well known, this negation-foundation is the basis of human freedom. See *ibid.*, p. 439.

47. Maurice Merleau-Ponty, *The Visible and the Invisible*, edited by Claude Lefort, translated by Alphonso Lingis (Evanston: Northwestern University Press, 1968), p. 54.

48. *Ibid.*, pp. 54–55.

49. Friedrich Nietzsche, *Beyond Good and Evil*, sec. 289, in *Basic Writings of Nietzsche*, translated and edited, with commentaries, by Walter Kaufmann (New York: Modern Library, 1968), p. 419.

50. Ludwig Wittgenstein, *The Big Typescript: TS 213*, edited and translated by C. Grant Luckhardt and Maximilian A.E. Aue (Oxford: Blackwell, 2005), sec. 88, p. 305e. The affinity between Wittgenstein's comment and the negative theology espoused by Maimonides in his crusade against the idolatrous capacity of the imagination to ascribe positive characteristics to God was already noted by Moshe Halbertal and Avishai Margalit, *Idolatry*, translated by Naomi Goldblum (Cambridge, MA: Harvard University Press, 1992), pp. 244–45. For an expanded analysis of the limits of language in the *Tractatus* of Wittgenstein and the *Guide* of Maimonides, see Donald McCallum, *Maimonides' Guide for the Perplexed: Silence and Salvation* (London: Routledge, 2007), pp. 72–85 and 123–30. The reflections of Maimonides on idolatry and representation are discussed by Halbertal and Margalit, *Idolatry*, pp. 54–66. On the two phases of purification of religious belief on the part of Maimonides, denying that God is a body and divesting God of all attribution, see Elliot R. Wolfson, "*Via Negativa* in Maimonides and Its Impact on Thirteenth-Century Kabbalah," *Maimonidean Studies* 5 (2008): 400–404.

51. Deleuze, *Expressionism in Philosophy*, p. 54.

52. Anton A. van Niekerk, "Postmetaphysical versus Postmodern Thinking:

Retaining the Baby without the Bathwater," *Philosophy Today* 39 (1995): 171–84; James R. Mensch, *Postfoundational Phenomenology: Husserlian Reflections on Presence and Embodiment* (University Park: Pennsylvania State University Press, 2001).

53. Here I depart from the course set by Henry, *The Essence of Manifestation*, pp. 138–39.

54. My thinking is aligned with the categorical rejection of theistic representations of the ultimate reality expressed in certain strands of Buddhism. Particularly relevant is the discussion in Richard P. Hayes, "Principled Atheism in the Buddhist Scholastic Tradition," in *Indian Philosophy: A Collection of Readings*, edited with introductions by Roy W. Perrett (New York: Garland Publishing, 2000), pp. 107–30. See also the analysis of theism and nontheism in Michael McGhee, *Transformations of Mind: Philosophy as Spiritual Practice* (Cambridge: Cambridge University Press, 2000), pp. 149–70.

55. Wyschogrod, "The Civilizational Perspective," pp. 61–62. See as well *idem*, "Intending Transcendence: Desiring God," in *Companion to Postmodern Theology*, edited by Graham Ward (London: Blackwell, 2001), pp. 349–65, reprinted in Edith Wyschogrod, *Crossover Queries: Dwelling with Negatives, Embodying Philosophy's Others* (New York: Fordham University Press, 2006), pp. 13–28. For an alternative approach to Heideggerian thinking on the topic of God as transcendent and the possible retrieval of the ontotheological, see Sonya Sikka, *Forms of Transcendence: Heidegger and Medieval Mystical Theology* (Albany: State University of New York Press, 1997).

56. It is worth recalling the statement of Paul Tillich, *The Courage to Be* (New Haven: Yale University Press, 1952), p. 185: "Theism in all its forms is transcended in the experience we have called absolute faith. It is the accepting of the acceptance without somebody or something that accepts. It is the power of being-itself that accepts and gives the courage to be. This is the highest point to which our analysis has brought us." It is noteworthy that Tillich's characterization of the absolute faith entails the transcendence of theism. For an extensive analysis of Tillich's worldview, see Roy D. Morrison, II, *Science, Theology and the Transcendental Horizon: Einstein, Kant and Tillich* (Atlanta: Scholars Press, 1994), pp. 113–92 and especially the section on detheification, pp. 173–81.

57. I am tacitly criticizing the phenomenology of the gift proffered by Marion and particularly its eucharistic implications. See *God Without Being*, pp. 161–82; *The Visible and the Revealed*, pp. 80–100 and p. 121; *Reduction and Givenness: Investigations of Husserl, Heidegger, and Phenomenology*, translated by Thomas A. Carlson (Evanston: Northwestern University Press, 1998), pp.

35–39, 42–43, 49–56; *Being Given*, pp. 71–118; "The Event, the Phenomenon, and the Revealed," in *Transcendence in Philosophy and Religion*, edited by James E. Faulconer (Bloomington: Indiana University Press, 2003), pp. 87–105, and the alternate translation "The Event or the Happening Phenomenon," in Marion, *In Excess*, pp. 30–53; and "The Reason of the Gift," in *Givenness and God*, pp. 101–34. For various discussions of this theme, particularly in Derrida and Marion, see Richard Kearney, "On the Gift: A Discussion between Jacques Derrida and Jean-Luc Marion," in *God, the Gift, and Postmodernism*, pp. 54–78; Thomas A. Carlson, *Indiscretion: Finitude and the Naming of God* (Chicago: University of Chicago Press, 1999), pp. 191–236; John D. Caputo, "Apostles of the Impossible: On God and the Gift in Derrida and Marion," in *God, the Gift, and Postmodernism*, pp. 185–222; Dominique Janicaud, "The Theological Turn of French Phenomenology," translated by Bernard G. Prusak, in *Phenomenology and the "Theological Turn": The French Debate* (New York: Fordham University Press, 2000), pp. 3–106; Robyn Horner, *Rethinking God as Gift: Marion, Derrida, and the Limits of Phenomenology* (New York: Fordham University Press, 2001); Gschwandtner, *Reading Jean-Luc Marion*, pp. 72–76, 140–45, 212–13; and Mark Manolopoulos, *If Creation Is a Gift* (Albany: State University of New York Press, 2009). See also the analysis of Nietzsche and Derrida on giving and being in Stephen H. Webb, *The Gifting God: A Trinitarian Ethics of Excess* (New York: Oxford University Press, 1996), pp. 58–81.

58. See Marlène Zarader, "Phenomenality and Transcendence," in *Transcendence in Philosophy and Religion*, pp. 106–19.

59. Here, too, my thinking is in dialogue with the likes of Marion, Caputo, Kearney, and a host of others who are part of the so-called "theological turn" in Continental philosophy. Specifically, I am interrogating the reversion to a theopoetic rendering of the self-giving. Poeticizing may well be an "act of constantly opening horizons of possibility," but there is no categorical need (unless one is predisposed to a theological pretense) to transpose those "gifts of possibility" into the "divine gift as creation" (Richard Kearney, "In Place of a Response," in *After God*, p. 375). Compare the astute assessment of Marion's notion of the gift in Verhack, "Immanent Transcendence," pp. 109–12. For a Lacanian critique of Marion along these lines, see Clayton Crockett, *Interstices of the Sublime: Theology and Psychoanalytic Theory* (New York: Fordham University Press, 2007), pp. 133–47. Givenness implies giving and the given, not necessarily a gift, especially if the latter is portrayed in postmodern theological terms as divinity liberated from the constriction of ontotheology. A sophisticated, although in my sense still inadequate attempt to utilize the image of the gift to effect the shift away from the God talk of theism and to serve as

the basis for a new grammar to think and write about the divine is found in Schrag, *God as Otherwise*, pp. 77–143. For another attempt to affirm transcendence without presuming divine being, see Mayra Rivera, *The Touch of Transcendence: A Postcolonial Theology* (Louisville: Westminster John Knox Press, 2007). Influenced by Levinas, Irigaray, Hispanic liberation theology, as well as the apophatic philosophical tradition in the West, Rivera's argument begins from the starting point that God is the irreducibly other always beyond our grasp, although perhaps not beyond our touch. The author employs the terms *relational transcendence* or *intracosmic transcendence* to denote a transcendence between creatures within creation, or more specifically, a transcendence that is encountered in the flesh of the other. God as the wholly other is the extreme illustration of interhuman difference, even as the author insists that her sense of transcendence avoids the "hard boundary" between the divine and the created (p. 133). For another attempt to reclaim *sacred transcendence* as the wholly other (in Rudolph Otto's expression) but yet accessible and immanent in the world, see Martin J. De Nys, *Considering Transcendence: Elements of a Philosophical Theology* (Bloomington: Indiana University Press, 2009), pp. 17–22.

60. Wilfrid Sellars, *Empiricism and the Philosophy of Mind*, with an introduction by Richard Rorty and a study guide by Robert Brandom (Cambridge, MA: Harvard University Press, 1997), p. 15. Needless to say, the main objective of this book is to criticize the assumption, which Sellars labels the "Myth of the Given," that direct and immediate experience is possible (pp. 33–34, 58–59, 64–65, 68–69, 77, 84–88, 112–13, 117).

61. Maurice Blanchot, *The Writing of Disaster*, translated by Ann Smock (Lincoln: University of Nebraska Press, 1986), p. 65: "Between the two falsely interrogative propositions—why is there something rather than nothing? and, why is there evil rather than good?—I do not recognize the difference which is supposed to be discernible, for both are sustained by a 'there is' [*un 'il y a'*] which is neither being nor nothingness, neither good nor evil, and without which the whole discussion collapses, or on account of which it has already collapsed. Above all, the *il y a*, because neutral, mocks the questions which bear upon it: when interrogated, it ironically absorbs the inquiry which cannot oversee it." For discussion of the *il y a* in Blanchot's thought and its relationship to Levinas, see Simon Critchley, "*Il y a*—Holding Levinas's Hand to Blanchot's Fire," in *Maurice Blanchot: The Demand of Writing*, pp. 10–22; Bruns, *Maurice Blanchot*, pp. 56–61.

62. See Edith Wyschogrod, *An Ethics of Remembering: History, Heterology, and the Nameless Others* (Chicago: University of Chicago Press, 1998), p. 16. Wyschogrod refers only to the *il y a* of Levinas, although she does mention that

just as mood is determinative of Heidegger's account of Dasein's relation to the world, so, too, for Levinas, the *il y a* is disclosed through horror. Without collapsing the important differences between the two thinkers, it seems to me correct to apply Wyschogrod's account of Levinas's *il y a* to Heidegger's *es gibt*. See also Wyschogrod, *Crossover Queries*, p. 69; Mark C. Taylor, *Altarity* (Chicago: University of Chicago Press, 1987), pp. 204–205. For a trenchant contrast of the two, based in part on Levinas's own efforts (see below, n. 64), see Dermot Moran, *An Introduction to Phenomenology* (London: Routledge, 2000), p. 334. For a list of other sources where the Heideggerian *es gibt* and the Levinasian *il y a* are discussed, see Alain P. Toumayan, *Encountering the Other: The Artwork and the Problem of Difference in Blanchot and Levinas* (Pittsburgh: Duquesne University Press, 2004), pp. 204–205 n. 5.

63. Paola Marrati, *Genesis and Trace: Derrida Reading Husserl and Heidegger* (Stanford: Stanford University Press, 2005), p. 99: "To think being not in relation to beings, but in relation to the *es gibt* whence it comes, means to think a history in which what takes place happens by way of an essential withdrawal, but a withdrawal that is no longer envisaged as something that would have taken place elsewhere, outside of the history that it produces and whose hidden ground it would be. This, if anything, is what is at stake in ontological difference." See *ibid.*, pp. 181–82: "It is the Husserlian problem of a genetic and non-static form of the transcendental, of a temporality of truth itself of which omnitemporality is but one form, that Derrida finds the possibility of a passivity that overflows the sphere of the transcendental, of a depth or profundity of genesis that complicates any purely phenomenological origin, of an alterity that cuts through all constitution. The empirical is a figure, a name for this alterity, the name of an 'already constituted' before any constitution (whether active or passive). The contamination of the empirical and the transcendental... points toward a double necessity. It justifies the transcendental demand of sense and of truth—of justice, even, if one shares Derrida's fears that the horizon of truth in our Western history is rather too epistemological to allow any scope for an ethics. It is a 'transcendental' demand because it is not immanent, identifiable or locatable, never present if the present is taken to refer to the synchrony of a manifestation or a recognition. It is the demand to *make* sense and to *make* truth... a sense and a truth neither of which is destined to disappear from the moment of their emergence but, as Celan writes of the poem, to forge a path toward eternity *through* time and not beyond it.... This 'transcendental' demand is already worked by the 'empirical'; the empirical already inscribes within the transcendental the singularity, the contingency, the fragility of every event, a contingency that does not merely signal resignation in the face of

the chaos and chance of the world . . . but points toward the ethical tensions of a temporality no longer centered on the present. The inscription of the empirical in the transcendental opens the latter to a constitutive alterity that can no longer function as an illusion or a protective strategy against anxiety" (emphasis in the original). I am not persuaded that the commingling of the empirical and the transcendental necessarily opens the latter to an alterity that occasions an ethical response, but this is a matter that I cannot pursue in detail here.

64. Emmanuel Levinas, *Existence and Existents*, translated by Alphonso Lingis, foreword by Robert Bernasconi (Pittsburgh: Duquesne University Press, 2001), pp. 51–60 (first published as "Il y a," *Deucalion* 1 [1946]: 141–54). On the attempt to differentiate his notion of *il y a* from the Heideggerian *es gibt*, see Emmanuel Levinas, *Ethics and Infinity: Conversations with Philippe Nemo*, translated by Richard A. Cohen (Pittsburgh: Duquesne University Press, 1985), pp. 47–52.

65. Emmanuel Levinas, *Otherwise Than Being or Beyond Essence*, translated by Alphonso Lingis (Dordrecht: Kluwer, 1991), pp. 5–7, 23, 45–48 (*Autrement qu'être ou au-delà de l'essence* [The Hague: Martinus Nijhoff, 1974], pp. 6–9, 29, 58–61). On saying as the silence that speaks through the "hyperbolic passivity of giving, which is prior to all willing and thematization," the "bearing witness of responsibility" that precedes every said, see Emmanuel Levinas, *Of God Who Comes to Mind*, translated by Bettina Bergo (Stanford: Stanford University Press, 1998), p. 74. Blanchot, *The Writing of Disaster*, p. 71, described suicide as "the effacement or destruction, or gift, which has always already been exposed in the precession of Speaking—Speaking separate from and outside of anything spoken, the sheer saying of writing—whereby this effacement, far from effacing itself in its turn, perpetuates itself without end, even in the interruption that is its mark." See Chapter 5 n. 128. The Levinasian distinction between the said and the saying has been discussed by numerous scholars. See Bernhard Waldenfels, "Levinas on the Saying and the Said," in *Addressing Levinas*, edited by Eric Sean Nelson, Antje Kapust, and Kent Still (Evanston: Northwestern University Press, 2005), pp. 86–97.

66. Emmanuel Levinas, *Entre Nous: On Thinking-of-the-Other*, translated by Michael B. Smith and Barbara Harshav (New York: Columbia University Press, 1998), pp. 123–32; *idem*, *Alterity and Transcendence*, translated by Michael B. Smith (New York: Columbia University Press, 1999), pp. 16–26; see John E. Drabinski, *Sensibility and Singularity: The Problem of Phenomenology in Levinas* (Albany: State University of New York Press, 2001), p. 146.

67. See Edith Wyschogrod, "Corporeality and the Glory of the Infinite in the Philosophy of Emmanuel Levinas," *Incarnation: Proceedings of the Conference*

of the Instituto di Studi Filosofici Enrico Castelli 63 (1998): 113–26, reprinted in *Crossover Queries*, pp. 29–44; *idem*, "Language and Alterity in the Thought of Levinas," in *The Cambridge Companion to Levinas*, edited by Simon Critchley and Robert Bernasconi (Cambridge: Cambridge University Press, 2002), pp. 195–98. Compare the examination of the face, the problem of appearance, the break with ontology, and the idea of the infinite in Edith Wyschogrod, *Emmanuel Levinas: The Problem of Ethical Metaphysics*, 2nd edition (New York: Fordham University Press, 2000), pp. 90–102. See also Etienne Feron, *De l'idée de transcendance à la question du langage: L'itinéraire philosophique de Levinas* (Grenoble: J. Millon, 1982); Adriaan T. Peperzak, *Beyond: The Philosophy of Emmanuel Levinas* (Evanston: Northwestern University Press, 1997), pp. 72–120, 162–170; Theodore de Boer, *The Rationality of Transcendence: Studies in the Philosophy of Emmanuel Levinas* (Amsterdam: J. C. Gieben, 1997); Catherine Chalier, *La trace de l'infini: Emmanuel Levinas et la source hébraïque* (Paris: Cerf, 2002), pp. 77–106 253–67; Philippe Crignon, "Figuration: Emmanuel Levinas and the Image," *Yale French Studies* 104 (2004): 100–125; Robert Bernasconi, "No Exit: Levinas' Aporetic Account of Transcendence," *Research in Phenomenology* 35 (2005): 101–17; Bettina Bergo, "Ontology, Transcendence, and Immanence in Emmanuel Levinas' Philosophy," *Research in Phenomenology* 35 (2005): 141–77; Samuel Moyn, *Origins of the Other: Emmanuel Levinas between Revelation and Ethics* (Ithaca: Cornell University Press, 2005), pp. 182–86; Merold Westphal, *Levinas and Kierkegaard in Dialogue* (Bloomington: Indiana University Press, 2008), pp. 58–111; and Sarah Allen, *The Philosophical Sense of Transcendence: Levinas and Plato on Loving Beyond Being* (Pittsburgh: Duquesne University Press, 2009). The approach of Levinas can be situated in the broader context of the Jewish philosophical aversion to the "lure of immanence" analyzed in detail by Steven Schwarzschild, *The Pursuit of the Ideal: Jewish Writings of Steven Schwarzschild*, edited by Menachem Kellner (Albany: State University of New York Press, 1990), pp. 61–81. See as well the analysis of the concept of the *Shekhinah* on pp. 235–50. I do not accept Schwarzschild's sharp contrast of the Jewish and Christian approaches to transcendence and immanence—the former views the will of God as the mechanism by which the divine is utterly separate from and yet intimately related to the world, whereas the latter posits a spatial model of incarnation, a "quasi-physical link" that, paradoxically, retains the "dichotomy between divinity and humanity" (p. 72)—but I do think that the portrait he paints (based, in no small measure, on the neo-Kantian idealism of Hermann Cohen) suitably applies to Levinas inasmuch as it is the ethical relation that both preserves the transcendence of God vis-à-vis nature and secures the possibility of the immanence of God in nature, especially in the sphere of interpersonal subjectivity.

68. Emmanuel Levinas, *The Levinas Reader*, edited by Seán Hand (Oxford: Blackwell, 1989), p. 148. For a more extended discussion of Levinas's critique of the Christian doctrine of incarnation, see Elliot R. Wolfson, "Secrecy, Modesty, and the Feminine: Kabbalistic Traces in the Thought of Levinas," in *The Exorbitant: Emmanuel Levinas between Jews and Christians*, edited by Kevin Hart and Michael A. Signer (New York: Fordham University Press, 2010), pp. 57–60, and compare the study of Gibbs cited below, n. 75.

69. Emmanuel Levinas, *Totality and Infinity: An Essay on Exteriority*, translated by Alphonso Lingis (Dordrecht: Kluwer, 1969), p. 171. I have also consulted *Totalité et infini: Essai sur l'extériorité* (The Hague: Martinus Nijhoff, 1961), p. 146.

70. *Ibid.*, p. 193 (*Totalité et infini*, p. 167).

71. *Ibid.*, p. 295 (*Totalité et infini*, p. 271).

72. Levinas, *Entre Nous*, p. 153. Compare Levinas, *Otherwise Than Being*, pp. 11–12 (*Autrement qu'être*, p. 14): "What is exceptional in this way of being signaled is that I am ordered toward the face of the other. In this order which is an ordination the non-presence of the infinite is not only a figure of negative theology. All the negative attributes which state what is beyond the essence become positive in responsibility, a response answering to a non-thematizable provocation and thus a non-vocation, a trauma." A similar criticism can be leveled against the later turn in Derrida's thinking; see the brief remarks on the passage from Marrati cited above, n. 63. For an attempt, unsuccessful in my judgment, to make sense of this dimension of Derrida's thought in relation to Levinas, see John D. Caputo, "*Adieu—sans Dieu*: Derrida and Levinas," in *The Face of the Other and the Trace of God: Essays on the Philosophy of Emmanuel Levinas*, edited by Jeffrey Bloechl (New York: Fordham University Press, 2000), pp. 276–311.

73. Emmanuel Levinas, *In the Time of the Nations*, translated by Michael B. Smith (London: Athlone, 1994), p. 171.

74. Most relevant is the lecture "Contempt for the Torah as Idolatry" in Levinas, *In the Time of the Nations*, pp. 55–75. See also the characterization of idolatry as the crossing of spatial transcendence by vision or as the rupture of transcendence, the secularization of which is identified further as the knowledge of the West, in Levinas, *God, Death, and Time*, p. 164. The emphasis on ontology—the nature of being comprehended by the intelligibility of the identification of being as being—is labeled by Levinas as the "transcendence of idolatry" or the "idolatrous transcendence" (p. 165).

75. Regarding this theme, see Robert Gibbs, "The Disincarnation of the Word: The Trace of God in Reading Scripture," in *The Exorbitant*, pp. 32–51.

76. My brief appraisal of Levinas can be compared profitably with the criticism of Jacques Derrida's seminal study "Violence and Metaphysics: An Essay on the Thought of Emmanuel Levinas" in *Writing and Difference*, translated with introduction and additional notes by Alan Bass (Chicago: University of Chicago Press, 1978), pp. 79–153, esp. 85–86, 114–17, 132–33, and see also Janicaud, "The Theological Turn," pp. 33–49; Todd May, *Reconsidering Difference: Nancy, Derrida, Levinas, and Deleuze* (University Park: Pennsylvania State University Press, 1997), pp. 90–94; Kas Saghafi, *Apparitions—Of Derrida's Other* (New York: Fordham University Press, 2010), pp. 7–28. See, by contrast, Schrag, *God as Otherwise*, p. 72, who is of the opinion that Levinas's "transposition of transcendence from an ontological into an ethical key opens new possibilities for thinking about God as the other than the other.... Levinas undermines the metaphysical, the ontological, the transcendental, and the existential notions of transcendence and recommends that we explore the meaning of transcendence as an event of the ethical." Based on the Levinasian critique and the turn from an ontological to an ethical notion of transcendence, Schrag advocates utilizing the image of the gift as the central component in the new grammar and new semantics in the discourse about the "God above God" (p. 143) that is appropriate to a postmodern era. Compare Hent de Vries, *Minimal Theologies: Critiques of Secular Reason in Adorno and Levinas*, translated by Geoffrey Hale (Baltimore: Johns Hopkins University Press, 2005), pp. 533–34. De Vries concludes that the perspective on transcendence to be elicited from the writings of Adorno and Levinas "is more paradoxical—indeed, is surreptitious—and permanently runs the risk of idolatry and blasphemy. This is not due to a lack of consistency or rigor in their philosophical projects: rather, of the *tertium datur* there can be neither truth or falsity, since this dimension is at once indestructible or irrepressible and undecidable or aporetic. It can only be 'said' through 'unsaying' and cannot be 'unsaid' without entangling it—once again—in the 'said' that the 'unsaying' interrupts, only immediately to betray itself in turn, ad infinitum." See *ibid.*, pp. 23–24, 33–36, 347–48. While de Vries acknowledges the "echo" or "resonance" of monotheistic religion in Levinas's characterization of the infinitely Other and thus accepts that this "central motif" in Judaism "in part determines the tone and texture of his philosophical thinking," he nonetheless insists that Levinas did not construct, reconstruct, or deconstruct "a religious philosophy in the systematic, let alone dogmatic, theological sense. Therefore, religious tradition cannot weigh decisively in an evaluation of the contribution of his figures of thought to a minimal theology whose modus operandi lies in the diminishing yet still remaining dimension of the almost invisible, the nearly untouchable, the scarcely audible, *in pianissimo*"

(p. 351). While I agree that one cannot elicit a systematic or dogmatic theology from Levinas, I do not concur that the impact of his Jewish faith was as limited as de Vries argues. On the contrary, it seems to me that it is precisely this commitment that renders his metaphysics of transcendence problematic and suspect of succumbing to theolatry, a theme that I explored in my lecture "Echo of the Otherwise: Erotic Transcendence and Overcoming Theolatry in Levinas and Wyschogrod," delivered in the Colloque International sur l'oeuvre de Emmanuel Levinas: Lectures de Difficile Liberté, held in Toulouse, France, July 4–9, 2010. I thus respectfully take issue with the conclusion reached by de Vries, *Minimal Theology*, p. 533: "Levinas's late work consistently explores a modality of transcendence which can dispense with the complementary false affirmatives of a complete negativity of the same (and hence absence of the other) or an unambiguous positivity (and hence presence) of the other. The trace makes plausible the diminishing but still remaining intelligibility of the discourse concerning transcendence in general and God in particular without once again burdening philosophy with a questionable ontotheology, the metaphysics of presence or absence to which theism and its analogues, yet likewise atheism with its naturalisms and humanisms, fall prey. A far more complicated relationship between infinity and fulfillment holds among all these historical, traditional and modern, dogmatic and enlightened, doctrines." For a similar approach to mark a shift from the affirmation of a metaphysical transcendence in *Totality and Infinity* to a transcendence without metaphysics in *Otherwise Than Being*, see Michael Fagenblat, *A Covenant of Creatures: Levinas's Philosophy of Judaism* (Stanford: Stanford University Press, 2010), pp. 101–106. In my judgment, the ethics of transcendence promulgated by Levinas may involve an irreconcilable tension between the metaphorical tropes of the face and the trace, the former demarcating the embodied corporeality demanded by the specificity of the other and the latter the disincarnation that is necessary to safeguard the glory of the infinite as that which remains other and forever beyond our grasp, but if spiritual optics culminates in an atheological showing, this should lead to an apophatic venturing beyond the theomorphic need to configure the transcendent even in the image of the nonmetaphorical metaphorization of the face as the nonappearing of the infinite other. It is for this reason that I also do not accept the surmise of de Vries (*Minimal Theologies*, p. 480) that Levinas's thought "touches profoundly on that of an open, that is to say, negative dialectical speculation: micrologically encircling a transcendence in immanence or immanence in transcendence that is, at the same time, a transcendence of transcendence and, hence, an immanence thought and experienced *otherwise*" (emphasis in the original). I do not see evidence for the transcendence of transcendence that would lead to the immanent positivity without recourse to the positing of the negative qua negative, that is, the negative that in no way is reduced to the positive, the transcendence that is immanent only by being transcendent. It seems to me this move is absolutely necessary to preserve Levinas's insistence that the "encounter in dialogue" is a "thought thinking beyond the world" (*Of God Who Comes to Mind*, p. 146). It is on this very point, moreover, that Levinas breaks with the correlation between thought and the world posited by Husserl and the phenomenological assumption that "appearing" is a "giving itself" to intentional consciousness. See *Of God Who Comes to Mind*, p. 139, and see *ibid.*, p. 100, where Levinas describes the "thought awakened to God" as a thought that "aspires to a beyond, to a deeper than oneself—aspiring to a transcendence different from the out-of-oneself that the intentional consciousness opens and traverses." Compare the passage cited below, n. 80.

77. Levinas, *Totality and Infinity*, p. 77 (emphasis in the original). I previously cited the end of this passage in "Secrecy," p. 58, but carelessly neglected to give the reference. Regarding this critical text, see also the comments of Dana Hollander, "Is the Other My Neighbor? Reading Levinas Alongside Hermann Cohen," in *The Exorbitant*, p. 98, and the reference to Purcell in the following note. The passage from *Totality and Infinity* should be compared with Levinas's observation in *Otherwise Than Being*, p. 5 (*Autrement qu'être*, p. 6): "Is not the inescapable fate in which being immediately includes the statement of being's *other* not due to the hold the *said* has over the *saying*, to the *oracle* in which the said is immobilized? Then would not the bankruptcy of transcendence be but that of a theology that thematizes the *transcending* in the logos, assigns a term to the passing of transcendence, congeals it into a 'world behind the scenes,' and installs what it says in war and in matter, which are the inevitable modalities of the fate woven by being in its interest?" (emphasis in the original). See also the bold formulation in Emmanuel Levinas, *God, Death, and Time*, translated by Bettina Bergo (Stanford: Stanford University, 2000), p. 207: "We then interpreted this breaking open of experience in witnessing, this agitation of the Same by the Other, as the *diachrony* of time. This is a time that would lend itself [*se donnerait*] to our understanding as a reference to God—as the *to-God* itself [l'*à-Dieu* même]—before being interpreted as a pure deficiency or as a synonym of the perishable or the noneternal. That is, what gives itself to be understood as that which is diametrically opposed to the traditional idea of God" (emphasis in the original).

78. Levinas, *Totalité et infini*, p. 50. Compare Levinas, *In the Time*, pp. 170–71: "To me, religion means transcendence, which, as proximity of the

absolutely other (i.e., of the one of the kind), is not a failed coinciding.... Religion is the excellence proper to sociality with the Absolute, or, if you will, in the positive sense of the expression, Peace with the other." See *idem*, *Alterity and Transcendence*, p. 35: "Obedience to the absolute order... to the word of God, on the condition of not naming God except on the basis of this obedience. An un-known God who does not take on a body, and who exposes himself to the denials of atheism!" On theology and the temptation of atheism in Levinas, see Michael Purcell, *Levinas and Theology* (Cambridge: Cambridge University Press, 2006), pp. 60–63. On Levinas's vision of divine transcendence as a form of "ontological atheism," see John Llewelyn, "Am I Obsessed by Bobby? (Humanism of the Other Animal)," in *Re-Reading Levinas*, edited by Robert Bernasconi and Simon Critchley (Bloomington: Indiana University Press, 1991), p. 239; Donald L. Turner and Ford Turrell, "The Non-Existent God: Transcendence, Humanity, and Ethics in the Philosophy of Emmanuel Levinas," *Philosophia* 35 (2007): 375–82, esp. 376–77. For Levinas's critique of theology, see also Richard A. Cohen, "Against Theology, or 'The Devotion of a Theology without Theodicy': Levinas on Religion," in *The Exorbitant*, pp. 74–89, esp. 78–83. For an innovative approach to this question, see Martin Kavka, "Levinas between Monotheism and Cosmotheism," in *Levinas Studies: An Annual Review* 2 (2007): 79–103, and the recent discussion in Fagenblat, *A Covenant of Creatures*, pp. 142–43.

79. For a critique of social utopianism, see Levinas, *Alterity and Transcendence*, pp. 111–17. On the lingering teleological dimension of Levinas's messianic speculation, see Graham Ward, "On Time and Salvation: The Eschatology of Emmanuel Levinas," in *Facing the Other: The Ethics of Emmanuel Levinas*, edited by Seán Hand (Surrey: Curzon, 1996), pp. 153–72. See also Bettina Bergo, "The Time and Language of Messianism: Levinas and Saint Paul," in *Levinas and the Ancients*, edited by Brian Schroeder and Silvia Benso (Bloomington: Indiana University Press, 2008), pp. 178–95. Bergo avoids the words "utopian" or "teleological," but her characterization of Levinas as a messianic thinker who believed that in the time that remains, that is, the time of the future, the "Good" will come to pass, justifies the use of these terms. For other accounts of eschatology in Levinas, see de Boer, *The Rationality of Transcendence*, pp. 33–55; Robert Bernasconi, "Different Styles of Eschatology: Derrida's Take on Levinas' Political Messianism," *Research in Phenomenology* 28 (1998): 3–19; Michael L. Morgan, *Discovering Levinas* (Cambridge: Cambridge University Press, 2007), pp. 208–27; Pierre Bouretz, *Witnesses for the Future: Philosophy and Messianism*, translated by Michael B. Smith (Baltimore: Johns Hopkins University Press, 2010), pp. 647–719.

80. Levinas, *Totality and Infinity*, pp. 77–78; (*Totalité et infini*, p. 50). For a more extensive analysis of dialogue, self-consciousness, and the proximity of the neighbor, see Levinas, *Of God Who Comes to Mind*, pp. 137–51, esp. 147: "Dialogue is thus not merely a way of speaking. Its significance has a general reach. It is transcendence. The saying involved in dialogue would not be one of the possible forms of transcendence but its original mode. Better again, transcendence has no meaning except by way of an I saying You. It is the *dia* of the dialogue. In the concrete context of the human, transcendence is thus a concept at least as valuable as that of immanence in the world, the ultimacy of which transcendence places in question." As Levinas makes clear in the continuation of this passage (pp. 147–48), speaking of that which is beyond the world does not signify the traditional metaphysical sense of "worlds behind the world" criticized by Nietzsche nor does it presuppose a notion of the self as a reified substance or subject. His notion of transcendence, in a word, is "beyond the anthropological and theological thematic." Compare the remarks on divine transcendence and ontological difference in Levinas, *Of God Who Comes to Mind*, pp. 125–26.

81. Levinas, *Totality and Infinity*, p. 78 (*Totalité et infini*, pp. 50–51).

82. Levinas, *Otherwise Than Being*, p. 3 (*Autrement qu'être*, pp. 3–4); Howard Caygill, *Levinas and the Political: Thinking the Political* (London: Routledge, 2002), p. 146. For discussion of Levinas's characterization of infinity as a *coincidentia oppositorum*, influenced by Kierkegaard's critique of Hegel's speculative infinite, see Taylor, *Altarity*, pp. 188–95. The engagement of Levinas's thought with Neoplatonism has been the emphasis of a number of studies, of which I will here mention a few of the relevant examples. See Jean-Marc Narbonne, *Levinas and the Greek Heritage* (Leuven: Peeters, 2006); John Izzi, "Proximity in Distance: Levinas and Plotinus," in *Levinas and the Ancients*, pp. 196–209, and in the same volume, the chapter by Brian Schroeder, "A Trace of the Eternal Return? Levinas and Neoplatonism," pp. 210–29. On the Platonic element in Levinas, see also Allen, *The Philosophical Sense of Transcendence*; Tanja Staehler, *Plato and Levinas: The Ambiguous Out-Side of Ethics* (New York: Routledge, 2010). For a critique of the Levinasian attempt to deploy phenomenology in the service of retrieving the Platonic metaphysics of transcendence, see Stella Sandford, *The Metaphysics of Love: Gender and Transcendence in Levinas* (London: Athlone, 2000), pp. 1–32. It goes without saying that Levinas himself would distinguish his conception of "transcendence in sociality" and the "proximity of the other" from the Plotinian notion of the ecstatic return of all things to the One beyond being and knowing. See *Alterity and Transcendence*, pp. 6–10, and p. 37: "Dis-interestedness of a responsibility for the other and for his *past*—a

past that for me is immemorial—on the basis of the *future* of prophesy—without which the un-known God would remain inaudible in his glory, breaking his negative theology without words—that is the temporality in which the intrigue of being and ontology is resolved in ethics" (emphasis in the original). Finally, it is worth noting that Levinas distinguished his critique of ontotheology from Heidegger's. See the author's "Note" appended to *Otherwise Than Being*, p. xlii (*Autrement qu'être*, p. x): "But to hear a God not contaminated by Being is a human possibility no less important and no less precarious than to bring Being out of the oblivion in which it is said to have fallen in metaphysics and in onto-theology." The reference to Heidegger is even more explicit in Levinas, *God, Death, and Time*, p. 160: "Onto-theo-logy consists in thinking of God as a being [*étant*] and in thinking being [*être*] on the basis of this superior or supreme being. The Heideggerian critique concerns this way of misunderstanding being and consists in saying that we must ultimately think of being, as all of metaphysics has done, on the basis of beings and only as the being of beings. The inquiry carried out here also begins from a critique of onto-theo-logy, but it seeks to think God without making being or beings intervene in the relation with God. It seeks to think God as a beyond-being" (emphasis in the original).

83. Levinas, *Otherwise Than Being*, p. 11 (*Autrement qu'être*, p. 13): "The non-present here is invisible, separated (or sacred) and thus a non-origin, an-archical. The Good cannot become present or enter into a representation."

84. Levinas, *Otherwise Than Being*, p. 8 (*Autrement qu'être*, pp. 9–10).

85. *Ibid.*, p. 100 (*Autrement qu'être*, p. 126).

86. *Ibid.*, pp. 88–90 (*Autrement qu'être*, pp. 112–14)

87. *Ibid.*, p. 152 (*Autrement qu'être*, p. 194).

88. *Ibid.*, p. 140 (*Autrement qu'être*, p. 179).

89. Levinas, *Totality and Infinity*, p. 78 (*Totalité et infini*, pp. 50–51). Compare *idem*, *Alterity and Transcendence*, p. 5: "Is not the face of one's fellow man the original locus in which transcendence calls an authority with a silent voice in which God comes to the mind? Original locus of the Infinite." And *ibid.*, pp. 32–35. See also Levinas, *Otherwise Than Being*, p. 12 (*Autrement qu'être*, p. 14): "This response answers, before any understanding, for a debt contracted before any freedom and before any consciousness and any present, but it does answer, as though the invisible that bypasses the present left a trace by the very fact of bypassing the present. That trace lights up as the face of the neighbor, ambiguously him *before whom* (or *to whom*, without any paternalism) and him *for whom* I answer. For such is the enigma or ex-ception of a face, judge and accused" (emphasis in original).

90. Levinas, *Of God Who Comes To Mind*, p. 166. Turner and Turrell, "The

Non-Existent God," pp. 377–78, go so far as to say that by humanizing divinity, or divinizing humanity, Levinas is in basic agreement with Feuerbach and Nietzsche. See, by contrast, Robert Erlewine, "Reclaiming the Prophets: Cohen, Heschel, and Crossing the Theocentric/Neo-Humanist Divide," *Journal of Jewish Thought and Philosophy* 17 (2009): 197–98.

91. Levinas, *Totality and Infinity*, p. 77 (*Totalité et infini*, p. 49).

92. Compare *ibid.*, p. 66 (*Totalité et infini*, pp. 37–38): "The face speaks. The manifestation of the face is already discourse.... The eyes break through the mask—the language of the eyes, impossible to dissemble. The eye does not shine; it speaks." Even if we were to accept the notion that the speaking ascribed to the face or to the eye is not a language made of words, but rather the linguistic marking of the relationship of proximity (Bruns, *Maurice Blanchot*, p. 109), it is still a mode of figuratively representing what is theoretically beyond any figuration. See Derrida, *Writing and Difference*, pp. 100–109. In his later work, Levinas embraces a more intensified apophatic language—what I would call an apophasis of apophasis—that exceeds his earlier articulations, even as they are conceptually on a par. See, for example, Levinas, *Otherwise Than Being*, p. 151 (*Autrement qu'être*, p. 193): "The refusal of presence is converted into my presence as present, that is, as a hostage delivered over as gift to the other. In proximity, in signification, in my giving of signs, already the Infinite speaks through the witness I bear of it, in my sincerity, in my saying without said, preoriginary saying which is said in the mouth of the very one that receives the witness.... It thus retains in its statement the trace of the excession of transcendence, of the beyond." In that context, Levinas contrasts his own apophatic formulations with the "propositions of negative theology." See also Levinas, *Of God Who Comes to Mind*, p. 69: "In this ethical turnabout, in this reference [*renvoi*] from the Desirable to the Undesirable, in this strange mission commanding the approach to the other, God is pulled out of objectivity, out of presence and out of being. He is neither object nor interlocutor. His absolute remoteness, his transcendence, turns into my responsibility—the non-erotic *par excellence*—for the other. And it is from the analysis just carried out that God is not simply the 'first other,' or the 'other *par excellence*,' or the 'absolutely other,' but other than the other, other otherwise, and other with an alterity prior to the alterity of the other, prior to the ethical obligation to the other and different from every neighbor, transcendent to the point of absence, to the point of his possible confusion with the agitation of the *there is* [*il y a*]." For a parallel formulation, see Levinas, *God, Death, and Time*, pp. 223–24. While I do not deny a shift in his thinking, this should not be overstated to the point of positing some fundamental turn on the path that ignores the continuity and

unity of vision (see the references to de Vries and Fagenblat above, n. 76). Consider the words of Levinas recorded in *Of God Who Comes to Mind*, p. 82: "The ontological language employed in *Totality and Infinity* is ontological because it wants above all not to be psychological. But in reality, it is already a search for what I call 'the beyond being,' the tearing of this equality to self which is always being—the *Sein*—whatever the attempts to separate it from the present." Concerning this passage, see the remarks of Jacques Derrida, *Adieu To Emmanuel Levinas*, translated by Pascale-Anne Brault and Michael Naas (Stanford: Stanford University Press, 1999), p. 143 n. 62. Finally, mention should be made of the comment of Levinas that his three works, *Totality and Infinity, Otherwise Than Being*, and *Of God Who Comes to Mind*, constitute a "whole." The remark is referred to in Salomon Malka, *Emmanuel Levinas: His Life and Legacy*, foreword by Philippe Nemo, translated by Michael Kigel and Sara M. Embree (Pittsburgh: Duquesne University Press, 2006), p. 285.

93. Emmanuel Levinas, *Collected Philosophical Papers*, translated by Alphonso Lingis (Dordrecht: Martinus Nijhoff, 1987), pp. 106–107: "The *illeity* of this He is not the it of things which are at our disposal, and to which Buber and Gabriel Marcel rightly prefer the Thou to describe a human encounter. The movement of an encounter is not something added to an immobile face; it is in the face itself. A face is of itself visitation and a transcendence. But a face, wholly open, can at the same time be in itself because it is in the trace of illeity.... The God who passed [Exodus 33:18–23] is not the model of which the face would be an image. To be in the image of God does not mean to be an icon of God, but to find oneself in his trace. The revealed God of our Judeo-Christian spirituality maintains all the infinity of his absence, which is the 'personal' order itself. He shows himself only by his trace.... To go toward Him is not to follow this trace which is not a sign; it is to go toward the others who stand in the trace of illeity. It is through this illeity, situated beyond the calculations and reciprocities of economy and of the world, that being has a sense. A sense which is not a finality." Compare Levinas, *Otherwise Than Being*, pp. 12–13 (*Autrement qu'être*, pp. 15–16), and see *ibid.*, pp. 93–94 (*Autrement qu'être*, pp. 119–20): "A face is not an appearance or sign of some reality, which would be personal like it is, but dissimulated or expressed by the physiognomy, and which would present itself as an invisible theme.... A face does not function in proximity as a sign of a hidden God who would impose the neighbor on me. It is a trace of itself, a trace in the trace of an abandon, where the equivocation is never dissipated ... a face as a trace, trace of itself, trace expelled in a trace, does not signify an indeterminate phenomenon; its ambiguity is not an indetermination of a noema, but an invitation to the fine risk of approach qua approach, to the exposure of one

to the other, to the exposure of this exposedness, the expression of exposure, saying. In the approach of a face the flesh becomes word, the caress a saying. The thematization of a face undoes the face and undoes the approach."

94. Levinas, *In the Time*, p. 171.

95. Anthony J. Steinbock, "Face and Revelation: Levinas on Teaching as Way-Faring," in *Addressing Levinas*, pp. 119–37.

96. The point I am raising seems to be implied in the remark of Levinas, *Of God Who Comes To Mind*, pp. 105–106: "Philosophical atheism, but also philosophical theism, refuse to accept even the originality of the psyche staking a claim beyond the world. They refuse to accept even the irreducibility of its noetic contours. In the remark about the *beyond*, one suspects an emphatic metaphor for intentional distance. Even if, in this suspicion, one risks having forgotten that the 'movement' beyond is the metaphor.... That is, even if one risks having forgotten that the elevation of meaning by the metaphor in what is *said* [*dit*] owes its height to the *transcendence* of the *saying* [*du dire*] to the other [*autrui*]" (emphasis in the original). On transcendence as the double movement of traversing and ascending, see Levinas, *God, Death, and Time*, p. 163.

97. The approach offered here should be contrasted with the more standard position of many post-Nietzschean philosophers and theologians, including Heidegger, Nancy, and Altizer, for whom the binaries transcendence and immanence, permanence and absence, continue to be understood as polar opposites. See the analysis of this matter in Thomas A. Carlson, "Unlikely Shadows: Transcendence in Image and Immanence," in *Transcendence: Philosophy, Literature, and Theology*, pp. 105–25. And compare Mark C. Taylor, *Tears* (Albany: State University of New York Press, 1990), p. 79: "What does the alternative of transcendence and immanence leave out? Is there a nondialectical third that lies *between* the dialectic of either/or and both/and? Might this third be neither transcendent nor immanent? Does this neither/nor open the time-space of a different difference and an other other—a difference and an other that do not merely invert but actually subvert the polarities of Western philosophical and theological reflection?" See as well the felicitous observation in Steven Heine, *Existential and Ontological Dimensions of Time in Heidegger and Dōgen* (Albany: State University of New York Press, 1985), p. 117: "Transcendence, according to Heidegger, is neither the speculatively claimed a-temporal or supra-temporal objectified realm beyond self and world nor the epistemologically analyzed perception of objects by a *vorhanden* subject. Rather, it represents the repetitive coming-towards of the thrownness or having-been of Being-in-the-world, that either loses itself in making entities present (inauthenticity) or resolutely encounters them in an active moment of vision

(authenticity)." Regarding Dōgen's view of temporality, see Chapter 5 n. 33.

98. Levinas, *Totality and Infinity*, p. 35 (*Totalité et infini*, p. 5). The author appropriates the term "transascendence" from Wahl to designate the "metaphysical movement" toward the transcendent, and as he openly acknowledges in n. 2 (in the original French, n. 1), he has "drawn much inspiration from the themes evoked" in *Existence humaine et transcendance*. Wahl is referred to as well in *Totality and Infinity*, p. 61 n. 6 (*Totalité et infini*, p. 32 n. 1). It is worth recalling as well that Levinas dedicated this work to Marcelle and Jean Wahl. The friendship between Levinas and Wahl is discussed by Malka, *Emmanuel Levinas*, pp. 149–51, 153–55, 158–60, 191–92. See also Levinas, *Collected Philosophical Papers*, p. 8; *idem*, "Jean Wahl et le sentiment," *Cahiers du Sud* 42 (1955): 453-59, English version in Emmanuel Levinas, *Proper Names*, translated by Michael B. Smith (Stanford: Stanford University Press, 1996), pp. 110-18, and the paper given by Levinas subsequent to Wahl's death, "Jean Wahl: Sans avoir ni être," in *Jean Wahl et Gabriel Marcel*, edited by Jeanne Hersch (Paris: Editions Beauchesne, 1976), pp. 13–31, English version in Emmanuel Levinas, *Outside the Subject*, translated by Michael B. Smith (Stanford: Stanford University Press, 1993), pp. 67–83. Levinas's indebtedness to Wahl's idea of transcendence and the quest for the "theological other" is discussed by Moyn, *Origins of the Other*, pp. 177–86.

99. Wahl, *Existence humaine et transcendance* (Neuchatel: Éditions de la Baconnière, 1944), p. 38. For a different interpretation of Wahl's passage and the comment of Deleuze and Guattari cited in n. 101, see Keller, "Rumors of Transcendence," pp. 140–42.

100. Jean Wahl, "Realism, Dialectic, and the Transcendent," *Philosophy and Phenomenological Research* 4 (1944): 498–500; *Existence humaine*, pp. 10–11.

101. Deleuze and Guattari, *What is Philosophy?* p. 45.

102. Ronald Hoy, "The Given and the Self-Presenting," *Noûs* 19 (1985): 347–64.

103. Quentin Meillassoux, *After Finitude: An Essay on the Necessity of Contingency*, translated by Ray Brassier (New York: Continuum, 2008), p. 28.

104. Alain Badiou, *Theoretical Writings*, edited and translated by Ray Brassier and Alberto Toscano (New York: Continuum, 2005), p. 197.

105. *Ibid.*, p. 198.

106. *Ibid.*, p. 201. For a more expansive discussion of the concept of appearing and the transcendental, see Alain Badiou, *Logics of Worlds: Being and Event, 2*, translated by Alberto Toscano (New York: Continuum, 2009), pp. 109–40.

107. An attempt to elicit the "theological promise" of an opening to God from Badiou's atheist ontology is offered by Frederiek Depoortere, *Badiou and*

Theology (New York: Continuum, 2009).

108. Caputo, *The Prayers and Tears*, p. xix. See the discussion on the "poetics of the impossible" in John D. Caputo, *The Weakness of God: A Theology of the Event* (Bloomington: Indiana University Press, 2006), pp. 101–12. On Derrida's interpretation of Heidegger's description of death as the possibility of an impossibility, see Marrati, *Genesis and Trace*, pp. 171–74. For reference to my own reflections on the constitution of temporality along these lines, see Wolfson, *Open Secret*, pp. 265–300.

109. Jacques Derrida, *Specters of Marx: The State of the Debt, the Work of Mourning, and the New International*, translated by Peggy Kamuf, introduction by Bernd Magnus and Stephen Cullenberg (New York: Routledge, 1994), p. 168. For creative elaborations of this dimension of Derridean deconstruction, see Mark C. Taylor, *Erring: A Postmodern A/theology* (Chicago: University of Chicago Press, 1984), and *idem*, *Tears*, pp. 73–85, and for discussion of atheology as transgressive syntax in Bataille, see Taylor, *Altarity*, pp. 135–48. On the possibility of a "deconstructive faith," see also Ian Edwards, "Derrida's (I)religion: A Theology (of Différance)," *Janus Head* 6 (2003): 142–53.

110. Hägglund, *Radical Atheism*, pp. 132–41. The author criticizes Caputo's theological misreading of the Derridean conception of the impossible that is central to his notion of the messianic without messianism. See John D. Caputo, "Temporal Transcendence: The Very Idea of *à-venir* in Derrida," in *Transcendence and Beyond*, pp. 188–203.

111. Merleau-Ponty, *The Visible and the Invisible*, p. 151.

112. I accept the argument that in Merleau-Ponty's phenomenological ontology, being is a process whereby what is simultaneously conceals (*cacher*) and reveals (*dévoiler*) itself, and thus his thought is not subject to the critique of ontological substantialism or metaphysical essentialism. See Atherton C. Lowry, "The Invisible World of Merleau-Ponty," *Philosophy Today* 23 (1979): 294–303. See also Véronique M. Fóti, "Chiasm, Flesh, Figuration: Towards a Non-Objective Ontology," in *Merleau-Ponty and the Possibilities of Philosophy: Transforming the Tradition*, edited by Bernard Flynn, Wayne J. Froman, and Robert Vallier (Albany: State University of New York Press, 2009), pp. 183–96. The conception of flesh and the chiasm of visibility espoused by Merleau-Ponty shares much with the Mahāyāna Buddhist reflection on the emptiness of form (see above, n. 30) as a number of scholars have noted. See, most recently, the collection of essays in *Merleau-Ponty and Buddhism*, edited by Jin Y. Park and Gereon Kopf (Lanham: Rowman & Littlefield, 2009), and especially the study in that volume by Glen A. Mazis, "The Flesh of the World Is Emptiness and Emptiness is the Flesh of the World, and Their Ethical Implications," pp. 183–208.

113. Alphonso Lingis, "Imperatives," in *Merleau-Ponty Vivant*, edited by Martin C. Dillon (Albany: State University of New York Press,1991), pp. 112–13.

114. Slavoj Žižek, *In Defense of Lost Causes* (London: Verso, 2008), p. 127: "The parallax Real is thus opposed to the standard (Lacanian) notion of the Real as that which 'always returns to its place,' namely, as that which remains the same in all possible (symbolic) universes: the parallax Real is rather that which accounts for the very multiplicity of appearances of the same underlying Real—it is not the hard core which persists as the Same, but the hard bone of contention which pulverizes the sameness into the multitude of appearances. In a first move, the Real is the impossible hard core which we cannot confront directly, but only through the lenses of a multitude of symbolic fictions, virtual formations. In a second move, this very hard core is purely virtual, actually non-existing, an X which be reconstructed only retroactively, from the multitude of symbolic formations which are 'all that there actually is.'" For an expanded discussion, see Slavoj Žižek, *The Parallax View* (Cambridge, MA: The MIT Press, 2006).

115. Žižek, *In Defense of Lost Causes*, p. 127 (emphasis in the original). See also pp. 288 and 319.

116. On rethinking the divine as possibility, see Richard Kearney, *The God Who May Be: A Hermeneutics of Religion* (Bloomington: Indiana University Press, 2001). In spite of Kearney's utilization of the dialectical speculation of Nicholas of Cusa (pp. 103–105), he continues to bifurcate the possible and the impossible in a manner that I find unsatisfactory. See also *idem*, "Enabling God," in *After God*, pp. 39–54. My own approach is marked by an overcoming of this polarity, and hence I speak of the "possible impossibility," terminology that is closer in spirit to Derrida's.

117. See, by contrast, Levinas, *Otherwise Than Being*, p. 106 (*Autrement qu'être*, pp. 134–35): "Prior to the return to itself proper to consciousness, this hypostasis, when it shows itself, does so under the borrowed mask of being. The event in which this unity or uniqueness of the hypostasis is brought out is not the grasping of self in consciousness. It is an assignation to answer without evasions, which assigns the self to be a self. Prior to the play of being, before the present, older than the time consciousness that is accessible in memory . . . the oneself is exposed as a hypostasis, of which the being it is as an entity is but a mask. . . . In itself, the oneself is the one or the unique separated from being." The self that is separated from being is that which Levinas usually marks as the face that is presumably behind the mask. It is the positing of something outside or beyond the mask that I find problematic and gratuitous.

CHAPTER ONE: IMAGINING OTHERWISE

1. Friedrich Nietzsche, *The Birth of Tragedy*, sec. 1, in *Basic Writings of Nietzsche*, p. 35.

2. *Ibid.*, sec. 9, p. 67.

3. *Ibid.*, sec. 1, p. 34.

4. *Ibid.*, sec. 4, p. 44.

5. *Ibid.*, sec. 8, p. 63. See Chapter 4 n. 102.

6. *Ibid.*, sec. 1, pp. 35–36.

7. Gordon C. F. Bearn, *Waking to Wonder: Wittgenstein's Existential Investigations* (Albany: State University of New York Press, 1997), p. 26.

8. Nietzsche, *The Birth of Tragedy*, sec. 4, p. 44. See *ibid.*, sec. 1, p. 35: "And perhaps many will, like myself, recall how amid the dangers and terrors of dreams they have occasionally said to themselves in self-encouragement, and not without success: 'It is a dream! I will dream on!' I have likewise heard of people who were able to continue one and the same dream for three and even more successive nights—facts which indicate clearly how our innermost being, our common ground, experiences dreams with profound delight and a joyous necessity." On the phenomenon of lucid dreaming, see the studies cited below, n. 217.

9. Nietzsche, *The Birth of Tragedy*, sec. 4, p. 45.

10. Friedrich Nietzsche, *Human, All Too Human, I*, translated, with an afterword, by Gary Handwerk (Stanford: Stanford University Press, 1995), pp. 22–23.

11. *Ibid.*, p. 18.

12. *Ibid.*, p. 24. On dreams as an "archaic inheritance," see Graham Parkes, *Composing the Soul: Reaches of Nietzsche's Psychology* (Chicago: University of Chicago Press, 1994), pp. 327–34. For discussion of the broader context to appreciate the genealogical approach to dreams, see John Richardson, "Nietzsche Contra Darwin," *Philosophy and Phenomenological Research* 65 (2002): 537–75, esp. 557–58.

13. Sigmund Freud, *The Interpretation of Dreams*, translated and edited by James Strachey, in collaboration with Anna Freud, assisted by Alix Trachey and Alan Tyson, *The Standard Edition of the Complete Psychological Works of Sigmund Freud* [hereafter *SE*], vol. 5 (London: Hogarth Press, 1953), p. 549; see Parkes, *Composing the Soul*, p. 329.

14. This indebtedness has been noted by various scholars. See, for instance, Ricouer, *Freud and Philosophy*, pp. 32–35 and 59–60, and the different approach offered by Tinneke Beeckman, "Reinterpreting Freud's Genealogy of Culture," in *Origins and Ends of the Mind: Philosophical Essays on Psychoanalysis*, edited by Christian Kerslake and Ray Brassier (Leuven: Leuven University Press, 2007),

pp. 117–34. The impact of Nietzsche is also readily discernible in the approach to the symbolism of dreams as the pictorial dramatization of an eternal struggle between the craving of primordial instincts and the demands of cultural inhibition advanced by Stekel, *Sex and Dreams*, pp. 18–21.

15. My use of the terms "irreality" and "irreal" reflects the connotation of *irreal* in the lexicon of Husserl and of *irréel* in the thought of Sartre. For a brief, but instructive discussion, see Jonathan Webber's comments in the "Notes on the Translation" in Jean-Paul Sartre, *The Imaginary: A Phenomenological Psychology of the Imagination*, revisions and historical introduction by Arlette Elkaïm-Sartre, translation and philosophical introduction by Jonathan Webber (London: Routledge, 2004), p. xxviii. In the older translation, Jean-Paul Sartre, *The Psychology of Imagination* (New York: Philosophical Library, 1948), *irréel* was rendered as "unreal" and "unreality." See Edwin L. Hersch, "Imagination and Its Pathologies: Domain of the Unreal or a Fundamental Dimension of Human Reality?" in *Imagination and Its Pathologies*, edited by James Phillips and James Morley (Cambridge, MA: The MIT Press, 2003), pp. 37–50.

16. Compare the view of Śaṅkara cited in Chapter 5 at n. 181.

17. Norman Malcolm, "Dreaming and Skepticism," *Mind* 72 (1973): 202–15, reprinted in *idem*, *Dreaming* (London: Routledge & Kegan Paul, 1959), pp. 101–107, and again in *Philosophical Essays on Dreaming*, edited by Charles E. M. Dunlop (Ithaca: Cornell University Press, 1977), pp. 64–80.

18. Jennifer Michelle Windt and Thomas Metzinger, "The Philosophy of Dreaming and Self-Consciousness: What Happens to the Experiential Subject during the Dream State?" in *The New Science of Dreaming*, edited by Deirdre Barrett and Patrick McNamara, vol. 3: *Cultural and Theoretical Perspectives* (Westport: Praeger, 2007), p. 194.

19. Jon Stewart, *Kierkegaard's Relation to Hegel Reconsidered* (Cambridge: Cambridge University Press, 2003), pp. 273–75.

20. Søren Kierkegaard, *Philosophical Fragments; Johannes Climacus*, edited and translated with introduction and notes by Howard V. Hong and Edna H. Hong (Princeton: Princeton University Press, 1987), p. 167 (emphasis in the original).

21. *Ibid.*, p. 168. For an examination of the notion of doubt in this work, see Stewart, *Kierkegaard's Relation*, pp. 261–68; Michael Strawser, *Both/And: Reading Kierkegaard From Irony to Edification* (New York: Fordham University Press, 1997), pp. 62–63, 68–76, 78–81.

22. Stewart, *Kierkegaard's Relation*, p. 274.

23. Kierkegaard, *Philosophical Fragments; Johannes Climacus*, pp. 167–68 and 255.

24. Compare the analysis of Husserl in John Sallis, *Delimitations: Phenomenology and the End of Metaphysics* (Bloomington: Indiana University Press, 1986), p. 66.

25. John Locke, *An Essay Concerning Human Understanding* (New York: Prometheus Books, 1994), IV.2.14, pp. 438–39. On the depiction of dreams as incoherent and irrational, see *ibid.*, II.1.16, p. 66.

26. *Ibid.*, IV.11.8, p. 540.

27. Gottfried Wilhelm Leibniz, *New Essays on Human Understanding*, translated and edited by Peter Remnant and Jonathan Bennett (Cambridge: Cambridge University Press, 1996), p. 375 (emphasis in the original). Compare the following assessment of Friedrich Heinrich Jacobi, *The Main Philosophical Writings and the Novel Allwill*, translated with an introductory study, notes, and bibliography by George di Giovanni (Montreal: McGill-Queen's University Press, 1994), p. 514: "In *contradiction* to the *true* being, towards which reason is exclusively directed as to its *ultimate* goal, reason posits the beings of the imagination. It does not just distinguish between some images and others—say, between necessary images and free ones—but distinguishes images [from the real] *absolutely*. It opposes *true* being to the being of the imagination, just as it opposes being awake to dreaming. On this immediate and apodeictic distinction between being awake and dreaming, between fiction and true being, reason stands or falls" (emphasis in the original).

28. Thomas Hobbes, *Leviathan*, edited with an introduction and notes by John Charles Addison Gaskin (Oxford: Oxford University Press, 1996), pt. 1, ch. 2, p. 13. See the editor's note on p. 478. When I briefly mentioned that I was working on this book to Moshe Halbertal, he mentioned Hobbes, which served as the catalyst for me to consider his views.

29. R. J. Zwi Werblowsky, *Joseph Karo: Lawyer and Mystic* (Philadelphia: Jewish Publication Society of America, 1977), pp. 9–24, esp. 21, and 266–75.

30. Joseph Karo, *Maggid Mesharim* (Jerusalem, 1960), p. 2.

31. *Midrash Tehillim*, edited by Solomon Buber (Vilna: Rom, 1891), 11:6, p. 102; *Pirqei Rabbi Eli'ezer* (Warsaw, 1852), ch. 34, 79a–b. For additional sources where the soul's ascent during sleep is emphasized without any mention of dreams, see *Midrash Bere'shit Rabba*, edited by Julius Theodor and Chanoch Albeck (Jerusalem: Wahrmann Books, 1965), 14:9, pp. 133–34; Louis Ginzberg, *The Legends of the Jews* (Philadelphia: Jewish Publication Society of America, 1968), 5:74–75 n. 18. See also Philo, *On Dreams*, translated by Francis H. Colson and George H. Whitaker (Cambridge, MA: Harvard University Press, 1968), I.2, p. 295, where the "second kind" of dream is described as one "in which our own mind, moving out of itself together with the Mind of the

Universe, seems to be possessed and God-inspired, and so capable of receiving some foretaste and foreknowledge of things to come." On the ascent of the soul, see *ibid.*, 1.138, p. 371. Compare Philo, *The Special Laws*, translated by Francis H. Colson (Cambridge, MA: Harvard University Press, 1968), 1.291, p. 227: "In consequence when the mind withdrawing from its daytime cares, with the body paralyzed in sleep and the obstruction of every sense removed, begins to turn itself about and concentrate upon the pure observation of its concepts, it looks into the liver as into a mirror where it gains a lucid view of all that mind can perceive and, while its gaze travels round the images to see whether they contain any ugly defect, it eschews all such and selects their opposites and so, well satisfied with all the visions presented to it, prophesies future events through the medium of dreams." For discussion of Philo's approach to dreams against the larger background of the philosophical views concerning divination, see Harry A. Wolfson, *Philo: Foundations of Religious Philosophy in Judaism, Christianity, and Islam*, 2 vols. (Cambridge, MA: Harvard University Press, 1947), 2:55–59, and 81–82, where the aforecited passage from *The Special Laws* is discussed. Of particular interest is the connection between the mechanics of dream interpretation (illustrated by the biblical figure of Joseph) and Philo's own attempt to interpret Scripture allegorically. See John R. Levison, "The Prophetic Spirit as an Angel According to Philo," *Harvard Theological Review* 88 (1995): 195 and 199–201.

32. *Zohar* 1:53b, 92a, 121b, 183a, 200a; 3:67a. All references in this work are based on *Sefer ha-Zohar*, edited and annotated by Reuven Margaliot, 3 vols. (Jerusalem: Mosad ha-Rav Kook, 1960). For discussion of the theme of sleep and dreams in the zoharic anthology, see Isaiah Tishby, *The Wisdom of the Zohar: An Anthology of Texts*, translated by David Goldstein (Oxford: Oxford University Press, 1989), pp. 809–14.

33. Marcel Détienne, *La notion de daïmon dans le pythagorisme ancien* (Paris: Les Belles Lettres, 1963), pp. 79–85; Jacques Le Goff, *The Medieval Imagination*, translated by Arthur Goldhammer (Chicago: University of Chicago Press, 1988), p. 198; Michel Foucault, *L'herméneutique du sujet: Cours au Collège de France (1981–1982)*, edited by Frédéric Gros under the direction of François Ewald and Alessandro Fontana (Gallimard: Le Seuil, 2001), pp. 48, 114, 460; Peter Struck, "Viscera and the Divine: Dreams as the Divinatory Bridge between the Corporeal and the Incorporeal," in *Prayer, Magic and the Stars in the Ancient and Late Antique World*, edited by Scott Noegel, Joel Walker, and Brannon Wheeler (University Park: Pennsylvania State University Press, 2003), pp. 125–36; Sarah Iles Johnston, *Ancient Greek Divination* (Chichester: Wiley-Blackwell Publishing, 2008), pp. 14–16.

34. *Zohar* 1:169b. In that context, it is also stated that since the soul separates from the body during sleep, a man is vulnerable to being tempted sexually in his dreams by impure female spirits. The nocturnal emission of semen that results from this male fantasy results in the birth of destructive forces that are designated as *nig'ei benei adam*, "the afflictions of human beings" (2 Samuel 7:14). See *Zohar* 2:130a; Tishby, *Wisdom*, p. 813.

35. Babylonian Talmud, Berakhot 57b.

36. Edward F. Pace-Schott, "Postscript: Recent Findings on the Neurobiology of Sleep and Dreaming," in *Sleep and Dreaming: Scientific Advances and Reconsiderations*, edited by Edward F. Pace-Schitt, Mark Solms, Mark Blagorve, and Stevan Harnad (Cambridge: Cambridge University Press, 2003), pp. 337–38.

37. As Jeffrey Kripal reminded me, prior to Corbin, the term "imaginal" in the modern study of religion was utilized by Frederic W. H. Myers, *Science and the Future Life with Other Essays*, 2nd edition (London: Macmillan, 1901), pp. 37–38.

38. James Hillman, *Re-Visioning Psychology* (New York: HarperCollins, 1992), pp. 36–38, 50–51, 237 n. 86 (Corbin is explicitly mentioned); *idem*, "Healing Fiction," in *Jungian Literary Criticism*, edited by Richard B. Sugg (Evanston: Northwestern University Press, 1993), pp. 129–38; Roger Brooke, *Jung and Phenomenology* (London: Routledge, 1991), pp. 157–58. For a comparative analysis of the imagination in Jung and Hillman, see Roberts Avens, *Imagination Is Reality: Western Nirvana in Jung, Hillman, Barfield and Cassirer* (Putnam: Spring Publications, 1980), pp. 31–47. The expression imaginal psychology is applied to Jung in Michael Vannoy Adams, *The Fantasy Principle: Psychoanalysis of the Imagination* (New York: Brunner-Routledge, 2004). See also Steven M. Joseph, "Jung and Kabbalah: Imaginal and Noetic Aspects," *Journal of Analytical Psychology* 52 (2007): 321–41.

39. Carl G. Jung, *Dream Analysis: Notes of the Seminar Given in 1928–1930*, edited by William McGuire (Princeton: Princeton University Press, 1984), p. 447. The bibliography on Jung's approach to dreams is enormous, and here I mention one exemplary study, which provides the historical and conceptual background as well as reference to other significant studies: Sonu Shamdasani, *Jung and the Making of Modern Psychology: The Dream of a Science* (Cambridge: Cambridge University Press, 2003), pp. 100–62.

40. Jung, *Dream Analysis*, p. 447.

41. See Elliot R. Wolfson, "Sacred Space and Mental Iconography: *Imago Templi* and Contemplation in Rhineland Jewish Pietism," in *Ki Baruch Hu: Ancient Near Eastern, Biblical, and Judaic Studies in Honor of Baruch A. Levine*,

edited by Robert Chazan, William Hallo, and Lawrence H. Schiffman (Winona Lake: Eisenbrauns, 1999), pp. 593–634; *idem*, "Seven Mysteries of Knowledge: Qumran E/sotericism Reconsidered," in *The Idea of Biblical Interpretation: Essays in Honor of James L. Kugel*, edited by Hindy Najman and Judith H. Newman (Leiden: Brill, 2003), pp. 173–213; *idem*, "Imago Templi and the Meeting of the Two Seas: Liturgical Time-Space and the Feminine Imaginary in Zoharic Kabbalah," *Res: Anthropology and Aesthetics* 51 (2007): 121–35.

42. *Odyssey* 19:560–67. See Le Goff, *The Medieval Imagination*, pp. 196–97 and 216–17 (discussing the distinction between true and false dreams in Augustine); Marcel Détienne, *The Masters of Truth in Ancient Greece*, translated by Janet Lloyd (New York: Zone Books, 1999), p. 73. See also Louise Pratt, "*Odyssey* 19.535–50: On the Interpretation of Dreams and Signs in Homer," *Classical Philology* 19 (1994): 147–52. For a more detailed account of Augustine's treatment of dreams, see Martine Dulaey, *Le rêve dans la vie et la pensée de Saint Augustin* (Paris: Études Augustiniennes, 1973). In accord with my own perspective, Moss, *The Secret History of Dreaming*, p. xii, maintains that the dream, or, more broadly, the imaginal realm, can be seen as the "origin of events and situations that are manifested in the surface world." See *ibid.*, p. xxi: "One of my aims in this book is to help renew our understanding that dreaming is a vital *understory* in the human odyssey—past, present, and future—and to incite others to restore it to its rightful place in the study of history" (emphasis in the original). And *ibid.*, p. 10: "By entering Dreamtime, we may be able to reach into the quantum soup of possibilities from which the events of the three-dimensional world bubble up." Another similarity between Moss and myself is his conception of the "spacious Now of the Dreamtime," a temporal coordinate through which "we may be able to re-envision the linear sequence of events from the standpoint of metahistory, an understanding that transcends linear time" (p. xiii). See *ibid.*, p. 24. I, too, elicit a nonlinear conception of temporality from the dream expressed in the compresence of the three modes of time in the ever-recurring moment that is differently the same, but I am loathe to refer to this alternate model as a metahistory. The reversibility of the time swerve of which I speak rests on taking seriously a scientific perspective that conflicts with the commonsensical view of time's irreversible linearity. See Wolfson, *Language, Eros, Being*, pp. xvii–xviii. Closer to my thinking is the formulation of Moss, *The Secret History of Dreaming*, p. 10: "Dreamtime is not long ago; in Dreamtime it is always *now*. Aborigines call Dreamtime the 'all-at-once.' Dreamtime is the seedbed of life, the origin of everything that is manifested in the world. It is not separate from the physical world; it is the inner pulse of the land" (emphasis in the original).

43. Husserl, *Ideas*, sec. 32, pp. 60–62, especially the conclusion of this section: "The whole prediscovered world posited in the natural attitude, actually found in experience and taken with 'freedom from theories' as it is actually experienced, as it clearly shows itself in the concatenations of experience, is now without validity for us; without being tested and also without being contested, it shall be parenthesized. In like manner all theories and sciences which relate to this world, no matter how well they may be grounded positivistically or otherwise, shall meet the same fate" (p. 62).

44. Edmund Husserl, *The Crisis of European Sciences and Transcendental Phenomenology*, translated, with an introduction, by David Carr (Evanston: Northwestern University Press, 1970), sec. 53, p. 180. For a thorough analysis of the phenomenological reduction in this text with special attention to the matter of the subjectivity of the world, see James Dodd, *Crisis and Reflection: An Essay on Husserl's Crisis of the European Sciences* (Dordrecht: Kluwer, 2004), pp. 175–206.

45. Eugen Fink, "The Phenomenological Philosophy of Edmund Husserl and Contemporary Criticism," in *The Phenomenology of Husserl: Selected Readings*, 2nd edition, edited with an introduction by R. O. Elveton (Seattle: Noesis Press, 2000), p. 113 (emphasis in the original).

46. An analysis of the matter of ontology in Husserlian phenomenology lies beyond the scope of this study. For a discussion that raises some of the major issues pertaining to this question and that challenges some of the established views, see Steven Galt Crowell, *Husserl, Heidegger, and the Space of Meaning: Paths Toward a Transcendental Phenomenology* (Evanston: Northwestern University Press, 2001), pp. 174–202. Consider the succinct summation in Janicaud, "The Theological Turn," p. 38: "For Husserl, the suspension of the natural attitude implies leaving behind all ontological realism.... Ontology is itself bracketed, whether on the level of the entity [*l'étant*] or on the level of the 'there is' ['*il y a*'] of being [*l'être*]."

47. Husserl, *Ideas*, sec. 88, pp. 214–15.

48. Husserl, *Crisis*, sec. 53, pp. 178–79.

49. Jean-Paul Sartre, *Imagination: A Psychological Critique*, translated with an introduction by Forrest Williams (Ann Arbor: University of Michigan Press, 1962), p. 134. The word "irreality" is used to translate *néant*, which conventionally connotes "nothing" or "nonbeing." The customary rendering, however, does not do justice to Sartre's intent; indeed, it actually obscures it. His point is that Husserl restored transcendence to the very unreality of mythical beings like the centaur, because they are intentional objects of consciousness, irrespective of their existence or nonexistence in the presumed real world.

50. Husserl, *Crisis*, sec. 54, p. 182; *idem*, *Die Krisis der Europäischen*

Wissenschaften und die Tranzendentale Phänomenologie, 2nd edition, edited by Walter Biemel, *Husserliana VI* (The Hague: Martinus Nijhoff, 1962), p. 186.

51. Husserl, *Crisis*, sec. 54, p. 183; *Die Krisis*, p. 187. See *idem*, *Cartesian Meditations*, sec. 58, pp. 134–36; W. R. Boyce Gibson, "The Problem of Real and Ideal in the Phenomenology of Husserl," *Mind* 34 (1925): 311–33; Lester Embree, "The Phenomenology of Representational Awareness," *Human Studies* 15 (1992): 301–11; Hans Blumberg, "The Life-World and the Concept of Reality," in *Life-World and Consciousness: Essays for Aron Gurwitsch*, edited by Lester E. Embree (Evanston: Northwestern University Press, 1972), pp. 425–44; Josef Seifert, *Back To Things Themselves: A Phenomenological Foundation for Classical Realism* (New York: Routledge & Kegan Paul, 1987). On Husserlian idealism and the construction of the dream, see the rich analysis of Pierre Carrique, *Rêve, vérité: Essai sur la philosophie du sommeil et de la veille* (Paris: Éditions Gallimard, 2002), pp. 173–242.

52. Husserl, *Ideas*, sec. 70, p. 160 (emphasis in the original). Obviously aware of the far-reaching implications of his assertion, Husserl added the following footnote: "A sentence which, as a quotation, should be especially suitable for a naturalistic ridiculing of the eidetic mode of cognition." For a detailed analysis of the role of fancifulness in Husserl's phenomenology, see Donald B. Kuspit, "Fiction and Phenomenology," *Philosophy and Phenomenological Research* 29 (1968): 16 –33. See also Brian Elliott, *Phenomenology and Imagination in Husserl and Heidegger* (London: Routledge, 2005), pp. 7–80. Elliott's analysis turns on this key statement where Husserl speaks of the primacy of free fantasy over and against perception.

53. Shigeto Nuki, "Phenomenology as Calculus?" in *Phenomenology: Japanese and American Perspectives*, edited by Burt C. Hopkins (Dordrecht: Kluwer, 1999), pp. 1–14, esp. 10–12; Elliott, *Phenomenology and Imagination*, p. 9.

54. Husserl, *Ideas*, sec. 88, p. 214: "Corresponding in every case to the multiplicity of Data pertaining to the really inherent noetic content, there is a multiplicity of Data, demonstrable in actual pure intuition, in a correlative '*noematic content*' or, in short, in the '*noema*'.... Perception, for example, has its noema, most basically its perceptual sense, i.e., the *perceived as perceived*. Similarly, the current case of remembering has its *remembered as remembered*, just as its <remembered>, precisely as it is 'meant,' 'intended to' in <the remembering>; again, the judging has the *judged as judged*, liking has the liked as liked, and so forth. In every case the noematic correlate, which is called 'sense' here... is to be taken *precisely* as it inheres 'immanentally' in the mental process of perceiving, of judging, of liking, and so forth, that is, just as it is offered to us when we *inquire purely into this mental process itself*" (emphasis in the original).

55. Sartre, *Imagination*, p. 139.

56. Sartre, *The Imaginary*, pp. 125–75.

57. For discussion of the Husserlian notion of the irreal and the oneiric presence in Sartre, see Carrique, *Rêve, vérité*, pp. 84–93. On the phenomenology of irreality in the thought of Fink and Husserl, see *ibid.*, pp. 208–42. On the structure of intentionality in dreams, see Anthony Rudd, *Expressing the World: Skepticism, Wittgenstein, and Heidegger* (La Salle: Open Court, 2003), pp. 19–27.

58. The statement of Heraclitus, reported by Plutarch (*De superstitione* 166c), is rendered in Charles H. Kahn, *The Art and Thought of Heraclitus: An Edition of the Fragments with Translation and Commentary* (Cambridge: Cambridge University Press, 1979), VI, p. 31: "The world of the waking is one and shared, but the sleeping turn aside into his private world." See Binswanger, *Dream and Existence*, pp. 98–99.

59. Foucault, "Dream, Imagination and Existence," p. 50.

60. *Ibid.*, p. 51.

61. *Ibid.*

62. *Ibid.*, p. 52.

63. *Ibid.*, p. 54.

64. *Ibid.*, p. 47.

65. *Ibid.*, p. 55.

66. Roger Caillois, "Logical and Philosophical Problems of the Dream," in *The Dream and Human Societies*, edited by Gustave Edmund von Grunebaum and Roger Caillois (Berkeley: University of California Press, 1966), p. 31.

67. Synesius of Cyrene, *On Dreams*, 1305b–c, cited in M. Andrew Holowchak, *Ancient Science and Dreams: Oneirology in Greco-Roman Antiquity* (Lanham: University Press of America, 2002), p. 111.

68. My comment, the full explication of which demands an essay of its own, bears some affinity with the drift of thinking attested in Pierre Fédida, *Le site de l'étranger: La situation psychanalytique* (Paris: Presses Universitaires de France, 1995).

69. Florence Dee Boodakian, *Tormenting Angel: A Psychoaesthetic Theory of Imagination* (New York: Peter Lang, 1999), p. 11.

70. Novalis, *Novalis: Philosophical Writings*, translated and edited by Margaret Mahony Stoljar (Albany: State University of New York Press, 1997), p. 25. Compare Novalis, *Notes for a Romantic Encyclopaedia: Das Allgemeine Brouillon*, translated, edited, and with an introduction by David W. Wood (Albany: State University of New York Press, 2007), sec. 237, p. 35: "THEORY OF THE FUTURE LIFE. Our life is no dream—however it should and perhaps will become one." And compare the statement in "Extracts from the *Freiberg*

Natural Scientific Studies (1798/99)," included the appendix, Novalis, *Notes for a Romantic Encyclopaedia*, sec. 31, p. 199: "To say that our life is a dream, is the same as saying that our life is a thought. Reflections on *dreams in the ordinary sense of the word*" (emphasis in the original).

71. Alexander Graham Cairns-Smith, *Evolving the Mind: On the Nature of Matter and the Origin of Consciousness* (Cambridge: Cambridge University Press, 1996), pp. 193–94. See also William C. Dement, *The Promise of Sleep* (New York: Delacorte Press, 1999), p. 301, cited in Frances Flannery-Dailey, *Dreamers, Scribes, and Priests: Jewish Dreams in the Hellenistic and Roman Eras* (Leiden: Brill, 2004), p. 108: "To certain parts of the brain, there is no difference between waking life and dreaming life. When we are dreaming of eating or fighting or thinking, the brain is sending out the same signals it would if we were awake and eating or fighting or thinking. In a way, all perception is dreaming." Flannery-Dailey invokes this passage in the context of noting that "modern science confirms the ancient view that dreams and visions exist along a continuum, by establishing that physiological dream states may occur in hypnagogic waking states, at the onset of sleep, in non-R.E.M. sleep or in R.E.M. sleep" (p. 107).

72. Caillois, "Logical," pp. 33, 34–35, 44–45. On the hallucinatory nature of dreaming, see Stekel, *Sex and Dreams*, p. 18.

73. Edward S. Casey, "Imagination, Fantasy, Hallucination, and Memory," in *Imagination and Its Pathologies*, pp. 65–91, esp. 72–79.

74. Jason W. Brown, *Mind and Nature: Essays on Time and Subjectivity* (London: Whurr, 2000), p. 109. Compare the discussion on dreaming, illusion, and reality in Stephen LaBerge, *Lucid Dreaming*, foreword by Robert Ornstein (Los Angeles: Jeremy P. Tarcher, 1985), pp. 205–28. The author argues that all experiences are mental representations and therefore of the same nature of dreams.

75. Aristotle, *De insomniis*, 458b27–28, translated by John I. Beare in *The Complete Works of Aristotle: The Revised Oxford Translation*, edited by Jonathan Barnes (Princeton: Princeton University Press, 1984), p. 729. See Aristotle, *De divinatione per somnum*, 464a25–26. In that context, Aristotle explains that "deranged" persons (*ekstatikon*) are likely to have the foresight or prevision (*prooran*) that some people are inclined to attribute to divinely inspired acts of prognostication (*Complete Works*, p. 738).

76. *De insomniis*, 459a21–22, in *Complete Works*, p. 730. But compare *ibid.*, 459a8–10, where it is stated emphatically that dreaming is not an "exercise of opinion or thought" and also "not an affection of the faculty of perception in a simple sense." In *De somno et vigilia* 456a26, in *Complete Works*, p. 725, Aristotle writes that "a dream is in a certain way a sense-impression." On the conflicting

views espoused by Aristotle with respect to the dream and its relation to sense perception, see Daniel Heller-Roazen, *The Inner Touch: Archaeology of Sensation* (New York: Zone Books, 2007), pp. 70–71.

77. *De insomniis*, 461a27–b10, in *Complete Works*, p. 733.

78. David Gallop, *Aristotle on Sleep and Dreams: A Text and Translation with Introduction, Notes and Glossary* (Peterborough, Ontario: Broadview Press, 1990), p. 19. For discussion of the Aristotelian psychobiological perspective and its influence in the Greco-Roman era, see Patricia Cox Miller, *Dreams in Late Antiquity: Studies in the Imagination of a Culture* (Princeton: Princeton University Press, 1994), pp. 42–51, and Holowchak, *Ancient Science*, pp. 39–52. See also the discussion on naturalistic explanations of dreams in William V. Harris, *Dreams and Experience in Classical Antiquity* (Cambridge, MA: Harvard University Press, 2009), pp. 229–78.

79. Sartre, *The Imaginary*, p. 152.

80. René Descartes, *Meditations on First Philosophy*, in *The Philosophical Writings of Descartes*, translated by John Cuttingham, Robert Stoothoff, and Dugald Murdoch, vol. 2 (Cambridge: Cambridge University Press, 1984), pp. 61–62. For discussion of the perspective of Descartes and citation of the pertinent sources, see O.K. Bouwsma, "Descartes' Skepticism of the Senses," *Mind* 54 (1945): 313–22, reprinted in *Philosophical Essays on Dreaming*, edited by Charles E.M. Dunlop (Ithaca: Cornell University Press, 1977), pp. 52–63, and the Jungian approach in Marie Louise Von Franz, *Dreams*, foreword by Robert Hinshaw (Boston: Shambhala, 1991), pp. 107–91; Robert Withers, "Descartes' Dreams," *Journal of Analytic Psychology* 53 (2008): 691–709. See also the study by Malcolm cited above, n. 17; Alice Browne, "Descartes's Dreams," *Journal of the Warburg and Courtauld Institutes* 40 (1977): 256–73; Brann, *The World of the Imagination*, pp. 338–40.

81. Sartre, *The Imaginary*, p. 159.

82. *Ibid.*, p. 163.

83. Malcolm, *Dreaming*, pp. 41–42.

84. Alexander of Aphrodisias, *On Aristotle's Metaphysics* 5, translated by William E. Dooley, S.J. (Ithaca: Cornell University Press, 1993), p. 120 (emphasis in the original).

85. Ludwig Wittgenstein, *Remarks on the Philosophy of Psychology*, edited by Gertrude E.M. Anscombe and Georg H. Wright, translated by Gertrude E.M. Anscombe (Oxford: Basil Blackwell, 1980), vol. 1, sec. 932, p. 165.

86. *Ibid.*, sec. 934, p. 165.

87. Robert M. Yost, Jr. and Donald Kalish, "Miss MacDonald on Sleeping and Waking," *Philosophical Quarterly* 5 (1955): 118.

88. For a different perspective, see Kelly Bulkeley, *Dreaming in the World's Religions: A Comparative History* (New York: New York University Press, 2008), pp. 27–28.

89. Daniel M. Wegner, *The Illusion of Conscious Will* (Cambridge, MA: The MIT Press, 2002), pp. 229–30. The example of the dream—the "completely unreal experience that often seems resoundingly real"—is offered by Wegner to illustrate the futility of drawing a hard and fast distinction between imagined and actual: "When we're in the middle of the dream, it may be difficult to distinguish the dream world from the real world. No matter how fantastic or strange, the dream world is real at the time we are in it."

90. Plato, *Theaetetus* 158c–d, in *The Collected Dialogues of Plato Including the Letters*, edited by Edith Hamilton and Huntington Cairns (Princeton: Princeton University Press, 1980), p. 863. On the dreamlike quality of newly aroused opinions without the substantiation of knowledge, see the remark of Socrates in Plato's *Meno* 85c, in *Collected Dialogues*, p. 370.

91. Wendy Doniger O'Flaherty, *Dreams, Illusion and Other Realities* (Chicago: University of Chicago Press, 1984), p. 198. See also Miller, *Dreams*, pp. 4–5.

92. Peter Gärdenfors, "The Detachment of Thought," in *The Mind as a Scientific Object: Between Brain and Culture*, edited by Christina E. Erneling and David Martcl Johnson (Oxford: Oxford University Press, 2005), p. 326.

93. Sigmund Freud, *The Interpretation of Dreams*, translated by Joyce Crick, with an introduction and notes by Ritchie Robertson (Oxford: Oxford University Press, 1999), p. 83.

94. *Ibid.*, p. 402 (emphasis in the original).

95. *Ibid.*, p. 189. See also Freud's 1899 essay "Screen Memories," in *SE*, 3:319–320. See also the extensive analysis of the dream and neurosis in Emil A. Gutheil, *The Language of the Dream* (New York: Macmillan, 1939), pp. 142–229.

96. Carl G. Jung, *Psychology of the Unconscious: A Study of the Transformations and Symbolisms of the Libido*, with a new foreword by Eugene Taylor (Princeton: Princeton University Press, 2001), pp. 23–24. Compare *idem*, *The Practice of Psychotherapy: Essays on the Psychology of the Transference and Other Subjects*, translated by R. F. C. Hull, 2nd edition (Princeton: Princeton University Press, 1966), pp. 151–52: "Since dreams provide information about the hidden inner life and reveal to the patient those components of his personality which, in his daily behavior, appear merely as neurotic symptoms, it follows that we cannot effectively treat him from the side of consciousness alone, but must bring about a change in and through the unconscious. In the light of our present knowledge this can be achieved only by the thorough and conscious assimilation of unconscious contents."

97. Carl G. Jung, *The Red Book: Liber Novus*, edited and introduced by Sonu Shamdasani (New York: W. W. Norton, 2009), p. 238. On the notion of divine folly, see pp. 292–93. For the historical background of the Platonic discussion of madness, see Dodds, *The Greeks and the Irrational*, pp. 64–101. On the theme of philosophical madness and political rhetoric in the *Phaedrus*, see Michael L. Morgan, *Platonic Piety: Philosophy and Ritual in Fourth-Century Athens* (New Haven: Yale University Press,1990), pp. 158–87. See also Josef Pieper, *Enthusiasm and Divine Madness: On the Platonic Dialogue Phaedrus*, translated by Richard and Clara Winston (New York: Harcourt, Brace & World, 1964); *idem*, *"Divine Madness": Plato's Case against Secular Humanism*, translated by Lothar Krauth (San Francisco: Ignatius Press, 1995); Silke-Maria Weineck, *The Abyss Above: Philosophy and Poetic Madness in Plato, Hölderlin, and Nietzsche* (Albany: State University of New York Press, 2002). For the influence of the Platonic idea on the Christian notion of the holy fool, see Guy G. Stroumsa, "Madness and Divinization in Early Christian Monasticism," in *Self and Self-Transformation in the History of Religions*, edited by David Shulman and Guy G. Stroumsa (Oxford: Oxford University Press, 2002), pp. 73–88. On the related Socratic comparison of poetic inspiration to the rhapsodic possession by the divine spirit, see Grace M. Ledbetter, *Poetics before Plato: Interpretation and Authority in Early Greek Theories of Poetry* (Princeton: Princeton University Press, 2003), pp. 88, 90–95.

98. Jung, *The Red Book*, p. 298: "My soul spoke to me in a whisper, urgently and alarmingly: 'Words, words, do not make too many words. Be silent and listen: have you recognized your madness and do you admit it?... You wanted to accept everything. So accept madness too. Let the light of your madness shine, and it will suddenly dawn on you. Madness is not to be despised and not to be feared, but instead you should give it life.... Be glad that you recognize it, for you will thus avoid becoming its victim. Madness is a special form of the spirit and clings to all teachings and philosophies, but even more to daily life, since life itself is full of craziness and at bottom utterly illogical. Man strives toward reason only so that he can make rules for himself. Life itself has no rules. That is its mystery and its unknown law. What you call knowledge is an attempt to impose something comprehensible on life.'"

99. Carl G. Jung, *The Psychogenesis of Mental Disease*, translated by R. F. C. Hull (Princeton: Princeton University Press, 1960), p. 241. For an analysis of dreams and madness in Jung and some of the thinkers that may have influenced him, see Shamdasani, *Jung and the Making of Modern Psychology*, pp. 113–14 and 133–37. For an application of the psychoanalytic suppositions about individual consciousness to the collective consciousness, see Walter Benjamin, *The*

Arcades Project, translated by Howard Eiland and Kevin McLaughlin, prepared on the basis of the German volume edited by Rolf Tiedmann (Cambridge, MA: Harvard University Press, 1999), p. 389: "The new, dialectical method of doing history presents itself as the art of experiencing the present as waking world, a world to which that dream we name the past refers in truth. To pass through and carry out *what has been* in remembering the dream! — Therefore: remembering and awaking are most intimately related. Awakening is namely the dialectical, Copernican turn of remembrance. The nineteenth century a spacetime <*Zeitraum*> (a dreamtime <*Zeit-traum*>) in which the individual consciousness more and more secures itself in reflecting, while the collective consciousness sinks into ever deeper sleep. But just as the sleeper—in this respect like the madman—sets out on the macrocosmic journey through his own body, and the noises and feelings of his insides, such as blood pressure, intestinal churn, heartbeat, and muscle sensation (which for the waking and salubrious individual converge in a steady surge of health) generate, in the extravagantly heightened inner awareness of the sleeper, illusion or dream imagery which translates and accounts for them, so likewise for the dreaming collective, which, through the arcades, communes with its own insides" (emphasis in the original). On the use of the dream image to characterize the experience of the dialectical movement in history, see also *ibid.*, p. 838: "Awakening as a graduated process that goes on in the life of the individual as in that of the generation. Sleep its initial stage. A generation's experience of youth has much in common with the experience <*Erfahrung*> of dreams. Its historical configuration is a dream-configuration. Every epoch has such a side turned toward dreams, the child's side. For the previous century, it is the arcades. But whereas the education of earlier generations explained these dreams for them in terms of tradition, of religious doctrine, present-day education simply amounts to the 'distraction' of children. What follows here is an experiment in the technique of awakening. The dialectical — the Copernican — turn of remembrance < *Wendung des Eingedenkens*> (Bloch)." See Elissa Marder, "Walter Benjamin's Dream of 'Happiness,'" in *Walter Benjamin and the Arcades Project*, edited by Beatrice Hanssen (London: Continuum, 2006), pp. 184–200; Michael Calderbank, "Surreal Dreamscapes: Walter Benjamin and the Arcades," *Papers of Surrealism* 1 (2003), available at http://www.surrealismcentre.ac.uk/papersofsurrealism/journal1/acrobat_files/Calderbank.pdf. I am grateful to Jules Simon for reminding me of Benjamin's important reflections on the dream.

100. Freud, *Interpretation of Dreams*, *SE*, 5:608 (emphasis in the original).

101. *SE*, 5:569.

102. *SE*, 5:569 n. 2. On the relationship between dreams and insanity, see Bergson, *Mind-Energy*, p. 124.

103. Sigmund Freud, *An Outline of Psychoanalysis*, translated by James Strachey (New York: W. W. Norton, 1949), p. 29.

104. The passage from Shakespeare is cited in *The Complete Letters of Sigmund Freud to Wilhelm Fliess 1887–1904*, translated and edited by Jeffrey Moussaieff Masson (Cambridge, MA: Harvard University Press, 1985), p. 252 n. 1.

105. *Ibid.*, p. 251. For an alternative translation, see *SE*, 1:256.

106. *Complete Letters of Sigmund Freud to Wilhelm Fliess*, p. 338. See also *SE*, 1:276.

107. The nexus between dreaming, artistic creativity, and mental pathology is not unique to modern psychoanalysis. For instance, see the evidence adduced in Carol Schreier Rupprecht, "Divinity, Insanity, Creativity: A Renaissance Contribution to the History and Theory of Dream/Text(s)," in *The Dream and the Text: Essays on Literature and Language*, edited by Carol Schreier Rupprecht (Albany: State University of New York Press, 1993), pp. 112–32. For a discussion of "creative madness" that takes into account cognitive neuroscience, but still proffers a nonreductive approach to religious phenomena, see Kelly Bulkeley, *The Wondering Brain: Thinking about Religion with and beyond Cognitive Neuroscience* (New York: Routledge, 2005), pp. 101–41. A separate question is the relationship of dreaming and depression. According to Aristotle, *De memoria*, 2, 453a 19, there is a correlation between people with melancholic dispositions and the amplified stimulation of the imagination. On this basis, Averroës, *Epitome of Parva Naturalia*, translated with notes and introduction by Harry Blumberg (Cambridge, MA: Medieval Academy of America, 1961), pp. 50–51, wrote that people with melancholy are both more prone to have truer dreams and to perceive during waking hours what others perceive during sleep.

108. Jacques Lacan, *The Seminar of Jacques Lacan, Book II: The Ego in Freud's Theory and in the Technique of Psychoanalysis 1954–1955*, edited by Jacques-Alain Miller, translated by Sylvana Tomaselli, with notes by John Forrester (New York: W. W. Norton, 1988), pp. 103–104.

109. Murray L. Wax, *Western Rationality and the Angel of Dreams: Self, Psyche, Dreaming* (Lanham: Rowman & Littlefield, 1999), p. 140.

110. Michel Foucault, *History of Madness*, edited by Jean Khalfa, translated by Jonathan Murphy and Jean Khalfa (London: Routledge, 2006), p. 339. For an analysis of Foucault's discussion of Freud, see Jacques Derrida, *Resistances of Psychoanalysis*, translated by Peggy Kamuf, Pascale-Anne Brault, and Michaël Naas (Stanford: Stanford University Press, 1998), pp. 81–82 and the concise account on p. 124 n. 8: "*Discovery* is understood by Foucault, along with *return*

and *language*. Freud is the event of a *discovery*—the unconscious and psychoanalysis as a movement of *return*—and what relates the discovery to the return is language, the possibility of speaking with madness, 'the possibility of a dialogue with unreason'" (emphasis in the original). On the relationship of madness and dreaming, see especially Foucault's reflections on the Cartesian meditations in *History of Madness*, pp. 44–47, 327–29, 343, 348, and the comments in the appendix "My Body, This Paper, This Fire," pp. 550–74, which was added to the 1972 edition of *Histoire de la folie* as a response to Jacques Derrida's essay "Cogito et *Histoire de la folie*," in *L'écriture et la différence* (Paris: Seuil, 1967), pp. 61–97, translated as "Cogito and the History of Madness," in *Writing and Difference*, pp. 31–63; see the discussion in Edward F. McGushin, *Foucault's Askēsis: An Introduction to Philosophical Life* (Evanston: Northwestern University Press, 2007), pp. 185–90.

111. Foucault, *History of Madness*, p. 348.

112. Foucault, "Nietzsche, Freud, Marx," in *The Essential Works of Foucault, 1954–1984*, vol. 2: *Aesthetics, Method, and Epistemology*, pp. 274–75.

113. Carl G. Jung, *The Archetypes and the Collective Unconscious*, translated by R. F. C. Hull, 2nd edition (Princeton: Princeton University Press, 1969), p. 160.

114. Hillman, *Re-Visioning Psychology*, pp. 74–75.

115. See J. Allan Hobson, *The Dreaming Brain: How the Brain Creates both the Sense and the Nonsense of Dreams* (New York: Basic Books, 1988), and the discussion in Kelly Bulkeley, *Visions of the Night: Dreams, Religion, and Psychology* (Albany: State University of New York, 1999), pp. 67–75.

116. J. Allan Hobson, *Dreaming as Delirium: How the Brain Goes Out of Its Mind* (Cambridge, MA: The MIT Press, 1999); *idem*, *The Dream Drugstore: Chemically Altered States of Consciousness* (Cambridge, MA: The MIT Press, 2001); *idem*, *Dreaming: An Introduction to the Science of Sleep* (Oxford: Oxford University Press, 2002), pp. 97–105.

117. Norman O. Brown, "Apocalypse: The Place of Mystery in the Life of the Mind," in *Interpretation: The Poetry of Meanings*, p. 8. The context in which Brown offers this comment is a brief discussion on the age-old distinction between holy and unholy madness.

118. One of the better-known examples to support the argument that other mammals dream is the oneiric behavior of cats mentioned frequently in the neuroscientific literature. See, for instance, Michel Jouvet, *The Paradox of Sleep: The Story of Dreaming*, translated by Laurence Garey (Cambridge, MA: The MIT Press, 1993), pp. 41–45, 82–88. On the conjecture that all mammals have the potential to dream, see also the brief comment of Robert Ornstein,

The Evolution of Consciousness: Of Darwin, Freud, and Cranial Fire—The Origins of the Way We Think (New York: Prentice-Hall, 1991), p. 197, and the review of the research of Matthew Wilson in the press release from the Massachusetts Institute of Technology News Office, "Animals Have Complex Dreams, MIT Researcher Proves," available at http://web.mit.edu/newsoffice/2001/dreaming.html, as well as the account of Wilson's later experiments together with Daoyun Ji in Deborah Halber, "Memory Experts Show Sleeping Rats May Have Visual Dreams," available at http://web.mit.edu/newsoffice/2006/visual-cortex.html. See also Chris Frith, Richard Perry, and Erik Lumer, "The Neural Correlates of Conscious Experience: An Experimental Framework," *Trends in Cognitive Sciences* 3 (1999): 105–14. For a brief but sober recounting of this theoretical issue, see Bulkeley, *Dreaming*, pp. 14–15.

119. For a cogent presentation, see Eric R. Kandel, *Psychiatry, Psychoanalysis, and the New Biology of Mind* (Washington, D.C.: American Psychiatric Publishing, 2005), pp. 263–307.

120. Aristotle, *De divinatione per somnum*, 463b12; Holowchak, *Ancient Science*, pp. 40–52, esp. 47. This idea circulated in the Middle Ages, for example, in Solomon ben Moses of Laguiri's *Sefer ha-Sheinah we-ha-Yeqiṣah* (*Book on Sleep and Waking*), a Hebrew translation of a Latin compilation based on Aristotle's treatises on sleep and dreams, erroneously attributed to Avicenna, a text cited as well in Shem Ṭov Ibn Falaquera's *De'ot ha-Filosofim* (*Opinions of the Philosophers*), in order to dismiss the claim, affirmed genuinely by Avicenna in the ninth chapter of *al-Risāla al-manāmiyyah* (*Epistle concerning Dreams*), that dreams are of a divine origin. Concerning the work of Solomon ben Moses of Laguiri, see now Hagar Kahana-Smilansky, "Aristotle on Sleep and Wakefulness: A Medieval Hebrew Adaptation of an Unknown Latin Treatise," *Aleph* 10 (2010): 67–118. The Aristotelian perspective on animal dreams is found as well in Gershon ben Solomon, *Sha'ar ha-Shamayim* (Rödelheim, 1801), 69a. See Ruth Glasner, "The Hebrew Version of De celo et mundo attributed to Ibn Sīnā," *Arabic Sciences and Philosophy* 6 (1996): 94–96; James T. Robinson, "Gershom ben Solomon's *Sha'ar ha-Shamayim*: Its Sources and Use of Sources," in *The Medieval Hebrew Encyclopedias of Science and Philosophy: Proceedings of the Bar-Ilan University Conference*, edited by Steven Harvey (Dordrecht: Kluwer, 2000), pp. 260–61; Steven Harvey, "Shem-Tov Ibn Falaquera's *De'ot ha-Filosofim*: Its Sources and Use of Sources," in *The Medieval Hebrew Encyclopedias*, pp. 231–32; Shlomo Pines, "The Arabic Recension of *Parva Naturalia* and the Philosophical Doctrine concerning Veridical Dreams according to *al-Risāla al-Manāmiyya* and Other Sources," *Israel Oriental Studies* 4 (1974): 120–21. See also Solomon Almoli, *Pitron Ḥalomot* (Warsaw, 1902), 8a. Almoli's book was first published

in Salonica in 1515 with the title *Mefasher Ḥalmin*, republished in Constantinople in 1518 and 1551, in Cracow in 1676, and many times thereafter. Regarding this figure, see Trachtenberg, *Jewish Magic*, pp. 236–38; Annelies Kuyt, "With one Foot in the Renaissance: Shlomoh Almoli and his Dream Interpretation," *Jewish Studies Quarterly* 6 (1999): 205–17.

121. There is an abundance of studies that outline the neurobiological approach. Here I mention a few that I have consulted in earnest: Hobson, *Dreaming Brain; idem, Dreaming: An Introduction to the Science of Sleep*; J. Allan Hobson, Edward F. Pace-Schott, and Robert Stickgold, "Dreaming and the Brain: Toward a Cognitive Neuroscience of Conscious States," in *Sleep and Dreaming*, pp. 1–50; Claude Gottesmann, "A Neurobiological History of Dreaming," in *The New Science of Dreaming*, edited by Deirdre Barrett and Patrick McNamara, vol. 1, *Biological Aspects* (Westport: Praeger, 2007), pp. 1–51. For an engaging criticism of both the psychoanalytic and the neurobiological approaches, see Ernest Hartmann, *Dreams and Nightmares: The Origin and Meaning of Dreams* (New York: Perseus Publishing, 2001).

122. The received acronym in the field of neuroscience to delineate "rapid eye movement," which serves as the central factor in correlating sleep and the mental activity of the brain that we demarcate as a state of dreaming. See Hobson, *Dreaming Brain*, pp. 134–53, and the critical evaluation offered by Mark Solms, "Dreaming and REM Sleep Are Controlled By Different Brain Mechanisms," in *Sleep and Dreaming*, pp. 51–58.

123. Mark Solms and Oliver Turnbull, *The Brain and the Inner World: An Introduction to the Neuroscience of Subjective Experience* (New York: Other Press, 2002), p. 184 (emphasis in the original). See also Mark Solms, *The Neuropsychology of Dreams: A Clinico-Anatomical Study* (Mahwah: Lawrence Erlbaum Associates, 1997), pp. 54–57.

124. See, for instance, the brief digest offered by G. William Domhoff, *The Scientific Study of Dreams: Neural Networks, Cognitive Development, and Content Analysis* (Washington, D.C.: American Psychological Association, 2003), p. 4.

125. Carl G. Jung, *The Practice of Psychotherapy: Essays on the Psychology of the Transference and Other Subjects*, translated by R. F. C. Hull, 2nd edition (Princeton: Princeton University Press, 1966), p. 148. See *idem*, *Dream Analysis*, p. 445, where Jung paraphrases the Latin proverb *Canis panem somniat, piscator pisces* in his response to the comment that an individual dreams in images derived from his vocation: "And his business occupation is a perfectly conscious thing to him, so we can safely assume that his dream has taken the language of that business, according to the old adage that the dog dreams of a bone and the fishes of water." The Latin proverb was invoked similarly by Jung

in correspondence with Wolfgang Pauli (May 4, 1953) to explain why the latter—a renowned physicist—had a tendency to have physical dreams, thereby hiding their psychological import. See *Atom and Archetype: The Pauli/Jung Letters, 1932–1958*, edited by Carl Alfred Meier, with the assistance of Charles Paul Enz and Markus Fierz, translated by David Roscoe, with an introductory essay by Beverley Zabriskie (Princeton: Princeton University Press, 2001), p. 113. In his letter of response (May 27, 1953), Pauli reacted negatively to Jung's explanation, insisting not only that there was a significant connection with physics in the dreams, but that for him the dreams "synthetically construct . . . a sort of *correspondentia* between psychological and physical facts. *In this process, the physical and mathematical terms are symbolically extended to the unconscious in general and to the individual psyche in particular*" (*Atom and Archetype*, pp. 118–19). Regarding this exchange, see David Lindorff, *Pauli and Jung: The Meeting of Two Great Minds* (Wheaton: Quest Books, 2004), pp. 153–63; Suzanne Gieser, *The Innermost Kernel: Depth Psychology and Quantum Physics: Wolfgang Pauli's Dialogue with C. G. Jung* (Berlin: Springer, 2005), pp 201–203.

126. See, however, Anthony Stevens, "Jungian Psychology, the Body, and the Future," *Journal of Analytic Psychology* 40 (1995): 353–64.

127. For an exemplary representation of such an approach, see Milton Kramer, *The Dreamer Experience: A Systematic Exploration* (New York: Routledge, 2007).

128. Edward F. Kelly, Emily Williams Kelly, Adam Crabtree, Alan Gauld, Michael Grosso, and Bruce Greyson, *Irreducible Mind: Toward a Psychology for the 21st Century* (Lanham: Rowman & Littlefield, 2007), pp. xx–xxi. My gratitude to Jeffrey Kripal for calling my attention to this book. The detailed analyses in this voluminous tome present a formidable challenge to the prevalent scientific view regarding the irreducible physical basis of human consciousness. See also the discussion of an immaterial mind in contrast to the material brain in Douglas M. Stokes, *The Nature of Mind: Parapsychology and the Role of Consciousness in the Physical World* (Jefferson: McFarland, 1997), pp. 131–61, and the study of Bulkeley, *The Wondering Brain*, pp. 13–52.

129. Allan Hobson in his foreword to Michel Jouvet, *The Castle of Dreams*, translated by Laurence Garey (Cambridge, MA: The MIT Press, 2008), pp. xvi–xvii.

130. Susan Parman, *Dream and Culture: An Anthropological Study of the Western Intellectual Tradition* (New York: Praeger, 1991), p. ix.

131. Solms and Turnbull, *Brain and the Inner World*, pp. 196–97.

132. Derek P. Brereton, "Dreaming, Adaptation, and Consciousness: The Social Mapping Hypothesis," *Ethos* 28 (2000): 379–409, esp. 380, where

dreaming is demarcated as "a pre-existing mammalian function that contributed to the development of hominid consciousness by providing the brain with virtual scenarios pertinent to the individual's success in an intensely social milieu. Individuals more capable of such risk-free scenario building, especially scenarios not wholly bound by the constraints of external reality, enjoyed a selective advantage. They were able to keep more neuronal options open, and thus locate themselves more effectively in a fluid, and manipulable, social milieu." See also Alan T. Lloyd, "Evolution and the Interpretation of (REM Sleep) Dreams," in *The New Science of Dreaming*, vol. 3, pp. 249–75.

133. Parman, *Dream and Culture*, p. 2.

134. Patricia A. Kilroe, "The Dream as Text, The Dream as Narrative," *Dreaming* 10 (2000): 125–37.

135. Wax, *Western Rationality*, p. 3.

136. Windt and Metzinger, "The Philosophy of Dreaming," pp. 194–95.

137. For a similar argument, see Erika Bourguignon, "Dreams That Speak: Experience and Interpretation," in *Dreaming and the Self: New Perspectives on Subjectivity, Identity, and Emotion*, edited by Jeannette Marie Mageo (Albany: State University of New York Press, 2003), pp. 133–53.

138. For discussion of the neural basis for the internal narratives generated by the activity of the brain's language, which serve as a basis for the representation of self, see John Bickle, "Empirical Evidence for a Narrative Concept of Self," in *Narrative and Consciousness: Literature, Psychology, and the Brain*, edited by Gary D. Fireman, Ted E. McVay, Jr., and Owen J. Flanagan (Oxford: Oxford University Press, 2003), pp. 195–208.

139. Gillian Einstein and Owen Flanagan, "Sexual Identities and Narratives of Self," in *Narrative and Consciousness*, p. 229. Brann, *The World of the Imagination*, p. 346, depicts dreams as the "inward epiphanies of passion," the "visual or musical precipitations of feeling."

140. Hobson, *Dreaming Brain*, pp. 257–69; Bert O. States, *Dreaming and Storytelling* (Ithaca: Cornell University Press, 1993), pp. 13–45. See also Bulkeley, *Dreaming*, pp. 2 and 17–18; Jeannette Marie Mageo, "Subjectivity and Identity in Dreams," in *Dreaming and the Self*, pp. 26–28.

141. For a highly technical discussion of this topic, see Katsuhiro Nakamura, *Quantum versus Chaos: Questions Emerging from Mesoscopic Cosmos* (Dordrecht: Kluwer, 1997).

142. Steven Guccione, "Can a Non-Computable Physical Law Be Considered Able to Predict?" in *The Foundations of Quantum Mechanics: Historical Analysis and Open Questions*, edited by Claudio Garola and Arcangelo Rossi (Singapore: World Scientific Publishing, 2000), pp. 261–66.

143. Kandel, *Psychiatry*, pp. 73–78.

144. See Henry P. Stapp, "Quantum Interactive Dualism: An Alternative to Materialism," http://www-physics.lbl.gov/~stapp/QID.pdf, and see discussion in Jeffrey J. Kripal, *Esalen: America and the Religion of No Religion* (Chicago: University of Chicago Press, 2007), pp. 309–12.

145. Bulkeley, *Dreaming*, p. 13.

146. Anthony Stevens, *Private Myths: Dreams and Dreaming* (Cambridge, MA: Harvard University Press, 1995), pp. 154–55.

147. Bert O. States, *The Rhetoric of Dreams* (Ithaca: Cornell University Press, 1988), pp. 58–79. For an historical study of the poem as a product of the dream vision in Middle English poets of the fourteenth century, see Constance B. Hieatt, *The Realism of Dream Visions: The Poetic Exploitation of the Dream-Experience in Chaucer and his Contemporaries* (The Hague: Mouton, 1967).

148. The comparison of dreaming to artistic creativity, and especially to the crafting of poetry, has been made by many thinkers from multiple disciplinary perspectives. See the brief discussion and citation of other sources in Anthony Shafton, *Dream Reader: Contemporary Approaches to the Understanding of Dreams* (Albany: State University of New York Press, 1995), pp. 56–57.

149. The metaphor employed to depict the structure of metaphor is based on the hermeneutical assumption of the rabbis regarding the interconnection of all parts of Scripture. See the further discussion in Chapter 3.

150. In this regard, my own thinking has kinship with the work of Bert O. States, who draws an analogy between dream making and the production of art, but who is nevertheless sympathetic to neuroscientific research. See States, *Rhetoric of Dreams*. The dream, writes States, "manifests strategies of thought that if traced upward into language would eventuate in the master tropes. So dreams are a kind of proto-rhetoric, not yet language. Hence, one way to study them might be to see how the principles of rhetoric—the four master tropes, in this case—could be traced back into the dream-work, bearing in mind that in applying verbal structures to preverbal structures we are already speaking an odd sort of metaphor. All in all, I might sum up my perspective as a phenomenological rhetoric of dreaming" (p. 6, emphasis in the original). For an alternate synopsis of his methodology, see *idem*, *Seeing in the Dark: Reflections on Dreams and Dreaming* (New Haven: Yale University Press, 1997), pp. 3–6. In *Dreaming and Storytelling*, pp. 43–44, States compares the bizarre nature of dream imagery to images deployed in poetry and fiction. See also *idem*, "Dreaming and Storytelling," *Hudson Review* 43 (1990): 571–86; *idem*, "Bizarreness in Dreams and Other Fictions," in *The Dream and the Text*, pp. 13–31; *idem*, "Dream Bizarreness and Inner Thought," *Dreaming* 10 (2000): 179–92.

Bulkeley, *Dreaming*, p. 18, similarly concludes that "at least some of the bizarre elements of dreaming can be understood as expressions of a *different kind of intelligence* whose natural language consists primarily of image, metaphor, and allegory" (emphasis in the original). For another attempt to articulate a theory of literary imagination, with a particular emphasis on the poetic, based on the psychoanalytic approach to dreams as well as on more current physiological studies, see the creative study of Boodakian, *Tormenting Angel*.

151. Bachelard, *Poetics of Reverie*, p. 16.

152. *Ibid.*, p. 49.

153. *Ibid.*, pp. 21–22.

154. Mageo, "Subjectivity and Identity in Dreams," p. 23.

155. David Edwards and Michael Jacobs, *Conscious and Unconscious* (Maidenhead, UK: Open University Press, 2003), pp. 102–20. See also Foulkes, *Dreaming*, pp. 45–49; Sibajiban Bhattacharyya, "Phenomenology and Indian Philosophy," in *Phenomenology and Indian Philosophy*, edited by Debi Prasad Chattopadhyaya, Lester Embree, and Jitendranath Mohanty (Albany: State University of New York Press, 1992), pp. 48–49; David Shulman, "Dreaming the Self in South India," in *Dream Cultures: Explorations in the Comparative History of Dreaming*, edited by David Shulman and Guy G. Stroumsa (New York: Oxford University Press, 1999), pp. 43–73.

156. Peter T. Struck, "The Self in Artemidorus' *Interpretation of Dreams*," in *Religion and the Self in Antiquity*, edited by David Brakke, Michael L. Satlow, and Steven Weitzman (Bloomington: Indiana University Press, 2005), pp. 109–22, esp. 119, argues that the dialectic of selfhood and alterity can be elicited from this classical work of late antiquity.

157. Georg Wilhelm Friedrich Hegel, *Lectures on the Philosophy of Spirit 1827–8*, translated with an introduction by Robert R. Williams (Oxford: Oxford University Press, 2007), pp. 106–107.

158. *Ibid.*, p. 108. On madness, see also Georg Wilhelm Friedrich Hegel, *Phenomenology of Spirit*, translated by Arnold V. Miller with analysis and foreword by John N. Findlay (Oxford: Oxford University Press, 1977), sec. 376, pp. 225–26, and the speculation on dreaming and derangement in *idem*, *Philosophy of Mind*, translated by William Wallace and Arnold V. Miller, revised with introduction and commentary by Michael Inwood (Oxford: Oxford University Press, 2007), sec. 405, p. 91 and sec. 408, pp. 117–20, and the exposition on pp. 384–85 n. 3. See discussion in Daniel Berthold-Bond, *Hegel's Theory of Madness* (Albany: State University of New York Press, 1995), pp. 25–28, 33–35, 44–45, 67–68, 100–101. For discussion of reason, imagination, and madness in Hegel, see John Sallis, *The Gathering of Reason*, 2nd edition (Albany: State University

of New York Press, 2005), pp. 141–55.

159. Hegel, *Phenomenology of Spirit*, sec. 740, p. 448. See *ibid.*, sec. 10, p. 6, where Hegel asserts that the minds that "give themselves up to the uncontrolled ferment of [the divine] substance, imagine that, by drawing a veil over self-consciousness and surrendering understanding they become the beloved of God to whom He gives wisdom in sleep; and hence what they in fact receive, and bring to birth in their sleep, is nothing but dreams." And compare Hegel, *Philosophy of Mind*, sec. 398, pp. 62–67.

160. Arthur Schopenhauer, *The World as Will and Representation*, translated by E. F. J. Payne, 2 vols. (Indian Hills: Falcon's Wing Press, 1958), 1:390–91.

161. *Ibid.*, 2:134–35. The priority accorded to dreams that occur in the morning is based on the older idea that once the previous night's meal was fully digested, the soul could see things more clearly. See Johnston, *Ancient Greek Divination*, pp. 14–15. Compare Gershon ben Solomon, *Sha'ar ha-Shamayim*, 69b, who records such an opinion in the name of Isaac Israeli's commentary on *Sefer Yeṣirah*, "The majority of dreams that a person dreams in the morning are veridical for the digestion is completed already by that time." The text is cited similarly in Almoli, *Pitron Ḥalomot*, 11a. The view is found in *Sefer Yezirah with Commentary by Dunash Ben Tamim*, edited by Menasche Grossberg (London: R. W. Rabinowicz, 1902), p. 38, and see the more recent version (based on the translation of Moses ben Joseph ben Moses ha-Dayyan from the twelfth or thirteenth century) published in Georges Vajda, *Le commentaire sur le "Livre de la création" de Dūnaš ben Tāmīm de Kairouan (Xe siècle)*, new edition, edited and augmented by Paul B. Fenton (Paris-Louvain: Peeters, 2002), p. 223. The French translation by Vajda appears on pp. 71–72, and on p. 72 n. 110 reference is made to both Gershon ben Solomon's *Sha'ar ha-Shamayim* and Almoli's *Pitron Ḥalomot*. For discussion of Israeli and his student, Dunash ben Tamim, see the introduction of the Fenton edition, pp. 3–10. On the status of dreams in the work of Isaac Israeli, see Chapter 2 n. 85.

162. John Warrack, *Richard Wagner: Die Meistersinger von Nürnberg* (Cambridge: Cambridge University Press, 1994), pp. 33–35.

163. Foucault, "Dream, Imagination and Existence," p. 59.

164. Anthony Damiani, *Standing in Your Own Way* (Burdett: Larson, 1993), p. 21 (emphasis in the original), as cited in Shimon Malin, *Nature Loves to Hide: Quantum Physics and Reality, a Western Perspective* (Oxford: Oxford University Press, 2001), p. 232.

165. Windt and Metzinger, "The Philosophy of Dreaming," p. 198.

166. Freud, *Interpretation of Dreams*, p. 246.

167. Hobson, *Dreaming: An Introduction to the Science of Sleep*, p. 142.

168. Friedrich Nietzsche, *Unpublished Writings from the Period of Unfashionable Observations*, translated, with an afterward, by Richard T. Gray (Stanford: Stanford University Press, 1995), 19 [167], p. 53.

169. Blanchot, *Friendship*, pp. 141–42.

170. *Ibid.*, p. 142.

171. *Ibid.*, p. 143.

172. *Ibid.*, p. 144.

173. *Ibid.*, p. 146. Regarding this passage, see Kevin Hart, *The Dark Gaze: Maurice Blanchot and the Sacred* (Chicago: University of Chicago Press, 2004), p. 124. A comparable point, it seems to me, is implied in the comments of Levinas, *Collected Philosophical Papers*, p. 4: "To be 'among things' is different from Heidegger's 'being-in-the-world'; it constitutes the pathos of the imaginary world of dreams—the subject is among things not only by virtue of its density of being, requiring a 'here,' a 'somewhere,' and retaining its freedom; it is among things as a thing, as part of the spectacle. It is exterior to itself, but with an exteriority which is not that of a body, since the pain of the I-actor is felt by the I-spectator, and not through compassion. Here we have really an exteriority of the inward." On the depiction of anonymity as the "non-unity and non-presence of the nameless," see Maurice Blanchot, *The Step Not Beyond*, translated by Lycette Nelson (Albany: State University of New York Press, 1992), p. 35, and Bruns, *Maurice Blanchot*, pp. 181–91, esp. 187.

174. Michael Talbot, *Mysticism and the New Physics* (London: Penguin Books, 1993), p. 2: "I may dream that I am sitting at a table having breakfast and talking with my friends, but when I awake, I know that both I and my friends are part of the continuum of the dream. To say that they are many 'consciousnesses' in the dream is merely a semantic distinction. All the people in the dream are maya. They are constructions of consciousness."

175. Danah Zohar, *The Quantum Self: Human Nature and Consciousness Defined by the New Physics* (New York: Quill, 1990), pp. 154–70, esp. 159.

176. Maurice Merleau-Ponty, *Phenomenology of Perception*, translated by Colin Smith (New York: Humanities Press, 1962), p. 168.

177. Ricoeur, *Freud and Philosophy*, p. 502.

178. Žižek, *In Defense of Lost Causes*, p. 293.

179. The position taken by Merleau-Ponty is also to be distinguished from the important Jungian modification of the Freudian psychoanalytic approach. See, for instance, Jung, *Mysterium Coniunctionis*, p. 443. In the context of discussing the phallic symbolism associated with what is conventionally the ninth of the ten emanations in kabbalistic theosophy, Jung notes: "Such comparisons mislead the modern mind into one-sided interpretations, for instance that

Yesod is simply the penis, or, conversely, that the obviously sexual language has no basis in real sexuality. But in mysticism one must remember that no 'symbolic' object has only one meaning; it is always several things at once. Sexuality does not exclude spirituality nor spirituality sexuality, for in God all opposites are abolished." Jung demonstrates a far more nuanced grasp of the phallic symbols employed by kabbalists than most of the contemporary experts, who have doggedly criticized my views by mistaking references to the phallus as if I were simplistically speaking of the penis. I would not acquiesce to the archetypal underpinning of Jung's remarks, but I do accept his views that the symbolic object is multivalent and that spirituality and sexuality are not antithetical. My preference, however, is to think of the phallus as a semiotic marker as opposed to the penis, which is an anatomical entity, but I would accept Jung's caution against interpreting phallic symbols in physiological terms. See Wolfson, *Language, Eros, Being*, p. 128.

180. See especially the section on the libidinal body and intercorporeity in Maurice Merleau-Ponty, *Nature: Course Notes from the Collège de France*, compiled and with notes by Dominique Séglard, translated by Robert Vallier (Evanston: Northwestern University Press, 2003), pp. 224–26.

181. On Merleau-Ponty's discussion of incarnation, see O'Sullivan, *The Incarnation of Language*, pp. 48–54.

182. Merleau-Ponty, *Phenomenology of Perception*, p. 166 (emphasis in the original).

183. *Ibid.*, p. 168 (emphasis in the original).

184. There is sizeable bibliography on the status of the body, sense perception, and the visual field in Merleau-Ponty's thought. For a representative list, see Remy C. Kwant, *Phenomenology of Language* (Pittsburgh: Duquesne University Press, 1965); Elizabeth Grosz, *Volatile Bodies: Toward a Corporeal Feminism* (Bloomington: Indiana University Press, 1994), pp. 86–111; Françoise Dastur, "Word, Flesh, Vision," in *Chiasms: Merleau-Ponty's Notion of Flesh*, edited by Fred Evans and Leonard Lawlor (Albany: State University of New York Press, 2000), pp. 23–49; James B. Steeves, *Imagining Bodies: Merleau-Ponty's Philosophy of Imagination* (Pittsburgh: Duquesne University Press, 2004). The influence of Merleau-Ponty on my thinking is well attested in previous publications. See Wolfson, *Language, Eros, Being*, pp. xxi–xxxi, 24–25, 190–96; *idem*, *Alef, Mem, Tau: Kabbalistic Musings on Time, Truth, and Death* (Berkeley: University of California Press 2006), pp. 13, 166–67. My engagement here, however, was inspired by the lecture of Michael O'Donovan-Anderson, "Merleau-Ponty and the Fourth Dogma of Empiricism," available at http://www.cs.umd.edu/~anderson/papers/apa2000.pdf. The interpretation of Merleau-Ponty

proffered in this essay is a continuation of the orientation outlined in Michael O'Donovan-Anderson, *Content and Comportment: On Embodiment and the Epistemic Availability of the World* (Lanham: Rowman & Littlefield, 1997).

185. Roy Wood Sellars, "Referential Transcendence," *Philosophy and Phenomenological Research* 22 (1961): 1–15.

186. Merleau-Ponty, *Phenomenology of Perception*, p. 214 (emphasis in the original).

187. *Ibid.*, p. 215.

188. *Ibid.*, pp. 265, 304, 415–16, 423, 451.

189. Patrick Burke, "Merleau-Ponty's Appropriation of Husserl's Notion of '*Präsenzfeld*,'" in *Husserl in Contemporary Context: Prospects and Projects for Phenomenology*, edited by Burt C. Hopkins (Dordrecht: Kluwer, 1997), pp. 37–58. As Burke adduces on the basis of Merleau-Ponty's *The Visible and the Invisible*, the notion of the *Präsenzfeld* presented in the *Phenomenology of Perception* was "still too much polarized by the here-there distinction in which primacy is given to the subject, the absolute here, the absolute present, as though 'thereness' is reduced to the fact that I perceive, that the world is there because I perceive it rather than my perceiving it being based on the fact that it is there" (p. 58). For an extended analysis of the phenomenological and transcendental fields in Merleau-Ponty, see Stefan Bucher, *Zwischen Phänomenologie und Sprachwissenschaft: Zu Merleau-Pontys Theorie der Sprache* (Münster: Nodus Publikationen, 1991), pp. 55–85.

190. Hans Wagner, "Critical Observations Concerning Husserl's Posthumous Writings," in *The Phenomenology of Husserl*, p. 223: "Corporeality is as constitutive of me as I (within the context of primordial transcendence) am constitutive of it. If, however, corporeality is constitutive, the primordial world is also constitutive. Hence primordial worldliness is constitutive of my subjectivity. The world is constitutive of me to the same degree as it is constituted by myself and others." On the affinity between Merleau-Ponty's view and the interdependence of subjectivity and objectivity implied in Husserl's notion of constitution, see also Dan Zahavi, *Husserl's Phenomenology* (Stanford: Stanford University Press, 2003), p. 73. To be more precise, Zahavi argues that Husserl "conceives of constitution as a process involving several intertwined transcendental constituents, both subjectivity and world.... Husserl takes the process of constitution to presuppose an element of *facticity*, a passive pregivenness without any active participation or contribution by the ego.... Obviously, this should not be taken as a new form of dualism, on the contrary, the idea is exactly that subjectivity and world cannot be understood in separation from each other." A similar approach to Husserl is offered by Dodd, *Crisis*

and Reflection, pp. 190–91.

191. Edmund Husserl, *Psychological and Transcendental Phenomenology and the Confrontation With Heidegger (1927–1931)*, translated and edited by Thomas Sheehan and Richard E. Palmer (Dordrect: Kluwer, 1997), p. 244.

192. Eugen Fink, *Sixth Cartesian Meditation: The Idea of a Transcendental Theory of Method*, with textual notations by Edmund Husserl, translated with an introduction by Ronald Bruzina (Bloomington: Indiana University Press, 1995), p. 136 (emphasis in the original).

193. James Dodd, *Idealism and Corporeity: An Essay on the Problem of the Body in Husserl's Phenomenology* (Dordrecht: Kluwer, 1997), p. 81 (emphasis in the original).

194. Dodd, *Crisis and Reflection*, pp. 185–86 (emphasis in the original).

195. Merleau-Ponty, *Phenomenology of Perception*, pp. 52–53.

196. Steeves, *Imagining Bodies*, pp. 89–102; James Morley, "The Texture of the Real: Merleau-Ponty on Imagination and Psychopathology," in *Imagination and Its Pathologies*, pp. 93–108, esp. 98–99. It is important to recall here the connection between Foucault's preoccupation with the experience of madness and the phenomenologist's preoccupation with getting back to the things themselves noted by Allan Megill, *Prophets of Extremity: Nietzsche, Heidegger, Foucault, Derrida* (Berkeley: University of California Press, 1987), p. 200.

197. Merleau-Ponty, *Phenomenology of Perception*, p. 215.

198. Merleau-Ponty, *The Visible and the Invisible*, pp. 5–7. Compare Fóti, "Chiasm, Flesh, Figuration," p. 186: "Since dream accomplishes a spontaneous *epokhè* of the positivity of body and world, it allows phenomenalization to come about in releasement from reification; and, although dream does not give one access to 'true negativity' or the emptiness at the heart of phenomenalization, it frequents, as Richir notes, 'the edge of being,' the jointure 'where the multiple entries upon the world intercross.' Richir concludes that this very multiplicity of registers of phenomenalization (with which dream—though not uniquely—puts one in touch) orients one away from any substantial ontology." See *ibid.*, p. 191. The essay cited by Fóti is Marc Richir, "Le sensible dans le rêve," in *Merleau-Ponty: Notes de cours sur l'origine de la géométrie de Husserl; suivi de Récherches sur la phénoménologie de Merleau-Ponty*, edited by Renaud Barbaras (Paris: Presses Universitaires de France, 1998), pp. 239–54, esp. 251.

199. Merleau-Ponty, *Phenomenology of Perception*, pp. x–xi.

200. *Ibid.*, p. 284.

201. *Ibid.*, pp. 284–85. The passage cited by Merleau-Ponty corresponds to Binswanger, *Dream and Existence*, p. 82.

202. *Ibid.*, p. 285. For an analysis of this passage with a different emphasis,

see Glen A. Mazis, *Emotion and Embodiment: Fragile Ontology* (New York: Peter Lang, 1993), pp. 82–83.

203. Merleau-Ponty, *Phenomenology of Perception*, p. 451 (emphasis in the original).

204. Maurice Merleau-Ponty, *The Incarnate Subject: Malebranche, Biran, and Bergson on the Union of Body and Soul*, preface by Jacques Taminiaux, translation by Paul B. Milan, edited by Andrew G. Bjelland Jr. and Patrick Burke (Amherst: Humanity Books, 2001) p. 46.

205. See the analysis of Patrick Burke, "The Flesh as *Urpräsentierbarkeit* in the Interrogative: The Absence of a Question in Derrida," in *Écart & Différance: Merleau-Ponty and Derrida on Seeing and Writing*, edited by Martin C. Dillon (Atlantic Highlands: Humanities Press, 1997), pp. 60–70, esp. 64–66. The view I am expressing reverberates as well with the attempt of Jacques Lacan, *The Seminar of Jacques Lacan, Book XI: The Four Fundamental Concepts of Psychoanalysis*, edited by Jacques-Alain Miller, translated by Alan Sheridan (New York: W. W. Norton, 1981), p. 20, to explain the "linguistic structure" of the unconscious: "The important thing, for us, is that we are seeking here—before any formation of the subject, of a subject who thinks, who situates himself in it—the level at which there is counting, things are counted, and in this counting he who counts is always included. It is only later that the subject has to recognize himself as such, recognize himself as he who counts." See Ricouer, *Freud and Philosophy*, pp. 395–406; Hermann Lang, *Language and the Unconscious: Lacan's Hermeneutics of Psychoanalysis* (Atlantic Highlands: Humanities Press, 1997); Dany Nobus, "Lacan's Science of the Subject: Between Linguistics and Topology," in *The Cambridge Companion to Lacan*, edited by Jean-Michel Rabaté (Cambridge: Cambridge University Press, 2003), pp. 50–68; Joel Dor, *Introduction to the Reading of Lacan: The Unconscious Structured Like a Language* (New York: Other Press, 1998); Russell Grigg, *Lacan, Language, and Philosophy* (Albany: State University Press of New York, 2008), pp. 43, 55–68, 151–69. See also Paul Verhaeghe, "The Dream between Drive and Desire: A Question of Representability," in *The Dreams of Interpretation: A Century down the Royal Road*, edited by Catherine Liu, John Mowitt, Thomas Pepper, and Jakki Spicer (Mineapolis: University of Minnesota Press, 2007), pp. 135–45.

206. Von Franz, *Dreams*, pp. 1–20; Charles Hanly, "On Being and Dreaming," in *Psychoanalysis and Philosophy*, edited by Charles Hanly and Morris Lazerowitz (New York: International Universities Press, 1970), pp. 155–87, esp. 163–64. Based on my assumptions regarding the nature of the dreamer and the dream laid out in detail in this chapter, I would respectfully take issue with the following observation of Bulkeley, *Dreaming*, p. 2: "A dream is an imagined

world of sights, sounds, thoughts, feelings, and activities that you (either as a character in the dream or a disembodied observer of it) experience during sleep." I cannot accept the distinction between being a character in the dream and a disembodied observer of it. Within the dreamscape, this is an untenable distinction—even the disembodied observer of the dream is a character in the dream.

207. Husserl, *Crisis*, sec. 53, p. 178. Needless to say, the problem of subjectivity in Husserlian phenomenology has been discussed by numerous scholars. Here I note a few more relatively recent analyses from which I have benefited: David Carr, *The Paradox of Subjectivity: The Self in the Transcendental Tradition* (New York: Oxford University Press, 1999); Søren Overgaard, *Husserl and Heidegger on Being in the World* (Dordrecht: Kluwer, 2004), pp. 131–63; James Mensch, "Manifestation and the Paradox of Subjectivity," *Husserl Studies* 21 (2005): 35–53.

208. Husserl, *Crisis*, sec. 53, p. 179.

209. The question was already raised by Husserl, *Ideas*, sec. 53, p. 124: "The complete world is not merely physical; it is also psychophysical.... Thus, *on the one hand consciousness is said to be the absolute* in which everything transcendent and, therefore, ultimately the whole psychophysical world, becomes constituted; and, *on the other hand*, consciousness is said to be a *subordinate real event within that world*" (emphasis in the original).

210. Husserl, *Crisis*, sec. 53, pp. 179–80.

211. *Ibid.*, sec. 53–54, pp. 181–82 (emphasis in the original).

212. *Ibid*, sec. 54, pp. 183–84.

213. See the brief, but insightful study by Samuel Hugo Bergman, "Metaphysical Implications of Husserl's Phenomenology," *Scripta Hierosolymitana* 2 (1955): 220–30.

214. Husserl, *Crisis*, sec. 42, p. 153 (*Die Krisis*, pp. 155–56); see also p. 113. I have benefited from the discussion in Mensch, "Manifestation," pp. 37–38.

215. My formulation is indebted to Herbert W. Guenther, *Wholeness Lost and Wholeness Regained: Forgotten Tales of Individuation from Ancient Tibet* (Albany: State University of New York Press, 1994), p. 108.

216. For a succinct discussion of Sartre's view on dreaming, see Kathleen V. Wider, *The Bodily Nature of Consciousness: Sartre and Contemporary Philosophy of Mind* (Ithaca: Cornell University Press, 1997), pp. 94–97.

217. Tracey L. Kahan and Stephen LaBerge, "Lucid Dreaming as Metacognition: Implications for Cognitive Science," *Consciousness and Cognition* 3 (1994): 246–64. See also Celia E. Green, *Lucid Dreams*, with a foreword by H. H. Price (London: Hamiosh Hamilton, 1968); LaBerge, *Lucid Dreaming*; Celia E. Green

and Charles McCreery, *Lucid Dreaming: The Paradox of Consciousness during Sleep* (London: Routledge, 1994); Hobson, *Dreaming as Delirium*, pp. 172–74. On the problem of consciousness and metacognition related to the dream, see Tracey L. Kahan and Stephen LaBerge, "Cognition and Metacognition in Dreaming and Waking: Comparisons of First and Third-Person Ratings," *Dreaming* 6 (1996): 235–49, and Tracey L. Kahan, "Consciousness in Dreaming: A Metacognitive Approach," in *Dreams: A Reader on the Religious, Cultural, and Psychological Dimensions of Dreaming*, edited by Kelley Bulkeley (New York: Palgrave, 2001), pp. 333–60.

218. Blanchot, *Friendship*, p. 141.

219. See the post of Chris Crawford on dreams (May 25, 1998), available at http://www.erasmatazz.com/page78/page175/page176/Dreams.html.

220. Freud, *Interpretation of Dreams*, pp. 12–13: "The first thing to emerge is that material appears in the dream-content which, when subsequently awake, we do not recognize as part of our knowledge or experience. We may well remember that we dreamed this or that, but not that we ever experienced it." See also Malcolm, *Dreaming*, and Daniel C. Dennett, "Are Dreams Experiences?" *Philosophical Review* 85 (1976): 151–71, reprinted in *Philosophical Essays on Dreaming*, pp. 227–50.

221. Hartmann, *Dreams and Nightmares*, pp. 11–13 and 95–117. There are many similarities between my approach and that of Hartmann, whose work became known to me only after I had already conceptualized and formulated my argument. There is, however, one crucial difference: I do not accept Hartmann's argument that dreams partake of "picture metaphors" and not "words or formulas" (p. 99). On the metaphorical quality of the production of dream imagery and the explicit comparison to the poetic process, see also States, *Dreaming and Storytelling*, pp. 26–27. The demarcation of dreaming as a social event offered by Wax, *Western Rationality*, rests on the comparison of the dream to an aesthetic or ritual performance: "Dreaming can only be appreciated and understood when viewed in relationship to the range of activities of psyche-and-soma (mind-and-body), which include the aesthetic, visionary, ritual, and ceremonial aspects of group living. Dreams are most akin to the plastic and narrative arts" (p. 3).

222. I have appropriated the notion of the "formal property" of dreams from Elaine Scarry, *Resisting Representation* (New York: Oxford University Press, 1994), p. 72.

223. Ricoeur, *Freud and Philosophy*, p. 15.

224. Cicero, *On Divination: Book 1*, translated with introduction and commentary by David Wardle (Oxford: Oxford University Press, 2006), p. 59.

On the comparison between literary and divinatory interpreters in Cicero, see Struck, *Birth of the Symbol*, pp. 169–70.

225. Sigmund Freud, *Collected Papers*, authorized translation under the supervision of Joan Riviere, vol. 4 (London: Hogarth Press, 1953), pp. 173–83. See also Sigmund Freud, *The Complete Introductory Lectures on Psychoanalysis*, translated and edited by James Strachey (New York: W. W. Norton, 1966), p. 99, where daydreams are referred to as the "raw material of poetic composition."

226. Freud, *Interpretation of Dreams*, p. 79.

227. For discussion of the preconditions that culminate in poetry and dreaming, see Moses Ulrich, "Paper Clips and Black Cows: On Poetry and Dreams," *The Psychoanalytic Quarterly* 69 (2000): 28–49.

228. Freud, *Interpretation of Dreams*, pp. 189–90. For an alternative perspective, see Shafton, *Dream Reader*, pp. 57–58, who argues that even though Freud recognized the "poetic speech" of dream images, his "commitment to straightforwardly communicated, consensual waking reality precluded complete appreciation of poetic means. But apart from that . . . a dream is unartlike in the Freudian scheme because art has form, has integrity, while dreams have not. Or more precisely, what form dreams have is an aspect of disguise, and is therefore antagonistic to communication or honest expression. Freud strongly disparaged '"symbolic" dream-interpreting,' by which the entire structure of the dream's surface—the *manifest dream*—is thought to convey the dream's real meaning as an allegory or metaphor. To the contrary, each item of the manifest dream comes to birth out of its own psychic resources and each undergoes its own distortion by the censorship" (emphasis in the original). I am not persuaded by Shafton's argument that the dream is so utterly dissimilar to the poem or to the artistic creation more generally according to the Freudian interpretation. On the correlation of the "primary purpose" in Freud's mapping of the mind and poetic thinking, see Harold Bloom, "Freud and the Poetic Sublime," in *Freud: A Collection of Critical Essays*, edited by Perry Meisel (Englewood Cliffs: Prentice-Hall, 1981), pp. 211–31. On the depiction of Freud as a "frustrated" poet, see Graham Frankland, *Freud's Literary Culture* (Cambridge: Cambridge University Press, 2000), pp. 162–233. See also Robert J. C. Young, "Freud's Secret: *The Interpretation of Dreams* Was a Gothic Novel," in *Sigmund Freud's The Interpretation of Dreams: New Interdisciplinary Essays*, edited by Laura Marcus (Manchester: Manchester University Press, 1999), pp. 206–31. See also R. R. Thomas, "The Narrative of Theory: The Novel in the 'Interpretation of Dreams,'" *Psychohistory Review* 18 (1989): 1–31.

229. Michael Maltby, "Wordless Words: Poetry and the Symmetry of

Being," in *Acquainted with the Night: Psychoanalysis and the Poetic Imagination*, edited by Hamish Canham and Carole Satyamurti (London: Karnac, 2003), pp. 49–70, esp. 51–55.

230. Ella Freeman Sharpe, *Dream Analysis: A Practical Handbook for Psycho-Analysts* (London: Hogarth, 1937), p. 19, cited in Maltby, "Wordless Words," p. 52.

231. To be exact, in the term "poetry," the author includes lyrical, dramatic, and narrative productions. See Hanns Sachs, *The Creative Unconscious: Studies in the Psychoanalysis of Art*, edited by Abraham A. Roback, 2nd edition (Cambridge, MA: Sci-Art Publishers, 1951), p. 12.

232. *Ibid.*, pp. 13–14.

233. Boodakian, *Tormenting Angel*, pp. 9–12.

234. Sachs, *The Creative Unconscious*, p. 13.

235. Kenneth Burke, "Freud—and the Analysis of Poetry," in *Freud: A Collection of Critical Essays*, p. 79.

236. *Ibid.*, p. 85.

237. *Ibid.*, pp. 85–86.

238. Grigg, *Lacan, Language, and Philosophy*, pp. 42–43.

239. Ricoeur, *Freud and Philosophy*, pp. 16–18. See *ibid.*, pp. 165–66: "Freud brings together the two ends of the chain of the fantastic—dreams and poetry. Both are manifestations of the same fate, the fate of unhappy, unsatisfied man."

240. *Ibid.*, p. 162.

241. Jacques Lacan, *The Seminar of Jacques Lacan, Book I: Freud's Papers on Technique 1953–1954*, edited by Jacques-Alain Miller, translated with notes by John Forrester (New York: W. W. Norton, 1991), p. 155.

242. Joan Copjec, *Read My Desire: Lacan against the Historicists* (Cambridge, MA: The MIT Press, 1994), p. 121.

243. Shoshana Felman, *Jacques Lacan and the Adventure of Insight: Psychoanalysis in Contemporary Culture* (Cambridge, MA: Harvard University Press, 1987), p. 54. On the question of translation and dream interpretation, see Lydia Marinelli and Andreas Mayer, *Dreaming by the Book: Freud's The Interpretation of Dreams and the History of the Psychoanalytic Movement*, translated by Susan Fairfield (New York: Other Press, 2003), pp. 127–37.

244. Ricoeur, *Freud and Philosophy*, p. 162.

245. *Ibid.*, p. 175 (emphasis in the original).

246. I have written at length about this topic in previous studies. See especially Elliot R. Wolfson, "Occultation of the Feminine and the Body of Secrecy in Medieval Kabbalah," in *Rending the Veil: Concealment and Revelation of Secrets in the History of Religions*, edited by Elliot R. Wolfson (New York:

Seven Bridges Press, 1999), pp. 113–54, reprinted with corrections in Elliot R. Wolfson, *Luminal Darkness: Imaginal Gleanings From Zoharic Literature* (London: Oneworld Publications, 2007), pp. 258–94; *idem*, *Language, Eros, Being*, pp. 25–32, 128–41, 223–33.

247. Freud, *Interpretation of Dreams*, p. 88 n. 4.

248. *Ibid.*, p. 341.

249. *Ibid.*, p. 340. See Laura Marcus, "Introduction: Histories, Representations, Autobiographics in *The Interpretation of Dreams*," in *Sigmund Freud's The Interpretation of Dreams: New Interdisciplinary Essays*, p. 20.

250. James Hillman, *The Dream and the Underworld* (New York: Harper & Row, 1979), pp. 123–27. See also the remark of Stekel cited in the Introduction, n. 6.

251. A number of scholars have explored Freudian psychoanalysis and mysticism. For a representative list, see Edwin R. Wallace, "Freud's Mysticism and Its Psychodynamic Determinants," *Bulletin of the Menninger Clinic* 42 (1978): 203–22; Ralph W. Hood Jr., "Mysticism, Reality, Illusion, and the Freudian Critique of Religion," *International Journal for the Psychology of Religion* 2 (1992): 141–59; William B. Parsons, *The Enigma of the Oceanic Feeling: Revisioning the Psychoanalytic Theory of Mysticism* (New York: Oxford University Press, 1999).

252. Sigmund Freud, *Totem and Taboo: Some Points of Agreement between the Mental Lives of Savages and Neurotics*, translated and edited by James Strachey (New York: W. W. Norton, 1950), pp. 118–19. This is discussed in more detail in *Interpretation of Dreams*, pp. 271–98, esp. p. 291: "we will understand that the dream-work had every cause to create *an indisputable refutation of an absurd demand* after the model contained in the dream-thoughts. However, the analysis shows us that it is not for the dream-work to create this simulacrum freely; rather, it is obliged to use material from the dream-thoughts for it. It is though an algebraic equation, in addition to the numbers, contained a plus and a minus sign for indicating a higher power or a root, and as though someone were to copy down this equation blindly, transferring the operative signs as well as the numerals into his copy and jumbling both sorts up together" (emphasis in the original). On the admission that the meaning of certain dreams could not be ascertained on account of their apparent absurdity, see also Sigmund Freud, *Leonardo da Vinci and a Memory of His Childhood*, translated by Alan Tyson, edited by James Strachey (New York: W. W. Norton, 1964), pp. 46–47.

253. For various perspectives on this theme, see *Le silence en psychoanalyse*, edited by Juan-David Nasio (Paris: Désir/Payot, 1998).

254. On the phenomenon of *Verneinung* in Freud, see Wilfried ver Eecke, *Denial, Negation, and the Forces of the Negative: Freud, Hegel, Lacan, Spitz, and*

Sophocles (Albany: State University of New York Press, 2006), pp. 7–23.

255. Ludwig Wittgenstein, *Lectures and Conversations on Aesthetics, Psychology and Belief*, compiled from notes taken by Yorick Smythies, Rush Rhees, and James Taylor, edited by Cyril Barrett (Oxford: Blackwell, 1966), p. 45. See Paul-Laurent Assoun, *Freud et Wittgenstein* (Paris: Presses Universitaires de France, 1988), pp. 109–38.

256. See Thorsten Botz-Bornstein, "The Dream of Language: Wittgenstein's Concept of Dreams in the Context of Style and *Lebensform*," *Philosophical Forum* 34 (2003): 73–76.

257. Jung, *Practice of Psychotherapy*, p. 148.

258. Ross Woodman, *Sanity, Madness, Transformation: The Psyche in Romanticism*, edited and with an afterword by Joel Faflak (Toronto: University of Toronto Press, 2005), p. 24.

259. Plato, *Republic* 382c–d, in *Collected Dialogues*, p. 629, and see analysis in Ramona A. Naddaff, *Exiling the Poets: The Production of Censorship in Plato's Republic* (Chicago: University of Chicago Press, 2002), pp. 32–33.

260. Plato, *Symposium* 175e, in *Collected Dialogues*, p. 530. On Plato's skepticism concerning the supernatural and oracular status of dreams, see the evidence from the *Laws* and *Epinomis* adduced by Dodds, *The Greeks and the Irrational*, p. 108. See also Steven S. Tigner, "Plato's Philosophical Uses of the Dream Metaphor," *American Journal of Philology* 91 (1970): 204–12; David Gallop, "Dreaming and Waking in Plato," in *Essays in Ancient Greek Philosophy*, edited by John P. Anton and George L. Kustas (Albany: State University of New York Press, 1971), pp. 187–201.

261. Plato, *Theaetetus* 201e, in *Collected Dialogues*, p. 908. See Ronald M. Polansky, *Philosophy and Knowledge: A Commentary on Plato's Theatetus* (Lewisburg: Bucknell University Press, 1992), pp. 213–22.

262. Lacan, *The Seminar of Jacques Lacan, Book XI*, p. 23.

263. *Ibid.*, p. 57.

264. *Ibid.*, p. 60.

265. *Ibid.*, p. 58.

266. My analysis has benefited from the discussion in Andrea Hurst, *Derrida vis-à-vis Lacan: Interweaving Deconstruction and Psychoanalysis* (New York: Fordham University Press, 2008), pp. 221–23.

267. Lacan, *The Seminar of Jacques Lacan, Book XI*, p. 59.

268. *Ibid.*, p. 60.

269. Derrida, *Resistances of Psychoanalysis*, pp. 10–11 (emphasis in the original). Compare Hurst, *Derrida vis-à-vis Lacan*, pp. 174–81.

270. Jacques Derrida, *Dissemination*, translated, with an introduction and

additional notes, by Barbara Johnson (Chicago: University of Chicago Press, 1981), p. 160.

271. *Ibid.*, p. 161. On Plato's use of *metaxy* to designate this in-between realm that participates in both the temporal and the eternal, the mutable and the immutable, see Plato, *Gorgias* 468a; *Symposium* 203b–c; Aristotle, *Metaphysics* 987b.

272. *Timaeus* 52b–c, in *Collected Dialogues*, pp. 1178–79. See John Sallis, *Chorology: On Beginning in Plato's Timaeus* (Bloomington: Indiana University Press, 1999), pp. 118–24. The Platonic notion of the "third space" brings to mind the description of the dream state in the *Bṛhadāraṇyaka Upaniṣad* 4.3.9 as the "third place" or intermediate where this world and the next world meet. See Angela Sumegi, *Dreamworlds of Shamanism and Tibetan Buddhism: The Third Place* (Albany: State University of New York Press, 2008), pp. 43–44.

273. Gaston Bachelard, *Water and Dreams: An Essay on the Imagination of Matter*, translated by Edith R. Farrell (Dallas: Pegasus Foundation, 1983), p. 16.

274. Ralph Waldo Emerson, "The Poet," in *Essays and Lectures* (New York: Library of America, 1983), p. 452.

275. Hartmann, *Dreams and Nightmares*, p. 99.

276. The convergence of the visual and audible relates to the literary form of the poem, as well as to its oral performance. Consider the following observation of Elaine Scarry, *Dreaming by the Book* (New York: Farrar, Straus and Giroux, 1999), p. 7: "Poetry—again unlike narrative—even has immediate sensory content, since the visual disposition of the lines and stanzas provides an at once apprehensible visual rhythm that is a prelude to, or rehearsal for, or promise of, the beautiful regulation of sound to come." See, by contrast, Hieatt, *Realism of Dream Visions*, p. 18: "The form, as typified by the *Romance of the Rose*, is, however, very much a vision: the imagery and description of the poem are richly visual, and the poem is to a very large extent an account of what the poet sees rather than of what he hears or thinks. To this extent perhaps it can be considered dreamlike, for dreams tend to be largely visual" (emphasis in the original). Hieatt cites Freud (*Realism of Dream Visions*, p. 18 n. 20) as an authority to support the ocularcentric interpretation of dreams. I do not concur with the dichotomization of the verbal and the visual either with respect to the poem or to the dream vision.

277. For discussion of this philosophical theme with reference to previous scholars, see Bence Nanay, "Is Twofoldness Necessary for Representational Seeing?" *British Journal of Aesthetics* 45 (2005): 248–57.

278. Isaac Afik (Abecassis), "Hazal's Perception of the Dream," Ph.D. dissertation, Bar-Ilan University, 1990, pp. 334–424 (Hebrew); Monford Harris,

Studies in Jewish Dream Interpretation (Northvale: Jason Aronson, 1994), pp. 5–6 and 10–11; Galit Hasan-Rokem, *Web of Life: Folklore and Midrash in Rabbinic Literature*, translated by Batya Stein (Stanford: Stanford University Press, 2000), pp. 88–107; Alexander Samely, *Rabbinic Interpretation of Scripture in the Mishnah* (Oxford: Oxford University Press, 2002), pp. 145–47. See additional references cited in Chapter 3 nn. 5, 7, and 9.

279. Hartmann, *Dreams and Nightmares*, p. 99.

280. On the relation of the narrative fiction and interpretation of the lower form of dream, *insomnium* or *enhupnion*, caused by the faculties of soul rather than by a divine power, see Vered Lev Kenaan, "Delusion and Dream in Apuleius' *Metamorphoses*," *Classical Antiquity* 23 (2004): 247–84. The complex relationship of reporting dreams and their interpretation is analyzed succinctly by Brann, *The World of the Imagination*, pp. 342–46. See also Eileen Rizo-Patron, "On the Role of the Oneiric in Testimonial Narrative," in *Traversing the Imaginary: Richard Kearney and the Postmodern Challenge*, edited by Peter Gratton and John Panteleimon Manoussakis, foreword by Richard Kearney (Evanston: Northwestern University Press, 2007), pp. 152–64.

281. Kilroe, "Dream as Text," p. 127.

282. *Ibid.*, p. 128 (emphasis in the original). See also Philip Shields, "Dreaming and Interpretation: A Treatment of the Interpretation of Dreams as a Dream," *Psychoanalysis and Contemporary Thought* 13 (1990): 79–105; Martin Derksen, "Dream Interpretation as Test Case for Hermeneutics," *Journal of Phenomenological Psychology* 22 (1991): 134–41; Carol Schreier Rupprecht and Kelly Bulkeley, "Reading Yourself to Sleep: Dreams in/and/as Texts," in *The Dream and the Text*, pp. 1–12; Carol Schreier Rupprecht, "Dreaming, Language, Literature," in *The New Science of Dreaming*, vol. 3, pp. 1–34.

283. Benjamin Libet, *Mind Time: The Temporal Factor in Consciousness* (Cambridge, MA: Harvard University Press, 2004), p. 84.

284. *Ibid.*, p. 85.

285. Rodger Kamenetz, *The History of Last Night's Dream: Discovering the Hidden Path to the Soul* (New York: HarperCollins, 2007), p. 11. While I appreciate the author's acknowledging my *Through a Speculum That Shines* in a laudatory manner (pp. 242, 249 n. 13, and 255), his repeated insistence on the struggle between word and image (pp. 49, 50–51, 74–75, 87–88, 96–97, 98) bespeaks an inattentiveness to the thrust of that monograph. In that work, as well as in subsequent publications, I emphasize the dialectical intertwining of word and image, the revelatory nature of interpretation and the interpretive nature of revelation. See Wolfson, *Language, Eros, Being*, pp. 1–45, the chapter tellingly entitled "Showing the Saying: Laying Interpretative Ground,"

a formulation distinctly indebted to Heidegger, for whom word and image similarly cannot be easily separated (pp. 14–17). It should come as no surprise that I do not agree with Kamenetz's remark that "most kabbalah taught today is concerned not with direct experiences, but with the study of other people's experiences. It is text-based and somewhat dry and abstract" (*History*, p. 40). He goes on to say that the "direct engagement" with "personal images" promulgated by his teacher, Colette Aboulker-Muscat, represents the exception to the rule. Kamenetz also contrasts the text-based kabbalah, which, he says, has been promoted by men and is prominent amongst the Ashkenazim, and the visionary kabbalah, which has been transmitted by women and is more characteristic of the Sephardim—he adopts the verbiage of Madame Colette and refers to this brand as the "kitchen kabbalah" (*ibid.*, pp. 40–41). Leaving aside the factual inaccuracy of this historical appraisal and the somewhat unfortunate use of language to account for it, the binary distinction made by Kamenetz ignores the main contention in the *Speculum* regarding the visionary status of textual study. For the most part, my contribution has been eclipsed, but it seems that a gesture toward my thesis is discernible in Kamenetz's statement "In dreams all the old religious quests and drama are vividly real, including that most ancient and impossible mystical quest, to see the face of God. A quest, more than any other, where the image and the word collide" (*ibid.*, p. 6). The *collusion* (rather than collision) of word and image is fundamental to my hermeneutical phenomenology. On the distinction between "thinking abstractly," which involves reading and writing, and "direct experiencing," see *ibid.*, p. 234. In my judgment, abstract thought is the most concrete form of direct experience; the most tangible is suffered at the highest level of idealization.

286. Ricoeur, *Freud and Philosophy*, p. 15: "dreams in themselves border on language, since they can be told, analyzed, interpreted." For a psycholinguistic elaboration of this motif, see Frank Heynick, *Language and Its Disturbances in Dreams: The Pioneering Work of Freud and Kraepelin Updated* (New York: J. Wiley & Sons, 1993).

287. On the more restricted depiction of dreaming as a form of imaginative creation akin to the writing of poetry and fiction, see the work of States cited above, n. 147. For a comparison of the production of dreams and poetic inscription, see also Richard A. Russo, "Dream Poetry as Dream Work," *Dreaming* 13 (2003): 13–27; Rupprecht, "Dreaming, Language, Literature," pp. 8–12.

288. See Carl G. Jung, *The Structure and Dynamics of the Psyche*, 2nd edition, translated by R. F. C. Hull (Princeton: Princeton University Press, 1969), pp. 230–34. Jung relates this physical principle to his notion of synchronicity; see Chapter 5 n. 37. For the application of physics to the dream phenomenon,

see Fred Alan Wolf, *The Dreaming Universe: A Mind-Expanding Journey Into the Realm Where Psyche and Physics Meet* (New York: Simon & Schuster, 1994); *idem*, "The Quantum Mechanics of Dreams and the Emergence of Self-Awareness," in *Toward a Scientific Basis for Consciousness*, edited by S. R. Hameroff, A. W. Kaszniak, and A. C. Scott (Cambridge, MA: The MIT Press, 1996), pp. 451–67.

289. Anders Karlsson, "Descartes Prize Talk," available at http://ec.europa.eu/research/science-awards/pdf/anders_karlsson_prague_speech_en.pdf.

290. Christopher Norris, *Quantum Theory and the Flight from Realism: Philosophical Responses to Quantum Mechanics* (London: Routledge, 2000), pp. 6–71.

291. *Ibid.*, p. 195.

292. Bernard d'Espagnat, *Veiled Reality: An Analysis of Present-Day Quantum Mechanical Concepts* (Boulder: Westview Press, 2003), pp. 306–307, 360–400. I thank Catherine Keller for drawing my attention to this work.

293. *Ibid.*, pp. 2–5.

294. *Ibid.*, pp. 8–9 (emphasis in the original).

295. *Ibid.*, pp. 309–59.

296. *Ibid.*, pp. 318–21.

297. Junichi Murata, "The Indeterminacy of Images: An Approach to a Phenomenology of the Imagination," in *Phenomenology: Japanese and American Perspectives*, pp. 169–83.

298. Wolf, *Dreaming Universe*, pp. 161 and 171.

299. Terence McKenna, *The Archaic Revival: Speculations on Psychedelic Mushrooms, the Amazon, Virtual Reality, UFOs, Evolution, Shamanism, the Rebirth of the Goddess, and the End of History* (New York: HarperCollins, 1991), p. 34. I am grateful to Jeffrey Kripal for drawing this text to my attention.

300. Patrick McNamara, "Counterfactual Thought in Dreams," *Dreaming* 10 (2000): 237–46.

301. See the remark of Jung cited in Chapter 5 at n. 36.

302. McKenna, *The Archaic Revival*, p. 91.

303. Talbot, *Mysticism*, p. 59.

304. See above, n. 144.

305. For an elaborate account of the philosophical theory that mind is the primary element in all living and nonliving things, see David Skrbina, *Panpsychism in the West* (Cambridge, MA: The MIT Press, 2005).

306. Here I am disagreeing with the Jungian approach. See, for instance, Carl G. Jung, *Children's Dreams: Notes from the Seminar Given in 1936–1940*, edited by Lorenz Jung and Maria Meyer-Grass, translated by Ernst Falzeder with the collaboration of Tony Woolfson (Princeton: Princeton University Press, 2008), p. 2: "As you know, the dream is a natural phenomenon. It does

not spring from a natural intention. One cannot explain it with a psychology taken from *consciousness*. We are dealing with a particular way of functioning independent of the human ego's will and wishes, intention or aim. It is an unintentional occurrence, just like everything in nature. So we also cannot assume that the sky gets clouded only to annoy us; it simply is as it is. The difficulty is, however, to get a *handle* on that natural occurrence" (emphasis in the original). See, however, May, "Introduction," in *Dreams and Symbols*, p. 8: "What I am arguing is that unconscious life is also *intentional*. It is oriented in some direction: the dream or fantasy is saying, this is the way I see the world, and this is the way I see myself in it. That is quite different from what has generally been assumed in psychoanalysis, that by *interpreting* the dream we give it meaning; for interpreting has tended to be our transforming the dream into our symbols; interpreting it in our formulations, rationalizing it in terms of our particular school.... What I am proposing is something different: namely, that the unconscious experience *itself* is intentional, moves toward meaning. It is *protentive*, to borrow Husserl's term. This meaning will not, however, be in logical terms. As Freud made entirely clear, the unconscious brooks contradictions, denials, reversals, and every other thing that horrifies our logic" (emphasis in the original).

307. Uriah Kriegel, "Is Intentionality Dependent upon Consciousness?" *Philosophical Studies* 116 (2003): 271–307.

308. Ludwig Wittgenstein, *Philosophical Grammar*, edited by Rush Rees, translated by Anthony Kenny (Berkeley: University of California Press, 1974), p. 145.

309. *Ibid.*

310. *Ibid.*, p. 146.

311. *Ibid.*, p. 143.

312. *Ibid.*, p. 146. In some respect, the philosophical insight accords with the role of intentionality in the ancient rites of purification related to dream incubation. See Kimberley C. Patton, "'A Great and Strange Correction': Intentionality, Locality, and Epiphany in the Category of Dream Incubation," *History of Religions* 43 (2004): 194–223.

313. Foucault, "Dream, Imagination and Existence," pp. 74–75. Foucault's view is analyzed in Giorgio Agamben, *The Signature of All Things: On Method*, translated by Luca D'Isanto with Kevin Attell (New York: Zone Books, 2009), pp. 104–105.

314. Here it is worth noting the distinction on the basis of Artemidorus made by Michel Foucault, *The History of Sexuality, Volume 3: The Care of the Self*, translated by Robert Hurley (New York: Vintage Books, 1988), p. 11: "dreams

of desire" (*enypnia*) disclose the "soul's reality in its present state," whereas "dreams of being" (*oneiroi*) "tell the future of the event in the order of the world." Moreover, as recent studies have shown, whereas non-REM dreams are limited to reliving past experiences, REM dreams are expansive appropriations and quirky combinations of sense memories that test possible scenarios of the future and thus help a person to prepare for what is to come based on what has been. From the standpoint of biological evolution, dreams are a coping mechanism for human survival. In some respects, this corresponds to the distinction made in the thirteenth century by Gershon ben Solomon, *Sha'ar ha-Shamayim*, 68b, between the dream in which the imagination conjures images based on previous sense experiences and the dream in which the imagination conjures images that are not based on what has been experienced in waking hours, which he tellingly refers to as what "we are to remember in the future" (*she-anu attidim lizkor*).

CHAPTER TWO: SEEING-NOT

1. See the definition of a contradiction in Moses Maimonides, *Introduction to Logic in the Hebrew Version of Moses Ibn Tibbon*, edited by Leon Roth, collated with the manuscript fragments in Arabic by David H. Baneth, 2nd edition (Jerusalem: Magnes Press, 1965), IV.3, p. 21 (Hebrew). See also Maimonides, *Guide*, I.32, p. 70; I.52, p.114; II.6, p. 261; Josef Stern, "Maimonides on Language and the Science of Language," in *Maimonides and the Sciences*, edited by Robert S. Cohen and Hillel Levine (Dordrecht: Kluwer, 2000), pp. 173–226, esp. 185–86. For an extensive and philologically rich discussion of the Maimonidean distinction between true and false, on one hand, and good and evil, on the other, see Shlomo Pines, "Truth and Falsehood Versus Good and Evil: A Study in Jewish and General Philosophy in Connection with The Guide of the Perplexed, I.2," in *Studies in Maimonides*, edited by Isadore Twersky (Cambridge, MA: Harvard University Press, 1990), pp. 95–157. On the question of the authenticity of the Maimonidean authorship of the *Treatise on the Art of Logic* (*Maqāla fi ṣina'at al-manṭiq*), see Herbert A. Davidson, *Moses Maimonides: The Man and His Works* (Oxford: Oxford University Press, 2005), pp. 313–22, and for an alternative view, see Joel L. Kraemer, *Maimonides: The Life and World of One of Civilization's Greatest Minds* (New York: Doubleday, 2008), pp. 69–73.

2. Abraham Ibn Ḥasdai, *Ben ha-Melekh we-ha-Nazir* (Jerusalem, 2002), ch. 15, p. 81.

3. Abraham Abulafia, *Ḥayyei ha-Nefesh* (Jerusalem, 2001), p. 87; Baḥya ben Asher, *Rabbenu Baḥya: Be'ur al ha-Torah*, edited by Ḥayyim D. Chavel, 3 vols.

(Jerusalem: Mosad ha-Rav Kook, 1981), 2:406 (*ad* Leviticus 2:11).

4. Maimonides, *Guide*, 1. "Introduction," p. 7. On communicating truth in flashes, see 1.34, p. 78. Pines, "Translator's Introduction," pp. civ–cv, suggested that this image reflects the influence of Ibn Bājja.

5. See below, nn. 91 and 92.

6. The inability to distinguish darkness and light, which is applied positively to Moses, in another passage is applied negatively to the "ignorant and neglectful, who are pleased to regard their own deficiency and stupidity as perfection and wisdom, and the perfection and knowledge of others as a defection from Law" (1.32, p. 70).

7. Amos Funkenstein, *Theology and the Scientific Imagination From the Middle Ages to the Seventeenth Century* (Princeton: Princeton University Press, 1986), p. 65 n. 25.

8. Ibn Ḥasdai, *Ben ha-Melekh we-ha-Nazir*, pp. 81–82.

9. Foucault, "Dream, Imagination and Existence," pp. 44–45.

10. This influence has been well documented in scholarly literature. See, for example, Heidi M. Ravven, "Some Thoughts on What Spinoza Learned from Maimonides about the Prophetic Imagination, Part One: Maimonides on Prophecy and Imagination," *Journal of the History of Philosophy* 39 (2001): 193–214; *idem*, "Some Thoughts on What Spinoza Learned from Maimonides about the Prophetic Imagination, Part Two: Spinoza's Maimonideanism," *Journal of the History of Philosophy* 39 (2001): 385–406; Idit Dobbs-Weinstein, "The Ambiguity of the Imagination and the Ambivalence of Language in Maimonides and Spinoza," in *Maimonides and His Heritage*, edited by Idit Dobbs-Weinstein, Lenn E. Goodman, and James A. Grady (Albany: State University of New York Press, 2009), pp. 95–111. See also the insightful analysis of the limits of knowledge, the critique of transcendence, and the complex role of imagination in Maimonides and Spinoza in Nancy K. Levene, *Spinoza's Revelation: Religion, Democracy, and Reason* (Cambridge: Cambridge University Press, 2004), pp. 38–47.

11. The emphasis on vision is something the civilizations of the ancient Near East shared with the Greeks, who similarly spoke predominantly of *seeing* a dream. See Dodds, *The Greeks*, p. 105; A. Leo Oppenheim, "The Interpretation of Dreams in the Ancient Near East, with a Translation of an Assyrian Dream-Book," *Transactions of the American Philosophical Society* 46 (1956): 226.

12. Numerous scholars have weighed in on the relation of dreams and prophecy in the Hebrew Scripture in the context of other ancient Near Eastern cultures. See Oppenheim, "Interpretation of Dreams," pp. 186–91, 193, 209–11; Solomon Zeitlin, "Dreams and Their Interpretation From the Biblical

Period to the Tannaitic Time: An Historical Study," *Jewish Quarterly Review* 66 (1975): 1–18; Jean-Marie Husser, *Dreams and Dream Narratives in the Biblical World* (Sheffield, UK: Sheffield Academic Press, 1999); Shaul Bar, *A Letter That Has Not Been Read: Dreams in the Hebrew Bible* (Cincinnati: Hebrew Union College Press, 2001); Ruth Fidler, *"Dreams Speak Falsely?" Dream Theophanies in the Bible: Their Place in Ancient Israelite Faith and Tradition* (Jerusalem: Magnes Press, 2005) (Hebrew); Flannery-Dailey, *Dreamers, Scribes, and Priests*, pp. 17–56. The literature on the phenomenon of prophecy in biblical times is equally enormous. For representative studies, see Robert R. Wilson, *Prophecy and Society in Ancient Israel* (Philadelphia: Fortress Press, 1980); Joseph Blenkinsopp, *Sage, Priest, Prophet: Religious and Intellectual Leadership in Ancient Israel* (Louisville: Westminster John Knox Press, 1995), pp. 115–65; Ronald E. Clements, *Old Testament Prophecy* (Louisville: Westminster Press, 1996); Albert Cook, *The Burden of Prophecy: Poetic Utterance in the Prophets of the Old Testament* (Carbondale: Southern Illinois University Press, 1996).

13. Rebecca Gray, *Prophetic Figures in Late Second Temple Jewish Palestine: The Evidence of Josephus* (New York: Oxford University Press, 1993), p. 28, and reference to other scholars cited on p. 176 n. 70. On the divine status of dreams, see Dodds, *The Greeks*, pp. 108–10; Miller, *Dreams*, pp. 65–73.

14. David E. Aune, *Prophecy in Early Christianity and the Ancient Mediterranean World* (Grand Rapids: William B. Eerdmans, 1983), pp. 25–26. For a highly technical analysis of this phenomenon, see Gil H. Renberg, "'Commanded By the Gods': An Epigraphical Study of Dreams and Visions in Greek and Roman Religious Life," Ph.D. dissertation, Duke University, 2003.

15. See, for instance, Gray, *Prophetic Figures*, p. 27. On the rabbinic dogma concerning the cessation of prophecy, see Ephraim E. Urbach, *The Sages: Their Concepts and Beliefs*, translated by Israel Abrams (Jerusalem: Magnes Press, 1975), pp. 577–79.

16. Philip S. Alexander, "Bavil Berakhot 55a–57b: The Talmudic Dreambook in Context," *Journal of Jewish Studies* 46 (1995): 232.

17. Babylonian Talmud, Ḥagigah 5b. Compare Abraham J. Heschel, *Prophetic Inspiration After the Prophets: Maimonides and Other Medieval Authorities*, edited by Morris M. Faierstein, preface by Moshe Idel (Hoboken: Ktav, 1996), p. 3.

18. Gray, *Prophetic Figures*, pp. 27–28, suggests that Josephus similarly viewed dreams as a major source for prophetic revelation, a view that may have reflected his own revelatory experiences, which are read back into the ancient sources. On the attempt to distinguish ordinary and revelatory dreams on the part of Josephus, see Gray, *Prophetic Figures*, pp. 60–65. See also Louis H. Feldman, "Prophets and Prophecy in Josephus," *Journal of Theological Studies* 41

(1990): 386–422; *idem, Josephus's Interpretation of the Bible* (Berkeley: University of California Press, 1998), pp. 100–102, 349–51, 633.

19. Babylonian Talmud, Berakhot 55b, 57b. An echo of this rabbinic tradition can be detected in Isaac of Acre's report of citing certain verses when waking up that reflect the content of his dream. See *Oṣar Ḥayyim*, MS Günzberg 775, fols. 158b–159a, translated and analyzed in Eitan P. Fishbane, *As Light Before Dawn: The Inner World of a Medieval Kabbalist* (Stanford: Stanford University Press, 2009), pp. 106–107.

20. Babylonian Talmud, Berakhot 57b. See Galit Hasan-Rokem, "'A Dream Amounts to the Sixtieth Part of Prophecy': On Interaction between Textual Establishment and Popular Context in Dream Interpretation by the Jewish Sages," in *Studies in the History of Popular Culture*, edited by Benjamin Z. Kedar (Jerusalem: Zalman Shazar Center for Jewish History, 1996), pp. 45–54 (Hebrew).

21. *Midrash Bere'shit Rabba* 17:5, p. 157, 44:17, p. 439. See Maimonides, *Guide*, II.36, p. 370. On the juxtaposition of the difficult dream (*ḥalom qasheh*) and difficult prophecy (*nevu'ah qashah*) together with extreme mourning (*evel shoṭeh*), see the saying transmitted in the name of R. Yoḥanan in *Midrash Bere'shit Rabba* 64:5, p. 704, and the dictum ascribed to him in Babylonian Talmud, Baba Batra 12b, "From the day that the Temple was destroyed, prophecy was taken from the prophets and given to fools [*shoṭim*] and to infants [*tinoqot*]." In conjunction with this talmudic teaching, Ginzberg, *Legends*, 5:442 n. 26, mentioned the saying of Jesus in Matthew 21:16, "Have you not read, 'Out of the mouth of infants and nursing babes you have brought praise for yourself'?"

22. Harris, *Studies*, pp. 15–19; Gershom Scholem, *Origins of the Kabbalah*, edited by R. J. W. Werblowsky, translated by Allan Arkush (Princeton: Princeton University Press, 1987), p. 240, and see n. 22 where Scholem mentions both Jacob of Marvège and Moses of Coucy.

23. Heschel, *Prophetic Inspiration*, p. 4; Tamar Alexander-Frizer, *The Pious Sinner: Ethics and Aesthetics in the Medieval Hasidic Narrative* (Tübingen: J. C. B. Mohr, 1991), pp. 87–89 and 91–94; Moshe Idel, "On Še'elat Ḥalom in Ḥasidei Aškenaz: Sources and Influences," *Materia Giudaica* 10 (2005): 99–109. The Hebrew version of this study appears as the appendix in Moshe Idel, *Nocturnal Kabbalists* (Jerusalem: Carmel, 2006), pp. 91–119 (Hebrew). For discussion of this technique in works that contemporary scholars have called "ecstatic kabbalah," see Idel, *Nocturnal Kabbalists*, pp. 15–36 (compare the French translation, *Les Kabbalistes de la nuit* [Paris: Editions Allia, 2003], pp. 12–28). See also Trachtenberg, *Jewish Magic*, pp. 241–43; Moshe Idel, "Astral Dreams in Judaism: Twelfth to Fourteenth Centuries," in *Dream Cultures*, pp. 238 and 243–44;

idem, "Dream Techniques in Jewish Mysticism," in *Jewish Heritage Online Magazine*, available at http://www.jhom.com/topics/dreams/techniques.html; and Joseph Dan, *On Sanctity: Religion, Ethics and Mysticism in Judaism and Other Religions* (Jerusalem: Magnes Press, 1998), pp. 38–39 (Hebrew). The technique is attested as well in *Sefer ha-Ḥezyonot*, the celebrated diary of the sixteenth-century kabbalist Ḥayyim Viṭal. See *The "Book of Visions": The Diary of Rabbi Hayyim Vital*, edited with notes and an introduction by Morris M. Faierstein (Jerusalem: Ben-Zvi Institute, 2005), p. 73 (Hebrew), and the English version in *Jewish Mystical Autobiographies: Book of Visions and Book of Secrets*, translated and introduced by Morris M. Faierstein, preface by Moshe Idel (New York: Paulist Press, 1999), pp. 77–78. See also Ḥayyim Viṭal, *Sha'arei Qedushshah* (Jerusalem: Mishor, 2005), IV.3, p. 289; *idem*, *Sefer ha-Pe'ulot: Refu'ot, Segullot, Qabbalah Ma'asit, Kimeyah* (Jerusalem, 2010), pp. 5, 11–12, 193, 265, 276, 351–56. On Viṭal's learning Torah and kabbalistic secrets from his teacher, Isaac Luria, in dream visitations after the latter's physical demise, see *The "Book of Visions"*, pp. 83–84; *Jewish Mystical Autobiographies*, pp. 90–91. For discussion of the oneiric evidence adduced in this text, which relates to both the author's own dreams (second part) and the dreams of others that were about him (part three), see Werblowsky, *Joseph Karo*, pp. 47–48; J. Bazak, *Beyond the Senses: A Study of Extra-Sensorial Perception in Biblical, Talmudical, and Rabbinical Literature in Light of Contemporary Parapsychological Research* (Tel-Aviv, 1968), p. 40 (Hebrew); David Tamar, "The Messianic Dreams and Visions of R. Ḥayyim Viṭal," *Shalem* 4 (1984): 211–29 (Hebrew); Michal Oron, "Dream, Vision, and Reality in Ḥayyim Viṭal's *Book of Visions*," *Jerusalem Studies in Jewish Thought* 10 (1992): 299–309 (Hebrew); and Faierstein's comments in *Jewish Mystical Autobiographies*, pp. 14–16 and 24. On the comparable phenomenon of dream divination in Christian medieval texts, see Frank Klaassen, "Magical Dream Provocation in the Later Middle Ages," *Esoterica* 8 (2006): 111–35. For an anthropological study of visitational dreams in a more contemporary Jewish cultural setting, see Yoram Bilu, "Oneirobiography and Oneirocommunity in Saint Worship in Israel: A Two-Tier Model for Dream-Inspired Religious Revivals," *Dreaming* 10 (2000): 85–101, and compare *idem*, "Dreams and Wishes of the Saint," in *Judaism Viewed from Within and from Without: Anthropological Studies*, edited by Harvey E. Goldberg (Albany: State University of New York Press, 1987), pp. 285–313.

24. Isaac of Acre, *Oṣar Ḥayyim*, MS Günzberg 775, fols. 100b–101a. For discussion of dream reports and the transition from waking to sleeping, a liminal state that is designated by the rabbinic expression *nim we-lo nim*, "asleep, but not asleep" (see Chapter 3 n. 36) in Isaac of Acre's diary, see Fishbane, *As Light*

Before Dawn, pp. 103–14.

25. On the connection of prophets and the dream inquiry, see Abraham Abulafia, *Oṣar Eden Ganuz* (Jerusalem, 2000), p. 338. See also the citation from *Sefer Raziel* in Abraham Ibn Ezra, *Perushei ha-Torah le-Avraham Ibn Ezra*, edited by Asher Weiser, 3 vols. (Jerusalem: Mosad ha-Rav Kook, 1977), 2:93 (*ad* Exodus 14:19): "The one who wants to make a dream request [*she'elat ḥalom*] should recite at the beginning of the night the verse 'In the thirtieth year' (Ezekiel 1:1), for there are seventy-two letters." The fuller context of this remark indicates that the significance of the number of letters in the first verse of Ezekiel's chariot vision is related to the seventy-two letter name, which is derived from the 216 letters in Exodus 14:19–21 that are divided into seventy-two triplets. In the short version of Abraham Ibn Ezra's Torah commentary, *Perushei ha-Torah*, 2:245 (*ad* Exodus 3:13), the tradition is cited in the name of *Sefer ha-Razim*, rather than *Sefer Raziel*. I note, parenthetically, that the two works, *Sefer Raziel* and *Sefer ha-Razim*, are mentioned together in a list of esoteric compositions delineated by Abraham Abulafia, *Sheva Netivot ha-Torah*, in Adolph Jellinek, *Philosophie und Kabbala*, erstes Heft (Leipzig: Heinrich Hunger, 1854), p. 21. The connection between the dream vision, prophecy, and the seventy-two letter name is made explicit in the *Perush ha-Merkavah* of Jacob ben Jacob ha-Kohen. See *The Commentaries to Ezekiel's Chariot of R. Eleazar of Worms and of R. Jacob ben Jacob ha-Kohen*, edited and introduced by Asi Farber-Ginat and Daniel Abrams (Los Angeles: Cherub Press, 2004), p. 83 (Hebrew). I previously cited the passages from Ibn Ezra and Jacob ha-Kohen (as well as a passage from Isaac of Acre, *Oṣar Ḥayyim*, MS Günzberg 775, fol. 16b) in *Through a Speculum*, p. 236 n. 191. See also Abraham Axelrod of Cologne, *Keter Shem Ṭov*, in Adolph Jellinek, *Auswahl kabbalistischer Mystik*, erstes Heft (Leipzig: A.M. Colditz, 1853), p. 41 (Hebrew section), cited and discussed in Moshe Idel, "Ashkenazi Esotericism and Kabbalah in Barcelona," *Hispania Judaica Bulletin* 5 (2007): 96–97.

26. There is a wealth of scholarship on the doctrine of prophecy in the writings of Maimonides. For a relatively recent analysis, which takes into account many of the previous studies, see the extensive discussion in Howard Kreisel, *Prophecy: The History of an Idea in Medieval Jewish Philosophy* (Dordrecht: Kluwer, 2001), pp. 148–315.

27. William Eamon, *Science and the Secrets of Nature: Books of Secrets in Medieval and Early Modern Culture* (Princeton: Princeton University Press, 1994), p. 40.

28. Richard Walzer, "Al-Fārābī's Theory of Prophecy and Divination," *Journal of Hellenic Studies* 77 (1957): 142–48; *idem*, *Greek into Arabic* (Cambridge, MA: Harvard University Press, 1962), pp. 206–19; Fazlur Rahman,

Prophecy in Islam: Philosophy and Orthodoxy (Chicago: University of Chicago Press, 1979), pp. 11–14 and 30–31; Herbert A. Davidson, *Alfarabi, Avicenna, and Averroes, On Intellect: Their Cosmologies, Theories of the Active Intellect, and Theories of Human Intellect* (Oxford: Oxford University Press, 1992), pp. 44–73. Maimonides' indebtedness to al-Fārābī's views on prophecy and revelation has been well documented. See Colette Sirat, *Les théories des visions surnaturelles dans la pensée juive du moyen-âge* (Leiden: E. J. Brill, 1969), p. 142; Jeffrey Macy, "Prophecy in al-Farabi and Maimonides," in *Maimonides and Philosophy*, edited by Shlomo Pines and Yirmiyahu Yovel (Dordrecht: Martinus Nijhoff, 1986), pp. 185–201, and reference to other scholars noted therein. On the impact of al-Fārābī's psychology, see Dov Schwartz, "The Quadripartite Division of the Intellect in Medieval Jewish Thought," *Jewish Quarterly Review* 84 (1993–1994): 227–36. On the supposedly lost monograph of al-Fārābī on dreams, see Abū Naṣr al-Fārābī, *On the Perfect State (Mabādi' ārā' ahl al-madīnat al-fāḍilah)*, revised text with introduction, translation, and commentary by Richard Walzer (Oxford: Oxford University Press, 1985), pp. 414–15.

29. Helmut Gätje, "Philosophische Traumlehren im Islam," *Zeitschrift der Deutschen Morgenländischen Gesellschaft* 109 (1959): 262–64; Gerhard Endreß, "Al-Kindī über die Wiedererinnerung der Seele: Arabischer Platonismus und die Legitimation der Wissenschaften im Islam," *Oriens* 34 (1994): 197, 205–206, 210–12, 215; Peter Adamson, "Al-Kindī and the Reception of Greek Philosophy," in *The Cambridge Companion to Arabic Philosophy*, edited by Peter Adamson and Richard C. Taylor (Cambridge: Cambridge University Press, 2005), p. 47.

30. Al-Fārābī, *On the Perfect State*, p. 211. See Mu'tazid Wali Ur-Rahman, "Al-Fârâbî and his Theory of Dreams," *Islamic Culture* 10 (1936): 137–51; Gätje, "Philosophische Traumlehren," pp. 264–67.

31. Pines, "Arabic Recension," pp. 124–25. See the summary account in Alexander Altmann, "Gersonides' Commentary on Averroes' Epitome of *Parva Naturalia*, II.3: Annotated Critical Edition," *Proceedings of the American Academy for Jewish Research* 46 (1979–1980): 2–3.

32. Al-Fārābī, *On the Perfect State*, p. 221. See Muhsin S. Mahdi, *Alfarabi and the Foundation of Islamic Political Philosophy* (Chicago: University of Chicago Press, 2001), pp. 159–60. For discussion of cognate themes in medieval Christian sources, see Thomas Ricklin, *Der Traum der Philosophie im 12. Jahrhundert: Traumtheorien zwischen Constantinus Africanus und Aristoteles* (Leiden: Brill, 1998), pp. 48–82.

33. Maimonides, *Guide*, II.36, p. 369.

34. Moses Maimonides, *Mishnah im Perush Rabbenu Moshe ben Maimon: Seder*

Neziqin, translated and edited by Joseph Kafiḥ (Jerusalem: Mosad ha-Rav Kook, 1965), p. 142.

35. Moses Maimonides, *Mishneh Torah* (New York: Schlusinger, 1947), Yesodei Torah 7:1.

36. Maimonides, *Guide*, II.32, pp. 360–62. For discussion of the different interpretations of Maimonides on this point offered by his commentators, see Sirat, *Les théories*, pp. 137–39.

37. Isaac Ibn Laṭif, *Sha'ar ha-Shamayim*, MS Vatican, Biblioteca Apostolica 335, fol. 33a (Maimonides' name is mentioned explicitly). See *ibid.*, fol. 7b, where the author reworks Maimonides' language to describe the traditional view of prophecy in contrast to the philosophical position: "Prophecy rests on a person through the divine will consequent to the perfection of his intellectual and natural attributes." The philosophical account of prophecy offered on fol. 32b is basically a paraphrase of al-Fārābī, who is mentioned explicitly (*he-ḥakham ha-yishma''eli abū naṣr*); see below, n. 69. See Sara O. Heller Wilensky, "Isaac Ibn Laṭif—Philosopher or Kabbalist?" in *Jewish Medieval and Renaissance Studies*, edited by Alexander Altmann (Cambridge, MA: Harvard University Press, 1967), pp. 198–200; Abraham Melamed, *The Philosopher-King in Medieval and Renaissance Jewish Political Thought*, edited with a foreword by Lenn E. Goodman (Albany: State University of New York Press, 2003), pp. 84–85. See also Yossi Esudri, "Studies on the Philosophy of R. Isaac Ibn Latif: Profile, Knowledge and Prophecy," Ph.D. dissertation, Hebrew University, 2008, pp. 110–12 (Hebrew). On Maimonides and Ibn Laṭif, see Sara O. Heller Wilensky, "Isaac Ibn Latif's 'The Gate of Heaven': A Mystical Guide of the Perplexed," in *Perspectives in Jewish Learning*, vol. 2, edited by Moses A. Shulvass (Chicago: Spertus College of Judaica, 1966), pp. 17–25; *idem*, "Isaac Ibn Laṭif—Philosopher or Kabbalist?" pp. 204–205 and 212; *idem*, "The Guide and the Gate: The Dialectical Influence of Maimonides on Isaac Ibn Latif and Early Spanish Kabbalah," in *A Straight Path—Studies in Medieval Philosophy and Culture: Essays in Honor of Arthur Hyman*, edited by Ruth Link Salinger (Washington, D.C.: Catholic University of America Press, 1988), pp. 266–78; Deborah Schechterman, "Studies in the Short Version of Sha'ar ha-Shamayim of Isaac Ibn Laṭif," M.A. thesis, University of Haifa, 1980, pp. 22–28 (Hebrew); Ḥaviva Pedaya, *Nahmanides: Cyclical Times and Holy Text* (Tel-Aviv: Am Oved, 2003), pp. 267 n. 21, 268 n. 25. 275, 328 n. 3 (Hebrew); Shoey Raz, "Isaac Ibn Laṭif and the Guide of the Perplexed," M.A. thesis, Bar-Ilan University, 2004 (Hebrew), and *idem*, "Metaphysics and the Account of the Chariot: Maimonides and Iṣḥaq Ibn Laṭif," in *Maimonides and Mysticism*, pp. 133–64 (Hebrew). See also Esudri, "Studies on the Philosophy," pp. 118–30. For the influence of al-Fārābī's political

thought, including a Hebrew rendering of sections from *The Virtuous State*, in Ibn Laṭif's *Sha'ar ha-Shamayim*, see Melamed, *The Philosopher-King*, pp. 75–81. Melamed is of the opinion that Ibn Laṭif's paraphrase of al-Fārābī preceded that of Shem Ṭov Ibn Falaquera. See as well Abraham Melamed, "Ibn Laṭif and Falaquera on the Characteristics of the Philosopher-King," *Tura: Studies in Jewish Thought* 2 (1992): 162–77 (Hebrew). Finally, mention should be made of the fact that prophecy is enumerated in Isaac Ibn Laṭif, *Rav Pe'alim*, edited by Samuel Schoenblum (Lemberg: Anna Wajdowicz, 1885), secs. 80–86, 25b–27a, as the third of five "supernal mysteries of the Torah" (*ha-setarim ha-elyonim ha-toraniyyim*) that are not fathomed by the "philosophers" (*filosofim*) or the "masters of contemplative speculation" (*ba'alei meḥqar ha-iyyuni*), and not even by some of the "sages of our Torah" (*ḥakhmei torateinu*). The five mysteries consist of the unity of the divine comprehended through the name of ten letters (presumably the Tetragrammaton written out in full as *yod waw dalet he alef waw alef waw he alef*, יו"ד ה"א וא"ו ה"א); the connection of the eternal and the creation of the world; the form of prophecy and revelatory visions; the form of the earth and the seas; and the ostensible conflict between the literal meaning of Scripture and truths ascertained on the basis of demonstrative reason. At the conclusion of the delineation, Ibn Laṭif writes (*Rav Pe'alim*, sec. 86, 27a): "These five mysteries are not to be inquired about [*lo nitnu lidrosh bahem*] except exclusively through oral transmission [*be-yiḥud peh el peh*] by one who is wise and understands on one's own, one who has already [attained] the true and concealed rational speculation regarding the mysteries of the Torah, the prophecies, and the forms of the world [*ha-iyyun ha-sikhli ha-amitti ha-ne'lam be-sitrei ha-torah we-ha-nevu'ot u-ve-ṣurot ha-olam*]." For analysis of the five mysteries, see Esudri, "Studies on the Philosophy," pp. 227–32. See *Rav Pe'alim*, sec. 39, 14a, where the philosopher (*ḥakham*) is said to deal with timeless matters, in contrast to the kabbalist (*mequbbal*), who is concerned with the dimension of time. This passage was already noted by Wilensky, "Isaac Ibn Laṭif—Philosopher or Kabbalist?" p. 221. The temporal implications of Ibn Laṭif's theory of cosmic cycles have been explored in Sara O. Heller Wilensky, "Messianism, Eschatology, and Utopia in the Philosophic-Mystical Current of Kabbalah in the Thirteenth Century," in *Messianism and Eschatology: A Collection of Essays*, edited by Zvi Baras (Jerusalem: Zalman Shazar Centre, 1983), pp. 221–37 (Hebrew); Pedaya, *Nahmanides*, pp. 22–23, 216–17. Both Wilensky and Pedaya suggest that, with regard to this matter, Ibn Laṭif may have been influenced by Ismā'īlī theology. For a fuller treatment of this topic, see Sara O. Heller Wilensky, "The 'First Created Being' in Early Kabbalah and its Philosophical Sources," in *Studies in Jewish Thought*, edited by Sara O. Heller

Wilensky (Jerusalem: Magnes Press, 1989), pp. 261–76 (Hebrew) (English translation in *Jewish Intellectual History in the Middle Ages* [*Binah: Studies in Jewish History, Thought, and Culture*, volume 3], edited by Joseph Dan (Westport: Praeger, 1994), pp. 65–77). On the role of time and place in the short version of Ibn Laṭif's *Sha'ar ha-Shamayim*, see Schechterman, "Studies," pp. 107–13, and Esudri, "Studies on the Philosophy," pp. 208–14. See also Ibn Laṭif, *Sha'ar ha-Shamayim*, MS Vatican, Biblioteca Apostolica 335, fol. 11a, where the philosophers are described as lacking "knowledge of the secret of the glorious name unique to the essence of the Creator, blessed be he" (*yedi'at sod ha-shem ha-nikhbad ha-meyuḥad le-eṣem ha-bore yitbarakh*). The recent claim of Raz that Ibn Laṭif should not be considered a kabbalist is rendered suspect in light of these passages and others that could have been mentioned. Concerning this matter of classification, see Wilensky, "Isaac Ibn Laṭif—Philosopher or Kabbalist?" pp. 210–22; *idem*, "The Relations between Mysticism and Philosophy in the Teachings of Rabbi Isaac Ibn Latif," *Jerusalem Studies in Jewish Thought* 6, nos. 3–4 (1987): 36–82 (Hebrew); Schechterman, "Studies," pp. 1–17; Hannah Kasher, "On the Terms Kabbalah and Kabbalist in Laṭif's Treatises," *Da'at* 41 (1999): 5–12 (Hebrew); and Esudri, "Studies on the Philosophy," pp. 136–46.

38. See *Guide*, II.48, pp. 409–10: Maimonides begins by saying that everything produced in time has a proximate cause and that the ultimate causal agency is the First Cause, which is "God's will and free choice." But then he goes on to say that in the prophetic books, natural causes are ascribed to God even though there is no direct causality between God and the world. See II.4, pp. 257–58. See also II.6, p. 262. After identifying the biblical notion of angels with the medieval Aristotelian-Neoplatonic notion of the separate intellects, Maimonides writes: "As for his saying that these separate intellects are also intermediaries between God, may He be exalted, and the existents; and that it is through their intermediation that the spheres are in motion, which motion is the cause of the generation of the things subject to generation; this too is the textual teaching of all the books. For you never find therein that an act was performed by God otherwise than *through an angel*." The "angel" connotes the separate intellects, and God can be accorded causal agency for natural forces in the world only indirectly. Consider also the language regarding divine purpose versus necessity and the problem of the "stable nature" of the impossible in II.19, pp. 302–303, and in III.15, pp. 459–61 (cf. II.13, p. 283). And see III.25, p. 505. Where God is said to will "only what is possible, and not everything that is possible, but only that which is required by His wisdom to be such." The limitation on the will imposed by wisdom seems to me to be another way that Maimonides expresses his naturalistic conception of divine volition. See,

however, II.20, p. 313, where necessity and will are contrasted as contraries. See Alfred L. Ivry, "Maimonides on Possibility," in *Mystics, Philosophers, and Politicians: Essays in Jewish Intellectual History in Honor of Alexander Altmann*, edited by Jehuda Reinharz and Daniel Swetschinski, with the collaboration of Kalman P. Bland (Durham: Duke University Press, 1982), pp. 67–84. See especially Maimonides' gloss of "divine actions" as "natural actions" in *Guide*, III.32, p. 525, and compare the comments of Pines, "Translator's Introduction," p. xcvi n. 66, regarding the possibility that this passage from the *Guide* may have suggested the well-known dictum of Spinoza, *Deus sive natura*. See also Wolfson, "*Via Negativa*," pp. 406–407. If, in the final analysis, the will of God coincides with a natural process, there would be little room to speak of prophecy as a supernatural phenomenon.

39. Wolfson, "*Via Negativa*," pp. 397–415.

40. Alfred L. Ivry, "Providence, Divine Omniscience and Possibility: The Case of Maimonides," in *Divine Omniscience and Omnipotence in Medieval Philosophy*, edited by Tamar Rudavsky (Dordrecht: D. Reidel, 1985), pp. 143–59; Charles M. Raffel, "Providence as Consequent upon Intellect: Maimonides' Theory of Providence," *Association for Jewish Studies Review* 12 (1987): 25–71.

41. Maimonides, *Guide*, II.38, p. 377.

42. *Ibid.*, II.37, p. 374.

43. *Ibid.*, II.41, p. 386 (emphasis in the original).

44. *Midrash Qohelet Rabbah* 10:20. See also *Midrash Wayyikra Rabbah*, edited by Mordecai Margulies (New York: Jewish Theological Seminary of America, 1993), 32:2, p. 740.

45. Maimonides, *Guide*, II.6, pp. 264–65.

46. A resonance of the Maimonidean perspective can be heard in the statement in Joseph ben Shalom Ashkenazi, *A Kabbalistic Commentary by Rabbi Yoseph ben Shalom Ashkenazi on Genesis Rabbah*, edited with an introduction and notes by Moshe Hallamish (Jerusalem: Magnes Press, 1984), p. 223 (Hebrew): "The philosophic sages have already written about the matter of prophecy, and this is their language: It is not farfetched that there will be found someone for whom the matters will be imagined when awake as they are imagined by the dreamer in his dream, and all this is through the nullification of the senses and he is awake." The continuation of the passage describes the "slumber of prophecy" (*tardemat ha-nevu'ah*) as a contemplative visualization of the letters of the divine name enveloped in color. It is reasonable to assume that this is an interpolation of a mystical practice on the part of the kabbalist, and not part of the original philosophical opinion he is citing. Support for my conjecture may be culled from a similar meditational exercise of imagining the letters

of the Tetragrammaton to attain the "secret of the true conjunction" (*sod ha-dibbuq ha-amitti*) offered by Isaac of Acre, *Sefer Me'irat Einayim: A Critical Edition*, edited by Amos Goldreich (Jerusalem: Hebrew University, 1981), p. 217 (Hebrew), cited by Viṭal, *Sha'arei Qedushshah*, IV.3, p. 290. The passage of Isaac of Acre is discussed by Moshe Idel, *Kabbalah: New Perspectives* (New Haven: Yale University Press, 1988), p. 50 (the influence on Viṭal is duly noted there as well), and Fishbane, *As Light Before Dawn*, pp. 242–43. In his edition of Joseph ben Shalom Ashkenazi, *A Kabbalistic Commentary*, p. 223 n. 38, Hallamish acknowledges that he cannot identify the exact source for the dictum of the philosophical sages, but he suggests a parallel in Abraham bar Ḥiyya, *Megillat ha-Megalleh*, edited by Adolf Poznanski, revised with an introduction by Julius Guttmann (Berlin: Mekize Nirdamim, 1924), p. 43, and he notes that the text is cited anonymously by Viṭal, *Sha'arei Qedushshah*, IV.3, p. 303. For an alternate translation and analysis, see Idel, *Kabbalah: New Perspectives*, pp. 105–106, and see also Melila Hellner-Eshed, *A River Flows from Eden: The Language of Mystical Experience in the Zohar*, translated by Nathan Wolski (Stanford: Stanford University Press, 2009), p. 403 n. 17.

47. Maimonides, *Guide*, II.36, p. 370. See Alan Brill, "The Phenomenology of True Dreams in Maimonides," *Dreaming* 10 (2000): 43–54. For a critique of the philosophical interpretation based on the fact that "veridical dreams" appear to people who have not been engaged in scientific study or in the purification of their souls, see Judah Halevi, *Sefer ha-Kuzari*, translated by Yehudah Even Shmuel (Tel-Aviv: Dvir, 1972), I.4, p. 5. The standard philosophical position is presented in I.1, p. 4; see also I.87, p. 28. Compare II.60, p. 82, where Halevi writes about the pure souls, who are assisted in their desire to be conjoined to divinity by means of prophecy, veridical dreams, and the purified forms of the imagination. The possibility of ascertaining esoteric knowledge through prophecy, the divinatory practice of the Urim and Thummim, and "reliable dreams," as opposed to various forms of magic and sorcery, is affirmed in III.11, p. 105. On the pairing of "righteous dreams" and "wondrous signs," see III.53, p. 139. See the various remarks concerning Halevi's approach to dreams and dreaming in Yochanan Silman, *Philosopher and Poet: Judah Halevi, the Kuzari, and the Evolution of His Thought*, translated by Lenn J. Schramm (Albany: State University of New York Press, 1995), pp. 60, 62, 95 n. 41, 111–12, 171, 217–18, 225, 228 n. 1, 257, 259 n. 6, 322 n. 5, 335. Mention should also be made of the fact that in his poems, Halevi mentions his own dream visions as the means to attain the direct experience of the divine. See Aharon Komem, "Between Poetry and Prophecy: Studies in the Poetry of Judah Halevi," *Molad* 2 (1969): 676–98, esp. 683 (Hebrew); Raymond P. Scheindlin, *The Gazelle:*

Medieval Hebrew Poems on God, Israel, and the Soul (Philadelphia: Jewish Publication Society, 1991), pp. 110, 167–69, 200–201. See Chapter 4 n. 99.

48. See Abū Ḥāmid al-Ghazālī, *The Niche of Lights: A Parallel English-Arabic Text*, translated, introduced, and annotated by David Buchman (Provo: Brigham Young University Press, 1998), p. 29: "The science of dream interpretation makes known to you the way similitudes are struck, since dreams are a part of prophecy." Buchman, p. 64 n. 3, suggests that al-Ghazālī is referring to the *ḥadīth*, "The veridical dream is one forty-sixth part of prophecy," which can be fruitfully compared to the talmudic dictum cited above at n. 20. On the various versions of this *ḥadīth*, see Ibn Khaldûn, *The Muqaddimah: An Introduction to History*, translated by Franz Rosenthal, 3 vols., 2nd edition (Princeton: Princeton University Press, 1967), 1:208 and references cited in n. 302, 3:103 and 3:107. In a second passage, al-Ghazālī alludes more explicitly to this tradition: "This lets you know how the prophets see forms and how they witness the meanings behind the forms. In most cases, the meaning is prior to the inward witnessing. Then the meaning radiates from the witnessing upon the imaginal spirit, whereupon the imagination becomes imprinted with a form that parallels the meaning and resembles it. This type of revelation in wakefulness needs interpretation, just as in dreams it needs dream interpretation. That which occurs in dreams is related to the prophetic characteristics, just as [the number] one is related to forty-six, while that which occurs in wakefulness is more closely related than this" (*The Niche of Lights*, p. 35). The theme was enunciated in more detail in al-Ghazālī, *The Incoherence of the Philosophers: A Parallel English-Arabic Text*, translated, introduced, and annotated by Michael E. Marmura (Provo: Brigham Young University Press, 1997), pp. 158–59: "Hence, there is a need for interpreting what the imagination symbolizes.... The science of [dream] interpretation branches out from this principle.... [In addition,] they claimed that the prophet has knowledge of the unknown in this way, except that the prophetic psychological faculty can attain such strength that the external senses do not submerge it. No wonder, then, that he perceives while awake what others see in sleep. The imaginative faculty, moreover, makes for him representations of what he sees. Sometimes the very thing remains in his memory, sometimes [only] its symbol, whereby this inspiration requires [metaphorical] interpretation, just as that which resembles it in sleep requires [dream] interpretation." And compare the text of al-Ghazālī cited and criticized in Averroës, *Tahafut al-Tahafut* (*The Incoherence of the Incoherence*), translated with introduction and notes by Simon van der Bergh, 2 vols. (London: E. J. W. Gibb Memorial, 1969), 1:303–306. See also the passages from al-Ghazālī's *Book of Penitence* (*Kitāb al-tawba*) from his *Reviving Religious Knowledge* (*Iḥyā' 'ulūm al-dīn*), cited

in Timothy J. Gianotti, *Al-Ghazālī's Unspeakable Doctrine of the Soul: Unveiling the Esoteric Psychology and Eschatology of the Iḥyā'* (Leiden: Brill, 2001), pp. 161–62. On the depiction of dream-visions (*ru'yā*) as the opening of the door of the heart to the spiritual world of angelic spirits (*'ālam al-malakūt*), see al-Ghazālī, *Kitāb sharḥ 'ajā'ib al-qalb: The Marvels of the Heart*, translated with an introduction and notes by Walter J. Skellie, with a foreword by Timothy J. Winter (Louisville: Fons Vitae, 2010), pp. 60 and 73–74. A lengthy discussion of dreams as the unveiling (*mukāshafa*) of the states of being that the dead undergo appears in the *Kitāb dhikr al-mawt wa-mā ba'dahu*, the fortieth book of the *Iḥyā' 'ulūm al-dīn*. See al-Ghazālī, *The Remembrance of Death and Afterlife*, translated with an introduction and notes by T. J. Winter (Cambridge: Islamic Texts Society, 1995), pp. 149–69. The aforementioned *ḥadīth* is cited on p. 150, and see p. 267 n. 2 for other references. And compare *ibid.*, p. 153: "Thus it is that the interpreter of dreams needs to investigate the thing imagined as an 'imitation' [*ḥikāya*], that is, an abstraction, looking into its symbols according to the correspondence which exists between the dream and the abstraction." See R. J. McCarthy, S. J., trans., *Al-Ghazālī's Path to Sufism and His Deliverance From Error, An Annotated Translation of Al Munqidh min al-Dalal*, preface by David Burrell, C. S. C, and introduction by William A. Graham (Louisville: Fons Vitae, 2000), pp. 74–75. On the distinction between dream interpretation (*ta'bīr*) and textual exegesis based on the presumption that the symbolic nature of the former—with the exception of the truthful dreams (*al-manām al-ṣādiq*) of prophets—ignores the external sense (*ẓāhir*) to obtain the internal (*bāṭin*), whereas the latter requires the internal sense to be drawn from the external, see Frank Griffel, *Al-Ghazālī's Philosophical Theology* (Oxford: Oxford University Press, 2009), p. 114. The role of imagination and dreaming as a means to visualize the invisible in al-Ghazālī has been discussed in detail by Aaron W. Hughes, "Imagining the Divine: Ghazali on Imagination, Dreams, and Dreaming," *Journal of the American Academy of Religion* 70 (2002): 33–53. See also Davidson, *Alfarabi, Avicenna, and Averroes*, p. 141; Pierre Lory, *Le rêve et ses interpretations en Islam* (Paris: Albin Michel, 2003), pp. 63–68; and Ebrahim Moosa, *Ghazālī and the Poetics of Imagination* (Chapel Hill: University of North Carolina Press, 2005), pp. 74–78.

49. Ibn Khaldûn, *The Muqaddimah*, 1:207–208: "Real dream vision is an awareness on the part of the rational soul in its spiritual essence, of glimpse(s) of the form of events. While the soul is spiritual, the forms of events have actual existence in it, as is the case with all spiritual essences. The soul becomes spiritual through freeing itself from bodily matters and corporeal perceptions. This happens to the soul (in the form of) glimpse(s) through the agency of sleep....

When this process is weak and indistinct, the soul applies to it allegory and imaginary pictures, in order to gain (the desired knowledge). Such allegory, then, necessitates interpretation. When, on the other hand, this process is strong, it can dispense with allegory. Then, no interpretation is necessary, because (the process) is then free from imaginary pictures." The link between al-Ghazālī and Ibn Khaldūn is made explicitly in the following description of the human soul in *The Muqaddimah*, 3:75: "When it leaves the body in sleep or in death, or when a prophet, in the state of revelation, changes from human perceptions to angelic ones, the soul takes its means of perceptions along, but free of the limbs of the body. With (these means of perception), the soul perceives, on the (other) level, whatever perceptions it wants to perceive, but these perceptions are on a higher plane than those that the soul had while it was in the body. This was stated by al-Ghazzâlî, who added that the human soul has a form that it retains after its separation (from the body) and that, just like the body's own structure, includes two eyes, two ears, and the rest of the limbs of the body serving (man) to attain perception."

50. *Midrash Bere'shit Rabba* 21:9, p. 203.

51. Maimonides, *Guide*, 1.49, pp. 108–109.

52. *Ibid.*, p. 109.

53. Davidson, *Alfarabi, Avicenna, and Averroes*, pp. 10–12, 27, 84, 87, 90, 92, 94, 99–102, 124.

54. Falzur Rahman, *Avicenna's Psychology* (London: Oxford University Press, 1952), pp. 35–37; Davidson, *Alfarabi, Avicenna, and Averroes*, pp. 118–22; Dimitri Gutas, *Avicenna and the Aristotelian Tradition* (Leiden: E. J. Brill, 1988), pp. 159–76; *idem*, "Imagination and Transcendental Knowledge in Avicenna," in *Arabic Theology, Arabic Philosophy, from the Many to the One: Essays in Celebration of Richard M. Frank*, edited by James E. Montgomery (Leuven: Peeters, 2006), pp. 337–54; *idem*, "Intellect without Limits: The Absence of Mysticism in Avicenna," in *Intellect et imagination dans la Philosophie Médiévale: Actes du XIe Congrès International de Philosophie Médiévale de la Société Internationale pour l'Étude de la Philosophie Médiévale*, edited by Maria Cândida Pacheco and José Francisco Meirinhos, 4 vols. (Turnhout: Brepols, 2006), 1: 351–72; Peter Heath, *Allegory and Philosophy in Avicenna (Ibn Sînâ) with a Translation of the Book of the Prophet Muḥammad's Ascent to Heaven* (Philadelphia: University of Pennsylvania Press, 1992), pp. 89–90. The influence of Avicenna on Maimonides has been well noted in scholarship, especially in terms of the distinction between essence and existence, the characterization of the divine as the necessary of existence, and the negative theology that ensues therefrom. See, for instance, Pines, "Translator's Introduction," pp. xciv–cvii; Davidson, *Moses*

Maimonides, pp. 94–95, 102–104, 121; Wolfson, "Via Negativa," pp. 367–69 and other references cited on p. 368 n. 12.

55. Gutas, *Avicenna*, pp. 28 and 176–77; William E. Gohlman, *The Life of Ibn Sina: A Critical Edition and Annotated Translation* (Albany: State of New York University Press, 1974), pp. 30–31. On the related phenomenon of the "ghostly afterlife" of Aristotle appearing to Muslim sages in a dream, see Steven M. Wasserstrom, "Sharing Secrets: Inter-Confessional Philosophy as Dialogical Practice," in *New Directions in Jewish Philosophy*, edited by Aaron W. Hughes and Elliot R. Wolfson (Bloomington: Indiana University Press, 2010), pp. 206–207. See also the evidence adduced by Hughes, "Imagining the Divine," pp. 38–39. The appearance of Aristotle in dreams is complemented by the continued reports of the oneiric manifestation of Muḥammad and other saintly figures to communicate knowledge about supernal matters. See Ignaz Goldziher, "The Appearance of the Prophet in Dreams," *Journal of the Royal Asiatic Society* (1912): 503–506 (I thank Aaron Hughes for calling my attention to this study); Lory, *Le rêve*, pp. 149–62; Moosa, *Ghazālī*, pp. 73–74. On the "imaginary interlocutors" in the visionary encounter of the dream, see also Amira Mittermaier, "The Book of Visions: Dreams, Poetry, and Prophecy in Contemporary Egypt," *International Journal of Middle Eastern Studies* 39 (2007): 234–39. Here it is apposite to recall the narrative framing in the introduction to Judah Halevi, *Sefer ha-Kuzari,* p. 1: the Khazar king has a series of nocturnal dreams in which an angel informs him that while his religious intentions may be fine, he must still cultivate the proper actions ordained by God to instantiate those intentions. The recurring angelic visitations eventually lead him to summon various interlocutors, including a philosopher, a Muslim, a Christian, and a Jew, to participate in a dialogue to discuss matters of religious and philosophical import. Eventually the king is persuaded by the rabbinic sage (referred to as the *ḥaver*) of the superiority of the monotheistic path of Judaism, and the entire Khazar people convert. From the overall plot of the text we may assume that the Jew alone has the capacity to expound the true meaning of the king's dreams. See also *ibid.*, II.1, p. 47. In I.8, p. 8, Halevi places in the mouth of the king the mandate that belief in God must be based on direct experience of the miraculous and not on what one hears from reports of someone else's experience, including the dream, or from tradition. See I.98, p. 36, where the king affirms that the truth that one does not attain the divine matter (*inyan ha-elohi*) except through fulfilling the commandments—the stereotypical Jewish perspective advanced by Halevi—was confirmed for him in the "vision of the dream." For discussion of these various passages, see Silman, *Philosopher and Poet*, pp. 61 n. 24, 63 n. 29, 95 n. 41, 228, 230–31, 237–38, 257–58, 271 n. 30,

277, 338. On the role of the dialogical in Halevi's *Kuzari*, see the innovative analysis of Aaron W. Hughes, *The Art of Dialogue in Jewish Philosophy* (Bloomington: Indiana University Press, 2008), pp. 26–49. Finally, mention should be made of Abraham Ibn Ezra's *Iggeret Shabbat*, an epistle that he purportedly received in a dream on 15 Ṭevet 4919, which corresponds to December 13, 1158, in which he encountered the Sabbath personified as a woman. The letter was first edited and published by Samuel David Luzzatto in *Kerem Ḥemed* 4 (1839) and has appeared since in several other editions. See, most recently, *The Sabbath Epistle of Rabbi Abraham Ibn Ezra ('iggeret haShabbat)*, translated and annotated by Mordechai S. Goodman (Jersey City: Ktav, 2009), and compare Irene Lancaster, *Deconstructing the Bible: Abraham ibn Ezra's Introduction to the Torah* (London: RoutledgeCurzon, 2003), pp. 19–20. The figurative depiction of Sabbath in this document should be viewed against Ibn Ezra's view that on the Sabbath, the soul's power of discernment and intellection is augmented by its receiving a "surplus of wisdom" (*tosefet ḥokhmah*). See *Perushei ha-Torah le-Avraham Ibn Ezra*, 1:20 (*ad* Genesis 2:3), 2:136 (*ad* Exodus 20:8); Elliot K. Ginsburg, *The Sabbath in the Classical Kabbalah* (Albany: State University of New York Press, 1989), p. 122 and see p. 142 n. 30, where Ibn Ezra's *Iggeret Shabbat* is mentioned.

56. Text cited by Pines, "Arabic Recension," pp. 122–23. See Aviezer Ravitzky, "Hebrew Quotations From the Lost Arabic Recension of Parva Naturalia," *Jerusalem Studies in Arabic and Islam* 3 (1981–1982): 197–98, reprinted in *idem*, *History and Faith: Studies in Jewish Philosophy* (Amsterdam: J. C. Gieben, 1996), pp. 312–13, and Amira Eran, "Intuition and Inspiration—The Causes of Jewish Thinkers' Objection to Avicenna's Intellectual Prophecy (Ḥads)," *Jewish Studies Quarterly* 14 (2007): 43–44. The attitude of medieval Jewish thinkers with regard to Avicenna's view was complex, some rejecting or modifying it and others accepting it less ambivalently. In the former camp, we can include Judah Halevi and Abraham Ibn Daud, and in the latter camp, Moses Ibn Ezra and Shem Tov Ibn Falaquera, who even wrote a philosophical composition with the title *Treatise of the Dream*, since the ideas expressed therein were purportedly revealed to him in dream states. See Henry Malter, "Shem Tob ben Joseph Palquera: His Treatise of the Dream," *Jewish Quarterly Review* 1 (1910–1911): 456–57, 470; Eran, "Intuition and Inspiration," pp. 45–57; Sara Sviri, "Dreaming Analyzed and Recorded: Dreams in the World of Medieval Islam," in *Dream Cultures*, pp. 255–56; Ravitzky, *History and Faith*, pp. 313–15; Harvey, "Shem-Tov Ibn Falaquera's *De'ot ha-Filosofim*," pp. 232–33; Kreisel, *Prophecy*, pp. 109–10.

57. Compare Averroës, *Tahafut al-Tahafut*, 1:316: "The ancient philosophers

assert about revelation and dreams only that they proceed from God through the intermediation of a spiritual incorporeal being which is according to them the bestower of the human intellect, and which is called by the best authors the active intellect and in the Holy Law angel."

58. Averroës, *Epitome of Parva Naturalia*, pp. 39–43, 47–48, 50, and see Gutas, *Avicenna*, pp. 172–74; Rahman, *Avicenna's Psychology*, p. 93. See also Averroës, *Tahafut al-Tahafut*, 1:305–306. False dreams are discussed by Averroës, *Epitome of Parva Naturalia*, pp. 52–53. They are said to arise on account of one of two reasons, either "as a result of the activity of the imaginative faculty during sleep in connection with the impressions remaining in the common sense from the external sense-objects and also as a result of the activity of the imaginative faculty in connection with notions deposited in the memorative and cogitative faculties from the same sense-objects" or "as a result of the natural desires of the soul."

59. Averroës, *Epitome of Parva Naturalia*, p. 47, and see *ibid.*, p. 51, as well as Averroës, *Tahafut al-Tahafut*, 2:167–68. Compare Shem Ṭov ben Joseph Ibn Falaquera, *Moreh ha-Moreh*, critical edition, introduction, and commentary by Yair Shiffman (Jerusalem: World Union of Jewish Studies, 2001), p. 317, translated in Malter, "Shem Tob," p. 455.

60. Averroës, *Epitome of Parva Naturalia*, p. 43, and see *ibid.*, p. 52. The view of Averroës was criticized by Gersonides, who maintained that theoretical matters (*devarim ha-iyyuniyim*) can be revealed in a dream, an experience that he attests for himself. See Altmann, "Gersonides' Commentary," p. 24; Levi ben Gershom, *Milḥamot ha-Shem* (Riva di Trento, 1560), II.4, 17d–18b; *idem*, *The Wars of the Lord*, translated with an appendix and notes by Seymour Feldman, 3 vols. (Philadelphia: Jewish Publication Society, 1987–1999), 2:42–47, and see Feldman's remarks on pp. 9–10; Sirat, *Les théories*, pp. 169–70.

61. Pines, "Translator's Introduction," pp. ci–cii; Eran, "Intuition and Inspiration," pp. 57–71. It is of interest to recall that in his commentary on the *Guide*, II.36, the well-known admirer of Averroës, Moses Narboni, *Be'ur le-Sefer Moreh Nevukhim*, edited by Jacob Goldenthal (Vienna: K.K. Hof- und Staatsdruckerei, 1852), 43a, cites the crucial passage from the *Epitome on Parva Naturalia* to explain the Maimonidean view on prophecy and dreams; see Altmann, "Gersonides' Commentary," pp. 3–4. The similarity of Maimonides' approach to dreams and that of Averroës, even without the former knowing the latter's *Epitome Parva Naturalia*, was duly noted by Alexander Altmann, *Essays in Jewish Intellectual History* (Hanover: University Press of New England, 1981), p. 80. On the question of Maimonides and Averroës, see Pines, "Translator's Introduction," pp. cviii–cxxiii, and, more recently, the studies by Alfred L.

Ivry, "Moses Maimonides: An Averroist *Avant la Lettre?*" *Maimonidean Studies* 5 (2008): 121–39, and in the same volume, Sarah Stroumsa, "The Literary Corpus of Maimonides and Averroes," pp. 223–41, and *idem*, *Maimonides in His World: Portrait of a Mediterranean Thinker* (Princeton: Princeton University Press, 2009), pp. 67–68, 73–76, 92 n. 41, 124.

62. Mordechai Z. Cohen, *Three Approaches to Biblical Metaphor From Abraham Ibn Ezra and Maimonides to David Kimhi* (Leiden: Brill, 2003), pp. 140–41.

63. Maimonides, *Mishneh Torah,* Yesodei Torah 7:6, see Cohen, *Three Approaches*, p. 197. On Mosaic prophecy in Maimonides, see below, n. 88. Compare Levi ben Gershom, *Milḥamot ha-Shem*, II.6, 19a; *idem*, *The Wars of the Lord*, 2:54.

64. Maimonides, *Mishneh Torah*, Yesodei Torah 7:3. Compare Maimonides, *Mishnah im Perush Rabbenu Moshe ben Maimon: Seder Neziqin*, p. 137, where the philosophical sages (*ba'alei ḥokhmah*) are said to articulate sublime matters "through the way of riddle and parable" (*be-derekh ḥiddah u-mashal*), and thus there is an exoteric and an esoteric dimension. The gap between prophecy and philosophy is significantly narrowed to the extent that both necessitate the articulation of truth through dissimilitude, the art of revealing by concealing. See Maimonides, *Guide,* "Introduction," p. 8; I.18, p. 43; I.54, p. 78, and discussion in Elliot R. Wolfson, *Abraham Abulafia—Kabbalist and Prophet: Hermeneutics, Theosophy, and Theurgy* (Los Angeles: Cherub Press, 2000), pp. 38–52. Needless to say, the esoteric dimension of the Maimonidean hermeneutic has been the focus of many studies. A good typological survey is provided by Aviezer Ravitzky, "The Secrets of The Guide of the Perplexed: Between the Thirteenth and Twentieth Centuries," in *Studies in Maimonides*, pp. 159–207. For a relatively recent analysis that takes into account some of the major previous treatments, see Moshe Halbertal, *Concealment and Revelation: Esotericism in Jewish Thought and Its Philosophical Implications*, translated by Jackie Feldman (Princeton: Princeton University Press, 2007), pp. 49–68. An exhaustive analysis of the words *mashal* and *hash'alah*, rendering respectively the Arabic *mathal* and *isti'āra*, in Maimonides is provided by Cohen, *Three Approaches*, pp. 98–136, and on the "psychological function" of *mashal* specifically in prophecy, see *ibid.*, pp. 196–200.

65. Babylonian Talmud, Berakhot 55b. See Chapter 3 n. 32.

66. Maimonides, *Guide*, II.43, p. 391 (emphasis in the original).

67. Babylonian Talmud, Ḥullin 90b, Tamid 29a; Maimonides, *Guide*, II.47, p. 407. The original dictum of R. Ammi is that the Torah, the prophets, and the sages all used hyperbole. Compare Moses Maimonides, *Ma'amar Teḥiyyat ha-Metim* in *Iggerot ha-Rambam*, edited, translated, and annotated by Isaac Shilat

(Jerusalem: Ma'aliyyot, 1987), p. 361.

68. Isaac Ibn Laṭif, *Sha'ar ha-Shamayim*, MS Vatican, Biblioteca Apostolica 335, fol. 2b.

69. *Ibid.*, fol. 33b. The threefold distinction of al-Fārāblī, who is referred to as the "philosophical sage" (*he-ḥakham ha-filosof*), is cited to support the claim that vision and dream comprise all the gradations of prophecy. To be more specific, the three gradations of prophecy attributed to al-Fārāblī consist, in descending order, of the wakeful vision; contemplating things in the mind without seeing them, a state that involves both wakefulness and sleep; and seeing things when one is asleep. The last type of vision involves allusions, parables, riddles, and images that call for interpretation. Ibn Laṭif notes that the perfection of the imagination also accounts for the fact that some dreams disclose the future "plainly" (*be-ve'ur*) and some by "way of parable" (*derekh mashal*). Compare Ibn Laṭif, *Rav Pe'alim*, sec. 40, 14a: "The parables [*ha-meshalim*] are all signs [*simanim*] in the image of marks [*bi-demut ṣiyyunim*] to draw attention to the concealed matters to which the parables allude [*ha-nimshalim ha-ne'lamim*]." Concerning this work, see Hannah Kasher, "The *Rav Pe'alim* by Isaac Ibn Laṭif," M.A. thesis, Bar Ilan University, 1974 (Hebrew). For an articulation similar to the perspective of Ibn Laṭif, see the commentary on the *Zohar* by Simeon Lavi, *Ketem Paz* (Livorno, 1795), 285a, and compare *ibid.*, 356b; Almoli, *Pitron Ḥalomot*, 6a. On the use of the term *mashal* in Ibn Laṭif to denote the philosophical-allegorical method of exegesis, see Wilensky, "Isaac Ibn Laṭif—Philosopher or Kabbalist?" p. 219; Barry D. Walfish, "Typology, Narrative, and History: Isaac ben Joseph ha-Kohen on the Book of Ruth," in *With Reverence for the Word: Medieval Scriptural Exegesis in Judaism, Christianity, and Islam*, edited by Jane Dammen McAuliffe, Barry D. Walfish, and Joseph W. Goering (Oxford: Oxford University Press, 2003), p. 129 n. 34. For an extended discussion of the doctrine of prophecy, dreams, and visions in Ibn Laṭif, see Esudri, "Studies on the Philosophy," pp. 233–90, esp. 247–58.

70. Ibn Laṭif, *Rav Pe'alim*, sec. 78, 25a.

71. Abraham Abulafia, *Ḥayyei ha-Olam ha-Ba* (Jerusalem, 1999), pp. 48–49. See *idem*, *Sefer ha-Malmad* (Jerusalem, 2002), p. 18, and analysis in Elliot R. Wolfson, "Kenotic Overflow and Temporal Transcendence: Angelic Embodiment and the Alterity of Time in Abraham Abulafia," *Kabbalah: Journal for the Study of Jewish Mystical Texts* 18 (2008): 144–46.

72. For discussion of this dimension of Abulafia's prophetic kabbalah, see Wolfson, *Language, Eros, Being*, pp. 234–42. An almost identical perspective to Abulafia is found in Ibn al-'Arabī's depiction of the manifestation of Gabriel in human form in his *Fuṣūṣ al-ḥikam*. See Muḥyīddīn Ibn al-'Arabī, *The Bezels of*

Wisdom, translation and introduction by Ralph W. J. Austin, preface by Titus Burckhardt (New York: Paulist Press, 1980), p. 121: "the appearance of the Angel to him as a man was also from the plane of the Imagination, since he [Gabriel] is not a man but an angel who took on himself human form. This [form] was transposed by the beholder with gnosis to its own true form." On the role of Gabriel and prophetic dreams in medieval Islamic and Jewish sources, see Chapter 3 n. 92. The influence of the Maimonidean approach can also be detected in the passages of Phineḥas of Korzec, *Imrei Pinḥas ha-Shalem*, cited in Chapter 5 at nn. 219–20.

73. Maimonides and other philosophers were criticized by Gersonides for allegorizing biblical figures. See Charles Touati, *La pensée philosophique et théologique de Gersonide* (Paris: Les Éditions de minuit, 1973), p. 484. According to my reading, the view of Maimonides is essentially consonant with earlier rabbinic approaches to the biblical narrative as suspended between fiction and historiography. See Daniel Boyarin, *Sparks of Logos: Essays in Rabbinic Hermeneutics* (Leiden: Brill, 2003), pp. 89–113. Influenced by several theoreticians, but especially Hayden White and Michael Riffaterre, Boyarin responded to the debate between Robert Alter and Milton Steinberg on the role of fictionality in biblical narrative by proposing that historiography and fiction for the rabbinic readers should be seen as "different semiotic functions within the text" rather than as "alternative genres" (p. 112). To my mind, his approach can be applied to Maimonides. See the pertinent discussion on the *majāz-ḥaqīqa* dichotomy in Cohen, *Three Approaches*, pp. 44–46. The question of Maimonides and the ancient midrashic method is a large one that has commanded a good deal of attention. See, for instance, James A. Diamond, *Maimonides and the Hermeneutics of Concealment: Deciphering Scripture and Midrash in The Guide of the Perplexed* (Albany: State University of New York Press, 2002). A separate, though not completely unrelated issue is Maimonides' attitude to rabbinic aggadah. This topic, too, has been discussed by many scholars. For a recent assessment, see the two studies by Yair Lorberbaum, "Changes in Maimonides' Approach to Aggadah," *Tarbiz* 78 (2009): 81–122 (Hebrew) and "'Incline Thy Ear, and Hear the Words of the Wise, and Apply Thy Heart Unto My Knowledge': Criticism of Aggadah in *The Guide of the Perplexed*," *Tarbiz* 78 (2009): 203–30 (Hebrew).

74. Maimonides, *Guide*, II.45, pp. 402–403 (emphasis in the original).

75. *Ibid.*, I.21, pp. 50–51. A possible echo of Saadya's related doctrine of the "created glory" (*kavod nivra*) can be heard in the depiction of the indwelling of the divine presence (*Shekhinah*) as a "created light" in I.25, p. 55. For discussion of Saadya's views, see Alexander Altmann, *Studies in Religious Philosophy and Mysticism* (Ithaca: Cornell University Press, 1969), pp. 140–60. On

the metaphorical explanation of the notions of hearing and seeing as modes of apprehension when attributed to God, see Maimonides, *Guide*, I.48, pp. 106–107.

76. *Ibid.*, I.65, p. 158.

77. *Ibid.*, pp. 158–59. See I.66, p. 160, I.67, p. 161.

78. *Ibid.*, I.4, pp. 27–28. On the interpretation of the vision of prophecy attained by Moses as intellectual apprehension, see I.21, p. 51.

79. *Midrash Bere'shit Rabba* 27:1, pp. 255–56.

80. Maimonides, *Guide*, I.46, p. 103 (emphasis in the original).

81. *Ibid.*, I.38, p. 87.

82. *Ibid.*, I.27, p. 58. Compare II.41, p. 387.

83. *Ibid.*, II.46, p. 404 (emphasis in the original).

84. The view proffered by Maimonides is on a par with the interpretation of prophecy as the externalization of the self expressed in the school of Abraham Abulafia. See Gershom Scholem, *Major Trends in Jewish Mysticism* (New York: Schocken Books, 1954), p. 142; Wolfson, *Language, Eros, Being*, pp. 238–42. Scholem does not mention Maimonides, but he does note the remark of Abraham Ibn Ezra in his commentary to Daniel 10:21 to the effect that "the one who speaks is a human and the one who hears is a human as well" (this is a more accurate translation than the one provided by Scholem). On the function of the imagination in Ibn Ezra, see Aaron W. Hughes, *The Texture of the Divine: Imagination in Medieval Islamic and Jewish Thought* (Bloomington: Indiana University Press, 2004), pp. 95–99. On the intellectual relationship of Maimonides and Ibn Ezra, see the review of the issue by Isadore Twersky, "Did R. Abraham Ibn Ezra Influence Maimonides?" in *Rabbi Abraham Ibn Ezra: Studies in the Writings of a Twelfth-Century Jewish Polymath*, edited by Isadore Twersky and Jay M. Harris (Cambridge, MA: Harvard University Press, 1993), pp. 21–48 (Hebrew section).

85. Compare the excerpt from the *Book on the Elements (Kitāb al-usṭuquṣṣāt)* in Alexander Altmann and Samuel M. Stern, *Isaac Israeli: A Neoplatonic Philosopher of the Early Tenth Century* (Oxford: Oxford University Press, 1958), p. 136, and discussion on pp. 140–45 and 211–14. Compare Heller-Roazen, *The Inner Touch*, pp. 146–47.

86. Avencebrolis, *Fons vitae ex arabico in latinum translatus ab Iohanne Hispano et Dominico Gundissalino*, edited by Clemens Baeumker (Münster: Aschendorff, 1895), III.42, p. 174: "quod substantia animae recipit formam intelligibilem a substantia intelligentiae in somnis animaliter, id est [exemplariter] imaginabiliter, et post somnum sentit eas anima corporaliter et materialiter." See *ibid.*, IV.16, p. 247: "etiam sume exemplum ad hoc ex aliqua forma corporali

qua uidetur a uigilanti, quia hae formae corporales exemplum sunt animalium formarum apprehensarum in somno; similiter formae animales apprehensae in somno exemplum sunt formarum intelligibilium interiorum." For the Hebrew version, see Solomon Ibn Gabirol, *Meqor Ḥayyim*, translated by Jacob Blubstein, edited by Abraham Zifroni (Tel-Aviv: Maḥbarot le-Sifrut, 1926), pp. 221 and 318, and see analysis in Sirat, *Les théories*, pp. 61–62 and 67–69. Interestingly, the reference to dreams is missing in the corresponding passages in the fragments from *Fons vitae* translated by Shem Ṭov Ibn Falaquera and published as *Liqquṭim min Sefer Meqor Ḥayyim* by Salomon Munk, *Mélanges de philosophie juive et arabe* (Paris: A. Franck, 1857), pp. 16 and 19 (Hebrew section); the French translation of the relevant passages appears on pp. 62–63 and 75.

87. Ibn Khaldûn, *The Muqaddimah*, 3:71–72, notes that human perceptions, which occur in dream visions while one is asleep, are the same as the external sense perceptions, and even though the limbs of the body are not used, the dreamer ascertains everything "without any doubt or misgiving." He goes on to contrast the views of the philosophers and speculative theologians. The former "assume that the imaginary pictures are transmitted by the imagination through the motion of thinking to the 'common sense' which constitutes the connecting link between external and inner sensual perception. As a result, (these pictures) are represented as something perceived in the external (world) by all the senses." The latter, by contrast, insist that the dream vision is created by God and "thus takes place in the same way that (perception) takes place in the waking state."

88. Maimonides, *Guide*, I.21, pp. 50–51; I.37, p. 86; II.37, p. 373; II.41, pp. 385–386; II.34, p. 367. The distinctiveness of Mosaic prophecy in Maimonides' writings has been the focus of many studies of which I here offer a modest sampling: Harry A. Wolfson, *Studies in the History of Philosophy and Religion*, edited by Isadore Twersky and George H. Williams, 2 vols. (Cambridge, MA: Harvard University Press, 1973–1977), 2:112–15; Altmann, *Essays in Jewish Intellectual History*, pp. 88–89; Menachem Kellner, "Maimonides and Gersonides on Mosaic Prophecy," *Speculum* 52 (1977): 65–66; Kreisel, *Prophecy*, pp. 172–74, 189–90. On the question of the divine/angelic versus human status of Moses in Maimonides, see Alfred L. Ivry, "Ismāʿīlī Theology and Maimonides' Philosophy," in *The Jews of Medieval Islam: Community, Society, and Identity*, edited by Daniel Frank (Leiden: E. J. Brill, 1995), pp. 288–91; *idem*, "The Image of Moses in Maimonides' Thought," in *Maimonides after 800 Years: Essays on Maimonides and His Influence*, edited by Jay M. Harris (Cambridge, MA: Harvard University Press, 2007), pp. 113–34, esp. 129–33. See also Kalman P. Bland, "Moses and the Law According to Maimonides," in *Mystics, Philosophers, and Politicians*,

pp. 49–66, esp. 50–53. On the Maimonidean depiction of Mosaic prophecy as the model of intellectual conjunction, see Alvin Reines, "Maimonides' Concept of Mosaic Prophecy," *Hebrew Union College Annual* 40–41 (1969–1970): 325–62, and the varied approach on the superiority of the prophecy of Moses in Maimonides as an illustration of his intellectualist mysticism in David R. Blumenthal, *Philosophic Mysticism: Studies in Rational Religion* (Ramat-Gan: Bar Ilan University Press, 2006), pp. 73–95.

89. Maimonides, *Guide*, III.51, p. 620.

90. David R. Blumenthal, "Maimonides' Philosophic Mysticism," in *Maimonides and Mysticism Presented to Moshe Hallamish On the Occasion of his Retirement*, edited by Avi Elqayam and Dov Schwartz [*Da'at* 64–66] (Ramat-Gan: Bar-Ilan University Press, 2009), pp. x–xvi, xxii (English section).

91. Maimonides, *Guide*, I.1, p. 7, I.13, p. 40, III.51, p. 623. For an interesting reverberation of the Maimonidean view in an important kabbalistic text from the late thirteenth or early fourteenth century, see Elliot R. Wolfson, "The Anonymous Chapters of the Elderly Master of Secrets: New Evidence for the Early Activity of the Zoharic Circle," *Kabbalah: Journal for the Study of Jewish Mystical Texts* 19 (2009): 186–89 and 196.

92. See Diamond, *Maimonides*, pp. 65–70. Maimonides' interpretation of the word "standing" is enhanced by the much older idea (with roots in the biblical canon) that the typical posture of the angels is to stand, and not to sit. For references, see Elliot R. Wolfson, "Yeridah la-Merkavah: Typology of Ecstasy and Enthronement in Ancient Jewish Mysticism," in *Mystics of the Book: Themes, Topics, and Typologies*, edited and with an introduction by Robert A. Herrera (New York: Peter Lang, 1993), p. 37 n. 70.

93. *Mishneh Torah*, Yesodei Torah 7:6.

94. Maimonides, *Mishnah im Perush Rabbenu Moshe ben Maimon: Seder Neziqin*, pp. 142–43.

95. *Ibid.*, pp. 259–60.

96. Kreisel, *Prophecy*, p. 173 n. 53, suggests that the image of rending a veil (*ḥijāb*) is reminiscent of the Ṣūfi description of prophetic illumination. For the use of the motif of removing the veil in depicting seeing God with the mind's eye, see Baḥya Ibn Paquda, *Sefer Torat Ḥovot ha-Levavot*, edited and translated by Joseph Kafiḥ (Jerusalem, 1973), VIII.4, pp. 379–80.

97. This view is briefly repeated in Maimonides' commentary to Kelim 30:2, in *Mishnah im Perush Rabbenu Moshe ben Maimon: Seder Ṭaharot*, translated and edited by Joseph Kafiḥ (Jerusalem: Mosad ha-Rav Kook, 1968), p. 145.

98. Maimonides, *Guide*, III.9, pp. 436–37.

99. *Ibid.*, I.37, p. 86. Cf. I. 64, pp. 156–57.

100. As noted by Pines in Maimonides, *Guide*, I.37, p. 86, nn. 23–24.

101. *Ibid.*, I.37, p. 86.

102. *Ibid.*, I.54, pp. 124–25.

103. Diamond, *Maimonides*, pp. 58–59.

104. Compare Maimonides, *Guide*, I.54, p. 126: "It behooves the governor of a city, if he is a prophet, to acquire similarity to these attributes, so that these actions may proceed from him according to a determined measure and according to the deserts of the people who are affected by them and not merely because of his following a passion." Note how this clashes with the statement of Maimonides in III.23 in his account of Elihu's response to Job. On the face of it, it seems that he merely repeats the views of the others, affirming that God is just, that Job suffers because he has done wrong, and that God does not care either for the obedience of those who obey or for the disobedience of those who disobey, that is, God is not effected one way or the other by human action. But the element that he adds is expressed parabolically by his referring to the intercession of an angel. Maimonides sums up the view of Elihu in the following terms: the ways of divine providence are not comparable to the ways of human providence, just as divine knowledge is not comparable to human knowledge. On the notion of *imitatio dei* and the model of communal leadership, see Howard Kreisel, *Maimonides' Political Thought: Studies in Ethics, Law, and the Human Ideal* (Albany: State University of New York Press, 1999), pp. 125–58, esp. 128–32; Melamed, *The Philosopher-King*, pp. 35–40 and 45–46.

105. This view is proffered by al-Fārābī in *The Opinions of the People of the Virtuous City, The Political Regime*, and *Epistle on the Intellect*, which is referred to explicitly in one passage in the *Guide* and implicitly elsewhere; see Maimonides, *Guide*, II.18, p. 299.

106. Pines, "Translator's Introduction," in Maimonides, *Guide*, pp. lxxx–lxxxiii, points out that al-Fārābī was not consistent. Thus, in his lost commentary on the Ethics, he argued that the corporeal human being is not capable of uniting with the incorporeal Active Intellect. In this later work, al-Fārābī affirms that the Active Intellect performs only as an efficient cause to foster the actualization of the potential intellect. This position concurs with Averroës, who maintained that al-Fārābī denied the possibility of union with the Active Intellect. Similarly, Ibn Bājja proposed the possibility of an individual's conjunction with the Active Intellect and he was critical of al-Fārābī's denial of this possibility. Pines suggests that the intellectual supremacy of Moses proffered by Maimonides has to be viewed in terms of the position of Ibn Bājja and al-Fārābī.

107. For a lucid articulation of this epistemological principle, see Alexander

of Aphrodisias, *On the Cosmos,* edited and translated by Charles Genequand (Leiden: Brill, 2001), p. 99: "For that which is actually intelligible is itself actually intellect, because perceiving by the intellect occurs by grasping the intelligible thing to which an intellect is assimilated when it grasps it by thinking it and thereby becomes that itself. Therefore, it is said that that which thinks, in the state of thinking, thinks itself, because in that state it becomes one and the same with itself... the thing thought in actuality is the intellect, since it is itself the intellect which is in actuality, by which I mean that the intellect in the state of thinking is the intelligible itself. The intellect, then, is actually thinking because of the intelligible thing, since the intellect which is in actuality, by its relation with the actually intelligible, is itself the actuality proceeding from the intellect."

108. Maimonides, *Guide*, 1.68, pp. 163–66. For a relatively recent discussion of this crucial chapter, see Josef Stern, "The Enigma of the *Guide of the Perplexed* 1, 68," in *Maimonides: Conservatism, Originality, Revolution*, 2 vols., edited by Aviezer Ravitzky (Jerusalem: Zalman Shazar Center for Jewish History, 2008), 2:437–51 (Hebrew).

109. Maimonides, *Guide*, 1.74, p. 221. It is worth recalling that Judah Halevi, *Sefer ha-Kuzari*, v.14, pp. 214–16, rejects the perspective of Ibn Bājja, which was also accepted by Averroës, but he acknowledges that it is the most logical conclusion to follow from the Aristotelian premises.

110. Many scholars have weighed in on the question of Maimonides' epistemology and the possibility of metaphysics or the knowledge of what is immaterial. As a representative list, see Shlomo Pines, "The Limitations of Human Knowledge according to Al-Farabi, Ibn Bajja, and Maimonides," in *Studies in Medieval Jewish History and Literature*, edited by Isadore Twersky (Cambridge, MA: Harvard University Press, 1979), pp. 82–109; *idem*, "Les limites de la métaphysique selon al-Farrabi, Ibn Bajja, et Maïmonide: sources et antitheses de ces doctrines chez Alexandre d'Aprodise et chez Themistius," *Miscellanea Mediaevalia* 13 (1981): 211–25; *idem*, "Dieu et l'être selon Maïmonide: Exégèse d'Exode 3, 14 et doctrine connexe," *Celui qui est: Interprétations juives et chrétiennes d'Exode 3, 14,* edited by Alain de Libera and Emile Zum Brunn (Paris: Cerf, 1986), pp. 15–24. All three essays are reprinted in *The Collected Works of Shlomo Pines: Studies in the History of Jewish Thought*, vol. 5, edited by Warren Zev Harvey and Moshe Idel (Jerusalem: Magnes Press, 1997), pp. 404–56. For an alternative perspective, see Alexander Altmann, *Von der mittelalterlichen zur modernen Aufklärung: Studien zur jüdischen Geistesgeschichte* (Tübingen: J. C. B. Mohr, 1987), pp. 60–129, and Josef Stern, "Maimonides on the Growth of Knowledge and the Limitations of the Intellect," in *Maïmonide, philosophie et*

savant (1138–1204), edited by Tony Lévy and Roshdi Rashed (Leuven: Peters, 2004), pp. 143–91.

111. Maimonides, *Guide*, "Introduction," p. 17.

112. Diane Lobel, *A Sufi-Jewish Dialogue: Philosophy and Mysticism in Baḥya Ibn Paqūda's Duties of the Heart* (Philadelphia: University of Pennsylvania Press, 2007), pp. 11, 19, 38–39, 255 n. 21.

113. Baḥya Ibn Paquda, *Sefer Torat Ḥovot ha-Levavot*, 1.10, p. 84.

114. Maimonides, *Guide*, 1.59, p. 139.

115. Joel L. Kraemer, "Maimonides' Use of Aristotelian Dialectic," in *Maimonides and the Sciences*, edited by Robert S. Cohen and Hillel Levine (Dordrecht: Kluwer, 2000), p. 123; *idem*, "Is There a Text in this Class?" *Aleph* 8 (2008): 257–58.

116. Kraemer, *Maimonides*, pp. 368–69. At p. 571 n. 62, Kraemer refers to the fact that the Arabic translators Eustathius, Mattā b. Yūnus and Naẓif b. Yumn al-Rūmī used *taḥayyur* and *ḥayra* for aporia in Aristotle's *Metaphysics*, and he cites Soheil M. Afnan, *Philosophical Terminology in Arabic and Persian* (Leiden: E. J. Brill, 1964), p. 84.

117. Alexander of Aphrodisias, *On Aristotle's Metaphysics 2 & 3*, translated by William E. Dooley, S. J., and Arthur Madigan, S. J. (Ithaca: Cornell University Press, 1992), p. 89.

118. See Gareth B. Matthews, *Socratic Perplexity and the Nature of Philosophy* (Oxford: Oxford University Press, 1999), and Mary-Jane Rubenstein, *Strange Wonder: The Closure of Metaphysics and the Opening of Awe* (New York: Columbia University Press, 2008).

119. See Warren Zev Harvey, "Three Theories of the Imagination in 12th-Century Jewish Philosophy," in *Intellect et imagination dans la Philosophie Médiévale*, 1:300–301.

120. Blanchot, *Friendship*, pp. 145–46.

121. Kendall L. Walton, *Mimesis as Make-Believe: On the Foundations of the Representational Arts* (Cambridge, MA: Harvard University Press, 1990), p. 43.

122. Foucault, "Dream, Imagination and Existence," p. 34.

123. *Ibid.*, pp. 34–35.

124. *Ibid.*, p. 35.

125. *Ibid.*, p. 39.

126. *Ibid.*, p. 40.

127. *Ibid.*, p. 44.

128. *Ibid.*, p. 45.

129. *Ibid.*, pp. 45 and 53.

130. *Ibid.*, p. 56.

131. Binswanger, *Dream and Existence*, p. 82.

132. Foucault, "Dream, Imagination and Existence," p. 57.

133. *Ibid.*, p. 58.

134. *Ibid.*, pp. 58–59.

135. *Ibid.*, p. 59. See *ibid.*, p. 64, where Foucault notes that time is not an "authentic temporality" in the opposition of light and dark, the conventional nocturnal and diurnal fluctuation.

136. *Ibid.*, pp. 60–61.

137. *Ibid.*, p. 67.

138. *Ibid.*, p. 68.

139. *Ibid.*, pp. 68–69.

140. *Ibid.*, p. 69.

141. *Ibid.*, p. 71.

142. Binswanger, *Dream and Existence*, p. 83, relates the "essential ontological structure" of rising and falling vis-à-vis the ground of our existence in the world to language, the poet's imagination, and the dream.

143. Foucault, "Dream, Imagination and Existence," p. 72.

144. *Ibid.*, p. 73.

145. *Ibid.*, pp. 73–74.

146. *Ibid.*, p. 74. Compare Agamben, *The Signature of All Things*, p. 105.

CHAPTER THREE: A LETTER OVER/WRITTEN

1. Scott B. Noegel, *Nocturnal Ciphers: The Allusive Language of Dreams in the Ancient Near East* (New Haven: American Oriental Society, 2007).

2. Compare the description of Hermes in *The Greek Magical Papyri in Translation, Including the Demotic Spells*, edited by Hans Dieter Betz (Chicago: University of Chicago Press, 1986), V.410–12, p. 108: "The prophet of events/ And Dream divine you're said to be, who send/Forth oracles by day and night." See Florian Ebeling, *The Secret History of Hermes Trismegistus: Hermeticism from Ancient to Modern Times*, foreword by Jan Assman, translated by David Lorton (Ithaca: Cornell University Press, 2007), pp. 24–25. For the equation of Hermes and the Armenian God Tīr, the heavenly messenger invested with the power to send dreams to human beings, see James R. Russell, "'Sleep' and 'Dreaming' in Armenian," in *Proceedings of the Fourth International Conference on Armenian Linguistics*, edited by John A. C. Greppin (Delmar: Caravan Books, 1992), p. 147, reprinted in James R. Russell, *Armenian and Iranian Studies* (Cambridge, MA: Harvard University Press, 2004), p. 477.

3. Carl G. Jung, *Psychology and Alchemy*, translated by R. F. C. Hull, 2nd

edition (Princeton: Princeton University Press, 1968), pp. 65, 132; *idem*, *Alchemical Studies*, translated by R. F. C. Hull (Princeton: Princeton University Press, 1967), p. 233.

4. *The Greek Magical Papyri*, v.401–402, p. 108, vii.669, p. 137. See Jung, *Psychology and Alchemy*, p. 132; Miller, *Dreams*, pp. 119–20.

5. Noegel, *Nocturnal Ciphers*, pp. 235–51. A comprehensive approach to rabbinic oneirology can be found in Afik, "Hazal's Perception." Afik delineates seven major ways that dreams are analyzed in rabbinic literature: psychological, quasi-prophetic, extrasensory, magical, educational, medical, and signifying an intermediate realm between the physical and intangible. See also Zeitlin, "Dreams," pp. 16–18; Brigitte Stemberger, "Der Traum in der rabbinischen Literatur," *Kairos: Zeitschrift für Religionswissenschaft und Theologie* 18 (1976): 1–42; Richard Kalmin, *Sages, Stories, Authors, and Editors in Rabbinic Babylonia* (Atlanta: Scholars Press, 1994), pp. 61–80; *idem*, "Talmudic Attitudes Toward Dream Interpreters: Preliminary Thoughts on their Iranian Cultural Context," in *The Talmud in Its Iranian Context*, edited by Carol Bakhos and M. Rahim Shayegan (Tübingen: Mohr Siebeck, 2010), pp. 83–99 (my thanks to Menachem Butler for drawing this essay to my attention); Avigdor Shinan, "The Dream in Midrash and the Midrash of the Dream," in *The Spectrum of Opinions and Worldviews about Dreams in Jewish Culture*, edited by Dror Kerem (Reḥovot, 1995), pp. 43–61 (Hebrew); Jeffrey L. Rubenstein, *The Culture of the Babylonian Talmud* (Baltimore: Johns Hopkins University Press, 2003), pp. 29–31; Ḥayyim Weiss, "'What This One Interpreted for Me That One Did Not Interpret for Me': A Cultural and Literary Reading of the 'Treatise on Dreams' in the Babylonian Talmud," Ph.D. dissertation, Hebrew University, 2007 (Hebrew). See also Dan, *On Sanctity*, pp. 35–41, who distinguishes between the ostensibly hyperlinguistic nature of the dream and its textual interpretation. In the dream itself, there is allegedly no fixed relation between sign and signified, whereas the interpretation is a form of verbal communication based on precisely such a relation. I concur that the act of interpreting seeks to make the nonsensical dream images sensible, but I do not accept the categorical distinction between the dream experience and its explication and the inference that they are independent domains of mental activity. I am also not persuaded by Dan's larger attempt to contrast the dream sharply with mystical vision on the semantic criteria he establishes. He seems to have been influenced especially by the Gadamerian approach of Derksen, "Dream Interpretation," a study that is cited by Dan, *On Sanctity*, p. 39 n. 20. On the essential textuality of the dream, connected particularly to the diaries penned by Jewish mystics, see Rachel Elior, "Reality in the Test of Fiction: Dreams in Mystical Thought—The Freedom of

Disassociation and Combination," in *The Spectrum of Opinions*, pp. 66, 68–74 (Hebrew). Although she makes no mention of it, Elior's thesis concurs with the argument I offered in *Through a Speculum That Shines* regarding the intertwining of experience and interpretation in Jewish mystical visions. See also Chapter 1 n. 285.

6. Saul Lieberman, *Hellenism in Jewish Palestine: Studies in the Literary Transmission, Beliefs, and Manners of Palestine in the I Century B.C.E.–IV Century C.E.* (New York: Jewish Theological Seminary, 1962), pp. 70–76. On sources in Late Antiquity that attest to the reputation of Jews as skilled in the art of interpreting dreams, see the evidence adduced by Feldman, *Josephus's Interpretation of the Bible*, p. 349 n. 34.

7. Philip S. Alexander, "Bavil Berakhot 55a–57b: The Talmudic Dreambook in Context," *Journal of Jewish Studies* 46 (1995): 236–41 and 243. See other references cited above in note 5, below in note 9, and in Chapter 1 n. 278.

8. Alexander, "Bavil Berakhot," pp. 232 and 246–47.

9. The name is vocalized alternatively as Bar Hadaya. In other contexts where this figure is mentioned, it appears that he was a member of the rabbinic establishment in Babylonia and then moved to Palestine. See Babylonian Talmud, Sukkah 43b; Giṭṭin 5b; Avodah Zarah 30a; Ḥullin 106b. Hasan-Rokem, *Web of Life*, p. 227 n. 25, suggests that *bar hedya* signifies the profession of dream interpreter based on the denotation of the terms *hedya* (clarity) and *be-hedya* (clearly) in the rabbinic lexicon. This seems to me to be a plausible explanation and fits well with the linguistic playfulness displayed by the rabbis more generally. A similar explication was offered by Abraham Isaac Kook, *Ein Ayah al Aggadot Ḥazal she-be-Ein Ya'aqov: Berakhot*, 2 vols. (Jerusalem: Makhon al shem ha-Rav Ṣevi Yehudah Quq, 1995–2000), 2:283, who added that this kind of vocation requires both proper training and autonomous aptitude. For an extended philological analysis of this narrative in light of the many textual variants, see Afik, "Hazal's Perception," pp. 219–63. See also Kalmin, *Sages*, pp. 67–69; *idem*, "Talmudic Attitudes," pp. 87–88; Ḥayyim Weiss, "'Twenty-Four Dream-Interpreters Were in Jerusalem . . .': On Dream-Interpreters and the Approaches to Dream-Interpretation in the 'Treatise on Dreams' in the Babylonian Talmud," *Madda'ei ha-Yahadut* 44 (2007): 46–50 (Hebrew); Simcha Fishbane, *Deviancy in Early Rabbinic Literature: A Collection of Socio-Anthropological Essays*, with an introduction by Nissan Rubin (Leiden: Brill, 2007), pp. 177–212; Yuval Harari, *Early Jewish Magic: Research, Method, Sources* (Jerusalem: Bialik Institute, 2010), pp. 330–40 (Hebrew); Holger M. Zellentin, "Late Antiquity Upside-Down: Rabbinic Parodies of Jewish and Christian Literature," Ph.D. dissertation, Princeton University, 2007, pp. 191–252.

10. Babylonian Talmud, Berakhot 56a.

11. Glen W. Bowersock, *Fiction as History: Nero to Julian* (Berkeley: University of California Press, 1994), pp. 80–81.

12. Yuval Harari, "The Sages and the Occult," in *The Literature of the Sages, Second Part: Midrash and Targum, Liturgy, Poetry, Mysticism, Contracts, Inscriptions, Ancient Sciences, and the Languages of Rabbinic Literature*, edited by Shmuel Safrai, Zeev Safrai, Joshua Schwartz, and Peter J. Tomson (Assen: Van Gorcum, 2006), pp. 553–54; *idem*, *Early Jewish Magic*, pp. 335–40.

13. David Stern, *Midrash and Theory: Ancient Jewish Exegesis and Contemporary Literary Studies* (Evanston: Northwestern University Press, 1996), p. 100 n. 17; Hasan-Rokem, *Web of Life*, p. 100. It is relevant to consider here the argument of Oppenheim, "The Interpretation of Dreams," pp. 220–25, that in the ancient Near East dream interpreters were of a lower social class, including especially women. See also Leo A. Oppenheim, "Mantic Dreams in the Ancient Near East," in *The Dream and Human Societies*, p. 350.

14. Alexander, "Bavli Berakhot," pp. 236 and 238.

15. *Ibid.*, p. 247. See also Harari, "The Sages and the Occult," pp. 555–58; Weiss, "'Twenty-Four Dream-Interpreters,'" pp. 50–53. Kalmin, "Talmudic Attitudes," argues that the opposition of the rabbis responsible for editing the Babylonian Talmud to professional dream interpretation may be related to their desire to differentiate themselves from the Magi and to minimize the influence of the latter over Babylonian Jews. In support of this argument, Kalmin notes that in Palestinian sources, the rabbis were portrayed more readily as professional dream interpreters (pp. 97–98). See also Zellentin, "Late Antiquity Upside-Down," pp. 237–41. For narratives that present rabbinic sages interpreting dreams, see Babylonian Talmud, Ta'anit 24b; Soṭah 31a; Sanhedrin 82a; Ḥullin 133a.

16. Freud, *Interpretation of Dreams*, p. 79. See also Bowersock, *Fiction as History*, pp. 81–82. On the dream interpretation in Artemidorus, see Foucault, *The History of Sexuality, Volume 3: The Care of the Self*, pp. 4–36; Miller, *Dreams*, pp. 77–91; Christine Walde, "Dream Interpretation in a Prosperous Age?: Artemidorus, the Greek Interpreter of Dreams," in *Dream Cultures*, pp. 121–42; Struck, *Birth of the Symbol*, pp. 183–84; Flannery-Dailey, *Dreamers*, pp. 97–99. On the role of dream interpreters as a professional class of specialists, see also Johnston, *Ancient Greek Divination*, pp. 134–37.

17. The argument here is corollary to the view offered by Saul Lieberman, *Greek in Jewish Palestine: Studies on the Life and Manners of Jewish Palestine in the II–IV Centuries C.E.* (New York: Philip Feldheim, 1965), pp. 100–14, that the rabbis did not fight against superstitions, but sanctioned them by endowing

them with a religious character. For more recent studies on attitudes to magic in the vast corpus of rabbinic litertaure, see Jacob Neusner, "Science and Magic, Miracle and Magic in Formative Judaism: The System and the Difference," in *Religion, Science, and Magic: In Concert and in Conflict*, edited by Jacob Neusner, Ernest S. Frerichs, and Paul Virgil McCracken Flesher (New York: Oxford University Press, 1989), pp. 61–81; Daniel Sperber, *Magic and Folklore in Rabbinic Literature* (Ramat-Gan: Bar-Ilan University Press. 1994); Jonathan L. Seidel, "Charming Criminals: Classification of Magic in the Babylonian Talmud," in *Ancient Magic and Ritual Power*, edited by Marvin Meyer and Paul Mirecki (Leiden: E. J. Brill, 1995), pp. 145–66; *idem*, "Studies in Ancient Jewish Magic," Ph.D. dissertation, University of California, Berkeley, 1996, pp. 157–221; Peter Schäfer, "Magic and Religion in Ancient Judaism," in *Envisioning Magic: A Princeton Seminar and Symposium*, edited by Peter Schäfer and Hans G. Kippenberg (Leiden: Brill, 1997), pp. 19–43, esp. 33–38; Giuseppe Veltri, *Magie und Halakha: Ansätze zu einem empirischen Wissenschaftsbegriff im spätantiken und frühmiitelalterlichen Judentum* (Tübingen: J. C. B. Mohr, 1997); Harari, "The Sages and the Occult," pp. 521–64; *idem, Early Jewish Magic*, pp. 272–352; Gideon Bohak, *Ancient Jewish Magic: A History* (Cambridge: Cambridge University Press, 2008), pp. 351–425. Finally, the rabbinic reference to professional oneiromancers suggests that the interpretation of dreams was not viewed as a democratic enterprise, as we find in the works of some Greek authors of the time, for example, the Neoplatonist Synesius of Cyrene (ca. 370–414). See Le Goff, *The Medieval Imagination*, p. 201.

18. The expression "structural homology" is appropriated from A. Kiarina Kordela, "Marx, Condensed and Displaced," in *The Dreams of Interpretation*, pp. 303–19. The author draws a parallel between the twofold notion of surplus in the respective domains of economics ("exchange-value" and "use-value" in Marxian terms) and semantics (metaphor and metonymy in the field of the signifier, condensation and displacement in the field of the Freudian subject, and enjoyment of meaning, *jouis-sens*, and enjoyment, *jouissance*, in the field of the Lacanian subject). Summing up her view, Kordela writes: "Hence, when we speak of a structural and functional homology between economic and semantic exchange, we are effectively speaking of a homology among three fields: economy, linguistics, and the constitution of the subject" (p. 305).

19. For discussion of the larger milieu in which this claim should be evaluated, see Yuval Harari, "Power and Money: Economic Aspects of the Use of Magic by Jews in Ancient Times and the Early Middle Ages," *Pe'amim: Studies in Oriental Jewry* 85 (2000): 14–42 (Hebrew).

20. Babylonian Talmud, Berakhot 10b. On the expression "master of the

dream" (*ba'al ha-ḥalom*), see also Babylonian Talmud, Sanhedrin 30a, and the remarks of Heschel, *Prophetic Inspiration*, pp. 4–5 n. 7.

21. Babylonian Talmud, Berakhot 55a. The relation of the principle "all dreams follow the mouth" and the aphorism that "a dream that is not interpreted is like a letter that is not read" was already noted by Trachtenberg, *Jewish Magic*, p. 236. See also Alexander, "Bavli Berakhot," pp. 234–35; Fishbane, *Deviancy*, pp. 184–85, 188–89. On the latter theme, see Maren R. Niehoff, "A Dream Which Is Not Interpreted Is Like a Letter Which Is Not Read," *Journal of Jewish Studies* 43 (1992): 58–84.

22. Alexander, "Bavli Berakhot," p. 236, remarks that he knows of "no convincing parallels from ancient dream-theory" to this notion. In his judgment, this idea "appears to be peculiar to rabbinic literature and to reflect distinctively rabbinic theories of textuality." On the reciprocal relation between the dream and its meaning, see also Weiss, "'Twenty-Four Dream-Interpreters,'" pp. 58–62. Kook, *Ein Ayah al Aggadot Ḥazal*, 2:266–67, emphasized that just as reading a letter facilitates the fulfillment of the desire of the one who wrote the letter on the part of the recipient, so the interpretation of the dream is instrumental in helping the individual realize the future eventuality hinted at within the dream. Kook's view is an elaboration of the interpretation of the talmudic teaching that "all dreams follow the mouth" found in Isaac ben Moses Arama, *Aqeidat Yiṣḥaq*, edited by Ḥayyim Yosef Pollak, 4 vols. (Pressburg: Victor Kittseer, 1849), 1:228b–229a, and see the partial rejoinder to the critical remarks of Arama offered by Samuel Eidels, referred to as the MaHaRShA, in his *Ḥiddushei Aggadot* to the relevant passage in the Babylonian Talmud, Berakhot 55b, s.v., *she-kol ha-ḥalomot*.

23. Alexander, "Bavli Berakhot," p. 237.

24. Babylonian Talmud, Shabbat 11a. For discussion of this ritual practice as it evolved in the medieval period, see Trachtenberg, *Jewish Magic*, pp. 245–47.

25. The process I have described here is in accord with the explication of the Sanskrit *svapna-siddha* offered by Jeffrey J. Kripal, *Roads of Excess, Palaces of Wisdom: Eroticism and Reflexivity in the Study of Mysticism* (Chicago: University of Chicago Press, 2001), pp. 299–304. Kripal renders the expression as "perfected in a dream" or as "a dream to perfect," which he characterizes as a mystically inspired hermeneutical practice of interpretation.

26. Palestinian Talmud, Ma'aser Sheni 4:12, 55c. Compare Babylonian Talmud, Berakhot 57a: "A tanna recited before R. Yoḥanan: All types of drink are good in a dream except for wine; sometimes one drinks it and it is good for him, and sometimes one drinks it and it is bad for him. Sometimes one drinks it and its good for him, as it says 'Wine that cheers the hearts of men' (Psalms

104:15), sometimes one drinks it and it is bad for him, as it says 'Give strong drink to the hapless and wine to the embittered' (Proverbs 31:6). R. Yoḥanan said to that tanna: It has been taught that for a scholar it is always good, as it says 'Come, eat my food and drink the wine that I have mixed' (*ibid.*, 9:5)." It also should be noted that in the aforecited context in the Palestinian Talmud there is a variant of this dictum, "the dream only follows its interpretation" (*ein ha-ḥalom holekh ella aḥar pitrono*). See also *Midrash Eikhah Rabbah* 1:18, "R. Yoḥanan said, 'The dream follows its interpretation [*ha-ḥalom holekh aḥar pitrono*] with the exception of wine." And in *Midrash Bere'shit Rabba* 89:8, pp. 1096–97: "R. Yoḥanan said, 'All the dreams follow the mouth [*kol ha-ḥalomot holkhin aḥar ha-peh*] with the exception of wine." According to a textual variant, however, the passage reads "all the dreams follow the interpretation" (*kol ha-ḥalomot holkhin aḥar ha-pitron*). Concerning this midrashic tradition and its proximity to the psychoanalytic approach, see Roger Caillois, *Images, Images . . . : Essais sur le rôle et les pouvoirs de l'imagination* (Paris: Librairie José Corti, 1966), pp. 72–73.

27. *Midrash Bere'shit Rabba* 68:12, p. 785.

28. On the *status quaestionis* of this topic, see the thorough analysis of Daniel Abrams, "The Invention of the *Zohar* as a Book: On the Assumptions and Expectations of the Kabbalists and Modern Scholars," *Kabbalah: Journal for the Study of Jewish Mystical Texts* 19 (2009): 7–142.

29. Judah ben Samuel he-Ḥasid, *Sefer Ḥasidim*, edited by Jehuda Wistinetzki and Jacob Freimann (Frankfurt am Main: Wahrmann Verlag, 1924), sec. 387, p. 118; *Zohar* 1:183a, 200a. The instruction to rehearse a dream before a friend is based on a passage in the Babylonian Talmud, Berakhot, 55b (according to the reading preserved in MS Oxford 366, cited in Harari, *Early Jewish Magic*, p. 331; see also Kalmin, "Talmudic Attitudes," p. 89) that counsels that a person report a dream that has made him sad in front of three people who are fond of him (*she-ohavim oto*). The printed version simply mandates that one should have the dream interpreted in the presence of three people, without any further specification. In the second zoharic context mentioned above, the interpretation of the dream that ensues from recounting it before a friend is explained theosophically as fostering the perfection of the "supernal mystery" through the unification of will (*re'uta*) or thought (*maḥashavah*) and speech (*millah*), which correspond respectively to *Ḥokhmah*, "the commencement of everything" (*sheruta de-khola*), and *Malkhut*, "the termination of everything" (*siyyuma de-khola*). See Tishby, *Wisdom*, p. 823. For an attempt to interpret this passage in a Jungian fashion, see Sanford L. Drob, *Kabbalistic Visions: C. G. Jung and Jewish Mysticism* (New Orleans: Spring Journal Books, 2010), pp. 216–17, 293 n. 58.

30. Babylonian Talmud, Berakhot 19a.

31. Jacob of Marvège, *She'elot u-Teshuvot min ha-Shamayim*, edited by Reuven Margaliot (Jerusalem: Mosad ha-Rav Kook, 1957), sec. 22, pp. 61–62. For a different translation and brief analysis, see Harris, *Studies*, pp. 18–19.

32. Babylonian Talmud, Berakhot 55b. The full dictum of R. Yoḥanan is that three types of dream are fulfilled: a dream that comes in the morning, a dream dreamt about a person by a friend, and a dream that is interpreted within a dream. Oppenheim, "The Interpretation of Dreams," p. 205, mentions this talmudic passage together with a stele from the neo-Babylonian king Nabonidus in which there is a report of a dream in which another dream is reported and interpreted, as well as a passage from the Assyrian Dream Book preserved in the library of Assurbanipal (see pp. 305–306 n. 229), as evidence of the phenomenon of a dream occurring within a dream. See also Caillois, "Logical," p. 38, and Weiss, "'What This One Interpreted for Me,'" pp. 67–69.

33. Alexander, "Bavli Berakhot," p. 234, assumes that the common denominator, which guarantees the authenticity of the three kinds of dream mentioned by R. Yoḥanan, is "the distance or disassociation of the dreamer's mind from the content of the dream or from its outcome."

34. Steven M. Oberhelman, "Dreams in Graeco-Roman Medicine," *Aufstieg und Niedergang der römischen Welt* II.37.1 (1993): 124–25.

35. Maimonides, *Guide*, II.43, p. 391.

36. Babylonian Talmud, Pesaḥim 120b, Ta'anit 12b, Megillah 18b, Yevamot 54a, Niddah 63a.

37. Blanchot, *Friendship*, p. 141.

38. Stern, *Midrash and Theory*, pp. 22–23. The converse to this argument is offered by Hasan-Rokem, *Web of Life*, p. 98: "In principle, a dream has multiple meanings.... Unlike the riddle, therefore, it does not invite one single solution but a more complex interpretation. The authors of Midrash...held strong views concerning the limits of dream interpretation and its legitimate sources."

39. Emmanuel Levinas, "The Jewish Understanding of Scripture," *Cross Currents* 44 (1994): 497. For a different rendering, see Emmanuel Levinas, *Beyond the Verse: Talmudic Readings and Lectures*, translated by Gary D. Mole (London: Athlone, 1994), p. 110.

40. The point, which has been made by various scholars, is summarized succinctly by Samuel C. Wheeler III, *Deconstruction as Analytic Philosophy* (Stanford: Stanford University Press, 2000), p. 141.

41. Babylonian Talmud, Berakhot 55b. See Weiss, "'Twenty-Four Dream-Interpreters,'" pp. 39–40, 44–46.

42. Alexander, "Bavli Berakhot," p. 236 n. 13, remarks that the "possibility

of giving multiple interpretations to a dream text was not unknown in antiquity" (he mentions the example of the fifth-century sophist Antiphon cited by Cicero in *De divinatione* II, 70), but he finds no parallel to the idea that "the interpretation activates the meaning of the dream, still less that the various interpretations will all come to pass."

43. The radicalness of the rabbinic conviction may be seen from the comment in *Maḥzor Viṭry* that specifies that only the first interpretation of the dream is binding, a stipulation that became a generally accepted rule. See Trachtenberg, *Jewish Magic*, p. 236, and references cited on p. 310 n. 11.

44. Alexander, "Bavli Berakhot," pp. 234–35.

45. Palestinian Talmud, Ma'aser Sheni 4:12, 55b; Babylonian Talmud, Giṭṭin 52a; Sanhedrin 30a; Horayot 13b. For discussion of this idiom, see Yehuda Shaviv, "The Words of Dreams Do Not Raise Up or Bring Down," *Sinai* 111 (1993): 174–77 (Hebrew).

46. *Midrash Bere'shit Rabba* 68:12, p. 784; *Midrash Eikhah Rabbah* 1:18.

47. Alexander, "Bavli Berakhot," p. 236. My account of the rabbinic understanding of dream interpretation can be profitably compared to the depiction of Ibn al-'Arabī in the passage from *Futūḥāt al-makkiyya*, translated in William C. Chittick, *The Sufi Path of Knowledge: Ibn al-'Arabi's Metaphysics of Imagination* (Albany: State University of New York Press, 1989), p. 119: "Reporting (*ikhbār*) about things is called 'expression' (*'ibāra*) and interpreting dreams is called 'interpretation' (*ta'bīr*). This is because the expresser/interpreter 'crosses over' (*'ubūr*) by means of what he says. In other words, by means of his words he passes (*jawāz*) from the presence (*ḥaḍra*) of his own self to the self of the listener. Hence he transfers his words from imagination to imagination, since the listener imagines to the extent of his understanding. Imagination may or may not coincide (*taṭābuq*) with imagination, that is, the imagination of the speaker with that of the listener. If it coincides, this is called his 'understanding' (*fahm*); if it does not coincide, he has not understood." For a deconstructionist reading of this text to proffer the idea of interpretation as a "point of embarkation" as opposed to a "matter of extraction," see Ian Almond, *Sufism and Deconstruction: A Comparative Study of Derrida and Ibn 'Arabi* (London: Routledge, 2004), p. 80.

48. Sarah Kofman, *Nietzsche and Metaphor*, translated by Duncan Large (Stanford: Stanford University Press, 1993), p. 144.

49. James L. Kugel, "Two Introductions to Midrash," in *Midrash and Literature*, edited by Geoffrey H. Hartman and Sanford Budick (New Haven: Yale University Press, 1986), pp. 83–84 (emphasis in the original).

50. John Felstiner, "'*Ziv*, That Light': Translation and Tradition in Paul Celan," *in The Craft of Translation*, edited by John Biguenet and Rainer Schulte

(Chicago: University of Chicago Press, 1989), p. 93. Celan's coinage is based on the etymological meaning of *translatio*, to carry over or to transport to the other side. Every act of interpretation is a translation of thought into language. For the historical background, see Jean Grondin, "The Task of Hermeneutics in Ancient Philosophy," in *Proceedings of Boston Area Colloquium in Ancient Philosophy, Volume* VIII *1992*, edited by John J. Cleary (Lanham: University Press of America, 1994), pp. 211–230, esp. 219–21.

51. For an attempt to distinguish the interpretative approach to dreams in the rabbinic material and the prophetic approach of the biblical accounts, see Devorah Schoenfeld, "Madness and Prophecy: Dreams, Texts, and the Power of Rabbinic Interpretation," *Pastoral Psychology* 56 (2007): pp. 223–35.

52. The more conventional delineation is found in *Mishnat Rabbi Eli'ezer*, which contains thirty-two rules of scriptural interpretation accredited to R. Eliezer ben Yose ha-Galili.

53. *Midrash ha-Gadol on Genesis*, edited by Mordecai Margulies (Jerusalem: Mosad ha-Rav Kook, 1975), "Introduction," p. 39. The text is cited by Lieberman, *Hellenism*, p. 70, at the beginning of his discussion of the similarity between the methods of dream interpretation and the hermeneutical principles of textual study.

54. Babylonian Talmud, Berakhot 56a.

55. Babylonian Talmud, Berakhot 57b. See Chapter. 2 n. 20.

56. Judah he-Ḥasid, *Sefer Ḥasidim*, sec. 382, pp. 116–17. For an alternative translation and analysis of this passage, see Harris, *Studies*, pp. 20–22. On the role of dreams in the German Pietism, see Monford Harris, "Dreams in Sefer Hasidim," *Proceedings of the American Academy of Jewish Research* 31 (1963): 51–80, and *idem*, *Studies*, pp. 15–38; Joseph Dan, "On the Teaching Concerning the Dream in Ḥasidei Ashkenaz," *Sinai* 68 (1971): 288–93 (Hebrew); Tamar Alexander, "Dream Narratives in 'Sefer Hasidim,'" *Trumah* 12 (2002): 65–78 (Hebrew); Annelies Kuyt, "Hasidut Ashkenaz on the Angel of Dreams: A Heavenly Messenger Reflecting or Exchanging Man's Thoughts," in *Creation and Re-Creation in Jewish Thought: Festschrift in Honor of Joseph Dan on the Occasion of his Seventieth Birthday*, edited by Rachel Elior and Peter Schäfer (Tübingen: Mohr Siebeck, 2005), pp. 147–63. See also the studies of Alexander-Frizer and Idel cited in Chapter 2 n. 23. The views expressed by the pietists should be considered in light of the surmise of Le Goff, *The Medieval Imagination*, p. 234, that in the twelfth century there was an extension of the privilege of dreaming meaningful dreams to any Christian and not limited to the elite. After having completed this manuscript, a copy of Jean-Claude Schmitt, *The Conversion of Herman the Jew: Autobiography, History, and Fiction in the Twelfth Century*,

translated by Alex J. Novikoff (Philadelphia: University of Pennsylvania Press, 2010), came to my attention. In the third chapter of that study, the author draws interesting parallels between Jewish and Christian approaches to the dream and its interpretation.

57. See the passage in Babylonian Talmud, Berakhot 55b, according to which Rava is said to have resolved an apparent textual conflict between "I will speak with him in a dream" (Number 12:6) and "And dreamers speak lies" (Zechariah 10:2) by asserting that the former refers to dreams revealed through an angel and the latter to dreams revealed through a demon. The rabbinic statement accords with the Stoic view that divination comes from the gods or from the demons. See Harry A. Wolfson, *Philo: Foundations of Religious Philosophy in Judaism, Christianity, and Islam*, 2 vols. (Cambridge: Harvard University Press, 1947), 2:55, and references to primary and secondary sources cited in n. 1 *ad locum*. Regarding this typological classification of dreams in pagan and Christian sources, see also Le Goff, *The Medieval Imagination*, pp. 202 and 212. Urbach, *The Sages*, p. 165, attempts to explain the different dicta associated with Rava by referring to an idea expressed in Zoroastrian and Plotinian sources: the demon is a result of one's own life. This distinction, which prevailed through many generations, is the basis of the analysis of dreams in Yehudah Pedaya, *Minḥat Yehudah* (Jerusalem, 1990), pp. 17 and 61–70. Some of the relevant passages are translated and discussed in Harris, *Studies*, pp. 65–80, and see Yoram Bilu, "Sigmund Freud and Rabbi Yehudah: On a Jewish Mystical Tradition of 'Psychoanalytic' Dream Interpretation," *The Journal of Psychological Anthropology* 2 (1979): 443–63. See also Miller, *Dreams*, pp. 63–64, who mentions the talmudic passage in the larger context of discussing dreams and angels in the literature of late antiquity.

58. Babylonian Talmud, Berakhot 55b; see Chapter 4 at n. 18.

59. Compare Eleazar ben Judah of Worms, *Ḥokhmat ha-Nefesh* (Jerusalem: Sodei Razayya, 2006), pp. 5–7. Eleazar explains that there is no dream that is not partially false, since the dream consists of the thoughts of a person's heart, and no one's thoughts are completely truthful. See *ibid.*, p. 24.

60. See Wolfson, *Through a Speculum*, pp. 206 and 209–14, to which many more sources could have been added. See also Sirat, *Les théories*, pp. 96–104, and Kuyt, "Hasidut Ashkenaz," pp. 151–55. My approach, as I have explicitly stated on numerous occasions in my publications, is indebted to the imaginal angelology developed in the works of Corbin. See Chapter 4 n. 92. For a contemporary articulation of a similar view, which also betrays the Corbinian influence, see David L. Miller, "Theologia Imaginalis," in *The Archaeology of the Imagination*, edited by Charles E. Winquist, *Journal of the American Academy*

of Religion Thematic Studies 48, no. 2 (1981): 1–18, esp. 13–14.

61. Wolfson, *Through a Speculum*, pp. 198–203 and 206–207, and see especially the reference to the study of Asi Farber-Ginat cited there, p. 206 n. 65. For an interesting essay that presents a different approach to the visionary aspects of German Pietism, albeit without any specific reference to dreams, see Natasha Esther Zabolotnaya, "Cosmology and Color Symbolism in R. Eleazar of Worms," *Kabbalah: Journal for the Study of Jewish Mystical Texts* 12 (2004): 45–80.

62. Eleazar ben Judah of Worms, *Ḥokhmat ha-Nefesh*, p. 60. Needless to say, many more passages could have been mentioned, because this theme is repeated often in the pietistic corpus.

63. *Ibid.*, pp. 14, 24–25, 42.

64. Wolfson, *Through a Speculum*, pp. 209–11.

65. In *Sefer Ḥasidim*, sec. 1521, p. 373, the verse "the dream comes with much brooding" (Ecclesiastes 5:2) is cited in conjunction with the rabbinic maxim "words of dreams are of no consequence." See above, nn. 45–46.

66. A related topic, which I will not explore in detail in this book, is the correlation of one's astrological sign and the nature of one's dreams. See, for example, the passage from Abraham Ibn Ezra's *Sefer ha-Moladot* cited in Almoli, *Pitron Ḥalomot*, 10b. Almoli does not reject this perspective, but he qualifies it by saying that these factors increase the probability of a particular outcome, but they do not necessitate it.

67. See above, n. 41.

68. *Sefer Ḥasidim*, sec. 1522, p. 373.

69. Babylonian Talmud, Sanhedrin 34a.

70. Babylonian Talmud, Shabbat 63a, Yevamot 11b, 24a.

71. Abulafia, *Sheva Netivot ha-Torah*, p. 13. For discussion of the sevenfold exegetical method in Abulafia's kabbalah, see Moshe Idel, *Language, Torah, and Hermeneutics in Abraham Abulafia* (Albany: State University of New York Press,1989), pp. 82–124; *idem*, *Kabbalah: New Perspectives*, pp. 235–36; *idem*, *Absorbing Perfections: Kabbalah and Interpretation* (New Haven: Yale University Press, 2002), pp. 263–64,'269–70, 431–32. See also Wolfson, *Abraham Abulafia*, pp. 76–78, 107–108.

72. Babylonian Talmud, Sanhedrin 92b, and see Raphael Loewe, "The 'Plain' Meaning of Scripture in Early Jewish Exegesis," *Papers of the Institute of Jewish Studies* 1 (1964): 172–75, and Boyarin, *Sparks of the Logos*, pp. 92–93. The position taken by Boyarin is close to the view I proffered independently in *Language, Eros, Being*, pp. 335–36, with respect to the Song of Songs being commensurate with the entire Torah, since it is the biblical book whose literal

meaning is figurative. Thus, we can speak of the Song of Songs as the paradigm that paradigmatically signifies the nature of the paradigm and thereby illumines more generally the poetic nature of Torah as the revealed word of God. See also Elliot R. Wolfson, "Suffering Eros and Textual Incarnation: A Kristevan Reading of Kabbalistic Poetics," in *Toward a Theology of Eros: Transfiguring Passion at the Limits of Discipline*, edited by Virginia Burrus and Catherine Keller (New York: Fordham University Press, 2006), pp. 346–52. Boyarin, *Sparks of the Logos*, pp. 94 and 102–104, also notes the interpretive status of the Song of Songs connected to its inherent parabolic status. See also *ibid.*, pp. 157–59. On the relationship of "parable" and "truth" with respect to the belief in the resurrection of the dead, see the comments of Maimonides, *Ma'amar Teḥiyyat ha-Metim*, p. 357.

73. See especially, Abulafia, *Ḥayyei ha-Nefesh*, pp. 47–48, and *idem*, *Mafteaḥ ha-Ḥokhmot* (Jerusalem, 2001), p. 44.

74. Maimonides, *Guide*, "Introduction," pp. 11–12.

75. *Ibid.*, III.32, p. 525.

76. *Ibid.*, I.26, p. 56; I.29, p. 62; I.33, p. 71; I.46, p. 100; I.53, p. 120; I.59, p. 140; III.13, p. 453. See also Maimonides, *Ma'amar Teḥiyyat ha-Metim*, p. 347. The rabbinic maxim in its original setting signifies the view of the school of Ishmael, in contrast to the school of Aqiva, that redundancy in biblical verses should not be interpreted, since the Torah uses the rhetorical practices of human beings. See Babylonian Talmud, Berakhot 31b, Yevamot 27a, Baba Meṣi'a 31b; Abraham J. Heschel, *Heavenly Torah as Refracted through the Generations*, edited and translated by Gordon Tucker and Leonard Levin (New York: Continuum, 2005), pp. 47–49. In the medieval philosophical literature, this maxim was applied more specifically to explain anthropomorphic and anthropopathic representations of God in Scripture.

77. For the expression "true figures" I am indebted to Wheeler, *Deconstruction*, pp. 116–36. See also the citation of Nietzsche in Chapter 4 at n. 103.

78. See Moshe Idel, *The Mystical Experience in Abraham Abulafia* (Albany: State University of New York Press, 1988), pp. 140, 200–201; *idem*, *Language, Torah, and Hermeneutics*, pp. 28 and 159 n. 147.

79. Babylonian Talmud, Baba Meṣi'a 3b, and compare the commentary of Rashi to Babylonian Talmud, Yevamot 25b, s.v. *we-ein adam mesim*.

80. Abraham Abulafia, *Sefer ha-Edut*, in *Maṣref ha-Sekhel* (Jerusalem, 2001), p. 58. On the status of the secret and the dialectic of concealment and disclosure in Abulafia, see Wolfson, *Abraham Abulafia*, pp. 52–93. For a different approach to Abulafian esotericism, which is predicated on a more emphatic contrast between innovative and conservative tendencies, see Idel, *Kabbalah:*

New Perspectives, pp. 215–16 and 253–55; *idem, Absorbing Perfections*, pp. 398 and 400–402.

81. See above, n. 21.

82. Based on the dictum of Ameimar in Babylonian Talmud, Baba Batra 12a. See Alon Goshen-Gottstein, "'The Sage is Superior to the Prophet': The Conception of Torah through the Prism of the History of Jewish Exegesis," in *Study and Knowledge in Jewish Thought*, vol. 2, edited by Howard Kreisel (Beer Sheva: Ben-Gurion University of the Negev Press, 2006), pp. 37–77 (Hebrew); Elliot R. Wolfson, "'Sage is Preferable to Prophet': Revisioning Midrashic Imagination," in *Scriptural Exegesis: The Shapes of Culture and the Religious Imagination: A Festschrift in Honor of Michael Fishbane*, edited by Deborah A. Green and Laura S. Lieber (Oxford: Oxford University Press, 2008), pp. 186–210.

83. *Zohar* 1:183a–b. On the importance of the dream as a means by which the human can access the supernal realm and learn of the divine intention, see Elijah de Vidas, *Re'shit Ḥokhmah ha-Shalem*, 3 vols. (Jerusalem, 1984), Sha'ar ha-Ahavah, ch. 6, 1:471.

84. See below, n. 96.

85. To be precise, the opinion expressed in this passage, which is exhibited elsewhere in zoharic literature and in other kabbalistic texts, is that prophecy originates in the seventh and eight emanations, *Neṣaḥ* and *Hod*, but these are visible only through the intermediary of *Shekhinah*, the speculum that does not shine. See Wolfson, *Through a Speculum*, p. 352 n. 87.

86. See above, n. 55.

87. *Zohar* 1:183a. Compare *Zohar* 1:238a; Tishby, *Wisdom*, p. 812. On the designation of Gabriel as the angel appointed over dreams, see *Galya Razya*, edited by Rachel Elior (Jerusalem: Hebrew University, 1981), p. 16 (introduction), also cited in Elior, "Reality," p. 66; Karo, *Maggid Mesharim*, p. 2. In the latter context, Gabriel is said to dispense dreams even to the nations of the world. On the characterization of Gabriel as the angel appointed over the archons of the nations, see Eleazar ben Judah of Worms, *Sodei Razayya* (Tel-Aviv, 2004), p. 76. Related to this motif is the tradition in the Babylonian Talmud, Soṭah 33a, that Gabriel taught Joseph—the master of dreams par excellence—the seventy languages of humanity. See Heschel, *Prophetic Inspiration*, p. 5 n. 7.

88. Tishby, *Wisdom*, p. 825 n. 87.

89. *Zohar* 1:149a, 149b; Moses de León, *Shushan Edut*, edited by Gershom Scholem, "Shenei Quntresim le-R. Moshe di Li'on," *Qoveṣ al Yad* 8 (1976): 369; *The Book of the Pomegranate: Moses de León's Sefer ha-Rimmon*, edited by Elliot R. Wolfson (Atlanta: Scholars Press, 1988), p. 126 (Hebrew section).

90. Joseph Angeleṭ, *Livnat ha-Sappir* (Jerusalem, 1913), 43a. It is of interest

to note that after offering this explanation to the zoharic text, Angeleṭ writes *u-varukh yode'a ha-emet*, "and bless the one who knows the truth," a stipulation that indicates uncertainty about his own surmise. The passage of Angeleṭ is referred to in Meir Ibn Gabbai, *Avodat ha-Qodesh* (Jerusalem: Shevilei Orḥot ha-Ḥayyim, 1992), 4.27, p. 493.

91. This grouping of the six archangels, which constitute the camp of *Shekhinah*, may also be related to the motif of the six steps of the throne (linked exegetically to 1 Kings 10:19), since the latter is one of the symbolic names of the divine presence. See *Tiqqunei Zohar*, edited by Reuven Margaliot (Jerusalem: Mosad ha-Rav Kook, 1978), sec. 18, 31b. If the connection between the six archangels and the six steps of the throne is correct, then Gabriel would correspond to the phallic potency of *Yesod*. Consider the tradition recorded by Joseph ben Shalom Ashkenazi, *Perush Sefer Yeṣirah*, in *Sefer Yeṣirah* (Jerusalem: Yeshivat Kol Yehuda, 1990), p. 19, that Gabriel was the master of Joseph, identified parenthetically as *Yesod*. Based on this passage, Ya'aqov Ṣevi Yalles, *Qehillat Ya'aqov* (Lemberg, 1870), s.v. *gavri'el*, 28a, wrote, "Gabriel is the aspect of *Yesod* for he was the master of Joseph." The matter is repeated in the section that includes the additions to the text, *Qehillat Ya'aqov*, s.v. *yosef*. By contrast, see *Qehillat Ya'aqov*, s.v. *gemara*, 1d, where Gabriel is paired with *Hod* and Uriel with *Yesod*. It is of interest to note, finally, that, according to the aforementioned passage from the *Tiqqunim*, the six steps are hinted at in the letters *samekh* and *waw* (the numerical value of which is 66) in the word *yesod* (made up of the letters *yod*, *samekh*, *waw*, and *dalet*). See *Tiqqunei Zohar*, sec. 18, 35b.

92. See Henry Corbin, *Temple and Contemplation*, translated by Philip Sherrard, with the assistance of Liadain Sherrard (London: KPI Limited, 1986), p. 272, and the sources recorded by Gershom Scholem, *Devils, Demons, and Souls: Essays on Demonology by Gershom Scholem*, edited by Esther Liebes (Jerusalem: Ben-Zvi Institute, 2004), p. 126 n. 40 (Hebrew). In addition to the passage from *Sidrei de-Shimusha Rabba*, which Scholem thought was a pseudepigraphic work composed by kabbalists in southern France in the late twelfth or early thirteenth century, he mentioned Judah Halevi, Abraham Ibn Daud, Moses of Burgos, and Baḥya ben Asher. It goes without saying that the special status of Gabriel in the Muslim tradition is also enhanced by this angel's visionary encounter with Muḥammad, the primary revelation that is traditionally understood as the means of inspiration by which the Qur'ān was produced. For an evaluation of this well-known dogma in light of other accounts of dreams in early Islamic literature, see Nile Green, "The Religious and Cultural Roles of Dreams and Visions in Islam," *Journal of the Royal Asiatic Society* 13 (2003): 289–90. See also Lory, *Le rêve*, pp. 29–53, and other references cited in Chapter 4 n. 49.

93. Compare Yiṣḥaq Isaac Ḥaver, *Beit Olamim* (Warsaw, 1889), 132b: "Thus Gabriel, who comes from the aspect of judgment, is the one appointed to explain the vision of prophecy." In the continuation of the passage, Ḥaver explicates the zoharic contrast of prophecy from the world of the masculine and the dream from the world of the feminine (see below, n. 97).

94. Following the reading in the Mantua text and all subsequent editions based on it; in the Cremona text, the words *we-ḥelma bi-semo'la* ("and the dream is on the left"), are missing.

95. *Mitparsha*, which can also be translated as "explicated." See below, n. 105.

96. *Zohar* 1:149a. The view expressed in this passage was interpreted in various ways by the anonymous kabbalist responsible for what are considered to be the later strata of zoharic literature, *Ra'aya Meheimna* and *Tiqqunei Zohar*. In *Zohar* 3:222b (*Ra'aya Meheimna*), the author distinguishes the expressions "vision" (*mar'ah*) and "dream" (*ḥalom*) in Numbers 12:6 by correlating the former with the speculum that shines (*Tif'eret* or *Yesod*) and the latter with the speculum that does not shine (*Shekhinah*). Even more intriguing is the interpretation of the same verse in *Zohar* 3:280b (*Ra'aya Meheimna*), according to which the "vision" is identified as the "supernal mother" (*ima illa'ah*), a symbolic designation of *Binah*, and the "dream" as the final *he* of the Tetragrammaton, one of the standard semantic markers for *Shekhinah*. The former is linked to prophecy, the "vision of the open eyes" (*mar'ah bi-fetiḥu de-ayyenin*), which occurs when one is awake (*mar'eh ve-haqiṣ*), and the latter to the "vision of the dream" (*mar'eh va-ḥalom*), which is envisioned "through the closing of the eyes" (*bi-setimu de-ayyenin*) when one is asleep, and thus it is called the "speculum that does not shine." For a related, but somewhat varied explanation, see *The Hebrew Writings of the Author of Tiqqunei Zohar and Ra'aya Mehemna*, edited and annotated by Efraim Gottlieb (Jerusalem: Israel Academy of Sciences, 2003), p. 36 (Hebrew): "*Binah* is the Written Torah given from the right, and it is the prophetic dream [*nevu'ah va-ḥalom*], *Malkhut* is the Oral Torah given from the left, and it is the wakeful prophecy [*nevu'ah ve-haqiṣ*]." Also noteworthy is a passage from *Tiqqunei Zohar*, sec. 18, 31b, wherein *Shekhinah* is designated as both "imagination" (*dimyon*) and vision (*mar'eh*), and the latter is distinguished further as the "vision of the dream" (*mar'eh va-ḥalom*) when the eyes are closed (*setimu de-ayyenin*) [for an interesting variant *bi-setira de-ayyenin*, see MS University of Toronto, Friedberg 5-015, fol. 26a] and as the "wakeful vision" (*mar'eh ve-haqiṣ*) when the eyes are opened (*petiḥu de-ayyenin*). See the paraphrase of this passage in Yalles, *Qehillat Ya'aqov*, s.v. *mar'eh ve-haqiṣ*, 5d: "This *Malkhut* is called the vision of the dream in the closing of the eyes ... for from the aspect of

Tif'eret she is called a wakeful vision and from the aspect of *Yesod* she is called a dream vision." The matter of the open and closed eyes in zoharic texts, which probably served as the exegetical basis for the author of the aforementioned passages from the *Ra'aya Meheimna* and *Tiqqunim*, are discussed in Wolfson, *Through a Speculum*, pp. 380–83. On the symbolic association of *mar'eh* (or *mar'ah*) and *Shekhinah*, see *Tiqqunei Zohar*, sec. 53, 87b. See also Joseph ben Shalom Ashkenazi, *A Kabbalistic Commentary*, p. 220, where the source of both prophetic visions and nocturnal dreams (specified in Numbers 12:6) is identified as the imaginative faculty (*koaḥ ha-medammeh*) that is in *Malkhut*.

97. On this technical terminology, see Elliot R. Wolfson, *Circle in the Square: Studies in the Use of Gender in Kabbalistic Symbolism* (Albany: State University of New York Press, 1995), pp. 89, 99, 103, and reference to Scholem given on p. 205 n. 47.

98. Alternately, Angeleṭ, *Livnat ha-Sappir*, 43a, explained that Gabriel comes forth from *Shekhinah*, which is also associated with the left side.

99. See Chapter 2 n. 21.

100. The Hebrew is *bishshul*, literally "cooking," but it can also connote the ripening of fruit on the vine.

101. De León, *Shushan Edut*, p. 369.

102. *Ibid.*

103. Compare de León, *Shushan Edut*, p. 337; *R. Moses de Leon's Sefer Sheqel ha-Qodesh*, critically edited and introduced by Charles Mopsik (Los Angeles: Cherub Press, 1996), pp. 47–48 (Hebrew); and *R. Moses de Leon's Commentary to Ezekiel's Chariot*, edited by Asi Farber-Ginat and Daniel Abrams (Los Angeles: Cherub Press, 1998), p. 69 (Hebrew). On the identification of *Neṣaḥ* and *Hod* as the source whence the prophets were sustained, see Joseph Gikatilla, *Sha'arei Ṣedeq* (Cracow: Fischer & Deutscher, 1881), 15b; *idem*, *Sha'arei Orah*, edited with introduction and notes by Joseph Ben Shlomo, 2 vols. (Jerusalem: Bialik Institute, 1981), 1:149, 158–59, 160, 161, and compare Roland Goetschel, "The Conception of Prophecy in the Works of R. Moses de Leon and R. Joseph Gikatilla," *Jerusalem Studies in Jewish Thought* 8 (1989): 217–37, esp. 222–23 (Hebrew).

104. That is, the word *mar'eh* occurs four times in Ezekiel 43:3, and the word *mar'ot* occurs once, but since it is a plural, it minimally refers to a sum of at least two, which added to the four equals six.

105. Translating the reading of the Mantua text *mitparshin*; the Cremona edition has the variant *mitpashṭei*, which does not alter the meaning. It is possible, however, that the Mantua text preserves as well the connotation of "explicated."

106. *Zohar* 1:196a.

107. Regarding this numerology, see Jacob bar Asher, *Perush Ba'al ha-Ṭurim al ha-Torah* (Benei Beraq, 1985), p. 182 (*ad* Exodus 25:9), and the manuscript sources cited in *Tosafot ha-Shalem: Commentary on the Bible*, vol. 9, edited by Jacob Gellis (Jerusalem: Harry Fischel Institute, 1993), p. 26 (Hebrew). See below n. 113.

108. Gikatilla, *Sha'arei Orah*, 1:248. For elaborate discussion and analysis of other texts, see Wolfson, *Through a Speculum*, pp. 306–17.

109. Moses Cordovero, *Pardes Rimmonim* (Jerusalem, 1962), 23:8, 17b: "The angel Gabriel is called the night vision, that is, the vision in which the matter of *Malkhut*, which is called night, is seen."

110. To behold *Shekhinah* in a dream vision is not always accorded a positive valence. See Moses de León, "Sefer ha-Mishkal: Text and Study," edited by Jochanan H. A. Wijnhoven, Ph.D. dissertation, Brandeis University, 1964, p. 99: "The secret of the blue [*tekhelet*] is that it is a throne for the encompassing throne of David, and it is [the secret] of the consuming attribute of judgment... and concerning this matter the sages, blessed be their memory, said 'All colors are pleasing in a dream except blue' [Babylonian Talmud, Berakhot 57b], for according to its secret and its comportment, it prevails to destroy the enemies of God... and those who transgress his law." The text of de León has a parallel in *Zohar* 1:51b, and compare 1:256a, 2:135a, 139a, and the passage from the *Piqqudin* stratum in 3:175a.

111. *Zohar* 1:149a.

112. *Zohar* 1:149b.

113. The symbolic image appears frequently in zoharic texts and the works of Moses de León. See, for instance, MS Munich 47, fol. 338b. Compare Abraham Abulafia, *Ḥayyei ha-Olam ha-Ba*, p. 149: Gabriel is described both as the angel who instructs one about the "secret of the Tetragrammaton" (*sod yhwh*) and who makes visible the "wonders of prophecy" (*nifla'ot ha-nevu'ah*). Interpreting the verse "When a prophet of the Lord arises among you, I make myself known to him in a vision, I speak with him in a dream" (Numbers 12:6), Abulafia associates "vision" (*mar'ah*) with Gabriel (both equal 246) and "dream" (*ḥalom*) with Edi (derived from Job 16:19), who is Enoch (the words *ḥalom*, *edi*, and *ḥanokh* all have the numerical value of 84), the figure who ascended and was transformed into Metatron. This passage is cited and discussed in Idel, *The Mystical Experience*, p. 89. The vocalization "edo" is incorrect, but see p. 153 n. 86, where the correct form "edi" is given, although the numerology there needs to be amended from 74 to 84. Idel points out that the identification of Gabriel and the vision is found in the commentary on *Sefer Yeṣirah* by Abulafia's teacher,

Baruch Togarmi (the relevant extract is cited by Idel, *The Mystical Experience*, p. 88). See Abulafia, *Sefer Ḥayyei ha-Olam ha-Ba*, p. 90, where the secret of the "vision of prophecy" (*mar'eh ha-nevu'ah*) is linked to the name Shaddai, a name that is connected to Metatron (both equal 314), the archon of the face (*sar ha-panim*), who is also identified as Yefifiah, the archon of the Torah (*sar ha-torah*) and the archon of the world (*saro shel olam*), Geliṣur, Galya Razya, and Raziel. The litany of names constitutes Abulafia's mystical recasting of the Maimonidean theory of prophecy as the conjunction of the human intellect and the Active Intellect. See Scholem, *Major Trends*, pp. 138–39 and 143–44; Idel, *The Mystical Experience*, pp. 116–19 and 125–32. On the connection between Metatron and dreams, see Viṭal, *Sefer ha-Pe'ulot*, p. 12.

114. *Zohar* 1:191b. A likely source for this zoharic homily may have been the retelling of the scriptural narrative in *Pirqei Rabbi Eli'ezer* (Warsaw, 1852), ch. 39, 82b, wherein it is emphasized that Joseph interpreted the dream of Pharaoh when the holy spirit dwelt upon him, an idea supported exegetically by Genesis 41:38. Compare the reworking of the verse in Qur'ān 12:101.

115. Ḥayyim Viṭal, *Liqquṭei Torah* (Jerusalem: Yeshivat Kol Yehuda, 1995), p. 104. Compare *idem*, *Sha'ar ha-Pesuqim* (Jerusalem: Yeshivat Qol Yehudah, 1995), pp. 91–92. See the text of Dov Baer Schneersohn mentioned in Chapter 4 n. 177 and the passage of Valle cited in Chapter 5 at n. 84.

116. Alan Brill, *Thinking God: The Mysticism of Rabbi Zadok of Lublin* (New York: Yeshiva University Press, 2002), pp. 127–28, incorrectly assumed that in this passage R. Ṣadoq was citing from the *Liqquṭei Torah* of Shneur Zalman of Liadi. I surmise that the mistake was caused by his decoding the reference in R. Ṣadoq to the triad of wisdom (*ḥokhmah*), understanding (*binah*), and knowledge (*da'at*) as an allusion to Ḥabad. On p. 127 n. 121, Brill even calls the reader's attention to the section on *wa-yeshev* (Genesis 37:1–40:23) in Shneur Zalman of Liadi's *Liqquṭei Torah*, but in fact, that work does not contain homilies on the book of Genesis (as we find, for example, in the collection *Torah Or*). R. Ṣadoq is actually citing the work of Viṭal by the same name (see the previous note); the remark about *ḥokhmah*, *binah*, and *da'at* is not a technical designation of Ḥabad, but a demarcation of the three states of expanded consciousness. Notwithstanding Brill's error, there are interesting parallels between the approaches of Shneur Zalman (and the Lubavitch masters more generally) and R. Ṣadoq to the dream phenomenon and the role of imagination to combine truth and untruth, but this is not the place to elaborate. For citation of some of the relevant sources, see Chapter 5 at nn. 223 and 225.

117. Ṣadoq ha-Kohen of Lublin, *Ṣidqat ha-Ṣaddiq* (Jerusalem: Makhon Har Berakhah, 2005), p. 110.

118. Many scholars have written on this phenomenon. For a recent study that engages some of the previous scholarship, see Moshe Idel, "Prayer, Ecstasy, and 'Alien Thoughts' in the Religious Experience of the Besht," in *Let the Old Make Way for the New: Studies in the Social and Cultural History of Eastern European Jewry Presented to Immanuel Etkes*, edited by David Assaf and Ada Rapoport-Albert, vol. 1: *Hasidism and the Musar Movement* (Jerusalem: The Zalman Shazar Center for Jewish History, 2009), pp. 57–120 (Hebrew).

119. Ricoeur, *Freud and Philosophy*, pp. 88–102. On the hermeneutics of the dream life, see Ferguson, *Lure of Dreams*, pp. 61–90.

120. Freud, *Interpretation of Dreams*, p. 334. Reference to the German text is based on Sigmund Freud, *Gesammelte Werke*, Band II/III (London: Imago Publishing, 1948), p. 518. In the Strachey translation, *Interpretation of Dreams*, p. 514, the critical expression *einen heiligen Text* is rendered as "Holy Writ." Freud's comparison of the dream to a text does imply the presumption of a general meaning, but not at the expense of the specific case histories. Just as a text's meaning will reflect the situation of the particular interpreter, so the meaning of the dream images has to be calibrated in accord with the individual dreamer's existential conditions.

121. Freud, *Interpretation of Dreams*, p. 247.

122. Jung, *Dream Analysis*, p. 457. Jung goes on to say that he influenced Freud to use the concept of "image" in analyzing the content of dreams.

123. Jung, *Practice of Psychotherapy*, p. 149. On the critique of Freud's notion of the dream as a façade, see *ibid.*, p. 32, and Carl G. Jung, *Aion: Researches Into the Phenomenology of Self*, 2nd edition, translated by R. F. C. Hull (Princeton: Princeton University Press, 1969), p. 203 n. 63. See also Carl G. Jung, *Memories, Dreams, Reflections*, recorded and edited by Aniela Jaffé, translated by Richard and Clara Winston (New York: Vintage Books, 1965), pp. 161–62: "I was never able to agree with Freud that the dream is a 'façade' behind which its meaning lies hidden—a meaning already known but maliciously, so to speak, withheld from consciousness. To me dreams are a part of nature, which harbors no intention to deceive, but expresses something as best it can, just as a plant grows or an animal seeks its food as best it can. These forms of life, too, have no wish to deceive our eyes, but we may deceive ourselves because our eyes are shortsighted.... Long before I met Freud I regarded the unconscious, and dreams, which are its direct exponents, as natural processes to which no arbitrariness can be attributed, and above all no legerdemain."

124. Jung, *Practice of Psychotherapy*, p. 149. See Steven Kings, "Jung's Hermeneutics of Scripture," *Journal of Religion* 77 (1997): 233–51, esp. 236–41 and 249–50.

125. Jung, *Psychology of Religion*, p. 26. For the talmudic reference, see above, n. 26.

126. Jung, *Psychology of the Unconscious*, p. 9.

127. Jung, *Alchemical Studies*, p. 301.

128. Jung, *Practice of Psychotherapy*, pp. 156–57.

129. Jung, *Alchemical Studies*, pp. 300–301.

130. Tomoko Masuzawa, *In Search of Dreamtime: The Quest for the Origins of Religion* (Chicago: University of Chicago Press, 1993), p. 12.

131. Jung, *Practice of Psychotherapy*, pp. 149–50.

132. *Midrash Shir ha-Shirim Rabbah*, edited by Shimon Dunaski (Jerusalem: Dvir, 1980), 1:52, p. 42, where the rabbis are described as stringing together (*ḥorzin*) words from the Torah, Prophets, and Writings, an idea connected to the scriptural expression *ḥaruzim*, a "string of jewels" (Song of Songs 1:10), and compare Palestinian Talmud, Ḥagigah 2:1, 77b (assuming that *ḥozrin be-divrei torah* should be corrected to *ḥorzin*, as was suggested by Wilhelm Bacher, *Die exegetische Terminologie der jüdischen Traditionsliteratur,* part 1*: Die bibelexegetische Terminologie der Tannaiten* [Leipzig: Hinrichs, 1905; reprint Darmstadt: Wissenschaftliche Buchgesellschaft, 1965], p. 65). Robert A. Paul, *Moses and Civilization: The Meaning Behind Freud's Myth* (New Haven: Yale University Press, 1996), p. 41, cites and builds upon the observation of Daniel Boyarin, *Intertextuality and the Reading of Midrash* (Bloomington: Indiana University Press, 1990), pp. 93–104, that the midrash may be compared to the "unconscious" of the biblical text. Also noteworthy is Paul's observation (pp. 228–29 n. 5) that Jacques Lacan, "Radiophonie," *Scilicet* 2/3 (1970): 81, had already called attention to the affinity between midrashic exegesis and Freud's method of interpretation. For possible Jewish influences on Freud, see below, n. 139.

133. Michael Fishbane, *The Exegetical Imagination: On Jewish Thought and Theology* (Cambridge, MA: Harvard University Press, 1998), p. 13. For a similar idea expressed in terms of the process of exemplification by the linking together of concrete images, see Boyarin, *Sparks of the Logos*, p. 99.

134. I am drawing here on the study of Martin Gliserman, *Psychoanalysis, Language, and the Body of the Text* (Gainesville: University Press of Florida,1996).

135. Alfred North Whitehead, *Science and the Modern World* (New York: Free Press, 1967), p. 51.

136. Paul Ricoeur, *Interpretation Theory: Discourse and the Surplus of Meaning* (Fort Worth: Texas Christian Press, 1976), pp. 58–59.

137. *Ibid.*, p. 59.

138. Compare the suggestion made by Jonathan Lear, *Freud* (New York:

Routledge, 2005), p. 89: "*The Interpretation of Dreams* is like the Talmud of Freudian psychoanalysis: it contains within itself a running commentary about how it should be read." For an attempt to relate the psychoanalytic approaches to dream interpretation in ancient religious cultures more broadly, see James Gollnick, *Dreams in the Psychology of Religion* (Lewiston: Edwin Mellen Press, 1987).

139. David Bakan, *Sigmund Freud and the Jewish Mystical Tradition* (Boston: Beacon Press, 1975), pp. 246–70, esp. 250–52. For other discussions comparing the Freudian and rabbinic approaches to the dream, see references cited below, n. 144. It is of interest to recall the assessment of Jung in a letter to Edith Schröder from April 1957 in Carl G. Jung, *Letters*, selected and edited by Gerhard Adler in collaboration with Aniela Jaffé, translated by R. F. C. Hull, 2 vols. (Princeton: Princeton University Press, 1973), 2:358–59: "For a real understanding of the Jewish component in Freud's outlook, a thorough knowledge would be needed of the specifically Jewish assumptions in regard to history, culture and religion. Since Freud calls for an extremely serious assessment on all these levels, one would have to take a deep plunge into the history of the Jewish mind. This would carry us beyond Jewish orthodoxy into the subterranean workings of Hasidism (e.g., the sects of Sabbatai Zwi), and then into the intricacies of the Kabbalah, which still remains unexplored psychologically." On the comparison of Jung's theories of dreams and kabbalistic approaches, see Drob, *Kabbalistic Visions*, pp. 222–25. See Chapter 4 n. 156. The more general question of the Jewish influence on Freud has been the focus of various scholarly analyses. Especially notable are the following studies: Reuben M. Rainey, *Freud as Student of Religion: Perspectives on the Background and Development of His Thought* (Missoula: Scholars Press, 1975); Marthe Robert, *From Oedipus to Moses: Freud's Jewish Identity* (London: Routledge & Kegan Paul, 1977); Justin Miller, "Interpretations of Freud's Jewishness, 1924–1974," *Journal of the History of the Behavioral Sciences* 17 (1981): 357–74; Dennis B. Klein, *Jewish Origins of the Psychoanalytic Movement* (Chicago: University of Chicago Press, 1985); Emanuel Rice, *Freud and Moses: The Long Journey Home* (Albany: State of New York Press, 1990); Yosef H. Yerushalmi, *Freud's Moses: Judaism Terminable and Interminable* (New Haven: Yale University Press, 1991); Richard J. Bernstein, *Freud and the Legacy of Moses* (Cambridge: Cambridge University Press, 1998).

140. Bakan, *Sigmund Freud*, p. 257.

141. *Ibid.*, p. 258.

142. Erich Fromm, *The Forgotten Language: An Introduction to the Understanding of Dreams, Fairy Tales, and Myths* (New York: Rinehart, 1951), p. 129.

143. A distinction along these lines is made between the traditional Muslim

oneirocriticism and psychoanalysis in John C. Lamoreaux, *The Early Muslim Tradition of Dream Interpretation* (Albany: State University Press of New York, 2002), pp. 4–5.

144. Bilu, "Sigmund Freud and Rabbi Yehudah;" Ken Frieden, *Freud's Dream of Interpretation*, foreword by Harold Bloom (Albany: State University of New York Press, 1990), pp. 73–93; *idem*, "Talmudic Dream Interpretation, Freudian Ambivalence, Deconstruction," in *The Dream and the Text*, pp. 103–11; Douglas M. Snyder, *Freud, Einstein, and Marx: The Influence of Judaism on Their Work* (Beverly Hills: Tailor Press, 1998), pp. 39–48; Murray L. Wax, "Interpreting Dreams: Joseph, Freud and the Judaic Tradition," *Journal of Psychology and Judaism* 22 (1998): 21–32; *idem*, *Western Rationality*, pp. 45–57; Miriam Huttler, "Jewish Origins of Freud's Interpretation of Dreams," *Journal of Psychology and Judaism* 23 (1999): 5–48; Sanford L. Drob, "'This Is Gold': Freud, Psychotherapy and the Lurianic Kabbalah," available at www.newkabbalah.com; Hasan-Rokem, *Web of Life*, p. 97. For a decidedly negative assessment, see Peter Gay, *A Godless Jew: Freud, Atheism, and the Masking of Psychoanalysis* (New Haven: Yale University Press, 1987). Another attempt to compare ancient Jewish dream interpretation (as mediated especially through the first part of Almoli's *Pitron Ḥalomot*) and a contemporary analytic method is made by Joel Covitz, *Visions in the Night: Jungian and Ancient Dream Interpretation*, 2nd revised edition (Toronto: Inner City Books, 2000). For a Jungian approach to dreams combined with kabbalistic imagery, see as well Lawrence Corey, "Kabbalah and the Interpretation of Dreams," in *A Modern Jew In Search of a Soul*, edited by J. Marvin Spiegelman and Abraham Jacobson (Phoenix: Falcon Press, 1986), pp. 47–84. For an application of kabbalistic teaching to the practice of dream visualization, see Catherine Shainberg, *Kabbalah and the Power of Dreaming: Awakening the Visionary Life* (Rochester: Inner Traditions, 2005), and Kamenetz, *History of Last Night's Dream*. Readers may find these works informative and even therapeutically beneficial, but they do not purport to be scholarly discussions of the interpretation of dreams according to Jewish mystical lore. In the same category, one can include the various monographs by Gerald Epstein, who proclaims himself, like Shainberg and Kamenetz, to be a disciple and translator of the teaching of Colette Aboulker-Muscat, which is based on the imaginal exercise of visualization proffered as a form of practical kabbalah (see Chapter. 1 n. 285).

145. Ricoeur, *Freud and Philosophy*, p. 15.

146. For a fuller discussion on the timeswerve and hermeneutic reversibility, see Wolfson, *Language, Eros, Being*, pp. xv–xxxi.

CHAPTER FOUR: *COINCIDENTIA OPPOSITORUM*

1. Edward S. Casey, *Imagining: A Phenomenological Study* (Bloomington: Indiana University Press, 1976), p. 211. Casey goes on to draw a more specific analogy between Freud's technique of free association and Husserl's method of free variation in the imagination.

2. This principle was formulated by Stekel, *Sex and Dreams*, pp. 139–42, as the "transposition into the opposite," or what he refers to as "symbolic parallelism" (*Gleichung*). See *ibid.*, p. 262: "*All effects in the dream are equal to each other and may substitute with one another*" (emphasis in the original). See also Harris, *Dreams and Experience*, pp. 136–39, and Foucault's account in *The History of Sexuality, Volume 3: The Care of the Self*, pp. 15–16, of the reversal of values between the dream image and its intended meaning according to Artemidorus.

3. Babylonian Talmud, Berakhot 56b. Consider the zoharic reworking of one of the rabbinic teachings from that source (see parallel with slight variants in *Midrash Tehillim*, 128:4, p. 514) that if one sees white grapes in a dream, whether in season or not, it is a good omen, whereas if one sees black grapes, if in season, it is good, and if not in season, it is bad. According to the medieval kabbalistic text, the duality is sharpened: "if one sees white grapes in a dream, it is a good sign, if black, no" (*Zohar* 1:192a).

4. Babylonian Talmud, Berakhot 56b.

5. Lieberman, *Hellenism in Jewish Palestine*, p. 71.

6. These expressions were used by Husserl in his 1936 essay "Die Frage nach dem Ursprung der Geometrie als intentional-historisches Problem," edited and published by Eugen Fink in *Revue international de Philosophie* 1 (1939): 201, and then appended as "Beilage III" in Husserl, *Die Krisis*, p. 369. The English translation appears in Husserl, *Crisis*, p. 358. For a critique of Husserl's notion of "linguistic flesh" or "linguistic incarnation" as a return to language as the "indispensable medium and condition of possibility for absolute ideal Objectivity, for truth itself," see Jacques Derrida, *Edmund Husserl's Origin of Geometry: An Introduction*, translated, with a preface and afterword, by John P. Leavey, Jr. (Lincoln: University of Nebraska Press, 1989), pp. 76–79, and compare the analysis of "Derrida's incarnational reading of Husserl" in O'Sullivan, *The Incarnation of Language*, pp. 15–30.

7. Husserl, *Crisis*, p. 359 (*Die Krisis*, p. 370). See analysis in Dodd, *Crisis and Reflection*, pp. 116–17.

8. Babylonian Talmud, Berakhot 56b.

9. *Ibid.*, 57a. Alexander, "Bavli Berakhot," p. 233, cites this passage and draws a parallel in the *Oneirocritica* I, 78 of Artemidorus: "To have sexual intercourse with a woman with whom one is familiar and on intimate terms, if the

dreamer is sexually attracted to and desirous of the woman, signifies nothing at all, because his desire for her has been aroused, But if he does not desire the woman, it is auspicious for him." The parallels between the *Oneirocritica* of Artemidorus and the dream interpretations of the rabbinic sages were demonstrated by Hans Lewy, "Zu dem Traumbuche des Artemidoros," *Rheinische Museum für Philologie*, Neue Folge 48 (1893): 398–413. See also Lieberman, *Hellenism in Jewish Palestine*, pp. 71–75. On the images of incestuous relations in dreams reported by Artemidorus, particularly sexual intercourse with one's mother, see Bowersock, *Fiction as History*, pp. 83–85; *Foucault, The History of Sexuality, Volume. 3: The Care of the Self*, pp. 21–23; and Moss, *The Secret History of Dreaming*, pp. 32–37. For a brief discussion of the erotic implications of the talmudic tradition that one who dreams of having sex with a betrothed maiden should expect greatness in Torah, see Rubenstein, *The Culture of the Babylonian Talmud*, p. 118. See *ibid.*, p. 30, where reference is made to another curious statement in Babylonian Talmud, Berakhot 57a: "He who sees a goose in his dream should expect to achieve wisdom, as it says 'Wisdom cries aloud in the street' (Proverbs 1:20), and the one who has sex with it will become the head of the academy (*rosh yeshivah*). Rav Ashi said, 'I saw it and had sex with it, and rose to greatness.'" Whatever else is underlying this tradition, it is reasonable to assume that the positive value accorded avian intercourse within the dreamscape should be interpreted as a reversal of the social mores generally accepted by the rabbinic sages.

10. See, for example, Malinowski, *The Sexual Life of Savages*, pp. 331–32.

11. Alexander, "Bavli Berakhot," p. 239.

12. Exodus 35:31, Proverbs 2:6. Compare *Pirqei Rabbi Eli'ezer*, ch. 3, 8b, where the ten sayings by means of which the world was said to be created are comprised in the triad of wisdom, understanding, and knowledge. This dictum had a significant impact on later kabbalistic speculation.

13. Judah he-Ḥasid, *Sefer Ḥasidim*, sec. 384, p. 117. The residual impact of this negative view of the dream state is reflected in the explanation of the biblical account of the sin in the Garden of Eden offered by Martin Buber, *Good and Evil: Two Interpretations* (New York: Charles Scribner's Sons, 1953), p. 69: the woman is described as yielding to the temptation of the serpent on account of being moved by "dream-longing" and the man yielding to the temptation of the woman on account of a "dream-lassitude." The shamefulness that arises as a consequence of their actions is lacking in the dream state. See Richard Kearney, *The Wake of Imagination: Toward a Postmodern Culture* (Minneapolis: University of Minnesota Press, 1988), pp. 41–42.

14. Babylonian Talmud, Pesaḥim 50a. According to this passage, R. Joseph

the son of R. Joshua ben Levi became ill and fell into a trance, and when he recovered, his father asked him what he had seen, to which replied "I saw a topsy-turvy world, the upper ones below and the lower ones above." R. Joshua ben Levi assured him, "My son, you saw a clear world [*olam barur*]." My gratitude to Daniel Boyarin for reminding me of this text.

15. See Jalal al-Din Rūmī, *The Mathnawí of Jalálu'ddin Rúmí*, edited and translated by Reynold A. Nicholson (London: Luzac, 1926–1940), 4:3098–99: "The oneiromancer, too, declares laughter in dreams to be (a presage of) weeping with regrets and griefs,/(While) for weeping in dreams joy and gladness are (presaged) in the interpretation, O gleeful man." See *ibid.*, 6:326: "If you dream of any one (being carried) on a bier, he will become a high-stirruped rider of (will rise to high eminence in) office."

16. Babylonian Talmud, Berakhot 55b. The teaching of R. Huna is supported by a baraita in which it is argued that during the course of his lifetime, David never saw a good dream and Aḥitophel, during the course of his lifetime, never saw a bad dream. The talmudic passage is explicated in the following way in *Zohar* 1:200a: since David was engaged all day with shedding blood and waging war, he dreamt of destruction and bloodshed, but he was not blessed with any dreams of peace. Extrapolating from the example of David, the zoharic author concludes that the phenomenon of a good person having a bad dream is to be explained as a premonition of the punishments that will be inflicted upon those who have transgressed the words of Torah. The bad dream, therefore, serves as a means by which the righteous person can inculcate the fear of God in potential sinners. For an alternative explanation, see Ḥayyim ben Bezalel, *Sefer ha-Ḥayyim* (Jerusalem, 1993), ch. 6, p. 72. The dream stands metaphorically for the transience of this world, and hence the meaning of the assertion that the righteous do not see good dreams means that for them, goodness is not constricted to a brief span of time, as it is for the wicked, who do not see a bad dream in their lifetime.

17. Babylonian Talmud, Berakhot, 57a. See Veltri, *Magie und Halakha*, p. 130.

18. Babylonian Talmud, Berakhot, 55b. The second part of Rava's statement concerning an elephant going through the eye of a needle brings to mind the comment attributed to Jesus, "For it is easier for a camel to go through the eye of a needle than for a rich man to enter the kingdom of God" (Luke 18:25). The comparison of the two dicta was made already by the Jewish apostate Heinrich Christian Immanuel Frommann, *Evangelium Lucae, Pars Posterior*, edited by Johann Heinrich Callenberg (Halle: Institutum Judaicum, 1737), 29a. For historical background on this figure, see Pinchas E. Lapide, *Hebrew in the Church:*

The Foundations of Jewish-Christian Dialogue (Grand Rapids: William B. Eerdmans, 1984), p. 77; Christopher M. Clark, *The Politics of Conversion: Missionary Protestantism and the Jews in Prussia 1728–1941* (Oxford: Oxford University Press, 1995), pp. 47–57; Holly Snyder, "A Tree with Two Different Fruits: The Jewish Encounter with German Pietists in the Eighteenth Century Atlantic World," *The William and Mary Quarterly* 58 (2001): 855–82, esp. 868–71; Elisheva Carlebach, *Divided Souls: Converts From Judaism in German, 1500–1750* (New Haven: Yale University Press, 2001), pp. 85–86; Christoph Rymatzki, *Hallischer Pietismus und Judenmission: Johann Heinrich Callenbergs Institutum Judaicum und dessen Freundeskreis* (Tübingen: Niemeyer, 2004), pp. 99–104, 140–42, 165–71; David Dowdey, *Jewish-Christian Relations in Eighteenth-Century Germany: Textual Studies on German Archival Holdings, 1729–1742* (Lewiston: Edwin Mellen Press, 2006), pp. 51–97. On the juxtaposition of the skin of the elephant and the skin of the camel, see also *Midrash Wayyikra Rabbah*, 6:3, p. 131.

19. See Chapter. 3 n. 58.

20. Babylonian Talmud, Berakhot 56a.

21. The insight expressed here is in accord with the observation of Elior, "Reality," pp. 67–68, that dreams (as we can infer from their literary accounts) are both rooted in the cultural tradition of the dreamer and open up new horizons that expand beyond it. Elior also emphasizes that the dream is a mixture of identities that shatters the boundaries of the world as we commonly experience it in wakeful states of consciousness. On the temporal and spatial reorientation in the dreams attested in Jewish mystical literature, see *ibid.*, pp. 74–75.

22. Sigmund Freud, "The Unconscious," *SE*, 14:186.

23. Freud, *Interpretation of Dreams*, p. 243, but see Freud's own qualification on the ability of dreams to express negation on pp. 248–49 and 254 and on the judgment of absurdity by which the dream work represents a contradiction on p. 277. Compare Brann, *The World of the Imagination*, p. 337.

24. Freud, *On Dreams*, pp. 28–29.

25. *Ibid.*, p. 29.

26. *Ibid.*, pp. 42–43 (emphasis in the original). Compare Freud, *Interpretation of Dreams*, p. 244.

27. Fromm, *The Forgotten Language*, p. 4. The interweaving of contradictory images in the dream state was also noted by Henri Bergson, *Time and Free Will: An Essay on the Immediate Data of Consciousness*, translation by F. L. Pogson (New York: Dover Publications, 2001), pp. 136–37.

28. Hieatt, *Realism of Dream Visions*, p. 18.

29. Hobbes, *Leviathan*, pt. 1, ch. 2, p. 13.

30. John R. Wikse, "Night Rule: Dreams as Social Intelligence," in *The*

Variety of Dream Experience: Expanding Our Ways of Working with Dreams, edited by Montague Ullman and Claire Limmer, 2nd edition (Albany: State University of New York Press, 1999), p. 145.

31. Malcolm, *Dreaming*, p. 57.

32. For a critique of Malcolm's view, see Vere C. Chappell, "The Concept of Dreaming," *Philosophical Quarterly* 13 (1963): 209–10, reprinted *in Philosophical Essays on Dreaming*, pp. 302–303.

33. Gaston Bachelard, *Water and Dreams: An Essay on the Imagination of Matter*, translated by Edith R. Farrell (Dallas: Pegasus Foundation, 1983), pp. 11–12 (emphasis in the original).

34. Hillman, *Dream and the Underworld*, p. 127. The citation is from Philostratus, *Imagines* 1.27.

35. *Ibid.* (emphasis in the original).

36. Gaston Bachelard, *Air and Dreams: An Essay on the Imagination of Movement*, translated by Edith R. Farrell and C. Frederick Farrell (Dallas: Dallas Institute Publications, 2002), pp. 263–64.

37. Jung, *Psychology and Alchemy*, pp. 33–34, 186, 346; *idem, Dream Analysis*, p. 704. For a critical assessment of the oppositionalism implicit in the Jungian approach, see James Hillman, *Dream and the Underworld*, pp. 74–85.

38. Bachelard, *Water and Dreams*, p. 35.

39. Bachelard, *The Poetics of Reverie*, p. 16, remarked that the "nocturnal dream can disorganize a soul and propagate, even during the day, the madness attempted during the night." I would not embrace Bachelard's language of madness, but I think the sense of disorganization he describes bears resemblance to what I have called "phenomenological disorientation."

40. Miller, *Dreams*, p. 6.

41. Bowersock, *Fiction as History*, pp. 1 and 17–18. On the Greek and Roman opinions about the truthfulness of dreams, see the extensive analysis in Harris, *Dreams and Experience*, pp. 123–228.

42. Babylonian Talmud, Berakhot 55a. The inherently false aspect of oneiric visions underlies the nexus between dreams and heresy attested in early attacks on the part of Church Fathers against what they considered heterodox views. and this includes Judeo-Christian and Gnostic sects. See Le Goff, *The Medieval Imagination*, pp. 205–207 and 212–13.

43. Tishby, *Wisdom*, pp. 812–13.

44. Babylonian Talmud, Berakhot 57b. See also Chapter 2 n. 20.

45. See Chapter 3 n. 87.

46. *Zohar* 1:183a. This passage is cited by Almoli, *Pitron Ḥalomot*, 6b, to support his claim that prophetic dreams, in contrast to ordinary dreams, do

not contain anything false or nonsensical. See Harris, *Studies*, pp. 39–63, esp. 41–43 and 60–62. See also the zoharic text cited below, n. 52. A similar distinction between prophecy and dreams is affirmed by Joseph Albo, *Sefer ha-Iqqarim* (Warsaw: Isaac Goldman, 1877), III.9, p. 222.

47. The word I have translated as "alluring demons" is *ṭehirin*, which is from the root *ṭhr*, "luster," "brilliance," or "purity." It is clear from several contexts that in the zoharic lexicon, the word connotes, inter alia, the nocturnal forces of destruction that allure human beings with their dazzle. See *Zohar* 1:94a, 125a–b, 130b, 198b, 203b, 232b; 2:56a, 130a–b, 198b, 205a, 207a; 3:62b, 213b, 266a, 286b. This terminology is likely based on the expression *ṭiharei* that appears in Targum on Song of Songs 4:6 to name a group of demonic forces. Compare the phrase *benei ṭiharerei* (or *ṭiharirei*) in Targum Jonathan ben Uziel to Numbers 6:24 and Deuteronomy 32:24. I surmise that the use of this locution in zoharic texts to designate demonic beings is equivalent to the Latin proverb "Non omne quod nitet aurum est"—"not all that shines is gold"—and the related saying made famous by Shakespeare in *The Merchant of* Venice (II. vii), "all that glisters is not gold," that is, at times, what is harmful can attract people with a superficial and deceptive glow.

48. *Zohar* 1:199b–200a.

49. *Zohar* 1:150b; 3:25a, 156b. See also *Zohar Ḥadash*, edited by Reuven Margaliot (Jerusalem: Mosad ha-Rav Kook, 1978), 88a. In several zoharic contexts (1:83a, 130a; 2:130a, 267a), the defiled soul is said to receive "deceptive words" from demonic beings during sleep. This theme may be based on the distinction in the Babylonian Talmud, Berakhot 55b, between the prophetic dream conveyed by an angel (*mal'akh*) and a false dream conveyed by a demon (*shed*). See *Zohar* 3:234b (*Ra'aya Meheimna*). Another possible source, which combines both talmudic dicta, is the passage cited in *Midrash Tanḥuma*, edited by Solomon Buber (Vilna: Rom, 1885), "Introduction," pp. 125–26. According to that text, a distinction is made between prophetic vision (*ḥezyon*) and a dream (*ḥalom*) based on the fact that the latter always contains "nonsensical matters" (*devarim beṭelim*). The sentiment expressed in the zoharic passages can also be compared to the Islamic *ḥadīth*, "the true dream (*ru'ya*) is from God, the bad dream (*ḥulm*) is from Satan," cited in Jonathan G. Katz, *Dreams, Sufism and Sainthood: The Visionary Career of Muhammad Al-Zawâwî* (Leiden: E. J. Brill, 1996), p. 209 n. 12, and see Menahem J. Kister, "The Interpretation of Dreams: An Unknown Manuscript of Ibn Qutayba's 'Ibârât al-Ru'yâ,'" *Israel Oriental Studies* 4 (1974): 72 n. 26. The division of dreams into false and truthful, which can be traced to the ancient Greeks, is known from the oneiric classification attested in other Muslim and Christian sources in the Middle Ages. See Gustave Edmund von

Grunebaum, "Introduction: The Cultural Function of the Dream as Illustrated by Classical Islam," in *The Dream and Human Societies*, pp. 7–9; Steven F. Kruger, *Dreaming in the Middle Ages* (Cambridge: Cambridge University Press, 1992), pp. 83–122; Katz, *Dreams*, pp. 208–10; John C. Lamoreaux, *The Early Muslim Tradition of Dream Interpretation* (Albany: State University of New York Press, 2002), pp. 35, 61–62, 65–66; Maria Mavroudi, *A Byzantine Book on Dream Interpretation: The Oneirocriticon of Achmet and Its Arabic Sources* (Leiden: Brill, 2002), pp. 160 and 166; Mittermaier, "The Book of Visions," pp. 239–43; *idem*, "(Re)Imagining Space: Dreams and Saint Shrines in Egypt," in *Dimensions of Locality: Muslim Saints, Their Place and Space*, edited by Georg Stauth and Samuli Schielke (Bielefeld: Transcript, 2008), pp. 47–66. For the rejection of the view that demons are responsible for divination, see the evidence adduced by Kreisel, *Prophecy*, p. 341. In spite of the irrefutable historical proof that systems of dream interpretation have been based on distinguishing true and false dreams, the philosophical import of this distinction is a complex matter that lies beyond the scope of this study. On dream visions and oneirocriticism in Muslim sources, see also Ibn Khaldûn, *The Muqaddimah*, 1:207–12, 3:103–10, and the critical assessments of Nathaniel Bland, "On the Muhammedan Science of Tabir, or Interpretation of Dreams," *Journal of the Royal Asiatic Society of Great Britain and Ireland* 16 (1856): 118–71; Leah Kinberg, *Morality in the Guide of Dreams: A Critical Edition of Kitāb al-Manām with Introduction* (Leiden: E. J. Brill, 1994), pp. 11–48; Marcia K. Hermansen, "Visions as 'Good to Think': A Cognitive Approach to Visionary Experience in Islamic Sufi Thought," *Religion* 27 (1997): 25–43; *idem*, "Dreams and Dreaming in Islam," in *Dreams: A Reader on Religious, Cultural and Psychological Dimensions of Dreaming*, edited by Kelly Bulkeley (New York: Palgrave, 2001), pp. 73–91; Annemarie Schimmel, *Die Träume des Kalifen: Träume und ihre Deutung in der islamischen Kultur* (Munich: C.H. Beck, 1998); Kelly Bulkeley, "Reflections on the Dream Traditions of Islam," *Sleep and Hypnosis* 4 (2002): 4–14; *idem*, *Dreaming*, pp. 192–212; Lory, *Le rêve*; Green, "The Religious and Cultural Roles," pp. 287–313.

50. *Zohar* 1:199b: "Some dreams are entirely true and in some of them there is truth and falsehood."

51. The possibility of demons having some premonition of the future is listed in a rabbinic passage as one of three things they have in common with the ministering angels. See Babylonian Talmud, Ḥagigah 16a; Moses Naḥmanides, *Perushei ha-Torah le-Rabbenu Moshe ben Naḥman*, edited by Ḥayyim D. Chavel (Jerusalem: Mosad ha-Rav Kook, 1984), 1:95 (*ad* Leviticus 17:7); *Zohar* 1:83a. 130a; 2:251b; 3:25a. See also the section from the *Midrash ha-Neʿlam* stratum in *Zohar* 2:17b, where it is stated that the way of the demons is to repeat to the soul

what they have received, and "if it is false, they inform it of false matters, and if it is true, all that they will say for a brief time will be true."

52. *Zohar* 1:238a.

53. Elliot R. Wolfson, *Venturing Beyond—Law and Morality in Kabbalistic Mysticism* (Oxford: Oxford University Press, 2006), pp. 43–44, 58–73, 131–32. Here it is worth recalling as well the following comment in the *Ma'amar Yiḥud ha-Yir'ah* appended to Moses Ḥayyim Luzzatto, *Adir ba-Marom*, part 2 (Jerusalem, 1988), p. 146: "There is also here the secret of the dream, which is the unification of the seventy-two [letter name] and the fifty-two [letter name], the coupling of *Arikh Anpin* and *Nuqba*, and this produces the secret of the dream [*sod ha-ḥalom*] and the secret of the dreamer [*sod ha-ḥolem*]. . . . And understand that the dream extends even to the Gentiles, for it stands in unity, and there is no fear." Luzzatto goes on to contrast Israel and the Gentiles insofar as in the case of the former the dream images are transposed into an actual prophetic vision. This, moreover, is the secret of the verse "When the Lord restores the fortunes of Zion, we will be as dreamers" (Psalms 126:1), "verily as dreamers, in the secret of the vowel of the *ḥolem* that surely rules over this."

54. *Zohar* 3:25a.

55. Compare the contrast between prophecy and the dream in *Zohar* 1:149a, cited in Chapter 3 at n. 96.

56. Tishby, *Wisdom*, pp. 468 and 591–94.

57. *Zohar* 2:264a.

58. *Zohar* 3:234b (*Ra'aya Meheimna*). For a similar use of the talmudic distinction between the angelic and demonic dreams, see Abraham Abulafia, *Mafteaḥ ha-Tokhaḥot* (Jerusalem, 2001), pp. 62–63. The gap between the two, however, is not so wide for Abulafia, since he recognizes that it is precisely when the sage enters into the gates of prophecy that the other spirit may take effect (pp. 68–69).

59. Cordovero, *Pardes Rimmonim* 26:2, 57a. See also the work of Cordovero's disciple, de Vidas, *Re'shit Ḥokhmah*, Sha'ar ha-Yir'ah, ch. 13, 1:258.

60. See Chapter 3 n. 57.

61. See above, n. 42.

62. Moses Ḥayyim Luzzatto, *Derekh ha-Shem* (Jerusalem, 1996), III.1.6, pp. 74–75.

63. Pedaya, *Minḥat Yehudah*, p. 62. See *ibid.*, p. 70, where a third category of dreams is affirmed: dreams that are confused and disorderly, but that do not cause agitation or fear. These dreams are said to come from the "image of the thought of the brain" (*ṣiyyur maḥashevet ha-moaḥ*), since the brain does not rest, even in the time of sleep. One need not be concerned about such dreams,

because they do not add or detract, and they are not omens of either good or evil.

64. *Zohar* 3:253a, 277a (*Ra'aya Meheimna*); *Zohar Ḥadash*, 47a, 48d, 78d. In the last of these passages, the "dregs of the Jewish demons" are identified as the source of the "other gods" (Exodus 20:2) connected with Ishmael and Esau, that is, Islam and Christianity. In the continuation of that passage, it is stated unequivocally that Christians and Muslims are "brothers" with the Jews from the body, but not from the soul in any of its gradations. However, it is also asserted that "with respect to every non-Jew who repents and separates from idolatry and transgression, the blessed holy One places a holy spirit and a holy soul within him, and thus he has a share in the world to come, not with the people of Israel, but a portion unto itself and a world unto itself." Following one opinion implied in rabbinic literature (Babylonian Talmud, Sanhedrin 105a) and expressed more explicitly by Maimonides (*Mishneh Torah*, Melakhim 8:11), this to some extent breaks down the inflexible ontological distinction between Jew and Gentile, because the matter of difference is more dependent on behavior—that is, if the non-Jew renounces the wayward path of idolatry and impiety, then he or she earns a stake in the afterlife. Notwithstanding the importance of this shift, even this text is clear that the status of the righteous Gentile is not on a par with the indigenous Jew, and hence some disparity is preserved.

65. Ḥayyim Viṭal, *Eṣ Ḥayyim* (Jerusalem, 1963), 50:7, 116a–b.

66. Pedaya, *Minḥat Yehudah*, p. 63.

67. *Ibid.*, p. 66.

68. The elevated status of the *ḥolem* is affirmed in the early work of Joseph Gikatilla, *Ginnat Egoz* (Jerusalem: Yeshivat ha-Ḥayyim we-ha-Shalom, 1989), pp. 434–35, but with a different symbolic connotation.

69. Joseph Gikatilla, *Sefer ha-Niqqud* (Jerusalem: Yerid ha-Sefarim, 1994), p. 16. For discussion of this text, see R. J. Zwi Werblowsky, "Kabbalistische Buchstabenmystik und der Traum (Joseph ben Abraham Gikatilas Exkurs über Herkunft und Bedeutung der Träume)," *Zeitschrift für Religion und Geistesgeschichte* 8 (1956): 164–69.

70. Gikatilla, *Sha'arei Ṣedeq*, 17a; *idem*, *Sha'arei Orah*, 1:161. And compare Ibn Gabbai, *Avodat ha-Qodesh*, IV.26, p. 489: "Because [the patriarchs] did not comprehend in the day, but only through the intermediary of the night, which is the barrier and the concealment of the face, their prophecy was mixed with parable, image, and allegory that is not translucent, like the matter through which they comprehended, which is called the speculum that does not shine and is not transparent. The secret is 'for she covered her face' (Genesis 38:15), and

this is the secret of 'in the hands of the prophets I was imaged' (Hosea 12:11)."

71. Babylonian Talmud, Berakhot 55b. See above n. 18.

72. *Zohar* 1:183a. See also 130a.

73. Piergabriele Mancuso, *Shabbatai Donnolo's Sefer Ḥakhmoni: Introduction, Critical Text, and Annotated Translation* (Leiden: Brill, 2010), p. 260 and sources mentioned there in n. 30. The corresponding Hebrew text appears on p. 153.

74. Ibn Gabbai, *Avodat ha-Qodesh*, IV.27, p. 495.

75. Viṭal, *Sha'arei Qedushshah*, III.5, pp. 253–55.

76. Luzzatto, *Derekh ha-Shem*, III.1.6, pp. 74–75.

77. Menasseh ben Israel, *Nishmat Ḥayyim* (Amsterdam, 1652), III.5, 104a–b. The dream is explained as a nullification of the corporeal faculties during sleep and the consequent strengthening of the rational soul. In support of his view, the author cites select zoharic passages (see above, n. 72).

78. Gikatilla, *Sha'arei Orah*, 2:89–90.

79. *Ibid.*, 2:84. In that context, Gikatilla links Jacob's dream vision of the ladder (Genesis 28:12) with this symbolism, arguing that he ascended by means of the median line, the aspect of knowledge (*da'at*), to the first emanation, the nothing (*ayin*), or the world of mercy (*olam ha-raḥamim*), whence he had a disclosure of the second emanation, the something (*yesh*), or wisdom (*ḥokhmah*), signified scripturally by the Tetragrammaton.

80. For an analysis of *Keter* as a coincidence of opposites in Gikatilla's kabbalistic thought, see Wolfson, *Venturing Beyond*, pp. 224–29.

81. The bibliography on the Beshṭ is enormous, so I will here only refer to some of the more recent works where one can find ample reference to other scholarship: Moshe Rosman, *Founder of Hasidism: A Quest for the Historical Ba'al Shem Tov* (Berkeley: University of California Press, 1996); Gershon D. Hundert, *Jews in Poland-Lithuania in the Eighteenth Century: A Genealogy of Modernity* (Berkeley: University of California Press, 2004), pp. 162–76; Immanuel Etkes, *The Besht: Magician, Mystic, and Leader*, translated by Saadya Sternberg (Waltham: Brandeis University Press, 2005); Ḥaviva Pedaya, "The Baal Shem Tov's Iggeret Hakodesh toward a Critique of the Textual Versions and an Exploration of Its Convergence with the World-Picture: Messianism, Revelation, Ecstasy, and the Sabbatean Background." *Zion* 70 (2005): 311–54 (Hebrew); Rachel Elior, *The Mystical Origins of Hasidism* (Oxford: Litman Library of Jewish Civilization, 2006), pp. 59–71; Netanel Lederberg, *Sod ha-Da'at: Rabbi Israel Ba'al Shem Tov, His Spiritual Character and Social Leadership* (Jerusaelm: Rubin Mass, 2007) (Hebrew).

82. Ḥabad follows a perspective that can be traced back to some thirteenth-century kabbalists, who began counting the ten *sefirot* with *Ḥokhmah* or

Maḥashavah, adding *Da'at* in place of *Keter*. This is not to say that *Keter* does not figure prominently in the teaching of Ḥabad. Briefly, it can be said that *Keter* is described variously as the nothing (*ayin*), the incomposite will (*raṣon pashuṭ*), and the infinite light (*or ein sof*) in which opposites coalesce.

83. The locus classicus for this terminology is Shneur Zalman of Liadi, *Liqquṭei Amarim: Tanya* (Brooklyn: Kehot, 1984), pt. 1, ch. 3, 7a–b.

84. See the passages cited in Chapter 2 n. 48; Hughes, "Imagining the Divine;" Chittick, *The Sufi Path of Knowledge*, p. 62, and for discussion of Ibn al-'Arabī's attitude toward and citation of key passages from al-Ghazālī, see Chittick, *The Sufi Path of Knowledge*, pp. 235, 405 n. 1, 409 n. 6. On the possibility that al-Ghazālī's use of the term *jabarūt* to name the intermediary world influenced Ibn al-'Arabī, see William C. Chittick, *The Self-Disclosure of God: Principles of Ibn al-'Arabī's Cosmology* (Albany: State University of New York Press, 1998), p. 260. For a comparative discussion of these two thinkers as representatives of the Neoplatonic current in medieval Ṣūfism, see Majid Fakhry, A *History of Islamic Philosophy*, 2nd edition (New York: Columbia University Press, 1983), pp. 246–56.

85. Corbin, *Creative Imagination*, pp. 179–95 and 216–20; *idem*, "The Visionary Dream in Islamic Spirituality," in *The Dream and Human Societies*, pp. 392–94 and 406–408. See also the independent analysis in the same volume by Fazlur Rahman, "Dream, Imagination, and 'Ālam al-mithāl," pp. 409–19; Sviri, "Dreaming," pp. 257–61; Green, "The Religious and Cultural Roles of Dreams," pp. 296–97; Samer Akkach, "The World of Imagination in Ibn 'Arabī's Ontology," *British Journal of Middle Eastern Studies* 24 (1997): 97–113, esp. 102: "The world of imagination . . . combines the characteristics of its two bordering domains: it is the place where the spirituality of the 'unseen' is integrated into the corporeality of the 'seen' to create the subtlety of imagination. It is the ontological level at which spirits manifest in sensible matrices, and abstract meanings take on their bodily forms. The world of imagination is the world of dreams where everything is real yet, like a phantom, untouchable and unreachable. Imaginable forms, like dreams, have an apparitional or phantasmal quality: they are perceivable, meaningful forms yet without physical presence. They are neither purely sensible nor purely abstract."

86. Henry Corbin, *Avicenna and the Visionary Recital*, translated by Willard R. Trask (New York: Pantheon Books, 1960), p. 35.

87. Chittick, *The Self-Disclosure of God*, p. 334.

88. Chittick, *The Sufi Path of Knowledge*, p. 119. See also Rachel Gordin, *Angels Don't Dream: The Teaching of Ibn 'Arabi—the Greatest Sufi Sheikh* (Jerusalem: Carmel, 2007), pp. 53, 115–16 (Hebrew). See also Chapter 3 n. 47 and

Chapter 5 at n. 226.

89. Chittick, *The Sufi Path of Knowledge*, pp. 115–18. On the depiction of Allāh as the one who brings opposites together, see *ibid.*, pp. 59, 67, 37, and Chittick, *The Self-Disclosure of God*, pp. 11, 73, 86, 184, 236–37. For a broader discussion of this theme, see Sara Sviri, "Fear and Hope: On the Coincidence of Opposites in Islamic Mysticism," *Jerusalem Studies in Arabic and Islam* 9 (1987): 316–49.

90. Chittick, *The Self-Disclosure of God*, p. 46.

91. *Ibid.*, pp. 54, 107, 332–33, 345, 358–59. Compare Rūmī, *The Mathnawí*, 2:2235–36: "Many a wonder is made manifest in sleep: in sleep the heart becomes a window. One that is awake and dreams fair dreams, he is the knower (of God): smear your eyes with his dust." See *ibid.*, 3:2333–40 and 4:3398–99, where the dreams of Joseph are upheld as a model for the noble saint. See the reference to the study of Subtelny cited in Chapter 5 n. 229. On visions and dreams in the Ṣūfi tradition, see also John Renard, *Friends of God: Islamic Images of Piety, Commitment, and Servanthood* (Berkeley: University of California Press, 2008), pp. 67–89, and the sources cited above, n. 49.

92. The influence of Corbin is discernible is much of my work. To mention some of the more prominent examples, see Wolfson, *Through a Speculum*, pp. 306–17; *Language, Eros, Being*, pp. xiii and 32–33; "Sacred Space;" and "*Imago Templi*." See also Chapter 3 n. 60. For an approach similar to my own, also informed by Corbin, see Jambet, *Le caché et l'apparent*, pp. 43–67.

93. On Corbin's indebtedness to phenomenology, especially as espoused in Heidegger's *Sein und Zeit*, see the dialogue between Corbin and Philippe Némo entitled "De Heidegger à Sohravardî," in Henry Corbin, *L'imâm caché* (Paris: Éditions de l'Herne, 2003), pp. 173–211. See also Roberts Avens, *The New Gnosis: Heidegger, Hillman, and Angels* (Dallas: Spring Publications, 1984); Daryush Shayegan, *Henry Corbin: La Topographie spirituelle de l'islam iranien* (Paris: Éditions de la Différence, 1990), pp. 41–47; Tom Cheetham, *The World Turned Inside Out: Henry Corbin and Islamic Mysticism* (Woodstock: Spring Journal Books, 2003), pp. 1–15. On Corbin's engagement with Jewish mysticism, see Paul B. Fenton, "Henry Corbin et la mystique juive," in *Henry Corbin: Philosophies et sagesses des religions du livre*, edited by Mohammad Ali Amir-Moezzi, Christian Jambet, and Pierre Lory (Turnhout: Brepols, 2005), pp. 151–64, and in the same volume, Maria E. Subtelny, "Le motif du trône et les rapports entre mystique islamique et mystique juive," pp. 195–212.

94. See, for example, the passages from the anonymous fifteenth-century *Sefer ha-Meshiv* and from the sixteenth-century Ovadiah Hamon of Barteniro cited and analyzed by Moshe Idel, "Enoch and Elijah: Some Remarks on

Apotheosis, Theophany and Jewish Mysticism," in *The Salt Companion to Harold Bloom*, edited by Roy Sellars and Graham Allen (Cambridge: Salt, 2007), pp. 360–66. For a more detailed analysis of the former text and the oneiric techniques attested therein, see Gershom Scholem, "The Maggid of R. Joseph Taitatzak," *Sefunot* 11 (1968): 47–112 (Hebrew), reprinted in *idem*, *Lurianic Kabbalah: Collected Studies by Gershom Scholem*, edited by Daniel Abrams (Los Angeles: Cherub Press, 2008), pp. 62–106 (Hebrew); Moshe Idel, "Inquiries in the Doctrine of Sefer ha-Meshiv," *Sefunot* 17 (1983): 185–266 (Hebrew); *idem*, "Nächtliche Kabbalisten," in *Die Wahrheit der Träume*, edited by Gartano Benedetti and Erik Hornung (Munich: Wilhelm Fink Verlag, 1997), pp. 85–117. See also Viṭal, *The "Book of Visions,"* p. 78; *Jewish Mystical Autobiographies*, p. 84. Viṭal utilizes a dream question (*she'elat ḥalom*) to attain comprehension of kabbalistic wisdom (*hassagat ḥokhmat qabbalah*). Concerning this technique, see Chapter 2 n. 23. Mention here should also be made of the oneiric and maggidic revelations of Mordecai Ashkenazi and their interpretations by his teacher Abraham Rovigo discussed and partially transcribed in Gershom Scholem, *The Dreams of R. Mordecai Ashkenazi: A Follower of Shabbetai Zevi* (Jerusalem: Schocken, 1938), pp. 13–100 (Hebrew). And compare Matt Goldish, *The Sabbatian Prophets* (Cambridge, MA: Harvard University Press, 2004), pp. 99–100 and 150. Also worthy of note are the angelic and spiritual visions (often in the form of dreams) experienced by Moses Ḥayyim Luzzatto and other members of his circle, such as Moses David Valle. See Meir Benayahu, "The 'Maggid' of R. Moses Ḥayyim Luzzatto," *Sefunot* 5 (1961): 297–36 (Hebrew); Isaiah Tishby, *Messianic Mysticism: Moses Hayim Luzzatto and the Padua School*, translated by Morris Hoffman (Oxford: Litman Library of Jewish Civilization, 2008), pp. 337–403.

95. Moses Ḥayyim Luzzatto, *Qelaḥ Pitḥei Ḥokhmah*, edited by Ḥayyim Friedlander (Benei Beraq, 1992), pp. 26–27. I am grateful to Jonathan Garb, who has drawn my attention to the suspicion regarding Luzzatto's authorship of this text, a matter that he is presently exploring in detail in a forthcoming study on the corpus of this figure. For the purposes of this analysis, the matter of authorship is not critical.

96. Yosef Ḥayyim of Baghdad, *Sod Yesharim* (Jerusalem, 1994), pt. 2, sec. 13, p. 128. See *idem*, *Da'at u-Tevunah* (Jerusalem, 2001), p. 9.

97. Barbara E. Galli, *Franz Rosenzweig and Jehuda Halevi: Translating, Translations, and Translators*, foreword by Paul Mendes-Flohr (Montreal: McGill-Queen's University Press, 1995), pp. 20–21; German original in Franz Rosenzweig, *Der Mensch und sein Werk: Gesammelte Schriften IV. Sprachdenken im Übersetzen*, vol. 1,*Hymnen und Gedichte des Jehuda Halevi*, edited by Reinhold

and Annemarie Mayer (Dordrecht: Martinus Nijhoff, 1984), p. 27.

98. Galli, *Franz Rosenzweig and Jehuda Halevi*, p. 187.

99. I have dedicated many of my studies to clarify the point, but none as extensively as Wolfson, *Through a Speculum*. Halevi is discussed on pp. 173–87, and see especially the role of the dream as the locus of a vision of God in the poem *Ye'iruni be-shimkha ra'ayonai* discussed on pp. 174–75. Compare the translation and analysis of this poem in Scheindlin, *The Gazelle*, pp. 164–69. Scheindlin perceptively noted that the poem "embodies the quasi-mystical paradox that true awakening occurs in the world of prophetic dreams" (p. 168). For the poet-seer, therefore, the genuine waking is not rising from sleep, but the spiritual awakening into the dream. See also Elliot R. Wolfson, "Light Does Not Talk But Shines: Apophasis and Vision in Rosenzweig's Theopoetic Temporality," in *New Directions in Jewish Philosophy*, pp. 87–88, and 101–104, where the texts of Rosenzweig on the vision of God as a state between dream and wakefulness are cited and analyzed.

100. I have taken the liberty to present here a slightly revised version of my discussion of metaphoricity in Wolfson, "Suffering Eros," pp. 342–43.

101. David B. Allison, *Reading the New Nietzsche: The Birth of Tragedy, The Gay Science, Thus Spoke Zarathustra, and On the Genealogy of Morals* (Lanham: Rowman & Littlefield, 2001), pp. 76–77.

102. Needless to say, there is a considerable bibliography on this topic, and here I mention only two relevant studies: Kofman, *Nietzsche and Metaphor*; Tim Murphy, *Nietzsche, Metaphor, Religion* (Albany: State University of New York Press, 2001).

103. Friedrich Nietzsche, *On Truth and Lying in a Non-Moral Sense*, in *The Birth of Tragedy and Other Writings*, edited by Raymond Geuss and Ronald Speirs, translated by Ronald Speirs (Cambridge: Cambridge University Press, 1999), pp. 144–46 (my emphasis). Consider as well Nietzsche's remark in *The Birth of Tragedy*, sec. 8, p. 63: "For a genuine poet, metaphor is not a rhetorical figure but a vicarious image that he actually beholds in place of a concept. A character is for him not a whole he has composed out of particular traits, picked up here and there, but an obtrusively alive person before his very eyes, distinguished from the otherwise identical vision of a painter only by the fact that it continually goes on living and acting." See Wheeler, *Deconstruction*, pp. 117–18.

104. Nietzsche, *Unpublished Writings*, 19 [178–80], pp. 56–57; *Sämtliche Werke: Kritische Studienausgabe*, edited by Giorgio Colli and Mazzino Montinari, 15 vols. (Berlin: Walter de Gruyter, 1999), 7:474–76.

105. Nietzsche, *Beyond Good and Evil*, sec. 289 (cited as the epigraph to the

Preface of this book).

106. Jane Love, "Appetite and Violability: Questioning a Platonic Metaphor," in *Crises in Continental Philosophy*, edited by Arleen B. Dallery, Charles E. Scott, with P. Holley Roberts (Albany: State University of New York Press, 1990), pp. 184–85.

107. Jacques Derrida, "The Retrait of Metaphor," in *The Derrida Reader: Writing Performances*, edited by Julian Wolfreys (Lincoln: University of Nebraska Press. 1998), p. 128.

108. On the collapse of the distinction between the literal and the figurative in Derrida's thinking about the inherent metaphoricity of language, see John Llewelyn, *Derrida on the Threshold of Sense* (New York: St. Martin's Press, 1986), pp. 74–80; Marian Hobson, *Jacques Derrida: Opening Lines* (London: Routledge, 1998), pp. 207–11; Christian Howells, *Derrida: Deconstruction from Phenomenology to Ethics* (Cambridge: Polity Press, 1999), pp. 60–64; Giuseppe Stellardi, *Heidegger and Derrida on Philosophy and Metaphor* (Amherst: Humanity Books, 2000), pp. 67–126. See also Gert-Jan van der Heiden, *The Truth (and Untruth) of Language: Heidegger, Ricoeur, and Derrida on Disclosure and Displacement* (Pittsburgh: Duquesne University Press, 2010), pp. 124–80. For discussion of other contemporary views on metaphor that resonate with this perspective, see C. A. Van Peursen, "Metaphor and Reality," *Man and World* 25 (1992): 165–80, esp. 169–71.

109. For a useful account of the seven masters, see Avrum M. Ehrlich, *Leadership in the HaBaD Movement: A Critical Evaluation of HaBaD Leadership, History, and Succession* (Northvale: Jason Aronson, 2000), and for a detailed study of the seventh rebbe, see *idem*, *The Messiah of Brooklyn: Understanding Lubavitch Hasidism Past and Present* (Jersey City: Ktav, 2004). In the last few years, there have been a number of important studies on Schneerson, many focusing on his messianic agenda and possible self-identification. For a representative list, see Wolfson, *Open Secret*, p. 303 nn. 8–10. In addition to the sources cited there, see also Naftali Loewenthal, "The Baal Shem Tov's Iggeret ha-Kodesh and Contemporary Habad 'Outreach,'" in *Let the Old Make Way for the New: Studies in the Social and Cultural History of Eastern European Jewry Presented to Immanuel Etkes*, edited by David Assaf and Ada Rapoport-Albert, vol. 1: *Hasidism and the Musar Movement* (Jerusalem: The Zalman Shazar Center for Jewish History, 2009), pp. 69–101 (English section); Samuel Heilman and Menachem Friedman, *The Rebbe: The Life and Afterlife of Menachem Mendel Schneerson* (Princeton: Princeton University Press, 2010).

110. I have elaborated on these dimensions of Ḥabad in "Revisioning the Body Apophatically: Incarnation and the Acosmic Naturalism of Habad

Hasidism," in *Apophatic Bodies*, pp. 147–99. A revised and expanded version appears in Wolfson, *Open Secret*, pp. 66–129. For previous discussions of Ḥabad cosmology variously designated as acosmism, pantheism, or panentheism, see Scholem, *Major Trends*, p. 341; Moshe Hallamish, "The Theoretical System of R. Shneur Zalman of Liady (Its Sources in Kabbalah and Hasidism)," Ph.D. dissertation, Hebrew University, 1976, pp. 56–60 and 127–32 (Hebrew); Yoram Jacobson, "The Doctrine of Creation in R. Shneur Zalman of Liadi," *Eshel Beer Sheva* 1 (1976): 307–68 (Hebrew); Joseph Weiss, *Studies in Eastern European Jewish Mysticism*, edited by David Goldstein (Oxford: Oxford University Press, 1985), pp. 45–46; Rachel Elior, "ḤaBaD: The Contemplative Ascent to God," in *Jewish Spirituality From the Sixteenth-Century Revival to the Present*, edited by Arthur Green (New York: Crossroad, 1987), pp. 163–64; *idem*, *The Paradoxical Ascent: The Kabbalistic Theosophy of Habad Hasidism*, translated by Jeffrey M. Green (Albany: State University of New York Press, 1993), pp. 49–58; *idem*, *The Mystical Origins*, pp. 115–25; Rivka Schatz-Uffenheimer, *Hasidism as Mysticism: Quietistic Elements in Eighteenth Century Hasidic Thought*, translated by Jonathan Chipman (Princeton: Princeton University Press, 1993), pp. 261–64. See also Seth Brody, "'Open to Me the Gates of Righteousness': The Pursuit of Holiness and Non-Duality in Early Hasidic Teaching," *Jewish Quarterly Review* 89 (1998): 3–44, esp. 39–43, where the nondual orientation of Aaron of Staroselye is discussed. My own taxon "apophatic embodiment" is meant to provide an alternative model. The approach I took to the Ḥabad material is, as I noted in *Open Secret* (p. 90), indebted to Catherine Keller, but it also resonates with the analysis of Alexei V. Nesteruk, "From the Unknowability of the Universe to the Teleology of Reason: A Phenomenological Insight into Apophatic Cosmology," in *Knowing the Unknowable: Science and Religions on God and the Universe*, edited by John Bowker (London: I.B. Tauris, 2009), pp. 63–86.

111. Shneur Zalman of Liadi, *Torah Or* (Brooklyn: Kehot, 1991), 28c-d.

112. For a negative assessment of the activity of the imagination conjuring dreams during sleep, a time that the intellect hypothetically is not functioning, see Shneur Zalman of Liadi, *Ma'amerei Admor ha-Zaqen: Ketuvim*, vol. 1 (Brooklyn: Kehot, 1985), pp. 35–44; Menaḥem Mendel Schneersohn, *Or ha-Torah: Bemidbar* (Brooklyn: Kehot, 1998), 3:1011; Menaḥem Mendel Schneerson, *Torat Menaḥem: Hitwwa'aduyyot 5714* (Brooklyn: Lahak Hanochos, 1998), 1:69. These themes are hardly unique to Ḥabad; on the contrary, they are found in many ḥasidic texts. See, for example, the reference to Naḥman of Bratslav cited below, n. 175.

113. It is necessary to point out that in Ḥabad thinking, the term *adam* applies most specifically to the Jews, a theme that is well attested in a plethora

of kabbalistic texts, including the zoharic and Lurianic sources, which influenced the Lubavitch masters. On the ethnocentric casting of *adam*, see the extensive documentation and analysis in Wolfson, *Venturing Beyond*, pp. 17–128. For an extended discussion of the Ḥabad perspective, see Wolfson, *Open Secret*, pp. 224–64.

114. On the comparison of the dream to exile based on the fact that both are vehicles for *berur*, see Shneur Zalman of Liadi, *Ma'amerei Admor ha-Zaqen: Al Ma'amerei Razal* (Brooklyn: Kehot, 1984), pp. 308–309 and 316. Compare Dov Baer Schneersohn, *Ma'amerei Admor ha-Emṣa'i: Hanaḥot* (Brooklyn: Kehot, 1994), p. 246: "Similarly it is understood with respect to the matter of exile that is compared to dream and sleep, for the length of the exile is for the sake of the purification of good from evil, and it is not only that the good will be by itself and the evil by itself, but rather that the good will be produced from the evil, and it is known that the benefit of dreams is to take out all the parts of the good that are in the evil until there remains nothing but the final limit of the evil." And see Menaḥem Mendel Schneersohn, *Or ha-Torah: Bere'shit*, vol. 5 (Brooklyn: Kehot, 1971), pp. 2018–19.

115. My use of the word "gnostic" does not necessarily imply any historical or even textual connection between late antiquity and the sixteenth-century Safed, although the possibility of some form of diffusion bridging the temporal gap cannot be ruled out categorically. Even in the absence of the latter, I am persuaded that the word "gnostic" is an appropriate way to characterize the worldview underlying Luria's mystical theosophy. See Scholem, *Major Trends*, p. 260; Isaiah Tishby, "Gnostic Doctrines in Sixteenth-Century Jewish Mysticism," *Journal of Jewish Studies* 6 (1955): 146–52; Lawrence Fine, *Physician of the Soul, Healer of the Cosmos: Isaac Luria and His Kabbalistic Fellowship* (Stanford: Stanford University Press, 2003), pp. 144–49.

116. For an exhaustive analysis of this principle, which takes into account previous scholarship, see Tsippi Kauffman, *In All Your Ways Know Him: The Concept of God and Avodah be-Gashmiyut in the Early Stages of Hasidism* (Ramat-Gan: Bar-Ilan University Press, 2009), pp. 173–392 (Hebrew).

117. See Yoram Jacobson, "The Love of God in the Teaching of R. Shneur Zalman of Liadi," *Te'udah* 7 (2001): 353–414 (Hebrew).

118. The point is made in a somewhat different terminological register in Shneur Zalman of Liadi, *Liqquṭei Torah* (Brooklyn: Kehot, 1996), Balaq, 1:71c. I do not accept the assumption of Schatz-Uffenheimer, *Hasidism as Mysticism*, p. 268, that the distinction made by Shneur Zalman between Torah and world as the locus of divine revelation is a tacit rejection of the ideal of corporeal worship as it was formulated by the Maggid of Międzyrzecz and his disciples (see

Hasidism as Mysticism, pp. 296–97). Schatz-Uffenheimer's view is accepted by Arthur Green, *Devotion and Commandment: The Faith of Abraham in the Hasidic Imagination* (Cincinnati: Hebrew Union College Press, 1989), pp. 64–65.

119. Shneur Zalman of Liadi, *Torah Or*, 25b.

120. *Ibid.*, 3b, 28c; *idem*, *Liqquṭei Torah*, Ha'azinu, 2:75d.

121. On the notion of *devequt* and self-annihilation in early ḥasidic literature, see Gershom Scholem, *The Messianic Idea in Judaism and Other Essays on Jewish Spirituality* (New York: Schocken Books, 1971), pp. 203–27, esp. 213–14, where the ideal of unification (*yiḥud*) and communion with the nothing, introduced by the Maggid of Międzyrzecz, is discussed. Scholem's referring to this phenomenon as an "abandonment to emotionalism" strikes me as misguided. For other discussions of *devequt*, mystical union, and self-annihilation (*biṭṭul ha-yesh*) in Ḥasidism, see Schatz-Uffenheimer, *Hasidism as Mysticism*, pp. 65–79; Jacobson, "The Doctrine of Creation," pp. 345–50; Elior, "ḤaBaD," pp. 181–91; *idem*, *The Paradoxical Ascent*, pp. 143–57; Naftali Loewenthal, *Communicating the Infinite: The Emergence of the Habad School* (Chicago: University of Chicago Press, 1990), pp. 188–94; Idel, *Kabbalah: New Perspectives*, pp. 49–51 and 62–73; *idem*, *Hasidism: Between Ecstasy and Magic* (Albany: State University of New York Press, 1995), pp. 107–27; Mendel Piekarz, *Between Ideology and Reality: Humility, Ayin, Self-Negation, and Devekut in the Hasidic Thought* (Jerusalem: Bialik Institute, 1994), pp. 55–81 and 104–78 (Hebrew); Ron Margolin, *The Human Temple: Religious Interiorization and the Structuring of Inner Life in Early Hasidism* (Jerusalem: Magnes Press, 2005), pp. 288–378 (Hebrew).

122. Shneur Zalman of Liadi, *Torah Or*, 111a.

123. Moshe Idel, "Universalization and Integration: Two Conceptions of Mystical Union in Jewish Mysticism," in *Mystical Union and Monotheistic Faith: An Ecumenical Dialogue*, edited by Moshe Idel and Bernard McGinn (New York: Macmillan, 1989), pp. 27–57, esp. 41–45; Elior, *The Paradoxical Ascent*, pp. 44–45; Loewenthal, *Communicating*, pp. 153 and 170; Leah Ornet, "Expressions of Mystical Union in R. Shneur Zalman of Liadi," *Tarbiz* 74 (2004): 585–611 (Hebrew); *idem*, "*Ratso va-shov, Running and Returning*": *Ethical and Mystical Perspectives in the Teaching of R. Shneur Zalman of Liadi—A Comparative Study* (Tel-Aviv: Hakibbutz Hameuchad, 2007), pp. 215–41(Hebrew).

124. The term *complexio oppositorum* to describe God or the ultimate reality was used by Jung as a synonym for Nicholas of Cusa's *coincidentia oppositorum*. See, for instance, Jung, *Aion*, p. 225; *idem*, *The Practice of Psychotherapy*, p. 320; *idem*, *Mysterium Coniunctionis*, pp. 104, 148, 166, 375; *idem*, *Memories, Dreams, Reflections*, pp. 334, 338, 341, 353; Steven M. Wasserstrom, *Religion After Religion: Gershom Scholem, Mircea Eliade, and Henry Corbin at Eranos* (Princeton:

Princeton University Press, 1999), p. 69. It is also of relevance to note that the expression *coincidentia oppositorum* was rendered as *complexio oppositorum* by Carl Schmitt in 1923 to characterize the Catholic Church. See Kam Shapiro, "Politics Is a Mushroom: Worldly Sources of Rule and Exception in Carl Schmitt and Walter Benjamin," *Diacritics* 37 (2007): 125, and *idem*, *Carl Schmitt and the Intensification of Politics* (Lanham: Rowman & Littlefield, 2008), p. 26.

125. Elior, "ḤaBaD," pp. 178–81. For a partial critique of Elior's dialectical approach and an alternative explanation based on positing two complimentary types of worship, see Idel, *Hasidism*, pp. 123–24. The position I have staked seeks the middle ground between Elior and Idel. Mention here should also be made of the characterization of the contemplative path of Ḥabad as a turning away from the world in Weiss, *Studies*, pp. 194–201. In my judgment, this depiction is inadequate, insofar as it fails to take into account the complicated question of the nature of worldliness in Ḥabad thought and the paradoxical relation of the cosmos to the infinite light.

126. On the principle of the *coincidentia oppositorum* in Ḥabad speculation, see Hallamish, "Theoretical System," pp. 163–74; Elior, *The Paradoxical Ascent*, pp. 25–31, 63–72, 97–100; *idem*, *The Mystical Origins*, pp. 106–14.

127. Palestinian Talmud, Berakhot 1:3, 3b; Babylonian Talmud, Eruvin 13b; Giṭṭin 6b.

128. Shneur Zalman of Liadi, *Torah Or*, 28d.

129. Shneur Zalman of Liadi, *Liqquṭei Torah*, Ki Tavo, 2:42d.

130. Dov Baer Schneersohn, *Perush ha-Millot* (Brooklyn: Kehot, 1993), 55d.

131. Shneur Zalman of Liadi, *Torah Or*, 98a.

132. Dov Baer Schneersohn, *Sha'arei Orah* (Brooklyn: Kehot, 1979), 111a and 134a; *idem*, *Torat Ḥayyim: Bere'shit* (Brooklyn: Kehot, 1993), 161b; *idem*, *Torat Ḥayyim: Shemot* (Brooklyn: Kehot, 2003), 96b, 229b, 298b; *idem*, *Perush ha-Millot*, 26c, 69d, 103d; *idem*, *Derushei Ḥatunah*, vol. 2 (Brooklyn: Kehot, 1991), p. 476; Shmuel Schneersohn, *Liqquṭei Torah: Torat Shmu'el 5627* (Brooklyn: Kehot, 2000), p. 412; *idem*, *Liqquṭei Torah: Torat Shmu'el 5632*, vol. 1 (Brooklyn: Kehot, 1999), pp. 136, 137; *idem*, *Liqquṭei Torah: Torat Shmu'el 5633*, vol. 2 (Brooklyn: Kehot, 1994), p. 510; Shalom Dovber Schneersohn, *Be-Sha'ah she-Hiqdimu 5672* (Brooklyn: Kehot, 1991), pp. 82, 404, 417, 420, 421, 460, 461, 474, 482, 586, 644, 663. 900, 905, 906, 1270, 1271, 1276, 1277, 1287, 1298, 1299; Yosef Yiṣḥaq Schneersohn, *Sefer ha-Ma'amarim 5689* (Brooklyn: Kehot, 1990), p. 64; Menaḥem Mendel Schneerson, *Torat Menaḥem: Hitwwa'aduyyot 5712*, vol. 2 (Brooklyn: Lahak Hanochos, 1997), p. 179; *idem*, *Torat Menaḥem: Hitwwa'aduyyot 5713*, vol. 1 (Brooklyn: Lahak Hanochos, 1997), p. 129; *idem*, *Torat Menaḥem: Hitwwa'aduyyot 5713*, vol. 2 (Brooklyn: Lahak Hanochos, 1997),

p. 113; *idem, Torat Menaḥem: Sefer ha-Ma'amarim 5714* (Brooklyn: Vaad Hanochos BLahak, 2006), pp. 9, 41–42.

133. Shneur Zalman of Liadi, *Torah Or*, 22d, 90a, 90b, 90c, 92b, 109a, 109d, 114d; *idem*, *Liqquṭei Torah, Behar*, 1:42b, 42d, Bemidbar, 12a, 12d; Dov Baer Schneersohn, *Sha'arei Orah*, 35b, 39a, 54b, 55a, 56a, 79b, 124b; *idem, Sha'arei Teshuvah* (Brooklyn: Kehot, 1995), 56d. On the concept of the nothing (*ayin*) in ḥasidic thought, see Schatz-Uffenheimer, *Hasidism as Mysticism*, pp. 67–79; Daniel C. Matt, "Ayin: The Concept of Nothingness in Jewish Mysticism," in *The Problem of Pure Consciousness: Mysticism and Philosophy*, edited by Robert K. C. Forman (New York: Oxford University Press, 1990), pp. 139–45.

134. On this technical term in earlier kabbalistic literature, see Scholem, *Origins of the Kabbalah*, pp. 312 and 439 n. 174, and Wolfson, *Language, Eros, Being*, pp. 99–105. For discussion of the term in Ḥabad speculation, see Rachel Elior, *The Theory of Divinity of Hasidut Habad: Second Generation* (Jerusalem: Magnes Press, 1982), pp. 37–48, 69–73, 106–107 (Hebrew); *idem*, *The Paradoxical Ascent*, pp. 25–31, 63–72.

135. Shneur Zalman's distinction between the circle and the line is based on Lurianic kabbalistic sources, where these geometric shapes were employed to delineate the two principal configurations of the divine emanations. Regarding this symbolism, see Ronit Meroz, "Redemption in the Lurianic Teaching," Ph.D. dissertation, Hebrew University, 1988, pp. 232–34 and 239–42 (Hebrew); Mordecai Pachter, *Roots of Faith and Devequt: Studies in the History of Kabbalistic Ideas* (Los Angeles: Cherub Press, 2004), pp. 131–84.

136. Compare Shneur Zalman of Liadi, *Liqquṭei Torah*, Shir ha-Shirim, 2:20a, where the enduement of darkness related to the dream is compared to the world of chaos in which there was a withdrawal of light that induced the breaking of the vessels and the scattering of the shards below.

137. See parallel in Shneur Zalman of Liadi, *Ma'amerei Admur ha-Zaqen 5565*, vol. 1 (Brooklyn: Kehot, 1980), p. 186: "As it is written 'I will clothe the heavens in blackness' (Isaiah 50:3), that is, the 'heavens' refers to the aspect of the perimeters above, and they will be garbed in other garments, to be hidden and to be concealed in them in a great concealment and hiddenness."

138. Shneur Zalman of Liadi, *Liqquṭei Torah*, Shelaḥ, 1:37d.

139. The term *hitkallelut* is usually translated as "integration," inasmuch as it denotes the reincorporation of the differentiated self into the nondifferentiated oneness of the infinite (see above n. 123). I have rendered the term as "(dis)integration" to capture the sense that the integration into the One is at the same time a disintegration of the individual.

140. Dov Baer Schneersohn, *Torat Ḥayyim: Shemot*, 192a. The expression

shenei hafakhim be-nose eḥad recurs often in Ḥabad sources to mark the paradoxical junction of opposites. See, for example, Shneur Zalman of Liadi, *Liqquṭei Torah*, Neṣavim, 2:49a; Yiṣḥaq Aizak Epstein, *Ma'amar ha-Shiflut we-ha-Simḥah* (Jerusalem, 1996), p. 187; Dov Baer Schneersohn, *Torat Ḥayyim: Bere'shit*, 88d, 192d, 221d, 244d; *idem*, *Ner Miṣwah we-Torah Or* (Brooklyn: Kehot, 1995), 70a, 84b; *idem*, *Sha'arei Teshuvah*, 14c; Menaḥem Mendel Schneersohn, *Ma'amerei Admur ha-Ṣemaḥ Ṣedeq 5614–5615* (Brooklyn: Kehot, 1997), pp. 79–80, 87; Shalom Dovber Schneersohn, *Be-Sha'ah she-Hiqdimu 5672*, p. 728; Menaḥem Mendel Schneerson, *Sefer ha-Ma'amarim 5734–5735* (Brooklyn: Wa'ad Kitvei Qodesh, 1989), p. 74; *idem*, *Torat Menaḥem: Hitwwa'aduyyot 5743*, vol. 1 (Brooklyn: Lahak Hanochos, 1990), p. 293; Elior, *The Paradoxical Ascent*, pp. 69 and 97–100.

141. Shneur Zalman of Liadi, *Ma'amerei Admur ha-Zaqen 5565*, vol. 1, pp. 184–85.

142. Shneur Zalman of Liadi, *Liqquṭei Torah*, Hosafot, 1:51b. In that context, the oneiric potential to combine contradictory images is linked to the part of the prayer concerning dreams preserved in the Talmud that was uttered before the priests at the moment that they spread out their fingers to bless the people of Israel (the prayer was later affixed liturgically to the priestly blessing), "Just as you changed the curse of Balaam from curse to blessing, so may you change all my dreams to good" (Babylonian Talmud, Berakhot 55b). The priestly blessing (Numbers 6:22–26) is incorporated into the *seder haṭavat ḥalom*, the liturgical offering to be recited in the morning prayers after a night in which one has had a distressing dream. See *Seder Avodat Yisra'el*, edited by Seligman Baer (Berlin: Schocken, 1937), p. 579. It is of interest to mention in conjunction with this rabbinic passage that the interpreter of dreams in pre-Islamic Arabia was the *kāhin*, a word that is etymologically the same as the Hebrew *kohen*, the priest. See Jean Lecerf, "The Dream in Popular Culture: Arabic and Islamic," in *The Dream and Human Societies*, p. 369. The connection of priests and dream interpretation with other mantic practices, such as divination, conjuration, and necromancy, is attested in ancient Mesopotamian sources, as well. See Oppenheim, "The Interpretation of Dreams," pp. 221–24; Blenkinsopp, *Sage, Priest, Prophet*, pp. 81–82. For a similar shamanistic phenomenon attributed to Zoroastrian Magi, see Russell, "'Sleep' and 'Dreaming' in Armenian," pp. 154–55 (*Armenian and Iranian Studies*, pp. 484–85).

143. Scholem, *Major Trends*, pp. 266–67; Isaiah Tishby, *The Doctrine of Evil and the 'Kelippah' in Lurianic Kabbalism* (Jerusalem: Schocken, 1942), pp. 28–34 (Hebrew); *idem*, *Wisdom*, pp. 276–77, 289, 333 n. 263; *idem*, *Paths of Faith and Heresy: Essays in Kabbalah and Sabbateanism* (Jerusalem: Magnes Press, 1982),

pp. 23–29 (Hebrew); Joseph Ben-Shlomo, *The Mystical Theology of Moses Cordovero* (Jerusalem: Bialik Institute, 1965), pp. 230–38 (Hebrew); Yehuda Liebes, *Studies in the Zohar,* translated by Arnold Schwartz, Stephanie Nakache, and Penina Peli (Albany: State University of New York Press, 1993), pp. 65–67; Meroz, "Redemption," pp. 128–42, 203–208, 239–45; Pinchas Giller, *Reading the Zohar: The Sacred Text of the Kabbalah* (Oxford: Oxford University Press, 2001), pp. 95–98; Fine, *Physician*, pp. 135–38.

144. Tishby, *Doctrine of Evil,* p. 32 n. 5; Scholem, *Major Trends*, p. 265.

145. Shneur Zalman of Liadi, *Torah Or*, 39c, 49b, 61b, 97b; *idem*, *Liqquṭei Torah*, Shemini, 1:18d; Ki Tazr'ia; Emor, 23d, 34c, 37d, 39c; Beha'alotkha, 31c.

146. Shneur Zalman of Liadi, *Liqquṭei Torah*, Ṣaw, 1:13d. See, however, Shmuel Schneersohn, *Liqquṭei Torah: Torat Shmu'el 5633*, vol. 2, p. 607: "Therefore, Joseph was an interpreter of dreams, for the dream comprises the two opposites, that is, the aspects of chaos and rectification."

147. Yosef Yiṣḥaq Schneersohn, *Sefer ha-Ma'amarim 5689*, p. 244.

148. *Ibid.*

149. Yosef Yiṣḥaq Schneersohn, *Sefer ha-Ma'amarim 5692–5693* (Brooklyn: Kehot, 2004), p. 489. On the distinction between the lie that dissimulates as truth and the lie that covers the truth, see also Yosef Yiṣḥaq Schneersohn, *Sefer ha-Ma'amarim 5710–5711* (Brooklyn: Kehot, 1986), pt. 2, p. 159.

150. Wolfson, *Open Secret*, pp. 52, 93, 103–109, 128–29, 132, 215.

151. On the depiction of the seemingly autonomous world as the concealment that covers the truth that there is no reality but the divine, see Menaḥem Mendel Schneerson, *Liqquṭei Siḥot* (Brooklyn: Kehot, 1992), 39:158–59: "The complete truth is that there is no existence to anything in the world apart from him, may he be blessed (and if it does not appear so to the eyes it is only on account of the concealment of the face that covers the truth).... The entire reality of the adversary [*ha-menagged*] is merely due to the concealment that covers the truth, for 'there is none beside him' (Deuteronomy 4:35), and nothing in the world has existence apart from him, may he be blessed. Hence, if a man cleaves to God to the point that his true unity, may he be blessed, is revealed in him, the reality of the adversary is abolished as the darkness that is pushed away before the light, for, in truth, it has no existence at all." The view I have proposed here and expanded upon in the following chapter resonates with the observation of Drob, *Kabbalistic Visions*, p. 133, that the kabbalistic doctrine of divine withdrawal or concealment (*ṣimṣum*) coheres with the Hindu Vedāntic notion that the whole world is like a dream in the mind of the Absolute. The infinite's withdrawal from itself "creates an illusion of finitude and multiplicity that is our world, an illusion that is many ways akin to a human dream."

From the accompanying note (p. 274 n. 42) it is clear that Drob has in mind the interpretation of the kabbalistic concept of divine withdrawal according to the so-called acosmism of Ḥabad. Finally, it is worth noting here that the Ḥabad perspective is anticipated in the following passage from the *Ma'amar Yiḥud ha-Yir'ah* of Luzzatto, *Adir ba-Marom*, part 2, pp. 150–51: "All of the worlds are naught but the disclosure of what was already arrayed in the perfection of the Infinite, blessed be he . . . for the reality of all the worlds is naught but as one who dreams a dream and sees the matter in the imagination, and similarly the complete potency of the Infinite, blessed be he, which has no temporality, is seen according to the way of time. . . . Thus the matter of time is nothing at all but how we imagine nature as it appears to us in accord with the withdrawal [*lefi ha-ṣimṣum*]. As we see in the dream itself that days and years pass in one dream, and it seems to the dreamer that this is how it verily is, similarly, when we are awake, we imagine the matters of nature in accord with what we see, and we call this imagining time, as if there could be one hour or one moment like the years of a dream, which are in truth a single moment."

152. Yosef Yiṣḥaq Schneersohn, *Sefer ha-Ma'amarim 5689*, p. 245. Compare Menaḥem Mendel Schneerson, *Torat Menaḥem: Sefer ha-Ma'amarim 5722* (Brooklyn: Vaad Hanochos BLahak, 2001), pp. 87–93; *idem*, *Torat Menaḥem: Sefer ha-Ma'amarim 5724* (Brooklyn: Lahak Hanochos, 2010), pp. 75–76.

153. Louis Jacobs, *Dobh Baer of Lubavitch: Tract on Ecstasy*, translated with introduction and notes (London: Vallentine Mitchell, 1963), pp. 11–12; *idem*, *Seeker of Unity: The Life and Works of Aaron of Starosselje* (London: Vallentine Mitchell, 1966), pp. 115–18; Elior, *The Theory of Divinity*, pp. 299–300, 308–309, 314–15; *idem*, *The Paradoxical Ascent*, pp. 197–200; Loewenthal, *Communicating*, pp. 131–34; Jonathan Garb, "Mystics' Critiques of Mystical Experience," *Revue de l'histoire des religions* 221 (2004): 316–17. Garb's analysis comes closest to my own, including noting a parallel to the Buddhist distinction between "absolute" and "relative truth" (p. 317 n. 99)—or, to be more precise, the Mahāyāna principle of two orders of truth, the conventional (*lokasaṃvṛtisatya*) and the supreme (*paramārthasatya*)—but there are some important differences. See the reference to the study of Brody cited above, n. 110.

154. Aaron Halevi Horowitz of Staroselye, *Sha'arei Avodah* (Shklov, 1821), introduction, pp. 21–22.

155. Aaron Halevi Horowitz of Staroselye, *Sha'arei Avodah*, Sha'ar ha-Tefillah, ch. 38, 68a. For an extensive analysis of prayer in Aaron Halevi's writings, see Jacobs, *Seeker of Unity*, pp. 113–37.

156. Jung, in *Memories, Dreams, Reflections*, p. 341, expressed a similar sentiment from a Christological perspective: "The Word happens to us; we

suffer it, for we are victims of a profound uncertainty: with God as a *complexio oppositorum*, all things are possible, in the fullest meaning of the phrase. Truth and delusion, good and evil, are equally possible." In light of this affinity between Jung and Ḥabad, it is of interest to recall the tantalizing remark made by the former in an interview on his eightieth birthday with Michael Schabad on July 22, 1955, that his "entire psychology" was anticipated by Dov Baer, the Maggid of Międzyrzecz, the teacher of Shneur Zalman of Liadi. See *C. G. Jung Speaking: Interviews and Encounters*, edited by William McGuire and R F. C. Hull (Princeton: Princeton University Press, 1977), pp. 271–72. It is not clear from the context why Jung made this comparison, but see the explanation offered by Drob, *Kabbalistic Visions*, p. 213. Also relevant is Jung's own kabbalistic vision in 1944, which he experienced as he was recuperating from a heart attack. As he recounts the vision years later, he speaks of having found himself in the "garden of pomegranates" (*pardes rimmonim*)—a probable reference to the treatise by Moses Cordovero, but likely used by Jung as a symbolic cipher for the orchard of the divine pleroma—witnessing the wedding between *Tif'eret* and *Malkhut*. Alternatively, he suggests that he may have been experiencing his own mystical marriage in the afterlife, insofar as he was identified with Simeon ben Yoḥai. In the second phase of the vision, the Jewish symbolism is replaced by the Christian image of the marriage of the Lamb to Jerusalem, and this, in turn, gives way in the third phase to the *hieros gamos* of the pagan gods, Zeus and Hera. See Jung, *Memories, Dreams, Reflections*, p. 294, and analysis in Drob, *Kabbalistic Visions*, pp. 207–27. In *Mysterium Coniunctionis*, pp. 22–24, Jung elaborates on the sacred union in kabbalistic theosophy, and in that context (p. 22 n. 111), he refers to a passage from Cordovero's treatise as cited in Christian Knorr von Rosenroth's *Kabbala denudata*.

157. Wolfson, *Open Secret*, pp. 109–10.

158. Dov Baer Schneersohn, *Torat Ḥayyim: Bere'shit*, 243c–d. See *idem*, *Torat Ḥayyim: Shemot*, 37d–39a.

159. The attempt on the part of Scholem, *Major Trends*, pp. 340–41, to separate the theosophical and psychological in the case of Ḥabad (which is proffered as a specific example of a phenomenon he thought to be symptomatic of Beshṭian ḥasidism more generally) is not satisfactory. Scholem's statement that "the secrets of the divine realm are presented in the guise of mystical psychology" fails to appreciate the extent to which these two are mirrors that reflect one another through the difference of their identity. If we are to adopt the language of the secrets of the divine being presented in the guise of the secrets of the soul, then we must equally posit that the secrets of the soul are presented in the guise of the secrets of the divine. I would say this is the case for the history

of kabbalah, but it has a particular resonance in the mystical pietism of Ḥabad.

160. Compare Dov Baer Schneersohn, *Torat Ḥayyim: Bere'shit*, 216a: "The matter is that dreams are in the aspect of the perimeters of chaos [*maqqifim de-tohu*], for there two opposites can dwell as one, even though they are absolutely distinguished from one another."

161. To be precise, in the Ḥabad teaching, the aspect of soul called *yeḥidah* is unique to the Jewish people, and hence their conception of the consubstantiality of divine and human is limited ethnocentrically. For a more elaborate discussion, see Wolfson, *Open Secret*, pp. 231–40.

162. See, however, Dov Baer Schneersohn, *Torat Ḥayyim: Shemot*, 38b–c, where the dreams of prophets, who are completely removed from their carnal bodies, are said to be free of any lie or devious image. See also the view of Almoli cited above, n. 46.

163. See Shmuel Schneersohn, *Liqquṭei Torah: Torat Shmu'el 5632*, vol. 1, p. 257: "This is [the import] of what is written 'we were as dreamers' (Psalms 126:1), just as in the time of the dream one can combine two opposites together . . . so, too, in the exile, one can combine two opposites, because a person's longing can be for the divine and also have a desire for matters of this world. And it is also possible to act against his will, blessed be he, for this is the matter of the dream."

164. Dov Baer Schneersohn, *Torat Ḥayyim: Bere'shit*, 49c, 219c; *idem*, *Torat Ḥayyim: Shemot*, 292a.

165. Dov Baer elaborates the point in *Torat Ḥayyim: Shemot*, 38a–b.

166. Compare Menaḥem Mendel Schneerson, *Torat Menaḥem: Hitwwa'aduyyot 5713*, vol. 1, p. 200, where the dream is classified as a weakened form of vision (*re'iyyah be-ḥalishut*) by means of which "it is possible to see two opposite things."

167. Menaḥem Mendel Schneerson, *Torat Menaḥem: Hitwwa'aduyyot 5743*, vol. 2 (Brooklyn: Lahak Hanochos, 1993), p. 1060. See *idem*, *Torat Menaḥem: Hitwwa'aduyyot 5723*, vol. 1 (Brooklyn: Lahak Hanochos, 2007), pp. 322–23. Compare the text of Viṭal cited in Chapter 3 at n. 115; Shneur Zalman of Liadi, *Ma'amerei Admor ha-Zaqen 5562* (Brooklyn: Kehot, 1975), pp. 94–95.

168. A version of the story is related in a talk from Simḥat Torah 5698 (1937) given by Yosef Yiṣḥaq Schneersohn, *Sefer ha-Siḥot 5696–Ḥoref 5700* (Brooklyn: Kehot, 1989), p. 251.

169. Menaḥem Mendel Schneerson, *Torat Menaḥem: Hitwwa'aduyyot 5742*, vol. 1 (Brooklyn: Lahak Hanochos, 1990), p. 330. The moral of the story, according to Schneerson, is that the ḥasid must respond to the non-Jew, even though the latter has no conception of the matter of annihilation. The form

of the response, therefore, was "not normal," but the one who offered it was able to conceal the matter without lying overtly. See also Menaḥem Mendel Schneerson, *Torat Menaḥem: Hitwwa'aduyyot 5711*, vol. 1 (Brooklyn: Lahak Hanochos, 1994), p. 274 n. 42.

170. Menaḥem Mendel Schneerson, *Torat Menaḥem: Hitwwa'aduyyot 5746*, vol. 1 (Brooklyn: Lahak Hanochos, 1990), p. 75.

171. Menaḥem Mendel Schneerson, *Torat Menaḥem: Hitwwa'aduyyot 5742*, vol. 3 (Brooklyn: Lahak Hanochos, 1990), p. 1648. See also *idem*, *Sefer ha-Ma'amarim 5732–5733* (Brooklyn: Wa'ad Kitvei Qodesh, 1989), p. 366.

172. Menaḥem Mendel Schneerson, *Torat Menaḥem: Hitwwa'aduyyot 5748*, vol. 1 (Brooklyn: Lahak Hanochos, 1990), pp. 65–66.

173. The story is interpreted in this way in Menaḥem Mendel Schneerson, *Torat Menaḥem: Hitwwa'aduyyot 5712*, vol. 1 (Brooklyn: Lahak Hanochos, 1995), p. 247. In that context, the seventh rebbe used the expression *ḥasid idyoṭ*.

174. Menaḥem Mendel Schneerson, *Torat Menaḥem: Hitwwa'aduyyot 5751*, vol. 3 (Brooklyn: Lahak Hanochos, 1993), p. 405.

175. Menaḥem Mendel Schneerson, *Torat Menaḥem: Sefer ha-Ma'amarim 5724*, pp. 73–75. The dream is depicted as the "disclosure of light that is above the vessels," but that nevertheless enters into the interiority of the dreamer, and thus the "matter of the dream" is compared to a "miracle that is above nature," the "most impossible" (*nimna ha-nimna'ot*). In that context, moreover, the purpose of the dream is explained as the "rectification of the letters of thought and speech" (*tiqqun otiyyot ha-maḥashavah we-ha-dibbur*). Since the dream is "above the intellect," it has the capacity to effectuate this rectification by purifying these letters and restoring them to their supernal source (*ibid.*, p. 72). For a more detailed and technical account, see Shalom Dovber Schneersohn, *Sefer ha-Ma'amarim 5678* (Brooklyn: Kehot, 1984), pp. 130–32; Menaḥem Mendel Schneerson, *Torat Menaḥem: Sefer ha-Ma'amarim 5722*, pp. 87–90. On the linguistic nature of dreams, see also the comment of Naḥman of Bratslav, *Liqquṭei MoHaRaN* (Benei Beraq, 1972), 1.19:9, 27d: "He who has attained the perfection of Hebrew [*sheleimut leshon ha-qodesh*] knows how to interpret dreams [that occur] in sleep as Joseph...for dreams are in accord with the food that one eats...and in every matter there are letters.... When one reclines and sleeps, the vapors from the food one has eaten rise, and they ascend to the brain, and the letters contained in them are joined together and from that the dream is made.... He who has attained the perfection of Hebrew knows the letters in everything, and hence he is capable of interpreting dreams. Understand well how we are now explaining the matter of the interpretation of dreams by means of the perfection of Hebrew.... Through the perfection

of Hebrew the gleam of the letters, which are in everything, is illumined, and dreams are from the gleam of the letters that are in all edible things. By means of this the righteous one, who is the aspect of Joseph, knows how to interpret dreams [that occur] in sleep." The parenthetical remark immediately following this passage records that it was copied directly from a manuscript in Naḥman's own hand. See also *Liqquṭei MoHaRaN*, II.5:9, 9a–b, where a similar description of the dream is offered. In that context, however, it is specified that the oneiric vision, which is brought about through an angel, is constituted by the speech (*dibbur*) that is the trace (*reshimu*) engraved and inscribed in the brain as a result of the withdrawal of the mind (*histallequt ha-da'at*) or the removal of consciousness (*histallequt ha-moḥin*). Naḥman further distinguishes two kinds of dreams, the dream of the angel and the dream of the demon, which are correlated respectively with two aspects of the imaginative faculty (*koaḥ ha-medammeh*), the human and the beast. Compare the negative assessment of dream as an expression of the imaginative faculty (the scriptural example mentioned to illustrate the general point is Pharaoh's dream) in *Liqquṭei MoHaRaN*, I.54:6, 62b. On Naḥman's twofold attitude toward dreams and his complex view concerning the faculty of the imagination, see Zvi Mark, *Mysticism and Madness: The Religious Thought of Rabbi Nachman of Bratslav* (New York: Continuum, 2009), pp. 5–7, 15–16, 22. See also Chapter 5 n. 6. For discussion of the personal dreams of Naḥman, which were reported to his leading disciple and successor, Nathan of Nemirov, see Arthur Green, *Tormented Master: A Life of Rabbi Nahman of Bratslav* (University: University of Alabama Press, 1979), pp. 8, 28, 39, 48, 81, 111–12, 164–71, 198–200; Isaac Lewin, Dror Schlezinger, and Danny Derby, "The Personality of R. Nahman of Bratslav: Comparing Dream Content Analysis and Biography," *Journal of Psychology and Judaism* 22 (1998): 33–50.

176. Menaḥem Mendel Schneerson, *Torat Menaḥem: Hitwwa'aduyyot 5713*, vol. 3 (Brooklyn: Lahak Hanochos, 1998), p. 91. According to this passage, the manifestation of the essence as it is (*gilluy ha-aṣmut kemo she-hu*) occurs most specifically in the Holy of Holies of the Jerusalem Temple, the "gate of heaven," *sha'ar ha-shamayim* (Genesis 28:17) on earth, the place that is above place. See also Menaḥem Mendel Schneerson, *Torat Menaḥem: Hitwwa'aduyyot 5743*, vol. 1, p. 293. On the depiction of the Holy of Holies as the place that is beyond place and the time that is beyond time, see Menaḥem Mendel Schneerson, *Liqquṭei Siḥot* (Brooklyn: Kehot, 1962), 2:407–408; *idem*, *Torat Menaḥem: Hitwwa'aduyot 5712*, vol. 3 (Brooklyn: Lahak Hanochos, 1996), pp. 186–88.

177. It is of interest to note that Dov Baer Schneersohn, *Perush ha-Millot*, 54d, associates Joseph, the interpreter of dreams, with Hadar, the eighth of the

Edomite kings, "the root of the rectification of the purifications" (*shoresh ha-tiqqun shel ha-berurim*). The portrayal of Hadar as the beginning of the *tiqqun* can be traced to zoharic literature, especially the Idrot strata (1:223b; 3:135a–b, 142a, 292a), an idea related to the fact that he is the only one of the kings of Edom whose wife, Meheṭabel, is mentioned (Genesis 36:39), an exegetical point developed especially in Lurianic kabbalah. See Liebes, *Studies*, pp. 12–19; Elliot R. Wolfson, "Divine Suffering and the Hermeneutics of Reading: Philosophical Reflections on Lurianic Mythology," in *Suffering Religion*, edited by Robert Gibbs and Elliot R. Wolfson (London: Routledge, 2002), pp. 130–31; *idem*, *Language, Eros, Being*, pp. 311 and 387; Avishar Har Shefi, "Malchin Kadmain: The Myth of the Edomite Kings in the Idrot Literature—The First Appearance," M.A. thesis, Bar-Ilan University, 2006 (Hebrew). Significantly, in the passage from Dov Baer, the redemptive activity is linked to dream interpretation. Needless to say, the soteriological role assigned to Joseph also relates to his symbolic relationship to *Yesod*, the phallic potency, which is connected as well to the number eight. On the relevance of this symbolism in the messianic teachings of Ḥabad, see Wolfson, *Open Secret*, pp. 53–55, 97, 298–300, 313 n. 112, 318 n. 39, 342 n. 187, 403–404 nn. 150–52, 405 nn. 164–65.

178. Shneur Zalman of Liadi, *Torah Or*, 28d.

179. *Ibid.*

180. Shneur Zalman of Liadi, *Liqquṭei Amarim: Tanya*, pt. 1, ch. 36, 46a–b; *idem*, *Seder Tefillot mi-kol ha-Shanah* (Brooklyn: Kehot, 1986), 132a; Dov Baer Schneersohn, *Sha'arei Teshuvah*, 142d; Menaḥem Mendel Schneerson, *Liqquṭei Siḥot* (Brooklyn: Kehot, 2000), 9:63–64.

181. Ben-Shlomo, *Mystical Theology*, pp. 95–100; Bracha Sack, *The Kabbalah of Rabbi Moshe Cordovero* (Jerusalem: Bialik Institute, 1995), pp. 57, 67–68, 192, 256 (Hebrew); Meroz, "Redemption," pp. 105–106, 165; Wolfson, "Divine Suffering," pp. 110–15; *idem*, *Language, Eros, Being*, p. 27. For the impact of the dialectic of disclosure and concealment on Ḥabad, see Elior, *The Theory of Divinity*, 67–71, and *idem*, *The Paradoxical Ascent*, pp. 116–17 and 121–22.

182. For elaboration of this motif, see Wolfson, *Open Secret*, pp. 25–26, 114–29, 206–207. A more conventional and literal understanding of messianic redemption as the unimpeded revelation of the divine will is offered by Jacobs, *Seeker of Unity*, p. 109

183. Shneur Zalman of Liadi, *Torah Or*, 114c.

184. Menaḥem Mendel Schneersohn, *Or ha-Torah: Devarim*, vol. 6 (Brooklyn: Kehot, 1984), p. 2204; Shmuel Schneersohn, *Liqquṭei Torah: Torat Shmu'el 5627*, p. 413. The expression *afisat ha-ra'yon* as a designation of *Keter* is found in Cordovero, *Pardes Rimmonim*, 23:1, 7c, 23:8, 18c; *idem*, *Or Ne'erav* (Jerusalem,

1974), p. 57. But the source cited by both Menaḥem Mendel and his son Shmuel is Meir Poppers, *Me'orot Natan* (Frankfurt am Main, 1709), 10b: "*Efes* [is the name by which] the Infinite is called, for there is no comprehension of it [*ki ein bo tefisah*], and in it is the negation of thought [*u-vo afisat ha-ra'yon*]." The work of Poppers is referred to as *Me'orei Or*. The passage is mentioned as well in the addenda to Shneur Zalman of Liadi, *Torah Or*, 114c.

185. Shneur Zalman of Liadi, *Liqquṭei Torah*, Naso, 1:20c. On the depiction of silence as the nullification of existence (*biṭṭul bi-meṣi'ut*), see Shneur Zalman of Liadi, *Torah Or*, 113b; Dov Baer Schneersohn, *Torat Ḥayyim: Shemot*, 349d, 450c–d. And see *idem*, *Torat Ḥayyim: Bere'shit*, 141a, where silence is linked to the "essential nullification" (*biṭṭul ha-aṣmi*).

186. Menaḥem Mendel Schneersohn, *Or ha-Torah: Siddur Tefillah* (Brooklyn: Kehot, 1984), p. 364.

187. Yosef Yiṣḥaq Schneersohn, *Sefer ha-Ma'amarim 5689*, p. 64. The expression *he'lem ha-aṣmi* is used frequently by exponents of Ḥabad philosophy. See above, n. 132.

188. On the quietistic ideal of negation that ensues from being conjoined to the Infinite, see the characteristic formulation of Aaron Halevi Horowitz of Staroselye, *Sha'arei ha-Yiḥud we-ha-Emunah* (Shklov, 1820), pt. 2, 46b: "To give one's soul in the unification, that is, to nullify and to be bound to the Infinite, blessed be he, in his essence, in the manner of nullifying all the worlds, one's body, and one's soul to the essence of the Infinite, blessed be he, in the way that all the worlds are nullified entirely, and everything is considered as having no worth at all in relation to his essence." Compare Jacobs, *Seeker of Unity*, pp. 108–109, and see references cited above, n. 121.

CHAPTER FIVE: UNDOING TIME

1. Given the plethora of studies on time and temporality in Husserl, I will refrain from listing any here. Readers interested in my own account of this topic should consult Wolfson, *Alef, Mem, Tau*, pp. 12, 17–24.

2. Sartre, *The Imaginary*, pp. 129–30.

3. *Ibid.*, pp. 130–31 (emphasis in the original).

4. Numerous thinkers and philosophers have weighed in on this topic. For a learned survey from antiquity to the present, see Jan Johann Albinn Mooij, *Time and Mind: The History of a Philosophical Problem* (Leiden: Brill, 2005).

5. Maurizio Ferraris, "What is There?" in Jacques Derrida and Maurizio Ferraris, *A Taste for the Secret*, translated from the French and Italian by Giacomo Donis, edited by Giacomo Donis and David Webb (Cambridge: Polity

Press, 2001), p. 111: "Metaphysically speaking, it is not unlikely that there should be a dream lasting a lifetime (i.e. that a mental state should proceed coherently independently of constant references to an external world)." For a contrary opinion that calls attention to a closer proportionality between estimated time in dreams and the clock time of waking reality, see LaBerge, *Lucid Dreaming*, pp. 74–78. The author does not deny the sensation of extended passages of time in the dreamscape, and in that sense dream time may not equal clock time, but he insists that the evidence from experiments with oneironauts is that it takes as long to dream that one is doing something as it does to actually do it.

6. Abraham Shamsian, *Sod Pitron ha-Ḥalomot* (Tsfat, 2001), p. 11: "The time of the dream is the 'trifle that holds a lot' [*Midrash Shemot Rabbah* 11:5], for one can see many things and many places in a dream, which is not possible if the vision were to occur when one is awake (in reality); even a whole year would not suffice for what one dreams within a short time." On the experience in a dream of a small measure of time as it if were an extended period, see Naḥman of Bratslav, *Liqquṭei MoHaRaN*, II.61, 29a. According to Naḥman, the confusion in the temporal perception in the dream is due to the fact that during sleep the power of reason (*sekhel*) withdraws and the faculty of imagination (*koaḥ ha-medammeh*) prevails (see Chapter 4 n. 175). Concerning this passage, see Green, *Tormented Master*, pp. 321–22; Elliot R. Wolfson, "The Cut That Binds: Time, Memory, and the Ascetic Impulse," in *God's Voice from the Void: Old and New Studies in Bratslav Hasidism*, edited by Shaul Magid (Albany: State University of New York Press, 2002), pp. 106–107. See Bulkeley, *Dreaming*, p. 2: "What strikes most people about their dreams is how weird and bizarre they sometimes appear. A dream can put you in any place, with anyone, doing anything—the ordinary limitations of waking life are suspended, allowing for a seemingly infinite range of possible scenarios and interactions.... Oddities abound in dreams—sudden shifts of time and location, strange mixtures of people and personalities, inexplicable behavior and feelings, extraordinary abilities and powers. Nothing is impossible in dreams. Everything seems to be permissible."

7. See Hiroshi Kojima, "The Vertical Intentionality of Time-Consciousness and Sense-Giving," in *Husserl in Contemporary Context*, pp. 79–93. The nonsensical quality of the dream and the destabilization of time and space implied thereby may account for the phenomenon attested in many cultures regarding the appearance of the deceased in dreams. See Oppenheim, "The Interpretation of Dreams," p. 204. For examples in rabbinic literature, see Babylonian Talmud, Shabbat 152a–b, Mo'ed Qaṭan 28a; Galit Hasan-Rokem,

"Communication with the Dead in Jewish Dream Culture," in *Dream Cultures*, pp. 213–32; Weiss, "'What This One Interpreted for Me'," pp. 35–37; and Harari, *Early Jewish Magic*, pp. 320–21. See also the comment of Fromm cited below at n. 30 and other references mentioned in n. 224.

8. Foucault, "Dream, Imagination and Existence," p. 58. With respect to the construction of time and memory in the dream, there are interesting affinities between Foucault and Benjamin, but I cannot pursue them in this context. See Benjamin's engagement with the psychoanalytic theory of the unconscious and memory in Freud (as discussed by Theodor Reik) and the "involuntary memory" of Proust, in *The Arcades Project*, pp. 402–403. See the references to Benjamin cited in Chapter 1 n. 99 and the essays by Stathis Gourgouris, "The Dream-Reality of the Ruin," in *Walter Benjamin and the Arcades Project*, pp. 201–24, and Tyrus Miller, "'Glass Before Its Time, Premature Iron': Architecture, Temporality, and Dream in Benjamin's Arcades Project," *ibid*., pp. 240–58.

9. Freud, "The Unconscious," *SE*, 14:187.

10. Ferguson, *Lure of Dreams*, pp. 71 and 76.

11. Bulkeley, *Dreaming*, pp. 110–11.

12. My thinking coincides with the observation of Edith Wyschogrod, "Between Phenomenology and the Negative's Power," in *Portraits of American Continental Philosophers*, edited by James R. Watson (Bloomington: Indiana University Press, 1999), p. 225: "But a difficulty in the commonsense view of history that has gone unnoticed is the interpretation of time as most primordially future time. Heidegger's ecstatic view of time is in accord with this perspective in that he sees the past primarily in future terms. It is as if one were to say: 'Even then, in the past, what was of importance was that one always looked ahead, for even then one was always already thrown over the abyss of one's own future nonexistence.'" See as well Wyschogrod, *An Ethics of Remembering*, pp. 240–45.

13. Foucault, "Dream, Imagination and Existence," p. 64. These terms are used by Foucault to describe the "time of the epic," but I have taken the liberty to extend them more generally to our ordinary temporal experience.

14. The fragment, cited by Clement, *Stromateis* II.17.4, as rendered in Kahn, *The Art and Thought of Heraclitus*, VII, p. 31.

15. Almoli, *Pitron Ḥalomot*, 2b–3a.

16. Tracey Kahan, Raania Moshen, Jeanette Tandez, and Jennifer McDonald, "Discriminating Memories for Actual and Imagined Taste Experiences: A Reality Monitoring Approach," *American Journal of Psychology* 112 (1999): 97–112.

17. Bulkeley, *Dreaming*, pp. 10–11. On memory and dreams, see Henri

Bergson, *Matter and Memory*, translated by Nancy Margaret Paul and W. Scott Palmer (New York: Zone Books, 1991), pp. 153–54, and *idem*, *Mind-Energy*, pp. 89–94. For Bergson, the scope of memory is expanded in the "dream plane," since the whole of the dreamer's past is available, as opposed to a wakeful state in which memory is restricted to the perception of the actual. See Henri Bergson, *The Creative Mind*, translated by Mabelle L. Andison (New York: Philosophical Library, 1946), pp. 29 and 89. On the intensified sense of duration in dreams, see Bergson, *Time and Free Will*, p. 126.

18. Michele Stephen, "Memory, Emotion, and the Imaginal Mind," in *Dreaming and the Self*, pp. 97–129.

19. *Zohar* 1:197b.

20. *Midrash Eikhah Rabbah* 5:1; *Pesiqta Rabbati: A Synoptic Edition based upon All Extant Manuscripts and the Editio Princeps*, edited by Rivka Ulmer, vol. 1 (Atlanta: Scholars Press, 1997), 13:16, p. 206. On the related formulation that there is no forgetfulness before the throne of glory, see de León, *The Book of the Pomegranate*, p. 160 n. 15 (Hebrew section); Wolfson, *Luminal Darkness*, p. 223 n. 96.

21. See Chapter 3 n. 21.

22. *Zohar* 1:199b.

23. For discussion of this image in kabbalistic and Ṣūfi sources, see Wolfson, *Alef, Mem, Tau*, pp. 102–104.

24. Elliot R. Wolfson, "Re/membering the Covenant: Memory, Forgetfulness, and History in the *Zohar*," in *Jewish History and Jewish Memory: Essays in Honor of Yosef Hayim Yerushalmi*, edited by Elisheva Carlebach, David S. Myers, and John Efron (Hanover: Brandeis University Press, 1998), pp. 214–46, corrected and slightly revised version in Wolfson, *Luminal Darkness*, pp. 185–227.

25. Palestinian Talmud, Pe'ah 1:1, 16b; Qiddusin 1:10, 61d; Sanhedrin 10:1, 27c; *Pesiqta Rabbati*, vol. 1, 13:16, p. 206.

26. *Zohar* 1:200a.

27. My earliest formulation of this dimension of kabbalistic hermeneutics appeared in Elliot R. Wolfson, "Circumcision, Vision of God, and Textual Interpretation: From Midrashic Trope to Mystical Symbol," *History of Religions* 27 (1987): 189–215, and see the more expansive discussion in *idem*, *Through a Speculum*, pp. 326–92. With all the criticisms leveled against my work on gender construction and kabbalistic symbolism, not one person has been able to bring evidence that contradicts the seminal claim regarding the inherent connection between secrecy and the phallus in traditional Jewish mystical texts inspired by a deeper phallocentric element in the biblical-rabbinic sensibility, and as far as I am concerned, in the absence of such contradictory evidence, the

androcentric reading I have promoted has not been undermined. See below, n. 65.

28. Compare the commentary on this zoharic passage in Lavi, *Ketem Paz*, 378b. On the centrality of interpretation to the dream, see the extensive discussion in *ibid.*, 353b–56a.

29. *Midrash Bere'shit Rabba* 89:5, pp. 1091–92; *Midrash Tanḥuma*, Miqqeṣ, 2. The contrast is made between the depictions of the agitation related to the respective dreams of Pharaoh (Genesis 41:8) and Nebuchadnezzar (Daniel 2:1); the former did not know the interpretation of his dream, whereas the latter had forgotten the dream, as well as its interpretation.

30. Fromm, *Forgotten Language*, pp. 4–5.

31. Palestinian Talmud, Sheqalim 6:1, 49d; Megillah 1:4, 70d; Soṭah 3:1, 22d; Babylonian Talmud, Pesaḥim 6b; *Mekhilta de-Rabbi Ishmael*, edited by Ḥayyim S. Horovitz and Israel A. Rabin (Jerusalem: Wahrmann, 1970), p. 139; *Midrash Tanḥuma*, Terumah, 8. For discussion of this principle of rabbinic hermeneutics, see Heschel, *Heavenly Torah*, pp. 240–43; Margarte Schlüter, "The Creative Force of a Hermeneutic Rule: The Principle 'There Is No Earlier and Later in the Torah' in Midrashic and Talmudic Literature," in *Creation and Re-Creation in Jewish Thought: Festschrift in Honor of Joseph Dan on the Occasion of His Seventieth Birthday*, edited by Rachel Elior and Peter Schäfer (Tübingen: Mohr Siebeck, 2005), pp. 59–84; Wolfson, *Alef, Mem, Tau*, pp. 59–60.

32. Eihei Dōgen, *The Heart of Dōgen's Shōbōgenzō*, translated by Norman Waddell and Masao Abe (Albany: State University of New York Press, 2002), p. 42.

33. *Ibid.*, pp. 47–58. The nature of *uji* is illumined from the examples of climbing the mountain or crossing the river: "At the time the mountain was being climbed and the river being crossed, I was there [in time]. The *time* has to *be* in me. Inasmuch as I am there, it cannot be that time passes away. As long as time is not a modality of going and coming, that time on the mountain in the immediate present—right now—of 'the time being' (being-time). Yet as long as time takes upon itself a modality of going and coming, the *being* in me in the immediate *now* of 'the time being' is being-time" (p. 50, emphasis in the original). See the passage from the *Busshō* fascicle of the *Shōbōgenzō* cited below, n. 203. The correspondence of my conceptualization of temporality and the thought of Dōgen is noted in Wolfson, *Alef, Mem, Tau*, p. 71, and for references to other scholarly discussions, see *ibid.*, p. 216 n.102. See also Victor Mansfield, "Time and Impermanence in Middle Way Buddhism and Modern Physics," in *Buddhism and Science*, pp. 305–21.

34. Dōgen, *The Heart of Dōgen's Shōbōgenzō*, p. 42.

35. Borges, *Labyrinths*, p. 234.

36. Carl G. Jung, *Psychology and Religion: East and West*, 2nd ed., translated by R. F. C. Hull (Princeton: Princeton University Press, 1969), p. 503.

37. See the essays "Synchronicity: An Acausal Principle" and "On Synchronicity" included in Carl G. Jung, *The Structure and Dynamics of the Psyche*, 2nd ed., translated by R. F. C. Hull (Princeton: Princeton University Press, 1969), pp. 417–531, and especially the comments on the "psychic relativity of time," *ibid.*, p. 433. The bibliography on this Jungian theme is extensive. Here I note a relatively recent discussion that pays careful attention to the role of dreams in exemplifying the phenomenon: Roderick Main, *The Rupture of Time: Synchronicity and Jung's Critique of Modern Western Culture* (New York: Brunner-Routledge, 2004); and see *idem*, *Revelations of Chance: Synchronicity as Spiritual Experience* (Albany: State University of New York, 2007) and *Atom and Archetype*, p. 39 (from a letter of Pauli to Jung dated 28 June 1949).

38. I am here applying to the dream the sense of temporality I have discussed elsewhere in a number of published studies. Consider as well Boodakian, *Tormenting Angel*, pp. 95–110. On the description of the dream as a weaving together of the "temporal reality" (*mammashut ha-zemanit*) with the "supratemporal web" (*ma'arag al zemani*) and the different perspectives by which to view the three modes of time implied thereby, see Elior, "Reality," p. 66. See also the depiction of the dreamtime offered in the passage from Moss cited in Chapter 1 n. 42.

39. In light of this, it is of interest to recall the rabbinic ruling that if one recites in reverse order (*lemafre'a*) the biblical portions included in the Shema (Deuteronomy 6:4–9, 11:13–21, Numbers 15:37–41), the Tefillah, the standing prayer of the eighteen benedictions, Hallel, the chapters of praise and thanksgiving from Psalms 113–18, or the scroll of Esther on Purim, one's religious obligation is not fulfilled. See Mishnah, Berakhot 2:3, Megillah 2:1; Tosefta, Berakhot 2:3, Megillah 2:1. See also Babylonian Talmud, Soṭah 17b, where a scroll for the suspected woman (Numbers 5:23) written from back to front is decreed to be invalid. It is not clear to me what underlies these hypothetical scenarios and why someone would think of intentionally reciting a liturgical or scriptural text in the wrong way. Ludwig Blau, *Das Altjüdische Zauberwesen* (Strassburg: Karl J. Trübner, 1898), pp. 148–49, surmised that the backward reading may have been a magical practice by which the text is transposed into an incantational formula. Perhaps the expression simply denotes an accidental misreading in which one confuses the sequence of the verses, an explanation attested by medieval talmudic commentators. See the references listed in Saul Lieberman, *Tosefta Ki-Fshuṭah: A Comprehensive Commentary on the Tosefta, Order*

Zera'im, Part 1, 2nd augmented edition (Jerusalem: Jewish Theological Seminary of America, 1992), p. 15 n. 5 (Hebrew). Be that as it may, the important point for my purpose is that the halakhic position does not obviate the fact that one can recount a story coherently, even if the narrative sequence is inverted.

40. Artemidorus, *The Interpretation of Dreams*, p. 33. See S. R. F. Price, "The Future of Dreams: From Freud to Artemidorus," *Past and Present* 113 (1986): 3–37; Bowersock, *Fiction as History*, pp. 80–87

41. Wolfson, *Alef, Mem, Tau*, p. 59.

42. McKenna, *Archaic Revival*, p. 91. For a different approach to the nocturnal time of dreams, also referred to as macrochronos, and the diurnal time of wakefulness, or the microchronos, in Jewish texts, see Idel, "Astral Dreams in Judaism," pp. 235–38, 246–47, and *idem* "Astral Dreams in R. Yohanan Alemanno's Writings," *Accademia: Revue de la Societe Marsile Ficin* 1 (1999): 127–28.

43. Moshe Idel, "Ta'anug: Erotic Delights From Kabbalah to Hasidism," in *Hidden Intercourse: Eros and Sexuality in the History of Western Esotericism*, edited by Wouter J. Hanegraaff and Jeffrey J. Kripal (Leiden: Brill, 2008), pp. 111–51.

44. On Morgenstern's sustained engagement with Ḥabad material, see the commentaries on Shneur Zalman of Liadi's *Tanya* in Isaac Meir Morgenstern, *Yam ha-Ḥokhmah Erev Rosh ha-Shanah 5766* (Jerusalem: Makhon Yam ha-Ḥokhmah, 2005), pp. 201–43, and *idem*, *Yam ha-Ḥokhmah 5769* (Jerusalem: Makhon Yam ha-Ḥokhmah, 2009), pp. 455–66.

45. Morgenstern, *Yam ha-Ḥokhmah Erev Rosh ha-Shanah 5766*, p. 312. On the linking together of prayer and dream, see the passage of Phineḥas of Korzec cited below, n. 212.

46. I have translated *adam* as "person," but I am confident the author was limiting his comments to the Jewish male, who alone can embark on a path of prayer that leads to unification with *Yesod*, which then extends to *Keter*. In an effort to redeem the text from its androcentric and phallocentric shortcomings, I have broadened its anthropological conception.

47. Morgenstern *Yam ha-Ḥokhmah Erev Rosh ha-Shanah 5766*, p. 312.

48. Morgenstern, *ibid.*, makes the point that if one who prays does not feel the light of pleasure, then the worship has not reached the aspect of prayer communicated by *wa-ani tefillah*.

49. See Introduction n. 93.

50. Wolfson, *Open Secret*, pp. 145–46. As I noted there, p. 356 n. 76, the source that influenced my formulation was Shneur Zalman of Liadi, *Torah Or*, 28d. A good portion of the text is cited above, Chapter 4 at n. 128.

51. Morgenstern, *Yam ha-Ḥokhmah Erev Rosh ha-Shanah 5766*, p. 312.

52. This idea is anchored in the description of God as "not human," *ki lo*

adam hu, in 1 Samuel 15:29.

53. This notion is substantiated by the derivation of *adam* from *eddammeh le-elyon*, "I will be likened to the most high," in Isaiah 14:14, the characterization of the image of the glory of God as the "semblance of the appearance of a human," *demut ke-mar'eh adam*, in Ezekiel 1:26, and the declaration of the divine "through the prophets I was imaged," *u-ve-yad ha-nevi'im adammeh*, in Hosea 12:11. See the extended analysis in Wolfson, *Open Secret*, pp. 240–48.

54. Compare the language of Blanchot cited below at n. 127.

55. On this understanding of the term *rega*, see Wolfson, *Open Secret*, pp. 277–80.

56. For the background of this spiritualized interpretation of liturgical worship as conjunction with the nothing in the teachings of the Besht and the Maggid of Międzyrzecz, see Rivka Schatz, "Contemplative Prayer in Hasidism," in *Studies in Mysticism and Religion Presented to Gershom G. Scholem on His Seventieth Birthday* (Jerusalem: Magnes Press, 1967), pp. 209–26.

57. Scholem, *Origins*, p. 438 n. 170. It is relevant to recall a passage from Isaac of Acre, *Oṣar Ḥayyim*, MS Günzberg 775, fol. 87b, where he reports reading in a dream the following four words ויקללם אין באין סוף. Upon waking he interprets them as alluding to a curse (*qelalah*) cast on the rebellious ones who believe only in the Infinite, for such a belief cannot sustain the liturgical and ritual practices demanded by a theistic conception of God. Regarding this text, see Sandra Valabregue-Perry, *Concealed and Revealed: 'Ein Sof' in Theosophic Kabbalah* (Los Angeles: Cherub Press, 2010), p. 228 (Hebrew). And compare another passage from *Oṣar Ḥayyim* cited and discussed in Wolfson, *Language, Eros, Being*, pp. 124–25. According to that text, the goal of contemplation is to be bound to the Infinite that is beyond names and images, but the only way to achieve that goal is through meditation on the image of the ineffable name, YHWH, which is compared to a ladder.

58. Morgenstern, *Yam ha-Ḥokhmah Erev Rosh ha-Shanah 5766*, p. 312.

59. *Ibid.*, pp. 312–13.

60. *Ibid.*, pp. 313–14.

61. Babylonian Talmud, Ḥagigah 13b, and for other sources and commentary, see Wolfson, *Through a Speculum*, p. 264; *idem*, *Along the Path: Studies in Kabbalistic Myth, Symbolism, and Hermeneutics* (Albany: State University of New York Press, 1995), pp. 34 and 155 n. 221.

62. On the identification of *Keter*, the encompassing light (*or maqqif*), as the source of the imagination (*shoresh ha-dimyon*), see Itamar Shwartz, *Qol Demamah Daqqah* [*Bilevavi Mishkan Evneh*, vol. 10] (Jerusalem, n.d.), p. 119: "The light of the imagination is the most elevated and it is rooted in

Keter... and this is the aspect of the human, who is called *adam* from the phrase *eddammeh le-elyon* (Isaiah 14:14), the aspect of the imagination [*dimyon*], for this is his entire worship, to conjoin himself to the imagination that is above the grasp of created being and, as it were, to become comparable to the blessed holy One, *eddammeh le-elyon*." The matter of the dream is not mentioned in this passage, but the supremacy accorded the imagination and its being linked to *Keter* is the basis for the identification of this gradation as the source of dreams.

63. For a more detailed discussion, see Wolfson, *Open Secret*, pp. 66–129.

64. This complex of symbolism was expounded independently at roughly the same time by Liebes and myself. See Yehuda Liebes, "Zohar and Eros," *Alpayyim* 9 (1994): 80 (Hebrew); Elliot R. Wolfson, "Woman—The Feminine as Other in Theosophic Kabbalah: Some Philosophical Observations on the Divine Androgyne," in *The Other in Jewish Thought and History: Constructions of Jewish Culture and Identity*, edited by Laurence J. Silberstein and Robert L. Cohn (New York: New York University Press, 1994), pp. 179–82; *idem*, *Through a Speculum*, p. 389 n. 236; *idem*, *Circle in the Square*, pp. 60–69. Note the passage from Erich Neumann's *Origins of the History of Consciousness* about the "higher phallus" and the head cited in Wolfson, *Language, Eros, Being*, pp. 571–72 n. 200.

65. Unfortunately, my detractors have not understood the use of the term "phallomorphism" to characterize the traditional kabbalistic symbolism, and thus they have felt the need to correct me by pointing out that the kabbalists were aware that there are women in the world with their own anatomy. Typical of this is the ongoing criticism of my work by Moshe Idel, epitomized, for instance, in the brief comment in *Absorbing Perfections*, pp. 580–81 n. 135. My perspective is described as assuming "a tendency to obliterate the difference between male and female divine powers, as part of the absorption of the female by and within the male. This thesis, which is sometimes helpful in understanding texts of Zoharic Kabbalah and those influenced by it, does not hold, however, for numerous other Zoharic treatments of the sexual polarity." For a more extensive, but equally flawed presentation of my views, see Moshe Idel, *Kabbalah and Eros* (New Haven: Yale University Press, 2005), pp. 128–31. For a partial response to Idel's anachronistic characterization of my method as anachronistic for using contemporary gender theory to analyze medieval sources, as well as his homogenizing portrayal of my supposedly homogenous and pansymbolic approach, see Elliot R. Wolfson, "Structure, Innovation, and Diremptive Temporality: The Use of Models to Study Continuity and Discontinuity in Kabbalistic Tradition," *Journal for the Study of Religions and Ideologies* 18 (2007): 154–57. Naturally, I am aware, and I have never denied, that the binary of male

and female is a prevalent motif in kabbalistic literature and that much emphasis has been placed on the union of the two. The issue for me, however, is how the dimorphism is to be interpreted. To affirm sexual polarity on behalf of the kabbalists is an obvious platitude, but it proves nothing about the values assigned respectively to femininity and masculinity in the overall semiotic register that informed their worldview. That women yearn erotically for men and the men reciprocally for women goes without saying; heterosexuality is understood dynamically as a mutual interplay and transposition of opposites: the female can become male and the male female. However, the point to which I have tried to call attention is that the androgyny itself is conceived by kabbalists from the angle of the male, informed, as they were, by the biblical accounts of Adam's creation, the second chapter of Genesis read as a midrashic explication of the first. This is the point sorely missed by Idel and those who have been influenced by his tireless critique. A similarly distorted and simplified presentation of my thought is found in Hellner-Eshed, *A River Flows from Eden*, pp. 169–70. I am charged with drawing on the French feminist tradition in order to emphasize that the "Jewish male mystics have related to the feminine and femininity as void and emptiness, pure passivity with no essence and being of its own, save for its encompassing the masculine." In the author's own mind, "the Zohar's understanding of the feminine and femininity is much more complex, diverse, and nuanced. Alongside the Zohar's portrayal of the feminine as absence and lack, or as part of the masculine, we find also numerous passages describing the feminine as an autonomous, independent quality with which the masculine seeks to unite.... In contrast to Wolfson, I repeatedly discern in the Zohar's pages the positive, erotic, and reciprocal drama of the feminine's yearning to joyfully fill her living, spacious, and desiring womb with all the variegated qualities that flow into her. I do not find here lack and absence, ruthless penetration, negation, and submersion in the masculine, but rather—on the contrary—a total language of feminine erotics, which surprisingly was formulated so poetically and with such nuance by men." Despite the bluster of this oratory, Hellner-Eshed's depiction of my work is woefully inadequate, and it is frankly irresponsible both intellectually and morally to suggest that I do not recognize that in the zoharic symbolism (and in kabbalistic sources more generally) there is a feminine persona with which the masculine seeks to unite. The same error has been made by Hellner-Eshed's teacher, Yehuda Liebes, who has dismissed my work perfunctorily in several of his essays or, more typically, has ignored it completely. I accept that Hellner-Eshed may be more sensitive to aspects of what she calls a "feminine erotics" in zoharic homilies, but this does not mean that she has presented my views properly.

Furthermore, it is not difficult for me to understand or to explain how it is that male kabbalists could fantasize so vividly about the erotic sensibilities of women. This does not release their gender construction from the grip of phallomorphism. For three other attempts to deal critically with my approach to the problem of gender and kabbalistic symbolism, see Daniel Abrams, *The Female Body of God in Kabbalistic Literature: Embodied Forms of Love and Sexuality in the Divine Feminine* (Jerusalem: Magnes Press, 2004), pp. 3–7 (Hebrew); Jonathan Garb, "Gender and Power in Kabbalah: A Theoretical Investigation," *Kabbalah: Journal for the Study of Jewish Mystical Texts* 13 (2005): 79–107, esp. 83–84 and 99–104; and Dvorah Bat-David Gamlieli, *Psychoanalysis and Kabbalah: The Masculine and Feminine in Lurianic Kabbalah* (Los Angeles: Cherub Press, 2006), pp. 61–64 and 248–52 (Hebrew). None of these scholars has challenged the crux of my argument, for they are all guilty of ignoring that the autonomy and power they ascribe to the feminine would relate to what I have marked as the first stage of the redemptive process, the heterosexual pairing of male and female occasioned by the split of the male androgyne; the containment of the feminine in the masculine is the second stage, the rectification of that fissure. The same critique can be leveled against the emphasis on the bipolar union of male and female in the various studies of Charles Mopsik, many of which have been conveniently collected in *Sex of the Soul: The Vicissitudes of Sexual Difference in Kabbalah*, edited with a foreword by Daniel Abrams (Los Angeles: Cherub Press, 2005). When I spoke of the male mystic visualizing the male deity, the central thesis of *Through a Speculum That Shines*, I had in mind the latter phase, wherein the female is restored to the male, commonly designated by the images of the phallic corona (*aṭeret berit*) or the woman ascending as a crown on the head of her husband (*aṭeret ba'lah*). Idel's appeal to polychromatism and egalitarianism (points that Garb regurgitates in deference to his teacher) is a verbal smokescreen. The prevalence of the phallogocentric point of reference is illustrated by the following anecdote. I recently purchased an edition of Meshullam Shraga Feibush Heilperin of Brezin, *Sefat Emet* (Jerusalem: Makhon Sefat Emet, 2008), and the first time I examined the book, a volume of 682 pages, it opened to this passage: "It is said that *Yesod* is the aspect of the redeemer, and the intention, according to our way, is that it is known that one of the reasons for circumcision is to weaken the power of desire in the soul...and therefore the one who merits to rectify the attribute of *Yesod*, to guard the covenant, rectifies everything, for everything depends on it, and this is the root and foundation of the entire Jewish religion [*ha-shoresh we-ha-yesod le-khol dat ha-yehudit*]" (pp. 258–59). There is nothing novel in this comment—I could cite dozens of other examples—but the extreme language is astonishing: the *entire Jewish religion* rests on the enjoinder to protect the purity of the male organ by guarding against sexual sins. Surely, an open-minded person would not quarrel with my conclusion that this sentiment, which is affirmed in innumerable sources, exemplifies a phallomorphic orientation. The resistance to my work reveals that much of Jewish studies remains captivated by identity politics, and especially potent in that regard is the desire to empower women and to do so on the basis of the traditional canon. I am sympathetic to this need, even if my scholarly work has shown that such a reading is hard to defend by a close philological analysis of the traditional sources. Garb, "Gender and Power," p. 102 n. 123, suggests that in contrast to my view, he maintains that "structure itself is often fluid." No original text is cited in support of this claim, but only reference to studies by Idel, Liebes, and Mopsik—the reference to Idel is to his more general discussion on "symbolism and dynamism" in *Kabbalah: New Perspectives*, pp. 222–34, in which there is no specific mention of gender. Even more vexing is the problem that the scholars mentioned by Garb as providing an alternative to me are the ones I have criticized in my work. It will be readily acknowledged that what is required of Garb (or any other critic) is to adduce primary texts and/or to scrutinize the work of the aforementioned scholars to see if they have truly confronted and disputed my work, and not simply to rely on their authority, as if this were a meaningful appraisal. None of them, or anyone else for that matter, has cited one kabbalistic source where the act of overflowing is classified as feminine and the act of receiving as masculine. That there is fluidity of gender roles, the feminization of the male and the masculinization of the female, is something I have discussed myself on many occasions, but this does not undermine the claim that the dynamic is made possible by structural inflexibility. For my most recent examination, which interrogates and in some respects alters my previous work, see Wolfson, *Open Secret*, pp. 200–23. I do acknowledge that the Ḥabad sources, especially the teaching of the seventh rebbe, provide an alternative model whereby the female is accorded a higher status than the male, but even in this case, the rigidity of structure is to some degree preserved, inasmuch as the potency to overflow remains masculine and the capacity to receive feminine, so that at best, the feminine assumes the position atop the male by becoming male. For analyses that are more congenial to my own, see Pinchas Giller, *Shalom Shar'abi and the Kabbalists of Beit El* (Oxford: Oxford University Press, 2008), pp. 131–46, and Shaul Magid, *From Metaphysics to Midrash: Myth, History, and the Interpretation of Scripture in Lurianic Kabbala* (Bloomington: Indiana University Press, 2008), pp. 111–42.

66. In the appendix to Moses David Valle, *Sefer Megalleh Amuqot: Be'ur Sefer*

Iyyov al Derekh Pardes (Jerusalem, 2009), p. 3 n. 2, Joseph Spinner asserts that the biblical commentaries published as *Be'urei ha-Pesuqim* attributed to Luzzatto were "mostly copied" and perhaps even authored by his student, Michael Tirani. I thank Jonathan Garb of the Hebrew University in Jerusalem for calling this source to my attention.

67. Moses Ḥayyim Luzzatto, *Oṣerot Ramḥal*, edited by Ḥayyim Friedlander (Benei Beraq, 1986), pp. 57–58. In that context, the special link between *Arikh Anpin* and redemption is based on the verse "But there shall be a continuous day—only the Lord knows when" (Zechariah 14:7), since the highest aspect of the Godhead is marked as the "continuous day" (*yom eḥad*), the day that has no nocturnal correlate, the day (*yom*) that is truly one (*eḥad*) insofar as there is no genuine other. See below n. 153. On the gender implications of Luzzatto's eschatological teaching, see Elliot R. Wolfson, "*Tiqqun ha-Shekhinah*: Redemption and the Overcoming of Gender Dimorphism in the Messianic Kabbalah of Moses Hayyim Luzzatto," *History of Religions* 36 (1997): 289–332, and compare the summary in Wolfson, *Language, Eros, Being*, pp. 75–76.

68. Elliot R. Wolfson, "Eunuchs Who Keep the Sabbath: Becoming Male and the Ascetic Ideal in Thirteenth-Century Jewish Mysticism," in *Becoming Male in the Middle Ages*, edited by Jeffrey J. Cohen and Bonnie Wheeler (New York: Garland, 1997), pp. 151–85, and the revised version in Wolfson, *Language, Eros, Being*, pp. 296–332. For a comparison of kabbalistic and tantric views on sexual union, see Mopsik, *Sex of the Soul*, pp. 144–47. Mopsik acknowledges that in both traditions, the semen constitutes a "luminous energy," but he contrasts the two on the grounds that for the kabbalist, "the aim is to concentrate this semen from the brain and all the organs of the body in order to propel it with the greatest force and determination towards the female partner," whereas for the yogin, the goal is to elevate the semen to its source in the superior centers of the head (pp. 144–45). I have argued that one can find evidence in kabbalistic sources of a practice that is closer to the tantric ideal; the fusion of masculine and feminine can be achieved in the embodied mind (or mindful body) of the male kabbalist and therefore does not always require an actual female partner. For a comparative study of kabbalah and Hindu tantra, in part indebted to my work, see Paul C. Martin, "The Erotic Imaginary of Divine Realization in Kabbalistic and Tantric Metaphysics," available at http://espace.library.uq.edu.au/eserv/UQ:179374/Kabbalah_and_Tantra_wpv2.pdf.

69. For a thorough review of the topic, see the introduction in *The Book Bahir: An Edition Based on the Earliest Manuscripts*, edited by Daniel Abrams (Los Angeles: Cherub Press, 1994), pp. 1–54 (Hebrew).

70. This is clearly the meaning of *taḥalim gufkha*, a connotation attested,

for instance, in the biblical expression *yaḥlemu veneihem*, "their children are healthy" (Job 39:4). For an interesting misreading, see *The Book of Bahir: Flavius Mithridates' Latin Translation, the Hebrew Text, and an English Version*, edited by Saverio Campanini with a foreword by Giulio Busi (Torino: Nino Aragno Editore, 2005), p. 142: "somniabis corpus tuum," which is rendered into English, p. 262: "you will dream of your body."

71. I have rendered the Hebrew *be-ro'shah* literally, but consider the suggestion of Scholem, *Origins*, p. 56 n. 12, that this locution reflects the Arabic *rasiha*, and thus should be translated as "herself," referring back to the soul. On the basis of this example and the presence of other Arabisms in this section of the bahiric text, Scholem concluded that "the paragraphs making use of the mysticism of the vowels have their origin in the Arab-speaking Orient." See also Ronit Meroz, "The Resplendent Light is in the East: On the Time and Place of the *Sefer Bahir*," *Da'at* 49 (2002): 171–76 (Hebrew). Meroz deals with the passage about the *ḥolem* on pp. 173–74, and see the criticism of her stance in Busi's foreword to *The Book of Bahir*, p. 14 n. 9.

72. *The Book Bahir*, sec. 27, pp. 131–33.

73. Gerhard Scholem, *Das Buch Bahir: Ein Schriftdenkmal aus der Frühzeit der Kabbala auf Grund der kritischen Neuausgabe* (Leipzig: W. Druglin, 1923), pp. 30–31 n. 5.

74. Abraham Ibn Ezra, *Perushei ha-Torah*, 2:187 (*ad* Exodus 28:9). The explanation is repeated by David Kimḥi, *Sefer ha-Shorashim im ha-Nimmuqim me-Rabbi Eliyahu ha-Levi ha-Ashkenazi*, edited by Johann Heinrich Biesenthal and Fürchtegott Lebrecht (Berlin: Impensis G. Bethge, 1847), sv. *ḥlm*, p. 106.

75. *Tiqqunei Zohar*, sec. 70, 129b.

76. Cordovero, *Pardes Rimmonim*, 19:4, 88c. For an expansion of this symbolism, see *Galya Razya*, p. 107. See also Ya'aqov Qoppel Liphshitz, *Sha'arei Gan ha-Eden*, 2 vols. (Jerusalem: Yerid ha-Sefarim, 2004), 1:94. In that passage, the symbolic link between *Malkhut* and *ḥolem* is explained in terms of her elevation to the source in the central point that is hidden within the Infinite, the point whence all the other lights emanate. Regarding this motif, see Wolfson, *Open Secret*, p. 214.

77. *Zohar* 1:211a. Compare *Ma'arekhet ha-Elohut*, ch. 4, 71a–b.

78. *The Book Bahir*, sec. 23, p. 129.

79. This was also noted by Meroz, "The Resplendent Light," pp. 173–74.

80. Wolfson, *Through a Speculum*, pp. 359–61 and 368–69 n. 149; *idem*, "Coronation of the Sabbath Bride: Kabbalistic Myth and the Ritual of Androgynisation," *Journal of Jewish Thought and Philosophy* 6 (1997): 301–44, revised version in Wolfson, *Luminal Darkness*, pp. 144–84; *idem*, *Language, Eros, Being*,

pp. 73–74, 76, 133, 184, 254, 263, 452–53 n. 192, 487 n. 194.

81. For example, see *Zohar* 1:131a, where the cornerstone is also designated as the foundation stone or the central point whence the world is sustained and through which the Holy of Holies exists. These are all descriptions of *Shekhinah*, but in the state when she has been transformed from a passive vessel to an overflowing fount, a change that, in my judgment, should be interpreted as a gender metamorphosis. See also *Zohar* 1:246b.

82. *Tiqqunei Zohar*, introduction, 15b, sec. 5, 20b.

83. See Tishby, *Messianic Mysticism*, pp. 289–336.

84. Moses David Valle, *Sefer Or Olam: Be'ur Sefer Bere'shit*, vol. 2 (Jerusalem, 1994), p. 598.

85. The symbolic association is based on the fact that just as the *ḥolem* is marked by a dot positioned on top of the letter, so *Keter* occupies the top rung of the sefirotic tree. See the fragment of an untitled work by Moses de León, MS Munich 47, fols. 369a–b; *Zohar* 3:17a (*Ra'aya Meheimna*), 247b (*Ra'aya Meheimna*); *Zohar Ḥadash*, 73c; *Tiqqunei Zohar*, introduction, 7a, sec. 10, 25a, sec. 18, 32b, sec. 69, 104a; Shem Ṭov ben Abraham Ibn Gaon, *Baddei ha-Aron u-Migdal Ḥananel*, edited by Samuel Loewinger (Jerusalem: Orient and Occident, 1977), 51a–b. For other kabbalists, including Moses de León in most of his works, *ḥolem* symbolically corresponds to *Ḥokhmah*, enumerated as the second emanation, but often designated as the "first" (*re'shit*). See de León, *The Book of the Pomegranate*, pp. 329–30 (Hebrew section) and the different views delineated on p. 329 n. 2.

86. *Zohar* 3:17a (*Ra'aya Meheimna*) and compare Cordovero, *Pardes Rimmonim*, 9:5, 58c. See also the speculation on the three vowels, *ḥolem*, *shureq*, and *ḥireq*, positioned respectively on top, in the middle, and on the bottom, in de León, *The Book of the Pomegranate*, pp. 329–30 and 333–35 (Hebrew section). The three vowels are described as forming one unity, an idea that lends support to my conjecture that the dream (*ḥalom*) is connected to the *ḥolem* in its ascent from the last of the sefirotic gradations (*Malkhut*) through the median line (*Tif'eret*) to the first (*Keter*). The triune oneness of the three vowels is graphically portrayed as the three dots above, in the middle, and below the letter *waw*. See *Zohar Ḥadash*, 104d (*Tiqqunim*); Abraham Abulafia, *Sefer ha-Ḥesheq* (Jerusalem, 1999), p. 15. On the presumed unity of these three vowels, see also Abraham Abulafia, *Gan Na'ul* (Jerusalem, 1999), p. 18.

87. Blanchot, *Friendship*, p. 146. See Chapter 1 at n. 173.

88. *Sefer ha-Peli'ah* (Przemysl: Zupnik, Knoller, and Hammerschmidt, 1883), 4a.

89. See Wolfson *Alef, Mem, Tau*, pp. 39–40. Some of the relevant passages

from de León and Gikatilla are cited by Matt, "Ayin," p. 130.

90. From the last section of Gikatilla's *Sha'arei Ṣedeq*, edited and annotated by Efraim Gottlieb, *Studies in the Kabbala Literature*, edited by Joseph Hacker (Tel-Aviv: Tel-Aviv University Press, 1976), p. 140 (Hebrew). On the unknowability of the first emanation, see Gikatilla, *Sod Yod-Gimmel Middot ha-Nov'ot min ha-Keter Elyon we-Niqra'im Ma'yenei ha-Yeshu'ah*, in Gershom Scholem, *Catalogus Codicum Hebraicorum, Pars Prima: Cabbala* (Jerusalem: E Prelis Universitatis Hebraicae, 1930), p. 219.

91. The nexus between *ḥolem*, king of the world (*melekh olam*), and salt (*melekh*) is enunciated as well in the anonymous *Berit Menuḥah* (Amsterdam, 1648), 8b.

92. Gottlieb, *Studies*, p. 136.

93. On the application of the term "hypernomian" to the study of Jewish esotericism, see Elliot R. Wolfson, "Mystical Rationalization of the Commandments in the Prophetic Kabbalah of Abraham Abulafia," in *Perspectives on Jewish Thought and Mysticism*, edited by Alfred Ivry, Allan Arkush, and Elliot R. Wolfson (Reading: Harwood, 1998), pp. 345–59; *idem*, "Beyond Good and Evil: Hypernomianism, Transmorality, and Kabbalistic Ethics," in *Crossing Boundaries: Ethics, Antinomianism and the History of Mysticism*, edited by G. William Barnard and Jeffrey J. Kripal (New York: Seven Bridges Press, 2002), pp. 103–56. Greatly revised versions of these studies appear respectively in Wolfson, *Abraham Abulafia*, pp. 204–28, and *Venturing Beyond*, pp. 186–285. For my most recent discussion, see Wolfson, *Open Secret*, pp. 55–58 and 161–99. The term was also used, albeit with a different connotation, by Elliot K. Ginsburg, *The Sabbath in the Classical Kabbalah* (Albany: State University of New York Press, 1989), p. 222, and in a manner consonant with my own by Shaul Magid, *Hasidism on the Margin: Reconciliation, Antinomianism, and Messianism in Izbica/Radzin Hasidism* (Madison: University of Wisconsin Press, 2003), pp. 209–12, 220, 352 n. 20 (my coinage of the term is acknowledged), and *idem*, *From Metaphysics to Midrash*, pp. 112, 125, 227. For a similar application of the term to Islamic mystical piety, see Paul L. Heck, "Mysticism as Morality: The Case of Sufism," *Journal of Religious Ethics* 34 (2006): 277–78: "While the intoxicated side can see antinomian behavior as an end in itself, the sober side recognizes such behavior as merely temporary and only useful as a foil against which to draw out the hypernomian possibilities of Sufism in which moral action beyond justice—again, a loving kindness—is the result, not moral transgression. The goal is not rebellion against the tradition but its reformulation in light of a higher moral vision."

94. See Wolfson, *Venturing Beyond*, pp. 215–16 n. 101 and 217–18 n. 108.

95. Jacques Derrida, "To Forgive: The Unforgivable and the Imprescriptible," in *Questioning God*, edited by John D. Caputo, Mark Dooley, and Michael J. Scanlon (Bloomington: Indiana University Press, 2001), pp. 25–26.

96. Jacques Derrida, *On Cosmopolitanism and Forgiveness*, translated by Mark Dooley and Michael Hughes, with a preface by Simon Critchley and Richard Kearney (London: Routledge, 2001), p. 33.

97. Derrida, "To Forgive," p. 48. For an analysis of this dimension of Derrida's thought, see Mary-Jane Rubenstein, "Of Ghosts and Angels: Derrida, Kushner, and the Impossibility of Forgiveness," *Journal for Cultural and Religious Theory* 9 (2008): 79–95.

98. Derrida, *On Cosmopolitanism*, pp. 59–60; see Rubenstein, "Of Ghosts," p. 83.

99. Babylonian Talmud, Yoma 36b.

100. See above n. 75.

101. See Abraham J. Heschel, *The Circle of the Baal Shem Tov: Studies in Hasidism*, edited by Samuel H. Dresner (Chicago: University of Chicago Press, 1985), pp. 1–43, esp. 10–15. On the exceptional affection that Phineḥas of Korzec displayed toward the *Zohar*, see the evidence adduced by Heschel, *ibid.*, pp. 4–5.

102. A line from the *Aveinu Malkeinu* prayer that is recited on the ten days of repentance from Rosh ha-Shanah to Yom Kippur, as well as on public fast days. The words cited by Phineḥas of Korzec refer to the possibility of the divine changing the decree of judgment, but he applies them to the righteous person, as well as to any person who repents.

103. Phineḥas of Korzec, *Imrei Pinḥas ha-Shalem*, edited by Elimelekh Eleazar Frankel, 2 vols. (Benei Beraq: Yeḥezqel Shraga Frankel, 2003), 1:423–24.

104. Elliot R. Wolfson, "Fore/givenness on the Way: Nesting in the Womb of Response," *Graven Images: Studies in Culture, Law, and the Sacred* 4 (1998): 153–69, reprinted in *Luminal Darkness*, pp. 228–57. The discussion here is a reworking of the version in *Luminal Darkness*, pp. 229–30.

105. For other accounts of time and forgiveness, see John D. Caputo, "The Time of Giving, the Time of Forgiving," in *The Enigma of Gift and Sacrifice*, edited by Edith Wyschogrod, Jean-Joseph Goux, and Eric Boynton (New York: Fordham University Press, 2002), pp. 117–47; Caputo, *The Weakness of God*, pp. 146–50, 168–70, 208–35; Edith Wyschogrod, "Repentance and Forgiveness: The Undoing of Time," *International Journal for Philosophy of Religion* 60 (2006): 157–68; Karmen MacKendrick, *Fragmentation and Memory: Meditations on Christian Doctrine* (New York: Fordham University Press, 2008), pp. 55–83.

106. Derrida, "To Forgive," pp. 31–32.

107. *Ibid.*, p. 32.

108. Rubenstein, "Of Ghosts," pp. 85–87.

109. Gilles Deleuze, *Difference and Repetition*, translated by Paul Patton (New York: Columbia University Press, 1994), p. 91.

110. See, for example, Roland Goetschel, "'Ehyeh Asher Ehyeh' in the Works of the Gerona Kabbalists," *Jerusalem Studies in Jewish Thought* 6, nos. 3–4 (1987): 287–98 (Hebrew).

111. De León, *Sefer Sheqel ha-Qodesh*, p. 6.

112. Scholem, *Major Trends*, p. 25; *idem*, "Schöpfung aus Nichts und Selbstverschränkung Gottes," *Eranos Jahrbuch* 25 (1956): 87–119; *idem*, *Origins*, pp. 422–27. See also Matt, "Ayin," pp. 132–34.

113. Scholem enunciated his understanding of the symbol in kabbalistic thought in many places in his vast oeuvre. For a representative list of some of the sources, see Scholem, *Major Trends*, p. 27; *idem*, "The Name of God and the Linguistic Theory of the Kabbala," *Diogenes* 79 (1972): 61–65, 80 (1972): 165 and 193; *idem*, *On the Kabbalah and Its Symbolism*, translated by Ralph Manheim (New York: Schocken Books, 1969), pp. 8–11, 22–23, 35–36; *idem*, *On the Possibility of Jewish Mysticism in Our Time and Other Essays*, edited and with an introduction by Avraham Shapira, translated by Jonathan Chipman (Philadelphia: Jewish Publication Society of America, 1997), pp. 139–40. See also *idem*, *On Jews and Judaism in Crisis: Selected Essays*, edited by Werner J. Dannhauser (New York: Schocken Books, 1976), p. 48. In that context, Scholem contrasts his understanding of kabbalistic symbolism, which he compares to Whitman, with modern technology, since the latter "thinks it can banish the symbolic dimension from reality." Scholem's dichotomization is unwarranted; technological advancement, as that of science more generally, only enhances the sense of mystery in the world.

114. Tishby, *Paths of Faith and Heresy*, pp. 11–22; Nathan Rotenstreich, "Symbolism and Transcendence: On Some Philosophical Aspects of Gershom Scholem's Opus," *The Review of Metaphysics* 31 (1978): 604–14; David Biale, *Gershom Scholem: Kabbalah and Counter-History* (Cambridge, MA: Harvard University Press, 1979), pp. 89–92; Eliezer Schweid, *Judaism and Mysticism According to Gershom Scholem: A Critical Analysis and Programmatic Discussion*, translated with an introduction by David Avraham Weiner (Atlanta: Scholars Press, 1985), pp. 43–44 and 126–27; Joseph Dan, "Gershom Scholem's Reconstruction of Early Kabbalah," *Modern Judaism* 5 (1985): 45–53; *idem*, *Gershom Scholem and the Mystical Dimension of Jewish History* (New York: New York University Press, 1988), pp. 162–64; Idel, *Kabbalah: New Perspectives*, pp. 231–32; *idem*, "The Function of Symbols in G. G. Scholem," *Jewish Studies* 38 (1998): 43–72 (Hebrew), and

the German translation "Zur Funktion von Symbolen bei G. G. Scholem," in *Gershom Scholem: Literatur und Rhetorik*, edited by Stéphane Mosès and Sigrid Weigel (Köln: Böhlau Verlag, 2000), pp. 51–92; *idem*, *Absorbing Perfections*, pp. 274–80, Susan A. Handelman, *Fragments of Redemption: Jewish Thought and Literary Theory in Benjamin, Scholem, and Levinas* (Bloomington: Indiana University Press, 1991), pp. 83–84 and 104–109; Wasserstrom, *Religion After Religion*, pp. 94–97; Daniel Weidner, *Gershom Scholem: Politisches, esoterisches und historiographisches Schreiben* (Munich: Wilhelm Fink Verlag, 2003), pp. 174–96 and 360–63.

115. Scholem, *Major Trends*, p. 27. The work that Scholem cites is Friedrich Creuzer, *Symbolik und Mythologie der alten Voelker*, which was published in 1816.

116. *Zohar* 3:65b.

117. The phrase is taken from Franz Rosenzweig, *The Star of Redemption*, translation by Barbara E. Galli (Madison: University of Wisconsin Press, 2005), p. 411. For discussion of the temporal characteristics of *Keter* along these lines, see Wolfson, *Alef, Mem, Tau*, pp. 91–96, 104–105, 115–17.

118. I have not found *ana ma'n da-ana*, an Aramaic rendering of the Hebrew *ehyeh asher ehyeh,* preserved in earlier literature, even though it is cited in the zoharic text as if it were from some older source. See also de León, *The Book of the Pomegranate*, p. 380 (Hebrew section): "One should not inquire and investigate hidden matters, as [the sages], blessed be their memory, said in many places 'I am what I am' [*ana ma'n da-ana*], and you are not permitted to ask and to scrutinize." In my annotations to *The Book of the Pomegranate* (n. 4), I failed to mention the zoharic passage (see reference in following note) in which this phrase occurs. Even so, de León's referring to "many places" is perplexing. The passages from *Sefer ha-Rimmon* and the *Zohar* were duly recorded by Mopsik in his edition of *Sefer Sheqel ha-Qodesh*, p. 99 n. 725.

119. *Zohar* 3:11a. On the nexus between summoning (*hazmanah*) the efflux and the name *ehyeh*, see Moses de León, *She'elot u-Teshuvot le-Rav Moshe di Li'on be-Inyenei Qabbalah*, in Isaiah Tishby, *Studies in Kabbalah and Its Branches: Researches and Sources*, vol. 1 (Jerusalem: Magnes Press, 1982), p. 41 (Hebrew).

120. Elliot R. Wolfson, "Murmuring Secrets: Eroticism and Esotericism in Medieval Kabbalah," in *Hidden Intercourse*, pp. 83–84.

121. De León, *Sefer Sheqel ha-Qodesh*, pp. 4–6, and the other passages in de León's oeuvre marked by Mopsik, p. 4 n. 28, where the apophatic image of the incomprehensible pure ether is used in conjunction with the first emanation. For discussion of the apophatic and kataphatic elements in this treatise of de León, see Eitan P. Fishbane, "Mystical Contemplation and the Limits of the Mind: The Case of *Sheqel ha-Qodesh*," *Jewish Quarterly Review* 93 (2002): 1–27.

As the author acknowledges (pp. 14–15 n. 32), he has been influenced by my own analysis of this matter in early kabbalistic works.

122. See de León, *Sefer Sheqel ha-Qodesh*, pp. 19–20.

123. On the use of this expression to designate *Ḥokhmah*, see de León, *Sefer Sheqel ha-Qodesh*, p. 21, and *idem*, "Sefer ha-Mishkal," p. 110.

124. De León, *Sefer Sheqel ha-Qodesh*, pp. 98–99.

125. Wolfson, *Language, Eros, Being*, pp. 96–97. On the term *efes* in Azriel and the Aristotelian notion of privation (*steresis*), see also Matt, "Ayin," p. 133, a source that I neglected to mention in my previous discussion. For a more recent discussion of the concepts of infinity and nothingness in Azriel's theosophy, see Valabregue-Perry, *Concealed and Revealed*, pp. 66–83, 210–21, 244–52.

126. This expression is utilized by the Spanish kabbalist and biblical exegete Baḥya ben Asher. See Efraim Gottlieb, *The Kabbalah in the Writings of R. Baḥya ben Asher Ibn Ḥalawa* (Jerusalem: Kiryat Sefer, 1970), p. 229 (Hebrew), noted as well by Matt, "Ayin," p.134.

127. Blanchot, *The Writing of Disaster*, p. 78. Blanchot's characterization of the present as being outside of time has an affinity with his aphorism on the temporal comportment of the messianic future (see below, n. 157).

128. *Ibid.*, p.70, where Blanchot describes suicide as "*the impossibility of every possibility*," in contrast to Heidegger's notion of the nonevent of death as "*the possibility of impossibility*." See Critchley, "*Il y a*," pp. 108–11; Bruns, *Maurice Blanchot*, pp. 66–70.

129. Friedrich Hölderlin, *Essays and Letters on Theory*, translated and edited by Thomas Pfau (Albany: State University of New York Press, 1988), p. 97. Concerning this passage, see Blanchot, *Friendship*, p. 147; Weineck, *The Abyss Above*, p. 68.

130. Gikatilla, *Sha'arei Orah*, 2:107–108.

131. Compare *ibid.*, 1:231.

132. *Sifre on Deuteronomy*, edited by Louis Finkelstein (New York: Jewish Theological Seminary of America, 1969), sec. 49, p. 114.

133. *Sifre on Deuteronomy*, sec. 26, pp. 38–39; *Midrash Tanḥuma* (Jerusalem: Eshkol, 1972), Wa-etḥannan, sec. 3, p. 853.

134. On the nexus between time, the mystery of prayer, and the unwarranted gift of divine forgiveness connected to *Keter* in the works of David ben Yehudah he-Ḥasid, see Wolfson, "*Imago Templi*," pp. 132–33, which is an expansion of my analysis in *Alef, Mem, Tau*, pp. 104–105. On contemplative unknowing and forgetting in the work of David ben Yehudah he-Ḥasid, see the passage cited by Matt, "Ayin," p. 135. For the original text, see David ben Yehudah he-Ḥasid, *The Book of Mirrors: Sefer Mar'ot ha-Ẓove'ot*, edited by Daniel

C. Matt (Chico: Scholars Press, 1982), p. 227 (Hebrew section), and see the editor's comments in his introduction, pp. 25–26.

135. Gikatilla, *Sha'arei Orah*, 2:115–17. By contrast, the sixth emanation, *Tif'eret*, is marked by the second-person pronoun, "you" (*attah*), and the tenth emanation, *Malkhut*, by the first-person pronoun, "I" (*ani*). See *ibid.*, 2:117–18. Compare the passage from Gikatilla's *Sha'arei Ṣedeq* in Gottlieb, *Studies*, pp. 135–36.

136. Gikatilla, *Sha'arei Ṣedeq*, in Gottlieb, *Studies*, p. 135.

137. Gikatilla, *Sha'arei Orah*, 2:114.

138. *Ibid*, 2:117. Compare Gikatilla, *Sha'arei Ṣedeq*, in Gottlieb, *Studies*, p. 138.

139. See *Sha'arei Orah*, 2:118, where Gikatilla instructs the reader with respect to the esoteric knowledge surrounding the designation of *Keter* as "it" (*hu*), "With God's help, if you will merit more, you will receive the mysteries and secrets in these matters orally [*mi-peh el peh*]."

140. Based on Proverbs 11:13.

141. Gikatilla, *Sod Yod-Gimmel Middot*, p. 220.

142. For more extended discussion, see Wolfson, *Alef, Mem, Tau*, pp. 118–36.

143. Gikatilla, *Sha'arei Orah*, 2:121.

144. Gikatilla, *Sha'arei Ṣedeq*, in Gottlieb, *Studies*, p. 147.

145. I have translated the verse in accord with Gikatilla's reading. Contextually, *mi-qedem* means "from the east."

146. Gikatilla, *Sha'arei Orah*, 2:121.

147. *Ibid.*, 2:142.

148. *Ibid.*, 2:125–26.

149. Gikatilla, *Sha'arei Ṣedeq*, in Gottlieb, *Studies*, pp. 157–58 and 160.

150. Henry Corbin, *Cyclical Time and Ismaili Gnosis* (London: Kegan Paul International, 1983), p. 26, utilizes this expression to describe the Hermetic figure of the "good daemon" (*Agathos Daimōn*), also identified as the celestial partner (*daimōn paredros*), "the helping, tutelary angel—a gratuitous gift obtained by prayer."

151. Gikatilla, *Sod Yod-Gimmel Middot*, p. 225.

152. For a more extensive discussion of the two models of unity, identity of difference versus difference of identity, see Wolfson, *Language, Eros, Being*, pp. 99–105, and the briefer, but more recent assessment in *idem*, *Open Secret*, pp. 101–103. On the notion of indifference or equanimity (*hashwa'ah*), particularly in the thought of Azriel of Gerona, see Valabregue-Perry, *Concealed and Revealed*, pp. 232–44.

153. Compare *Zohar* 3:134b (*Idra Rabba*) and the analysis in Wolfson, *Alef,*

Mem, Tau, pp. 95–96. By contrast, the explanation of *yom eḥad* (Zechariah 14:7) as signifying the union of male and female, *Tif'eret* and *Malkhut*, is found in several other zoharic passages. See *Zohar* 1:107b; 3:96b, and the parallel in David ben Yehudah he-Ḥasid, *The Book of Mirrors*, p. 91 (Hebrew section). For a different interpretation, see *Zohar* 1:115b, 213a–b; 2:19b.

154. The expression I have translated as "governs" is *rakhiv al*, which literally means "rides upon." My rendering reflects a figurative meaning associated with the root *rkhb* in the time of the composition of this kabbalistic treatise. A feasible source could have been Maimonides, *Guide of the Perplexed*, 1.70, p. 171; see the discussion in Wolfson, *Abraham Abulafia*, pp. 44–45.

155. *Tiqqunei Zohar*, sec. 70, 122b. I have discussed this passage, together with the commentary on it attributed to Elijah ben Solomon, the Vilna Gaon, in Wolfson, *Alef, Mem, Tau*, pp. 92–93.

156. Both connotations, "ascend to" and "vanish in," are implied by the root *slq*.

157. Wolfson, *Open Secret*, pp. 265–300, esp. 284–89. In that context, I neglected to mention the following passage in Blanchot, *The Writing of Disaster*, pp. 141–42: "Jewish messianic thought (according to certain commentators), suggests the relation between the event and its nonoccurrence.... Both future and past (it is said at least once that the Messiah has already come), his coming does not correspond to any presence at all.... And if it happens that to the question 'When will you come?' the Messiah answers, 'Today,' the answer is certainly impressive: so, it is today! It is now and always now. There is no need to wait, although to wait is an obligation. And when is it now? When is the now which does not belong to ordinary time, which necessarily overturns it, does not maintain but destabilizes it? When?—especially if one remembers that this 'now' which belongs to no text, but is the now of a severe, fictitious narrative, refers to texts that make it once more dependent upon realizable-unrealizable conditions." See *ibid.*, p. 143: "Every just act...makes of its day the last day or—as Kafka said—the very last: a day no longer situated in the ordinary succession of days but one that makes of the most commonplace ordinary, the extraordinary." Blanchot is alluding to the paradoxical quip of Franz Kafka, *Parables and Paradoxes* (New York: Schocken Books, 1971), p. 81, that the Messiah "will come, not on the last day, but on the very last," a passage that I interpreted in a similar way in *Open Secret*, pp. 268 and 288. Another thinker that I neglected to mention is Steven Schwarzschild. Compare his "On Jewish Eschatology" in *The Pursuit of the Ideal*, pp. 209–28. Commenting on the twelfth of the thirteen Maimonidean principles, "I believe with full faith in the coming of the Messiah, and, though he tarry, I anticipate him, nonetheless,

on every day, when he may come," Schwarzschild writes: "the logic of this formulation entails that...the Messiah will always not yet have come, into all historical eternity. It is his coming, or rather the expectation of his coming, not his arrival, his 'advent,' that is obligatory Jewish faith.... Jewishly, the Messiah not only has not come but also will never have come—that he will always be coming" (pp. 209–11). As the author readily admits, he is influenced by Hermann Cohen's asymptotic notion of the messianic future, which involves the perpetual delay of the advent even as it secures its constant potentiality.

158. Emmanuel Levinas, *Time and the Other*, translation by Richard A. Cohen (Pittsburgh: Duquesne University Press, 1987), p. 122. I suspect that the view of Levinas is indebted to Rosenzweig. See Wolfson, "Light Does Not Talk," pp. 93–102 and 134 n. 92.

159. Merleau-Ponty, *Phenomenology of Perception*, p. 423. On the notion of the "field of presence," see Chapter 1 at n. 188.

160. Moses de León, *Mishkan ha-Edut*, MS Berlin Or. Quat. 833, fols. 2b. In the version of this text preserved in MS Vatican 283, fol. 144b, there is the additional line at the conclusion of the passage, "until his form ascends to be conjoined with its creator [*ad alot ṣurato lehitdabbeq bi-devequt yoṣrah*]."

161. Scholem, *Major Trends*, p. 194, records manuscript evidence that a copy of Maimonides' *Guide of the Perplexed* was copied for Moses de León. See also Tishby, *Wisdom*, p. 17. There is, however, some difficulty with this claim, because the colophon of the manuscript to which Scholem referred (*Major Trends*, p. 395 n. 131) proclaims that the scribe, Samuel ben Isaac, copied the work for Moshe di Li'on and completed it on Sunday, the 12th of Elul, in the year 1476 (MS Günzberg 777, fol. 177b). I thank Daniel Abrams, who passed on this information to me in the name of Tsvi Langermann. In spite of the dubious nature of this evidence, I think it is still safe to say that de León was conversant with some of the Maimonidean corpus. See my preliminary comments in de León, *The Book of the Pomegranate*, pp. 36–38 (introduction). Scholem, *Major Trends*, p. 203, again notes the influence of Maimonides on de León (based on evidence that has now been exposed to be erroneous), but he also mentions a passage from *Mishkan ha-Edut* that is ascribed to the "teacher of righteousness" (*moreh ṣedeq*), describing the "philosopher's ecstatic ascent into the world of pure intelligence and his vision of the One" (see *ibid.*, p. 398 n. 155). Scholem presumes the passage is from the *Enneads* of Plotinus, which circulated in the Middle Ages as the *Theology of Aristotle*. In my opinion, de León is actually paraphrasing Maimonides, and not Plotinus, and he is not describing a vision of the One per se. The exact context in which the citation appears is the spiritual interpretation of fasting (including on Yom Kippur) as

a means by which the soul divests itself of its material encasement and unites with the supernal realm. After making this point, de León writes, "And in this manner the teacher of righteousness said, when my soul is meditating [*be-hitbodedi im nafshi*], I will cast and remove my body from it, and I will dwell as a soul without a body [*we-eshev ke-nefesh be-lo guf*], and I will contemplate the supernal world [*we-etbonen ba-olam ha-elyon*], and I will experience spiritual delight [*et'anneg ta'anug ruḥi*], which is in the pattern of the delight of the world to come [*dugmat ta'anug olam ha-ba*]. Mouths tire of speaking about it and hearts as well from containing its form" (*Mishkan ha-Edut*, MS Berlin Or. Quat. 833, fol. 32a). Paul B. Fenton, *Philosophie et exégèse dans Le Jardin de la métha-phore de Moïse Ibn 'Ezra, philosophie et poète anadalou du XIIe siècle* (Leiden: E. J. Brill, 1997), pp. 218–19, compares the passage from *Mishkan ha-Edut* to a citation in the name of Aristotle from the *Sefer ha-Bedolaḥ* in Moses Ibn Ezra's *Arugat ha-Bosem* (I am grateful to my student Guadalupe Gonzalez Dieguez for reminding me of this reference). As Fenton commented (p. 218 n. 534), the passage from Moses de León's *Mishkan ha-Edut* was cited already by Moritz Steinschneider, *Hebräische Bibliographie: Blätter für neuere und ältere Literatur des Judenthums* 6 (1863): 107, as an illustration of citations from the selections from the *Enneads* of Plotinus that circulated as the *Theology of Aristotle*, but he neglected to mention that Steinschneider also referred to the text from *Sefer ha-Bedolaḥ* in Moses Ibn Ezra. See also Moritz Steinschneider, *Die hebräischen übersetzungen des mittelalters und die Juden als dolmetscher: Ein Beitrag zur literaturgeschichte des mittelalters, meist nach handschriftlichen quellen* (Berlin: Kommissionsverlag des Bibliographischen Bureaus, 1893), p. 243 n. 975, where he suggests that Ibn Ezra probably knew the text from its citation in the *Rasā'il Ikhwān al-Ṣafā'*. As Steinschneider noted in both contexts, a different version of this extract (which is based on *Enneads* IV.8.1) is quoted in the name of Aristotle in Shem Ṭov Ibn Falaquera's *Sefer ha-Ma'alot*. The passage is reproduced in Paul B. Fenton, "Shem Tov Ibn Falaquera and the Theology of Aristotle," *Da'at* 29 (1992): 31–32 (Hebrew), and see *idem*, "The Arabic and Hebrew Versions of the Theology of Aristotle," in *Pseudo-Aristotle in the Middle Ages: The* Theology *and Other Texts*, edited by Jill Kraye, W. F. Ryan, and C. B. Schmitt (London: Warburg Institute, 1986), pp. 257–58 and 260 n. 2. See also Moshe Idel, "Metamorphoses of a Platonic Theme in Jewish Mysticism," *Jewish Studies at the Central European University* 3 (2002–2003): 73 (see n. 16, where Moses de León is mentioned as one who quotes the Plotinian text), and *idem*, *Ascensions on High in Jewish Mysticism: Pillars, Lines, Ladders* (Budapest: Central European University Press, 2005), p. 41. On the paraphrase of Plotinus's portrayal of ecstasy in the *Theology of Aristotle*, see also Altmann and Stern, *Isaac Israeli*, pp.

190–91, and Altmann, *Studies*, pp. 32–33. Altmann, in *Studies*, p. 33 n. 151, offers a lengthy critique of Scholem's characterization of the passage cited in *Mishkan ha-Edut*, but he does not challenge the identification of it as a paraphrase of Plotinus from the *Theology of Aristotle* (although I note, parenthetically, that Altmann's remark that Scholem was the first to notice Moses de León's use of the *Theology* passage in *Mishkan ha-Edut* needs to be corrected in light of the fact that Steinschneider already made this observation). Altmann renders the expression *moreh ṣedeq* as "true Teacher" and assumes that it refers to Aristotle (or, to be more exact, Plotinus in the guise of Aristotle), but he does not provide any evidence to corroborate that the Greek philosopher received this epithet in medieval Jewish sources. On the possible translation of another passage from the *Theology* by Falaquera, see T. Zvi Langermann, "A New Hebrew Passage from the *Theology of Aristotle* and Its Significance," *Arabic Sciences and Philosophy* 9 (1999): 247–59. Following Steinschneider, Fenton contends that Moses Ibn Ezra is citing the *Theology*. Even though the similarities between the two passages cannot be denied, I am still doubtful that de León thought he was quoting from the work ascribed to Aristotle. More importantly, the passage is not about the vision of the One (as Scholem suggested), but about angelic transformation (*nikhnas im benei elohim*, literally, "entering with the sons of God") and the consequent vision of the splendor of the glory (*wa-er'eh az be-aṣmi mi-ziw ha-kavod*), an idea that is operative in some passages in Maimonides describing prophecy and the beatitude of the world to come, which is understood in rabbinic terms as enjoying or feasting on the splendor of the *Shekhinah* (Babylonian Talmud, Berakhot 17a, and compare the allegorical interpretation in Maimonides, *Mishneh Torah*, Teshuvah 8:2). This is the gist of the brief rendering of the passage from *Mishkan ha-Edut* in Viṭal, *Sha'arei Qedushshah*, IV.3, p. 299 (a reference mentioned by Fenton, *Philosophie et exégèse*, p. 219, albeit with a different interpretive stance). A scribal notation (mentioned already by Steinschneider, *Hebräische Bibliographie* 6 [1863]: 107) from a later hand in the margin of the manuscript, *ma'amar ha-moreh*, indicates that the anonymous reader understood that de León was alluding to a dictum of Maimonides, and not to the pseudo-Aristotelian text. In my judgment, a similar Maimonidean slant is evident in the two places in Nissim ben Moses of Marseilles, *Ma'aseh Nissim: Perush la-Torah*, edited by Howard Kreisel (Jerusalem: Mekize Nirdamim, 2000), pp. 99 and 407, where the passage from the *Theology* is cited (introduced in the former with the words "according to the dictum of the sage," *ke-ma'amar he-ḥakham*, and in the second, "as the sage said," *kemo she-amar he-ḥakham*). See Howard Kreisel, "Some Observations on Ma'aseh Nissim by R. Nissim of Marseilles," in *Perspectives on Jewish Thought and Mysticism*, edited by Alan Arkush, Alfred L, Ivry, and Elliot R. Wolfson (Australia: Harwood, 1998), p. 209 (for this reference I am again grateful to Guadalupe Gonzalez Dieguez). Altmann, *Isaac Israeli*, p. 191, remarked that the final stage of the experience described in the paraphrase of *Enneads* IV.8.1 in the *Theology of Aristotle* is not the soul's union with but adherence to (*muta'alliq*) the divine world, which results in a seeing of the light and splendor that is beyond language and comprehension. By contrast, the Plotinian text clearly expresses the soul's identity with the divine. The passage in *Mishkan ha-Edut* similarly places the emphasis on the divesting of the soul of the body, the ascent to the supernal realm, and the state of conjunction, which is framed as beholding the light that is ineffable and unfathomable, but even in the paraphrase, the claim that the soul is in the divine position is preserved, and this is not the case in the passage of de León. On balance, the experience depicted by de León accords with the Maimonidean perspective on prophecy and his spiritualized understanding of the world to come. My conjecture is supported by the fact that it was not uncommon for authors in the time of de León to refer to Maimonides or to his book as *moreh ṣedeq* (in the latter case, the meaning of the term is the "guide to righteousness"). For instance, see the introduction of the translator Samuel ben Judah Ibn Tibbon to Moses Maimonides, *Shemoneh Peraqim le-ha-Rambam im Perush Ḥesed Avraham* (Jerusalem: Yesodi, 1998), p. 10; Menaḥem ben Solomon Meiri, *Beit ha-Beḥirah al Massekhet Berakhot*, edited and annotated by Samuel Dikman (Jerusalem: Yad ha-Rav Herzog, 1965), pp. 21, 25, 27, 32, 33; Abba Mari of Lunel, *Sefer Minḥat Qina'ot*, in *Teshuvot ha-Rashba*, edited by Ḥayyim Z. Dimitrovski (Jerusalem: Mosad ha-Rav Kook, 1990), p. 228; Abraham Abulafia, *Sefer ha-Yashar*, in *Maṣref ha-Sekhel* (Jerusalem, 2001), p. 99; *idem*, *Mafteaḥ ha-Sefirot* (Jerusalem, 2001), p. 8; *idem*, *Mafteaḥ ha-Tokhaḥot*, pp. 31, 78; *idem*, *Shomer Miṣwah* (Jerusalem, 2001), p. 9; *idem*, *Mafteaḥ ha-Ra'yon* (Jerusalem, 2002), pp. 7 and 44; *idem*, *Sheva Netivot Torah*, p. 12; David Kimḥi, *Perush al Yirmeyahu*, in *Miqra'ot Gedolot* (New York: Abraham Isaac Friedman, 1961), pp. 213 (Jeremiah 7:22), 221 (Jeremiah 9:23), 230 (Jeremiah 13:1). I am not familiar with the title *moreh ṣedeq* being applied to Aristotle in medieval Jewish sources. It is noteworthy that Steinschneider (*Hebräische Bibliographie* 6 [1863]: 107) placed a parenthetical exclamation mark after referring to this reference in de León's *Mishkan ha-Edut*, which likely indicates that he, also, considered it to be unusual. Finally, I mention the remark of Hermann Cohen in his "Charakteristik der Ethik Maimunis" that for Maimonides and the other medieval Jewish philosophers Aristotle was considered one of the "pious of the nations of the world," *Frommer der Völker der Welt*, a translation of the Hebrew expression *ḥasidei ummot ha-olam*. See Hermann

Cohen, *Jüdische Schriften*, Dritter Band (Berlin: C. A. Schwetschke & Sohn, 1924), p. 243. I have found no earlier text to corroborate Cohen's assertion.

162. Altmann, *Studies*, p. 33 n. 155, mentions the text from *Mishkan ha-Edut* and a parallel in Moses de León's *Or Zaru'a*, which he explains as a "vision of the supernal world of pure intellect." Altmann suggests, moreover, that the supernal form seen by the prophet is the "supernal Matter," a concept that is known from Neoplatonic sources, including the fragments attributed erroneously to Empedocles. (Concerning this text, see Altmann and Stern, *Isaac Israeli*, pp. 159–64.) However, the passage from Moses de León, *Sefer Or Zaru'a*, edited by Alexander Altmann, *Qoveṣ al Yad* 9 (1980): 255–56, does not speak of a vision of a supernal form, let alone anything resembling the notion of the supernal matter. What is affirmed is the ability of the "enlightened one" (*maskil*) to ascend mentally and to reach the "gradation of the splendor of the unity" (*ma'alat zohar ha-yiḥud*) [or, according to the manuscript variant that Altmann cites, *ma'alat zohar ha-yesod*, the "gradation of the splendor of the foundation"]. The goal set forth is to apprehend through the "eye of the intellect" (*ein ha-sekhel*) that which "the tongue cannot describe and the lips cannot articulate," that is, the "supernal splendor" (*zohar elyon*) whose existence and unity are beyond comprehension. I think it is possible to explicate de León on the basis of Maimonidean principles. For other Neoplatonic-oriented passages in *Or Zaru'a*, which are compared to parallels in Moses Ibn Ezra, see Fenton, *Philosophie et exégèse*, pp. 220–22.

163. De León, *Mishkan ha-Edut*, MS Berlin Or. Quat. 833, fol. 3a.

164. Ibn Ḥasdai, *Ben ha-Melekh we-ha-Nazir*, ch. 26, p. 129. On the historical-literary background of this belletristic work, see Samuel M. Stern, "Ibn Ḥasdāy's Neoplatonist: A Neoplatonic Treatise and Its Influence on Isaac Israeli and the Longer Version of the Theology of Aristotle," *Oriens* 13–14 (1960–61): 59; *The Dream of the Poem: Hebrew Poetry from Muslim and Christian Spain 950–1492*, translated, edited, and introduced by Peter Cole (Princeton: Princeton University Press, 2007), pp. 221–22.

165. See references in Chapter 2 nn. 63, 88–89, 91, 93–95.

166. De León, *Mishkan ha-Edut*, MS Berlin Or. Quat. 833, fol. 3a.

167. *Ibid.*, fols. 3a–b. De León does not elaborate on this parable because, as he writes explicitly, he has dealt with it in another composition, the *Sefer Meshal ha-Qadmonim*. Thus far such a work by this author has not been discovered. The title, however, is reminiscent of Isaac Ibn Sahula's *Meshal ha-Qadmoni*, allegedly the first text to quote from the *Midrash ha-Ne'lam* stratum of zoharic literature. See Gershom Scholem, "Did Rabbi Moses de León Compose the Book of the Zohar?" *Madda'ei ha-Yahadut* 1 (1926): 26–27 (Hebrew);

idem, "The First Citation from the Midrash ha-Ne'lam," *Tarbiz* 3 (1932): 181–83 (Hebrew); *idem*, *Major Trends*, p. 187; Samuel M. Stern, "Rationalists and Kabbalists in Medieval Allegory," *Journal of Jewish Studies* 6 (1955): 73–86, esp. 74–75; Tishby, *Wisdom*, pp. 20 and 23; Arthur Green, "Rabbi Isaac Sahula's Commentary on the Song of Songs," *Jerusalem Studies in Jewish Thought* 6, nos. 3–4 (1987): 400–401 (Hebrew). On Ibn Sahula and the *Zohar*, see also Liebes, *Studies in the Zohar*, p. 196 n. 19; Ronit Meroz, "Zoharic Narratives and Their Adaptations," *Hispania Judaica* 3 (2000): 15–16.

168. Abraham Melamed, "The Image of India in Medieval Jewish Culture: Between Adoration and Rejection," *Jewish History* 20 (2006): 299–314, esp. 306–307. Melamed chronicles the history of the Hellenistic connection between Jewish and Indian wisdom, which provides the fuller context to understand the narrative recorded by de León, but he does not mention the kabbalistic sources (see below, n. 206) or the specific topic of comparing the world to a dream.

169. For a detailed exploration of this theme, see Arvind Sharma, *The World as Dream* (New Delhi: D.K. Printworld, 2006).

170. For an exacting analysis of this term in its Vedic and post-Vedic usage, see Jan Gonda, *Change and Continuity in Indian Religion* (The Hague: Mouton, 1965), pp. 164–97. According to Gonda, the central meaning that underlies all uses of the expression is an "incomprehensible wisdom and power enabling its possessor, or being able itself, to create, devise, contrive, effect, or do something." *Māyā* thus connotes a "creative wisdom-and-power" (p. 166).

171. Heinrich Zimmer, *Myth and Symbols in Indian Art and Civilization*, edited by Joseph Campbell (New York: Pantheon Books, 1946), pp. 39–40; *idem*, *Philosophies of India*, edited by Joseph Campbell (Cleveland: Meridian Books, 1956), p. 276; Alain Daniélou, *Hindu Polytheism* (New York: Bollingen Foundation, 1964), pp. 150–51.

172. For an elaboration of this point, see Wolfson, "Structure," pp. 149–54.

173. Compare the discussion of this topic as expounded by Asanga and Vasubadhu, scholastic thinkers of the Indian Yogācāra tradition, in Paul J. Griffiths, *On Being Mindless: Buddhist Meditation and the Mind-Body Problem* (La Salle: Open Court, 1986), pp. 80–84. For a recent study of this theme, wherein one can find reference to earlier scholarship, see Sthaneshwar Timalsina, *Consciousness in Indian Philosophy: The Advaita Doctrine of "Awareness Only"* (London: Routledge, 2009).

174. Zimmer, *Philosophies of India*, pp. 460–61. Consider the crucial difference between the Advaita systems of Śaṅkara and Rāmānuja analyzed in the introduction to *The Vedānta Sutras of Bādarāyana with the Commentary of*

Śaṅkara, translated by George Thibaut, 2 vols. (New York: Dover Publications, 1962), 1:xxx: "While, however, the advaita taught by Saṅkara is a rigorous, absolute one, Râmânuga's doctrine has to be characterized as visishta advaita, i.e. qualified non-duality, non-duality with a difference. According to Saṅkara, whatever is, is Brahman, and Brahman itself is absolutely homogeneous, so that all difference and plurality must be illusory. According to Râmânuga also, whatever is, is Brahman; but Brahman is not of a homogeneous nature, but contains within itself elements of plurality owing to which it truly manifests itself in a diversified world. The world with its variety of material forms of existence and individual souls is not unreal Mâyâ, but a real part of Brahman's nature, the body investing the universal Self. The Brahman of Saṅkara is in itself impersonal, a homogenous mass of objectless thought, transcending all attributes; a personal God it becomes only through its association with the unreal principles of Mâyâ, so that—strictly speaking—Saṅkara's personal God, his Îsvara, is himself something unreal. Râmânuga's Brahman, on the other hand, is essentially a personal God, the all-powerful and all-wise ruler of a real world permeated and animated by his spirit." See also Wendell Charles Beane, *Myth, Cult and Symbols in Śākta Hinduism: A Study of the Indian Mother Goddess* (Leiden: Brill, 2001), pp. 156–68; Pulasth Soobah Roodurmun, *Bhāmatī and Vivaraṇa Schools of Advaita Vedānta: A Critical Approach* (Delhi: Motilal Banarsidaas, 2002), pp. 133–70; Natalia Isayeva, *Shankara and Indian Philosophy* (Albany: State University of New York Press, 1993), pp. 213–15 and 222–24. The approaches assigned respectively to Śaṅkara and Rāmānuja have a striking affinity to two possibilities that may be elicited from reflections of Ḥabad masters on the relationship between the infinite essence and the concatenation of worlds. See Wolfson, *Open Secret*, pp. 93–96.

175. See O'Flaherty, *Dreams*, p. 114.

176. Sarvepalli Radhakrishnan, *Indian Philosophy*, 2 vols. (Oxford: Oxford University Press, 1929), 1:184–86 and 593–94; William M. Indich, *Consciousness in Advaita Vedānta* (Delhi: Motilal Banarsidass, 1980), pp. 5–6; Isayeva, *Shankara*, pp. 114–15; Arvind Sharma, *The Philosophy of Religion and Advaita Vedānta: A Comparative Study in Religion and Reason* (University Park: Pennsylvania State University Press, 1995), pp. 4, 170, 202–208, and, in greater detail, *The World as Dream*, pp. 53–113; Surendra Sheodas Barlingay, *Reunderstanding Indian Philosophy: Some Glimpses* (New Delhi: D.K. Printworld, 1998), pp. 195–213.

177. Cited in Indich, *Consciousness in Advaita Vedānta*, p. 63.

178. *Ibid.*, pp. 57–66 and 82–95. See also Daniélou, *Hindu Polytheism*, pp. 24–25; Zimmer, *Philosophies of India*, p. 452; Debabrata Sinha, *Metaphysic of*

Experience in Advaita Vedānta: A Phenomenological Approach (Delhi: Motilal Banarsidass, 1983), pp. 26–31; Jones, *Science and Mysticism*, pp. 60–70, 128, 163, 194; John Taber, "Reason, Revelation and Idealism in Śaṅkara's Vedānta," in *Indian Philosophy: A Collection of Readings*, edited with introductions by Roy W. Perrett (New York: Garland Publishing, 2000), pp. 172–73; George Gillespie, "Dreams and Dreamless Sleep," *Dreaming* 12 (2002): 199–207; Arvind Sharma, *Sleep as a State of Consciousness in Advaita Vedānta* (Albany: State University of New York Press, 2004), pp. 49–72. On the attribution of this fourfold classification to Gauḍapāda, a precursor of Śaṅkara, see Jeaneane Fowler, *Perspectives of Reality: An Introduction to the Philosophy of Hinduism* (Brighton: Sussex Academic Press, 2002), pp. 240–41. For discussion of the dream phenomenon in Hindu sources more generally, see O'Flaherty, *Dreams*, pp. 14–35; Bulkeley, *Dreaming*, pp. 20–49; Sharma, *The World as Dream*, pp. 115–30; Sumegi, *Dreamworlds*, pp. 35–48. On the role of Ayurvedic dream theory to awaken one to the reality that the predominant psychic activity in the waking state is dreaming, see Sudhir Kakar, *Shamans, Mystics, and Doctors: A Psychological Inquiry into India and Its Healing Traditions* (Chicago: University of Chicago Press, 1991), p. 246.

179. Thomas E. Wood, *The Māṇḍūkya Upaniṣad and the Āgama Śāstra: An Investigation into the Meaning of the Vedānta* (Honolulu: University of Hawaii Press, 1992), p. 6.

180. *Ibid.*, pp. 16–19.

181. *The Vedānta Sutras of Bādarāyana*, 1:324. On Śaṅkara's biography and bibliography, see Isayeva, *Shankara*, pp. 69–104.

182. *The Vedānta Sutras of Bādarāyana*, 1:325.

183. For an interesting discussion along these lines, see R. Balasubramanian, "Advaita Vedānta on the Problem of Enworlded Subjectivity," in *Phenomenology and Indian Philosophy*, pp. 77–93.

184. Surendranath Dasgupta, *Indian Idealism* (Cambridge: Cambridge University Press, 1969), pp. 158–59; Fowler, *Perspectives of Reality*, pp. 265–66; Yoshitsugu Sawai, "The Structure of Consciousness in Śaṅkara's Philosophy," in *Consciousness and Reality: Studies in Memory of Toshihiko Izutsu*, edited by Sayyid Jalāl al-Dīn Āshtiyānī, Hideichi Matsubara, Takashi Iwami, and Akiro Matsumoto (Leiden: Brill, 2000), pp. 333–38.

185. Paul Deussen, *The System of Vedânta*, translated by Charles Johnston (Chicago: Open Court, 1912), pp. 99–100. See *idem*, *The Philosophy of the Upanishads*, translated by Alfred S. Geden (New York: Dover Publications, 1966), pp. 228–39.

186. *Tibetan Yoga and Secret Doctrines*, edited by Walter Y. Evans-Wentz

(Oxford: Oxford University Press, 1958), p. 161. On the relation of *māyā* to the false appearance (*mithyādarśanam*) of dreams in both Hindu and Buddhist sources, see Gonda, *Change and Continuity*, pp. 171–89, and O'Flaherty, *Dreams*, pp. 114–26. See also Serinity Young, *Dreaming in the Lotus: Buddhist Dream Narrative, Imagery, and Practice*, foreword by Carol Schreier Rupprecht (Boston: Wisdom Publications, 1999), pp. 43–53, esp. 47; Sumegi, *Dreamworlds*, pp. 49–93.

187. *Tibetan Yoga*, p. 163.

188. *Ibid.*, p. 164.

189. *Ibid.*, p. 166. Compare the delineation of the four things to be achieved by the practitioner of yoga to become a *mahāyogin* in the Mahāyāna *Laṅkāvatāra-sūtra* in David J. Kalupahana, *A History of Buddhist Philosophy: Continuities and Discontinuities* (Honolulu: University of Hawaii Press, 1992), pp. 180–81. The fourth step, understanding that the realization of noble wisdom is within one's own self, is facilitated by the first three steps, cultivation of the idea that the visible (*dṛṣya*) is one's own mind (*svacitta*), renunciation of the view that arising, enduring, and ceasing are produced by external events, and the perception of the non-existence of the objective world. On Vasubandhu's refutation of commonsense realism in his *Vijñaptimātratāsiddhi* on the grounds that all experience is like a dream, see *ibid.*, p. 187, and the passages translated by Charles H. Hamilton in *A Sourcebook in Indian Philosophy*, edited by Sarvepalli Radhakrishnan and Charles E. Moore (Princeton: Princeton University Press, 1957), pp. 328, 331, 332. And compare the commentary on the critical passage from this sūtra in the *Bhāvanākrama* (*Stages of Meditation*) by the eighth-century Indian sage Kamalaśīla, translated in *Buddhist Scriptures*, edited by Donald S. Lopez Jr. (London: Penguin Books, 2004), pp. 367–69. See also Dasgupta, *Indian Idealism*, pp. 95–102, and the discussion on dreaming, death, and transcendence in LaBerge, *Lucid Dreaming*, pp. 229–47, esp. 236–39; *idem*, "Lucid Dreaming and the Yoga of the Dream State: A Psychophysiological Perspective," in *Buddhism and Science*, pp. 233–58; Wallace, *Contemplative Science*, pp. 124–30; *idem*, *Hidden Dimensions: The Unification of Physics and Consciousness* (New York: Columbia University Press, 2007), pp. 90–93 and 100–101.

190. An informative discussion of this term can be found in Timalsina, *Consciousness*, pp. 63–81. The author notes, inter alia, that for the classical Advaitins (Śaṅkara, Maṇḍana, Sureśvara, and Padmapāda), the terms *māyā* and *avidyā* functioned synonymously.

191. *Mahāparinirvāṇa Sūtra*, ch. 46, p. 490, available at http://www.nirvanasutra.net . The version on that site is the one translated by Kosho Yamamoto, edited, revised and copyrighted by Tony Page (London: Nirvana Publications,

1999–2000). In the continuation of this passage, it is acknowledged that the "sphere of neither ideation-nor-nonideation" is itself a state of ideation, indeed, the "ideation of nonideation," which is known when one awakens to the realization that all phenomena are devoid of defining attributes, even the characteristic of being or not being (pp. 490–91). Consider as well the reworking (apparently based on a philological misunderstanding) of the statement in *The Yoga-system of Patañjali; or, The Ancient Hindu Doctrine of Concentration of Mind, Embracing the Mnemonic Rules, Called Yoga-sūtras of Patañjali, and the Comment, Called Yoga-bhāshya, Attributed to Veda-Vyāsa, and the Explanation, Called Tattva-vāiçāradī, of Vāchaspati-Miçra*, translated by James Haughton Woods (Cambridge, MA: Harvard University Press, 1927), p. 29: "Sleep is a fluctuation [of mind-stuff] supported by the cause (*pratyaya*, that is *tamas*) of the [transient] negation [of the waking and the dreaming fluctuations]," in Shlomo Pines and Tuvia Gelblum, "Al-Bīrūnī's Arabic Version of Patañjali's *Yogasūtra*: A Translation of His First Chapter and a Comparison with Related Sanskrit Texts," *Bulletin of the School of Oriental and African Studies* 29 (1966): 316, "The fourth (faculty of the soul) is dream(ing), which is man's knowledge of things which are (in reality) other (than what he knows), which have no subsisting reality corresponding to the knowledge in question."

192. Talbot, *Mysticism*, pp. 99–100: "Control over one's dreams and the realization of the dreamlike nature of reality appears to have one major purpose in most mystical teachings—to loosen the hold the *tonal* has upon the way we construct our environment.... In the paradigm of reality presented by the new physics all categories of the real and unreal break down. Just as we can no longer consider Schrödinger's cat as being either alive *or* dead, we cannot consider the objective world as existing *or* not existing. This is exactly what is implied in the Buddhist proverb 'Is God dead?' If you say yes *or* no you lose your Buddha nature. In Buddhism, acquiring a Buddha nature is akin to finally becoming one with the *nagual*. The *tonals* drop from the eyes like ponderous cataracts and suddenly the interpenetrating universes spread out before the consciousness in dazzling splendor" (emphasis in the original). See also Jones, *Science and Mysticism*, pp. 128–29, and the expression of Christopher Norris mentioned in Chapter 1 at n. 290.

193. Nāgārjuna, *In Praise of the Incomparable*, in *Straight From the Heart: Buddhist Pith Instructions*, translated and introduced by Karl Brunnhölzl (Ithaca: Snow Lion Productions, 2007), p. 15. Compare the final discourse attributed to the Buddha in *The Diamond Sūtra* from the Mahāyāna *Prajñāpāramitā* in *Buddhist Wisdom Books, containing The Diamond Sutra and The Heart Sutra*, translated and explained by Edward Conze (London: George Allen & Unwin Ltd, 1975), p. 68:

"As stars, a fault of vision, as a lamp,/ A mock show, dew drops, or a bubble,/ A dream, a lightning flash, or cloud,/ So should one view what is conditioned." See as well the statements of Subhūti in *The Perfection of Wisdom in Eight Thousand Lines and Its Verse Summary*, translated by Edward Conze (Bolinas: Four Seasons Foundation, 1973), pp. 98–99: "All objective facts are like a magical illusion, like a dream. The various classes of saints, from Streamwinner to Buddhahood, also are like a magical illusion, like a dream.... Even Nirvana, I say, is like a magical illusion, is like a dream.... Even if perchance there could be anything more distinguished, of that too I would say that it is like an illusion, like a dream. For not two different things are illusion and Nirvana, are dreams and Nirvana."

194. On the ocularcentric privileging of perception in South Asian Mahāyāna texts and practices, see David L. McMahan, *Empty Vision: Metaphor and Visionary Imagery in Mahāyāna Buddhism* (London: RoutledgeCurzon, 2002).

195. Compare Vasubandhu, *Wei Shih Er Shih Lun: The Treatise in Twenty Stanzas on Representation-Only*, translated by Clarence H. Hamilton (New Haven: American Oriental Society, 1938), pp. 63–64. From stanza 16, "Before we have awakened we cannot know/That what is seen in the dream does not exist," the following is adduced: "Just as in the awakened state we do not know dream objects are not externally real, but do know it on awaking, even so the world's falsely discriminated recurrent impressions are confused and fevered as in the midst of a dream, all that is seen being wholly unreal; before the true awakening is attained [this] cannot be naturally known. [But] if there is a time when we attain that world-transcending knowledge, emancipatory and non-discriminative, then we call it the true awakening. After this, the purified knowledge of the world which is obtained takes precedence; according to the truth it is clearly understood that those objects are unreal." And see the comments on stanza 18, "The mind by sleep is weakened;/Dream and waking retributions are not the same," in *ibid*., pp. 67–68: "In the dream state the power of the mind, weakened by sleep, is reduced; but in the waking state it is not so. Therefore the acts which are performed ought to receive matured consequences, superior and inferior, which are not the same. [The difference] is not because of external objects."

196. *Nāgārjuna's Reason Sixty with Chandrakīrti's Commentary*, translated, with introduction, by Joseph Loizzo (New York: American Institute of Buddhist Studies, 2007), p. 124.

197. *Ibid*., p. 125.

198. Rangjung Dorje, *Luminous Heart: The Third Karmapa on Consciousness, Wisdom, and Buddha Nature*, translated and introduced by Karl Brunnhölzl

(Ithaca: Snow Lion Publications, 2009), p. 214.

199. Jamgön Kongtrul, *The Treasury of Knowledge: Esoteric Instructions*, translated and annotated by Sarah Harding (Ithaca: Snow Lion Publications, 2007), p. 242: "All double delusions arise without valid existence, so all the delusions of dreams just dissipate on their own in this special yoga. In these instructions, first one learns to recognize whatever dreams arise based on the vital point of lucid dreaming [or grasping that it is a dream while dreaming], by practicing the four empowerments of vital essences and the nine unerring vital points. Then one clears away the obstructions of excessive delusion, excessive wakefulness, excessive euphoria, and excessive emptiness through devotion, accumulation of merit, and so on.... When the skill with dreams is thus energetically refined, they are blended with luminous clarity." Compare *The Practice of the Six Yogas of Naropa*, translated, edited and introduced by Glenn H. Mullin (Ithaca: Snow Lion Publications, 1997), p. 37: "At night, strive to invoke the self-purification of confused dreams;/Guard the three doors with the hook of mindfulness./Retain, purify, increase and transform the contents of dreams,/And eliminate all obstacles to practice./One rides on the sun and moon, travels to all buddhafields,/And behold! All 'good' and 'bad' illusions become self-liberated."

200. Moss, *The Secret History of Dreaming*, p. xii, noted that in many cultures "dreaming is fundamentally about waking up." Compare the discussion of "dreaming of waking up" elicited from the thought of Zhuangzi (Chuang Tzu) and Nāgārjuna in David R. Loy, *Awareness Bound and Unbound: Buddhist Essays* (Albany: State University of New York Press, 2009), pp. 74–76. As Loy argues, the philosophical intent of the statements of Zhuangzi, including his well-known remark about Zhuang Zhou having dreamt that he was a butterfly and waking up uncertain if he is Zhou who dreamt he is a butterfly or a butterfly who dreamt he is Zhou (*The Complete Works of Chuang Tzu*, translated by Burton Watson [New York: Columbia University Press, 1968], p. 49), is on a par with the Buddhist insight, expressed incisively by Nāgārjuna, that to wake up is to realize that there is only a dream, and to dream of waking from that dream is to imagine falsely that there is some ultimate reality. Things of this world are both real and not real and therefore neither real nor not real.

201. Steven Heine, *A Dream Within a Dream: Studies in Japanese Thought* (New York: Peter Lang, 1991), pp. 39–42. See the analysis of Heine, pp. 33–37, and Taigen Dan Leighton, *Visions of Awakening Space and Time: Dōgen and the Lotus Sutra* (Oxford: Oxford University Press, 2007), pp. 32–34.

202. See William H. Grosnick, "The Zen Master Dogen's Understanding of the Buddha-Nature in Light of the Historical Development of the

Buddha-Nature Concept in India, China, and Japan," Ph.D. dissertation, University of Wisconsin-Madison, 1979, pp. 210–20; Paul Williams, *Mahāyāna Buddhism: The Doctrinal Foundations*, 2nd edition (London: Routledge, 2009), pp. 177–79.

203. Dōgen, *The Heart of Dōgen's Shōbōgenzō*, pp. 60–61 and 63. The identification of the differentiated world and the nondifferentiated ground is also implied in the statement cited by Dōgen in the name of the Buddha, *ibid.*, p. 65: "If you wish to know the Buddha-nature's meaning, you must contemplate temporal conditions. If the time arrives, the Buddha-nature will manifest itself." On Dōgen's conception of "being-time," see the references cited above, n. 33. The idea is also expressed in terms of the identification of the form of nature and the Buddhist sūtra in the *Sansuigyō* fascicle (*The Sūtra of Mountains and Water*). See Dōgen, *Shōbōgenzō: The True Dharma-Eye Treasury*, vol. 1, translated by Gudo Wafu Nishijima and Chodo Cross (Berkeley: Numata Center for Buddhist Translation and Research, 2007), pp. 217–34. Significantly, the Buddha dharma is characterized in that text primarily in the image of constant walking: "We should investigate the fact that just as the moment before the sprouting of creation, and since before the King of Emptiness, walking—in forward steps and backward steps—has never stopped even for an instant.... The moment of forward walking does not oppose backward walking, and the moment of backward walking does not oppose forward walking" (p. 218). The state wherein both self and world are beyond the dichotomy of the sentient and the insentient is also referred to by the paradoxical image of the "flowing mountains," obviously meant to destabilize the commonsense distinction between the solidity of the mountains and the fluidity of the river. Even so, the aspect of water is privileged in this text, although it is emphasized that it has no inherent nature, since the form it assumes is imparted to it by the perceiver: "Water is neither strong nor weak, neither moving nor still, neither cold nor warm, neither existent nor nonexistent, neither delusion nor realization.... In general, ways of seeing mountains and water differ according to the type of being [that sees them].... Now let us be wary of this. Is it that there are various ways of seeing one object? Or is it that we have mistakenly assumed the various images to be one object? At the crown of effort, we should make still further effort. If the above is so, then practice-and-experience and pursuit of the truth also may not be [only] of one kind or of two kinds; and the ultimate state also may be of thousands of kinds and myriad varieties. When we keep this point in mind, although there are many kinds of water, it seems that there is no original water, and no water of many kinds" (pp. 221–22).

204. Dōgen, *The Heart of Dōgen's Shōbōgenzō*, p. 41: "The moment you

begin seeking the Dharma, you move far from its environs. The moment the Dharma is been rightly transmitted to you, you become the Person of your original part." Compare the language in the *Sansuigyō* fascicle, *Shōbōgenzō: The True Dharma-Eye Treasury*, vol. 1, p. 221: "We should manifest in reality the path on which self encounters self. We should advance and retreat along the vigorous path on which the external world exhausts in practice the external world, and we should spring free." By abiding in place, all dharmas are liberated from place.

205. *Ibid.*, pp. 40–41. Compare the fascicle *Gyōbutsu-yuigi* in Dōgen, *Shōbōgenzō: The True Dharma-Eye Treasury*, vol. 2, translated by Gudo Wafu Nishijima and Chodo Cross (Berkeley: Numata Center for Buddhist Translation and Research, 2008), pp. 43–44. The "acting buddha" is described as one who is beyond "initiated enlightenment, "original enlightenment, "inherent enlightenment," and "non-existent enlightenment." Paradoxically, the mind enlightened "in the Buddha's state of truth" does "not expect enlightenment." The acting buddha is "released from the fetter of 'Buddha" and the fetter of 'Dharma.'... The meaning of the 'fetter of Buddha' is as follows: when we view and understand *bodhi* as '*bodhi*,' we have directly been fettered by the view itself and by that understanding itself. Passing instantaneously through the moment of consciousness, never expecting that it might be the period of liberation, we misunderstand [*Bodhi*] in vain." The truly awakened mind is not hampered by any constraint, even the constraint of having been liberated from all constraints. To arouse the dharma nature within the dharma nature, however, is to be bound to the unbound and thus to tie oneself more tightly by the rope of ignorance. The acting buddha is "neither in love with 'original enlightenment' nor in love with 'initiated enlightenment,' and is beyond 'not having enlightenment' and beyond 'having enlightenment'" (p. 50). Bodhi mind is attained by the practice of zazen and the letting go of the desire to take hold, but the continuous effort must be to reach the more advanced state of "taking hold in excess of 'taking hold'" and "letting go in excess of 'letting go'" (p. 52), that is, to be free of all attachment, including the attachment to being free from all attachment. As Dōgen remarked in the *Bendōwa* fascicle, *The Heart of Dōgen's Shōbōgenzō*, p. 12, the practitioner who undertakes the meditational technique of zazen "without fail casts off body and mind" and "severs all the hithertofore disordered and defiled thoughts and views emanating from his discriminating consciousness." In this manner, he "conforms totally with the genuine Buddha nature," but he also achieves the potential (*ki*) of "transcending Buddha, vigorously promoting the Dharma (*hō*) transcending Buddha." The implications of Dōgen's thinking are drawn by Uchiyama Roshi in *The Wholehearted Way: A*

Translation of Eihei Dōgen's Bendōwa, with Commentary by Kōshō Uchiyama Roshi, translated by Shohaku Okumura and Taigen Daniel Leighton (Tokyo: Tuttle Publishing, 1997), p. 115: "We should not separate practice and enlightenment into two. Since zazen is itself enlightenment, there is no way to think that I become enlightened as a result of zazen practice. To sit zazen is to be in the profound sleep of enlightenment. Therefore, to think that I am enlightened is the same to think that I sleep well within sound sleep. This is sham sleep. When we sleep really well, we cannot think that we sleep well. In the same way, within zazen, we cannot see if we are enlightened or not.... We sit right in that place where we can look at both enlightenment and delusion equally." The same outlook is found in the *Shōichi kokushi kana hōgo* (*A Vernacular Dharma Talk by the National Teacher Shōichi of Tōfuku*) by Enni (1202–1280), translated by Carl Bielefeldt in *Buddhism in Practice: Abridged Edition*, edited by Donald S. Lopez, Jr. (Princeton: Princeton University Press, 2007), p. 150: "The buddha mind is basically without delusion or awakening.... The buddha mind is without marks and without attachments.... Therefore, where we have no-mind and no-thought in the midst of the four attitudes of walking, standing, sitting, and reclining, this is the true employment of the mind, the true concerted effort." See as well verse 32 from the *Vaitathya-prakaraṇa* section of the Āgama Śāstra translated in Wood, *The Māṇḍūkya Upaniṣad*, p. 19: "There is no destruction, nor again origination; no one who is bound and no spiritual aspirant. There is no one longing for liberation, nor indeed any one who is liberated. This is the highest truth."

206. For discussion of the depiction of Indian wisdom in these terms in medieval Jewish texts, see Melamed, "The Image of India," pp. 304–11. On the phonetic resemblance of Abraham and Brahmin, see *ibid.*, p. 302. On the possibility that Indian mythology may have been known to Moses de León, see the brief. but tantalizing suggestion of Raphael Patai, *The Hebrew Goddess* (New York: Ktav, 1967), p. 183. For a wide-ranging, but largely speculative study, see Maurice Fluegel, *Philosophy, Qabbala, and Vedānta* (Baltimore: The Sun Printing Office, 1902). The author's approach, laudable though it may have been, does not meet the criteria of philological-historical scholarship. This does not mean, however, that there is nothing to be gained by the comparative perspective he outlined. Consider the passage in *Zohar* 3:10a, cited in the name of the "book of Rav Hamnuna Sava," concerning the spherical nature of the world and the impact this has on the different temporal zones. The insight, which is also attributed to "the books of the ancients" and to the "book of the first Adam," is a "mystery transmitted to the masters of wisdom [*ma'reihon de-ḥokhmeta*], and not to those who demarcate boundaries [*mefalgei teḥumin*]." The

depiction of the universe as a sphere is known from earlier sources, including rabbinic texts, but as some have suggested in the past, the zoharic account may reflect the ancient Indian view dealt with at length in the *Aryabhatiya* of Aryabhata (476–550). See also Isaac Ibn Laṭif, *Rav Pe'alim*, sec. 51, 16a. This is a matter that requires a careful investigation that lies beyond the scope of this study. Minimally, the passage from de León discussed in the body of this chapter provides textual evidence that one eminent medieval kabbalist was willing to think of Jewish esoteric wisdom in these terms. On the specific affinity between kabbalah and Vedānta related to the illusory nature of the phenomenal world and the infinite, see Fluegel, *Philosophy, Qabbala, and Vedānta*, pp. 231–32. For a commendable effort at a comparative analysis, albeit with an entirely different agenda, see Barbara A. Holdrege, *Veda and Torah: Transcending the Textuality of Scripture* (Albany: State University of New York Press, 1996).

207. Jacob Joseph of Polonnoye, *Toledot Ya'aqov Yosef* (Korzec, 1780), 25a–b. At the end of the passage, the author refers to the *Olelot Efrayim* of Ephraim Solomon ben Aaron of Luntshits, a text that he cites frequently (see *ibid.*, 99b, where it is mentioned again in conjunction with the matter of the ladder beheld by Jacob). Two sections of that homiletical work deal with Jacob's vision, but neither enunciates the view that the physical world as a whole is a dream. See *Olelot Efrayim* (Prague, 1619), sec. 166, 43a–b; sec. 269, 68c.

208. On the status of letters in the teaching of the Beshṭ and early Ḥasidism, especially as it relates to the experience of communion (*devequt*) through Torah study and prayer, see Scholem, *The Messianic Idea*, pp. 211–13; Weiss, *Studies*, pp. 58–59; Idel, *Hasidism*, pp. 92–94, 160–70, 215–21; Margolin, *The Human Temple*, pp. 186 and 202–203.

209. Jacob Joseph of Polonnoye, *Ketonet Passim*, critical edition with introduction and notes by Gedalyah Nigal (Jerusalem: Makhon Peri ha-Areṣ, 1985), p. 102. Elior, *The Mystical Origins*, p. 120, similarly describes the purpose of contemplative worship in ḥasidic thought as the striving of the human "to comprehend the divine unity of opposites: that the 'real' world one perceives is illusory, and the only reality is divinity."

210. Babylonian Talmud, Rosh ha-Shanah 28a.

211. Dov Baer, the Maggid of Międzyrzecz, *Or Torah* (Brooklyn: Kehot, 1972), 67d. This passage was also included in the compilation *Ṣawwa'at ha-Ribash* (Brooklyn: Kehot, 1998), sec. 90, p. 40.

212. Menaḥem Mendel of Viṭebsk, *Liqquṭei Amarim* (Lemberg, 1911), 38b. Compare Phineḥas of Korzec, *Imrei Pinḥas ha-Shalem*, 1:126. Prayer is described as being "above time [*lema'lah min ha-zeman*] like a dream in which one dreams something that happens for a quarter of an hour that in truth is a moment

[*rega*], for the dream is above time. So, too, the Torah and prayer can all be in one moment."

213. Concerning that figure, also referred to as Shmeril of Zwierzchowka, see *In Praise of the Baal Shem Tov [Shivḥei ha-Besht]: The Earliest Collection of Legends about the Founder of Hasidism*, translated and edited by Dan Ben-Amos and Jerome R. Mintz (Bloomington: Indiana University Press, 1970), pp. 3, 59, 132; Heschel, *The Circle of the Baal Shem Tov*, pp. 57 and 121.

214. Phineḥas of Korzec, *Imrei Pinḥas ha-Shalem*, 1:474–75.

215. *Ibid.*, 1:475.

216. *Ibid.*, 1:34–35, 121, 122, 452.

217. *Ibid.*, 1:122. The editor (n. 180) suggests that perhaps the expression *nequddah she-ba-ḥalom* should be emended to *nequddah she-ba-ḥolem*, that is, the point that is in the vowel. I prefer the former and thus am reluctant to correct the text.

218. Maimonides, *Mishneh Torah*, Yesodei ha-Torah 2:7.

219. Phineḥas of Korzec, *Imrei Pinḥas ha-Shalem*, 1:40.

220. *Ibid.*, 1:122.

221. Moses Ḥayyim Ephraim of Sudlykow, *Degel Maḥaneh Efrayim* (Jerusalem: Mir, 1995), p. 38. The figurative characterization of exile as sleep and redemption as wakefulness is an older motif that gained currency in ḥasidic sources. See, for instance, Phineḥas of Korzec, *Imrei Pinḥas ha-Shalem*, 1:471: "Exile is the secret of slumber, whence emerge many difficulties, but if it be the will of God, when the Messiah comes, all will be clear, and this is the meaning of 'your eyes will see your master' (Isaiah 30:20)."

222. Moses Ḥayyim Ephraim of Sudlykow, *Degel Maḥaneh Efrayim*, pp. 259–60. For reference to the oneiric practices of Moses Ḥayyim Ephraim of Sudlykow and other ḥasidic masters of his time, see Idel, *Hasidism*, pp. 54 and 274 n. 34. Several dreams of the Ba'al Shem Ṭov and his appearance in the dreams of others are transmitted in the legendary account of his life. See, for example, *In Praise of the Baal Shem Tov*, pp. 48–49, 53–54, 158–59, 175–76, 186, 246–47. On the distinction between the dream (*ḥalom*) and vision (*ḥezyon*) in the tale about R. Joseph Ashkenazi (*In Praise of the Baal Shem Tov*, pp. 48–49), see Ḥaviva Pedaya, "The Baal Shem Tov, R. Jacob Joseph of Polonnoye, and the Maggid of Mezhirech: Outlines for a Religious Typology," *Da'at* 45 (2000): 53–54 (Hebrew).

223. Ṣadoq ha-Kohen of Lublin, *Dover Ṣedeq* (Jerusalem: Makhon Har Berakhah, 2008), p. 114.

224. The oneiric blurring of the line between life and death is displayed as well in the possibility of a deceased person appearing to a living person in a

dream, a phenomenon hardly unique to Jewish sources. See, for instance, de Vidas, *Re'shit Ḥokhmah*, Sha'ar ha-Yir'ah, ch. 12, 1:238; Sha'ar ha-Ahavah, ch. 16, 1:471; Ṣevi Hirsch Kaidonover, *Qav ha-Yashar* (New York: Beit Sefer, 1974), ch. 12. See above, n. 7.

225. Ṣadoq ha-Kohen of Lublin, *Liqquṭei Ma'amarim* (Jerusalem: Makhon Har Berakhah, 2008), pp. 169–70. See also *idem*, *Resisei Laylah* (Jerusalem: Makhon Har Berakhah, 2003), pp. 195–96; *idem*, *Ṣidqat ha-Ṣaddiq*, pp. 109–10; *idem*, *Maḥashavot Ḥaruṣ* (Jerusalem: Makhon Har Berakhah, 2006), pp. 10–11 and 106. For an extended discussion of dreams and the unconscious in the writings of this ḥasidic master, see Brill, *Thinking God*, pp. 110–33.

226. Ibn al-'Arabī, *Bezels of Wisdom*, pp. 121–25.

227. *Ibid.*, pp. 123–24.

228. Muḥyīddīn Ibn al-'Arabi, *The Wisdom of the Prophets* (*Fusus al-Hikam*), translated from Arabic to French with notes by Titus Burckhardt, translated from French to English by Angela Culme-Seymour (Aldsworth: Beshara, 1975), pp. 62 n. 10 and 64 n. 17. See also the analysis of the motif of dream and reality in the thought of Ibn al-'Arabī in Toshihiko Izutsu, *Sufism and Taoism: A Comparative Study of Key Philosophical Concepts* (Berkeley: University of California Press, 1983), pp. 7–22.

229. Rūmī, *Mathnawí*, 3:1729–738. For analysis of this passage, see Maria Subtelny, "The Traces of the Traces: Reflections of the Garden in the Persian Mystical Imagination," in *Gardens and Imagination: Cultural History and Agency*, Dumbarton Oaks Colloquium on the History of Landscape Architecture, edited by Michael Conan (Washington, D.C.: Dumbarton Oaks Research Library and Collection, 2008), p. 28. I thank the author for drawing my attention to her study. Compare Rūmī, *Mathnawí*, 4:3633, where the world is compared to sleep.

230. *Ibid.*, 8:47.

231. *Ibid.*, 8:47–48.

232. *Ibid.*, 4:1370. I am indebted to Subtelny, "The Traces," pp. 27–29, who explicates this passage in conjunction with the other section of the *Mathnawí* wherein the prophetic tradition that the world is the sleeper's dream is cited.

233. Rūmī, *Mathnawí*, 8:48, and see Reynold A. Nicholson, *Studies in Islamic Mysticism* (Cambridge: Cambridge University Press, 1921), p. 118. See *ibid.*, pp. 90–92, and 97, where the author compares Jīlī's view in the *Insānu 'l-kāmil* to the Vedānta system. It is worth recalling the passing comment of Ur-Rahman, "Al-Fârâbî," p. 151, that "there is not much difference, regarding the nature of the ætiology of dreams, between Hindu and Muslim thinkers."

234. Foucault, "Dream, Imagination and Existence," p. 47. The citation

is from F. W. J. Schelling, *Werke*, edited by Otto Weiss (Munich: Biederstein, 1946), 4:217. Although Foucault links the dreamlike quality of the world to the German philosophers Novalis and Schelling, it is not impossible that he was also influenced in this matter by Buddhist sources, an interest that became more explicit at a later stage in his life. See Uta Liebmann Schaub, "Foucault's Oriental Subtext," *Proceedings of the Modern Language Association* 104 (1989): 306–16, reprinted in *Critical Essays on Michel Foucault*, edited by Karlis Racevskis (New York: G.K. Hall & Co., 1999), pp. 101–17. Regarding Foucault's particular interest in Zen Buddhism, including his visit to the Seionji temple in Uenohara, Japan, see the dialogical exchange "Michel Foucault and Zen: A Stay in a Zen Temple (1978)," in Michel Foucault, *Religion and Culture*, selected and edited by Jeremy R. Carrette (New York: Routledge, 1999), pp. 110–14. See also Didier Eribon, *Michel Foucault*, translated by Betsy King (Cambridge, MA: Harvard University Press, 1991), p. 310, and Robert Wicks, "Foucault," in *The Blackwell Guide to Continental Philosophy*, edited by Robert C. Solomon and David Sherman (Oxford: Blackwell Publishing Ltd, 2003), p. 258. Finally, the influence of Eastern thought on Schelling should also not be ignored. On this topic, see Wilhelm Halbfass, *India and Europe: An Essay in Understanding* (Albany: State University of New York Press, 1988), pp. 100–105, esp. 102, where Schelling's attraction to the Vedāntic tendency to see the world as an illusory being (*māyā*) is duly noted.

235. Allen Ginsberg, *Collected Poems 1947–1977* (New York: HarperCollins, 2006), p. 336.

236. For philosophical explorations of this theme in the Japanese Buddhist tradition, see Daisetz T. Suzuki, *The Zen Doctrine of No Mind: The Significance of the Sūtra of Hui-neng (Wei-Lang)*, edited by Christmas Humphreys (New York: Samuel Weiser, 1972), and Joan Stambaugh, *The Formless Self* (Albany: State University of New York Press, 1999). See the more recent and expansive analysis of the conceptual background of the Buddhist psychology in Jonardon Ganeri, *The Concealed Art of the Soul: Theories of Self and Practices of Truth in Indian Ethics and Epistemology* (Oxford: Oxford University Press, 2007), pp. 157–215.

237. A few weeks after writing these words, I came across the following remark of the Fifth Dalai Lama of the Gelug-pa sect cited in Jeffrey Hopkins, *Tantric Techniques*, edited by Kevin Vose (Ithaca: Snow Lion Publications, 2008), p. 14: "If both the self [that is the validly existent person] and [the self that is] the nonexistent object of negation are not intimately identified, it is like dispatching an army without knowing where the enemy is or like shooting an arrow without having sought out the target." Hopkins glosses this comment: "If

we do not have a fairly clear sense of an inherently existing 'I,' we will mistake the refutation as negating the 'I' itself rather than a specific reification of the 'I.' . . . If an image of the object of negation does not appear well to the mind, the meaning of the selflessness that negates it cannot be ascertained." This is precisely what I intended by my remarks "negating the affirmation of negation by affirming the negation of affirmation." See also the words of the *Genjōkōan* in Dōgen, *The Heart of Dōgen's Shōbōgenzō*, p. 41: "To learn the Buddha Way is to learn one's self. To learn one's self is to forget one's self. To forget one's self is to be confirmed by all dharmas. To be confirmed by all dharmas is to cast off one's body and mind and the bodies and minds of others as well." According to Uchiyama Roshi in *The Wholehearted Way*, p. 43 n. 2, the idea expressed in this passage corresponds to *jijuyū zammai*, the "concentration of self-fulfillment," mentioned toward the beginning of the *Bendōwa* fascicle of the *Shōbōgenzō*: "The enjoyment, fulfillment, or satisfaction is the samadhi of the self, of which there is no other. This is not an experience that is somewhere other than here and now, it is not something to be acquired or gained. . . . Everything becomes everything, all becomes all. *Jijuyū* samadhi is buddha's practice." See the comprehensive discussion of this topic in Zhihua Yao, *The Buddhist Theory of Self-Cognition* (London: Routledge, 2005).

238. For analysis of this matter from a clinical perspective, see Melvin E. Miller, "No-Self and the Emptying God: Dwelling in the Emptying Place," in *Self and No-Self: Continuing the Dialogue between Buddhism and Psychotherapy*, edited by Dale Mathers, Melvin E. Miller, and Osamu Ando (London: Routledge, 2009), pp. 79–91.

239. See the comments from Keller and Miller cited in the Introduction at nn. 35–36, and the remarks of Corbin at n. 43.

240. Elliot R. Wolfson, *Footdreams and Treetales: 92 Poems* (New York: Fordham University Press, 2007), p. 66. Fittingly, the title of the poem is "b/e," which conveys the difficulty of distinguishing sharply between dream and reality.

Bibliography

Abba Mari of Lunel. *Sefer Minḥat Qina'ot*. In *Teshuvot ha-Rashba*, edited by Ḥayyim Z. Dimitrovski. Jerusalem: Mosad ha-Rav Kook, 1990.

Abraham Axelrod of Cologne. *Keter Shem Ṭov*. In Adolph Jellinek, *Auswahl kabbalistischer Mystik*, erstes Heft, pp. 29–48. Leipzig: A. M. Colditz, 1853.

Abraham bar Ḥiyya. *Megillat ha-Megalleh*. Edited by Adolf Poznanski. Revised with an introduction by Julius Guttmann. Berlin: Mekize Nirdamim, 1924.

Abrams, Daniel. *The Female Body of God in Kabbalistic Literature: Embodied Forms of Love and Sexuality in the Divine Feminine*. Jerusalem: Magnes Press, 2004 (Hebrew).

——. "The Invention of the *Zohar* as a Book: On the Assumptions and Expectations of the Kabbalists and Modern Scholars." *Kabbalah: Journal for the Study of Jewish Mystical Texts* 19 (2009): 7–142.

Abulafia, Abraham. *Gan Na'ul*. Jerusalem, 1999.

——. *Ḥayyei ha-Nefesh*. Jerusalem, 2001.

——. *Ḥayyei ha-Olam ha-Ba*. Jerusalem, 1999.

——. *Mafteaḥ ha-Ḥokhmot*. Jerusalem, 2001.

——. *Mafteaḥ ha-Ra'yon*. Jerusalem, 2002.

——. *Mafteaḥ ha-Sefirot*. Jerusalem, 2001.

——. *Mafteaḥ ha-Tokhaḥot*. Jerusalem, 2001.

——. *Oṣar Eden Ganuz*. Jerusalem, 2000.

——. *Sefer ha-Edut*. In *Maṣref ha-Sekhel*. Jerusalem, 2001.

——. *Sefer ha-Ḥesheq*. Jerusalem, 1999.

——. *Sefer ha-Malmad*. Jerusalem, 2002.

——. *Sefer ha-Yashar*. In *Maṣref ha-Sekhel*. Jerusalem, 2001.

——. *Sheva Netivot ha-Torah*. In Adolph Jellinek, *Philosophie und Kabbala*, 1:1–25. Leipzig: Heinrich Hunger, 1854.

Adams, Michael Vannoy. *The Fantasy Principle: Psychoanalysis of the Imagination*. New York: Brunner-Routledge, 2004.

Adamson, Peter. "Al-Kindī and the Reception of Greek Philosophy." In *The Cambridge Companion to Arabic Philosophy*, edited by Peter Adamson and Richard C. Taylor, pp. 32–51. Cambridge: Cambridge University Press, 2005.

Adriannse, H. J. "After Theism." In *Religion: Beyond a Concept*, edited by Hent de Vries, pp. 392–412. New York: Fordham University Press, 2008.

Afik (Abecassis), Isaac. "Hazal's Perception of the Dream." Ph.D. dissertation, Bar-Ilan University, 1990 (Hebrew).

Agamben, Giorgio. *Potentialities: Collected Essays in Philosophy*. Edited, translated, and with an introduction by Daniel Heller-Roazen. Stanford: Stanford University Press, 1999.

———. *The Signature of All Things: On Method*. Translated by Luca D'Isanto with Kevin Attell. New York: Zone Books, 2009.

Akkach, Samer. "The World of Imagination in Ibn 'Arabī's Ontology." *British Journal of Middle Eastern Studies* 24 (1997): 97–113.

Albo, Joseph. *Sefer ha-Iqqarim*. Warsaw: Isaac Goldman, 1877.

Alexander of Aphrodisias. *On Aristotle's Metaphysics 2 & 3*. Translated by William E. Dooley, S. J. and Arthur Madigan, S. J. Ithaca: Cornell University Press, 1992.

———. *On Aristotle's Metaphysics 5*. Translated by William E. Dooley, S. J. Ithaca: Cornell University Press, 1993.

———. *On the Cosmos*. Edited and translated by Charles Genequand. Leiden: Brill, 2001.

Alexander, Philip S. "Bavil Berakhot 55a–57b: The Talmudic Dreambook in Context." *Journal of Jewish Studies* 46 (1995): 230–48.

Alexander, Tamar. "Dream Narratives in 'Sefer Hasidim.'" *Trumah* 12 (2002): 65–78 (Hebrew).

Alexander-Frizer, Tamar. *The Pious Sinner: Ethics and Aesthetics in the Medieval Hasidic Narrative*. Tübingen: J. C. B, Mohr, 1991.

Al-Fārābī, Abū Naṣr. *On the Perfect State (Mabādi' ārā' ahl al-madīnat al-fāḍilah)*. Revised text with introduction, translation, and commentary by Richard Walzer. Oxford: Oxford University Press, 1985.

Al-Ghazālī, Abū Ḥāmid. *Al-Ghazālī's Path to Sufism and His Deliverance From Error, An Annotated Translation of Al Munqidh min al-Dalal*. Translated by R. J. McCarthy, S. J. Preface by David Burrell, C. S. C. Introduction by William A. Graham. Louisville: Fons Vitae, 2000.

———. *The Incoherence of the Philosophers: A Parallel English-Arabic Text*. Translated, introduced, and annotated by Michael E. Marmura. Provo: Brigham Young University Press, 1997.

——. *Kitāb sharḥ 'ajā'ib al-qalb: The Marvels of the Heart*. Translated with an introduction and notes by Walter J. Skellie, with a foreword by Timothy J. Winter. Louisville: Fons Vitae, 2010.

——. *The Niche of Lights: A Parallel English-Arabic Text*. Translated, introduced, and annotated by David Buchman. Provo: Brigham Young University Press, 1998.

——. *The Remembrance of Death and Afterlife*. Translated with an introduction and notes by T. J. Winter. Cambridge: Islamic Texts Society, 1995.

Allen, Sarah. *The Philosophical Sense of Transcendence: Levinas and Plato on Loving Beyond Being*. Pittsburgh: Duquesne University Press, 2009.

Allison, David B. *Reading the New Nietzsche: The Birth of Tragedy, The Gay Science, Thus Spoke Zarathustra, and On the Genealogy of Morals*. Lanham: Rowman & Littlefield, 2001.

Almoli, Solomon. *Pitron Ḥalomot*. Warsaw, 1902.

Almond, Ian. *Sufism and Deconstruction: A Comparative Study of Derrida and Ibn 'Arabi*. London: Routledge, 2004.

Altmann, Alexander. *Essays in Jewish Intellectual History*. Hanover: University Press of New England, 1981.

——. "Gersonides' Commentary on Averroes' Epitome of *Parva Naturalia*, II.3: Annotated Critical Edition." *Proceedings of the American Academy for Jewish Research* 46 (1979–1980): 1–31.

——. *Studies in Religious Philosophy and Mysticism*. Ithaca: Cornell University Press, 1969.

——. *Von der mittelalterlichen zur modernen Aufklärung: Studien zur jüdischen Geistesgeschichte*. Tübingen: J. C. B. Mohr, 1987.

Altmann Alexander, and Samuel M. Stern. *Isaac Israeli: A Neoplatonic Philosopher of the Early Tenth Century*. Oxford: Oxford University Press, 1958.

Ames, William L. "Emptiness and Quantum Theory." In *Buddhism and Science: Breaking New Ground*, edited by B. Alan Wallace, pp. 285–302. New York: Columbia University Press, 2003.

Angeleṭ, Joseph. *Livnat ha-Sappir*. Jerusalem, 1913.

Arama, Isaac ben Moses. *Aqeidat Yiṣḥaq*. 4 vols. Edited by Ḥayyim Yosef Pollak. Pressburg: Victor Kittseer, 1849.

Artemidorus. *The Interpretation of Dreams: Oneirocritica*. Translation and commentary by Robert J. White, 2nd edition, revised and enlarged. Torrance: Original Books, 1990.

Assoun, Paul-Laurent. *Freud et Wittgenstein*. Paris: Presses Universitaires de France, 1988.

Atom and Archetype: The Pauli/Jung Letters, 1932–1958. Edited by Carl Alfred

Meier with the assistance of Charles Paul Enz and Markus Fierz. Translated by David Roscoe, with an introductory essay by Beverley Zabriskie. Princeton: Princeton University Press, 2001.

Aune, David E. *Prophecy in Early Christianity and the Ancient Mediterranean World*. Grand Rapids: William B. Eerdmans, 1983.

Avencebrolis (Solomon Ibn Gabirol). *Fons Vitae ex Arabico in Latinum Translatus ab Iohanne Hispano et Dominico Gundissalino*. Edited by Clemens Baeumker. Münster: Aschendorff, 1895.

——. *Meqor Ḥayyim*. Translated by Jacob Blubstein. Edited by Abraham Zifroni. Tel-Aviv: Maḥbarot le-Sifrut, 1926.

Avens, Roberts. *Imagination Is Reality: Western Nirvana in Jung, Hillman, Barfield and Cassirer*. Putnam: Spring Publications, 1980.

——. *The New Gnosis: Heidegger, Hillman, and Angels*. Dallas: Spring Publications, 1984.

Averroës. *Epitome of Parva Naturalia*. Translated with notes and introduction by Harry Blumberg. Cambridge, MA: Medieval Academy of America, 1961.

——. *Tahafut al-Tahafut* (*The Incoherence of the Incoherence*). Translated with introduction and notes by Simon van der Bergh. 2 vols. London: E. J. W. Gibb Memorial, 1969.

Bachelard, Gaston. *Air and Dreams: An Essay on the Imagination of Movement*. Translated by Edith R. Farrell and C. Frederick Farrell. Dallas: Dallas Institute Publications, 2002.

——. *The Poetics of Reverie: Childhood, Language, and the Cosmos*. Translated by Daniel Russell. Boston: Beacon Press, 1971.

——. *Water and Dreams: An Essay on the Imagination of Matter*. Translated by Edith R. Farrell. Dallas: Pegasus Foundation, 1983.

Bacher, Wilhelm. *Die exegetische Terminologie der jüdischen Traditionsliteratur*, part 1: *Die bibelexegetische Terminologie der Tannaiten*. Leipzig: Hinrichs, 1905. Reprint, Darmstadt: Wissenschaftliche Buchgesellschaft, 1965.

Badiou, Alain. *Logics of Worlds: Being and Event, 2*. Translated by Alberto Toscano. New York: Continuum, 2009.

——. *Saint Paul: The Foundation of Universalism*. Translated by Ray Brassier. Stanford: Stanford University Press, 2003.

——. *Theoretical Writings*. Edited and translated by Ray Brassier and Alberto Toscano. New York: Continuum, 2005.

Badiou, Alain, and Slavoj Žižek. *Philosophy in the Present*. Edited by Peter Engelmann. Translated by Peter Thomas and Alberto Toscano. Cambridge: Polity Press, 2010.

Baḥya ben Asher. *Rabbenu Baḥya: Be'ur al ha-Torah*. Edited by Ḥayyim D.

Chavel. 3 vols. Jerusalem: Mosad ha-Rav Kook, 1981.

Bain-Selbo, Eric. "A Review of Jürgen Habermas, *Religion and Rationality: Essays on Reason, God, and Modernity*." *Journal for Cultural and Religious Theory* 5 (2003): 139–43.

Bakan, David. *Sigmund Freud and the Jewish Mystical Tradition*. Boston: Beacon Press, 1975.

Balasubramanian, R. "Advaita Vedānta on the Problem of Enworlded Subjectivity." In *Phenomenology and Indian Philosophy*, edited by Debi Prasad Chattopadhyaya, Lester Embree, and Jitendranath Mohanty, pp. 77–93. Albany: State University of New York Press, 1992.

Bar, Shaul. *A Letter That Has Not Been Read: Dreams in the Hebrew Bible*. Cincinnati: Hebrew Union College Press, 2001.

Barlingay, Surendra Sheodas. *Reunderstanding Indian Philosophy: Some Glimpses*. New Delhi: D.K. Printworld, 1998.

Bazak, J. *Beyond the Senses: A Study of Extra-Sensorial Perception in Biblical, Talmudical, and Rabbinical Literature in Light of Contemporary Parapsychological Research*. Tel-Aviv, 1968 (Hebrew).

Beane, Wendell Charles. *Myth, Cult and Symbols in Śākta Hinduism: A Study of the Indian Mother Goddess*. Leiden: Brill, 2001.

Bearn, Gordon C.F. *Waking to Wonder: Wittgenstein's Existential Investigations*. Albany: State University of New York Press, 1997.

Beeckman, Tinneke. "Reinterpreting Freud's Genealogy of Culture." In *Origins and Ends of the Mind: Philosophical Essays on Psychoanalysis*, edited by Christian Kerslake and Ray Brassier, pp. 117–34. Leuven: Leuven University Press, 2007.

Benayahu, Meir. "The 'Maggid' of R. Moses Ḥayyim Luzzatto." *Sefunot* 5 (1961): 297–336 (Hebrew).

Benjamin, Walter. *The Arcades Project*. Translated by Howard Eiland and Kevin McLaughlin. Prepared on the basis of the German volume edited by Rolf Tiedmann. Cambridge, MA: Harvard University Press, 1999.

Ben-Shlomo, Joseph. *The Mystical Theology of Moses Cordovero*. Jerusalem: Bialik Institute, 1965 (Hebrew).

Benson, Bruce Ellis. *Graven Ideologies: Nietzsche, Derrida, and Marion on Modern Idolatry*. Downers Grove: InterVarsity Press, 2002.

Bergman, Samuel Hugo. "Metaphysical Implications of Husserl's Phenomenology." *Scripta Hierosolymitana* 2 (1955): 220–30.

Bergo, Bettina. "Ontology, Transcendence, and Immanence in Emmanuel Levinas' Philosophy." *Research in Phenomenology* 35 (2005): 141–77.

——. "The Time and Language of Messianism: Levinas and Saint Paul." In

Levinas and the Ancients, edited by Brian Schroeder and Silvia Benso, pp. 178–95. Bloomington : Indiana University Press, 2008.

Bergson, Henri. *The Creative Mind*. Translated by Mabelle L. Andison. New York: Philosophical Library, 1946.

——. *Matter and Memory*. Translated by Nancy Margaret Paul and W. Scott Palmer. New York: Zone Books, 1991.

——. *Mind-Energy*. Translated by H. Wildon Carr, edited by Keith Ansell Pearson and Michael Kolkman, with an introduction by Keith Ansell Pearson. New York: Palgrave Macmillan, 2007.

——. *Time and Free Will: An Essay on the Immediate Data of Consciousness*. Translation by F. L. Pogson. New York: Dover Publications, 2001.

Bernasconi, Robert. "Different Styles of Eschatology: Derrida's Take on Levinas' Political Messianism." *Research in Phenomenology* 28 (1998): 3–19.

——. "No Exit: Levinas' Aporetic Account of Transcendence." *Research in Phenomenology* 35 (2005): 101–17.

Bernstein, Richard J. *Freud and the Legacy of Moses*. Cambridge: Cambridge University Press, 1998.

Berthold-Bond, Daniel. *Hegel's Theory of Madness*. Albany: State University of New York Press, 1995.

Bhattacharyya, Sibajiban. "Phenomenology and Indian Philosophy." In *Phenomenology and Indian Philosophy*, edited by Debi Prasad Chattopadhyaya, Lester Embree, and Jitendranath Mohanty, pp. 44–76. Albany: State University of New York Press, 1992.

Biale, David. *Gershom Scholem: Kabbalah and Counter-History*. Cambridge, MA: Harvard University Press, 1979.

Bickle, John. "Empirical Evidence for a Narrative Concept of Self." In *Narrative and Consciousness: Literature, Psychology, and the Brain*, edited by Gary D. Fireman, Ted E. McVay, Jr., and Owen J. Flanagan, pp. 195–208. Oxford: Oxford University Press, 2003.

Bilu, Yoram. "Dreams and Wishes of the Saint." In *Judaism Viewed from Within and from Without: Anthropological Studies*, edited by Harvey E. Goldberg, pp. 285–313. Albany: State University of New York Press, 1987.

——. "Oneirobiography and Oneirocommunity in Saint Worship in Israel: A Two-Tier Model for Dream-Inspired Religious Revivals." *Dreaming* 10 (2000): 85–101.

——. "Sigmund Freud and Rabbi Yehudah: On a Jewish Mystical Tradition of 'Psychoanalytic' Dream Interpretation." *The Journal of Psychological Anthropology* 2 (1979): 443–63.

Binswanger, Ludwig. *Augewähtle Vorträge und Aufsätze*, vol. 1. Bern: A. Francke, 1947.

——. *Dream and Existence*. Translated by Jacob Needleman. In Michel Foucault and Ludwig Binswanger, *Dream and Existence*, edited by Keith Hoeller, pp. 79–105. Atlantic Highlands: Humanities Press, 1993.

——. *Le rêve et l'existence*. Translated by J. Verdeaux. Paris: Desclée de Brouwer, 1954.

Blanchot, Maurice. *Friendship*. Translated by Elizabeth Rottenberg. Stanford: Stanford University Press, 1997.

——. *The Infinite Conversation*. Translation and foreword by Susan Hanson. Minneapolis: University of Minnesota Press, 1993.

——. *Maurice Blanchot: The Demand of Writing*. Edited by Carolyn Bailey Gill. London: Routledge, 1996.

——. *The Step Not Beyond*. Translated by Lycette Nelson. Albany: State University of New York Press, 1992.

——. *The Writing of Disaster*. Translated by Ann Smock. Lincoln: University of Nebraska Press, 1986.

Bland, Kalman P. "Moses and the Law According to Maimonides." In *Mystics, Philosophers, and Politicians: Essays in Jewish Intellectual History in Honor of Alexander Altmann*, edited by Jehuda Reinharz and Daniel Swetschinski with the collaboration of Kalman P. Bland, pp. 49–66. Durham: Duke University Press,1982.

Bland, Nathaniel. "On the Muhammedan Science of Tabir, or Interpretation of Dreams." *Journal of the Royal Asiatic Society of Great Britain and Ireland* 16 (1856): 118–71.

Blau, Ludwig. *Das Altjüdische Zauberwesen*. Strassburg: Karl J. Trübner, 1898.

Blenkinsopp, Joseph. *Sage, Priest, Prophet: Religious and Intellectual Leadership in Ancient Israel*. Louisville: Westminster John Knox Press, 1995.

Blumberg, Hans. "The Life-World and the Concept of Reality." In *Life-World and Consciousness: Essays for Aron Gurwitsch*, edited by Lester E. Embree, pp. 425–44. Evanston: Northwestern University Press, 1972.

Blumenthal, David R. "Maimonides' Philosophic Mysticism." In *Maimonides and Mysticism Presented to Moshe Hallamish On the Occasion of his Retirement*, edited by Avi Elqayam and Dov Schwartz [*Da'at* 64–66], pp. v–xxv (English section). Ramat-Gan: Bar-Ilan University Press, 2009.

——. *Philosophic Mysticism: Studies in Rational Religion*. Ramat-Gan: Bar Ilan University Press, 2006.

Bohak, Gideon. *Ancient Jewish Magic: A History*. Cambridge: Cambridge University Press, 2008.

Boodakian, Florence Dee. *Tormenting Angel: A Psychoaesthetic Theory of Imagination*. New York: Peter Lang, 1999.

The Book Bahir: An Edition Based on the Earliest Manuscripts. Edited by Daniel Abrams. Los Angeles: Cherub Press, 1994.

The Book of Bahir: Flavius Mithridates' Latin Translation, the Hebrew text, and an English Version. Edited by Saverio Campanini, with a Foreword by Giulio Busi. Torino: Nino Aragno Editore, 2005.

Borges, Jorge Luis. *Labyrinths: Selected Stories and Other Writings*. Edited by Donald A. Yates and James E. Irby. Preface by André Maurois. New York: New Directions, 1964.

Botz-Bornstein, Thorsten. "The Dream of Language: Wittgenstein's Concept of Dreams in the Context of Style and *Lebensform*." *Philosophical Forum* 34 (2003): 73–89.

Bouretz, Pierre. *Witnesses for the Future: Philosophy and Messianism*. Translated by Michael B. Smith. Baltimore: Johns Hopkins Press, 2010.

Bourguignon, Erika. "Dreams That Speak: Experience and Interpretation." In *Dreaming and the Self: New Perspectives on Subjectivity, Identity, and Emotion*, edited by Jeannette Marie Mageo, pp. 133–53. Albany: State University of New York Press, 2003.

Bouwsma, O. K. "Descartes' Skepticism of the Senses." *Mind* 54 (1945): 313–22. Reprinted in *Philosophical Essays on Dreaming*, edited by Charles E. M. Dunlop, pp. 52–63. Ithaca: Cornell University Press, 1977.

Bowersock, Glen W. *Fiction as History: Nero to Julian*. Berkeley: University of California Press, 1994.

Boyarin, Daniel. *Intertextuality and the Reading of Midrash*. Bloomington: Indiana University Press, 1990.

———. *Sparks of Logos: Essays in Rabbinic Hermeneutics*. Leiden: Brill, 2003.

Brann, Eva T. H. *The World of the Imagination: Sum and Substance*. Lanham: Rowman & Littlefield, 1991.

Brereton, Derek P. "Dreaming, Adaptation, and Consciousness: The Social Mapping Hypothesis." *Ethos* 28: 379–409.

Brill, Alan. "The Phenomenology of True Dreams in Maimonides." *Dreaming* 10 (2000): 43–54.

———. *Thinking God: The Mysticism of Rabbi Zadok of Lublin*. New York: Yeshiva University Press, 2002.

Brody, Seth. "'Open to Me the Gates of Righteousness': The Pursuit of Holiness and Non-Duality in Early Hasidic Teaching." *Jewish Quarterly Review* 89 (1998): 3–44.

Brooke, Roger. *Jung and Phenomenology*. London: Routledge, 1991.

Brown, Jason W. *Mind and Nature: Essays on Time and Subjectivity*. London: Whurr, 2000.

Brown, Norman O. "Apocalypse: The Place of Mystery in the Life of the Mind." In *Interpretation: The Poetry of Meanings*, edited by Stanley R. Hopper and David L. Miller, pp. 7–13. New York: Harcourt, Brace and World, 1967.

Browne, Alice. "Descartes's Dreams." *Journal of the Warburg and Courtauld Institutes* 40 (1977): 256–73.

Bruns, Gerald L. "Anarchic Temporality: Writing, Friendship, and the Ontology of the Work of Art in Maurice Blanchot's Poetics." In *The Power of Contestation: Perspectives on Maurice Blanchot*, edited by Kevin Hart and Geoffrey H. Hartman, pp. 121–40. Baltimore: Johns Hopkins University Press, 2004.

———. *Maurice Blanchot: The Refusal of Philosophy*. Baltimore: Johns Hopkins University Press, 1997.

Buber, Martin. *Good and Evil: Two Interpretations*. New York: Charles Scribner's Sons, 1953.

Bucher, Stefan. *Zwischen Phänomenologie und Sprachwissenschaft: Zu Merleau-Pontys Theorie der Sprache*. Münster: Nodus Publikationen, 1991.

Buddhism in Practice: Abridged Edition. Edited by Donald S. Lopez, Jr. Princeton: Princeton University Press, 2007.

Buddhist Scriptures. Edited by Donald S. Lopez, Jr. London: Penguin Books, 2004.

Buddhist Wisdom Books, containing The Diamond Sutra and The Heart Sutra. Translated and explained by Edward Conze. London: George Allen & Unwin Ltd, 1975.

Bulhof, Ilse N. "Being Open as a Form of Negative Theology: On Nominalism, Negative Theology, and Derrida's Performative Interpretation of Khôra." In *Flight of the Gods: Philosophical Perspectives on Negative Theology*, edited by Ilse N. Bulhof and Laurens ten Kate, pp. 195–222. New York: Fordham University Press, 2000.

Bulkeley, Kelly. *Dreaming in the World's Religions: A Comparative History*. New York : New York University Press, 2008.

———. "Reflections on the Dream Traditions of Islam." *Sleep and Hypnosis* 4 (2002): 4–14.

———. *Visions of the Night: Dreams, Religion, and Psychology*. Albany: State University of New York, 1999.

———. *The Wondering Brain: Thinking about Religion with and beyond Cognitive Neuroscience*. New York: Routledge, 2005.

Burke, Kenneth. "Freud—and the Analysis of Poetry." In *Freud: A Collection of Critical Essays*, edited by Perry Meisel, pp. 73–94. Englewood Cliffs: Prentice-Hall, 1981.

Burke, Patrick. "Merleau-Ponty's Appropriation of Husserl's Notion of '*Präsenzfeld*'." In *Husserl in Contemporary Context: Prospects and Projects for Phenomenology*, edited by Burt C. Hopkins, pp. 37–58. Dordrecht: Kluwer, 1997.

Byrne, Richard W., and Andrew Whiten. "The Manipulation of Attention in Primate Tactical Deception." In *Machiavellian Intelligence: Social Expertise and the Evolution of Intellect in Monkeys, Apes and Humans*, edited by Richard W. Byrne and Andrew Whitten, pp. 211–23. Oxford: Oxford University Press, 1988.

Caillois, Roger. *Images, Images. . . : Essais sur le rôle et les pouvoirs de l'imagination*. Paris: Librairie José Corti, 1966.

——. *L'incertitude qui vient des rêves*. Paris: Gallimard, 1956.

——. "Logical and Philosophical Problems of the Dream." In *The Dream and Human Societies*, edited by Gustave Edmund von Grunebaum and Roger Caillois, pp. 23–52. Berkeley: University of California Press, 1966.

Cairns-Smith, Alexander Graham. *Evolving the Mind: On the Nature of Matter and the Origin of Consciousness*. Cambridge: Cambridge University Press, 1996.

Calderbank, Michael. "Surreal Dreamscapes: Walter Benjamin and the Arcades." *Papers of Surrealism* 1 (2003). Available at http://www.surrealismcentre.ac.uk/papersofsurrealism/journal1/acrobat_files/Calderbank.pdf.

Caligor, Leopold and Rollo May. *Dreams and Symbols: Man's Unconscious Language*. New York: Basic Books, 1968.

Caputo, John D. "Adieu—sans Dieu: Derrida and Levinas." In *The Face of the Other and the Trace of God: Essays on the Philosophy of Emmanuel Levinas*, edited by Jeffrey Bloechl, pp. 276–311. New York: Fordham University Press, 2000.

——. "Apostles of the Impossible: On God and the Gift in Derrida and Marion." In *God, the Gift, and Postmodernism*, edited by John D. Caputo and Michael J. Scanlon, pp. 185–222. Bloomington: Indiana University Press, 1999.

——. *The Prayers and Tears of Jacques Derrida: Religion without Religion*. Bloomington: Indiana University Press, 1997.

——. "Shedding Tears Beyond Being: Derrida's Experience of Prayer." In *Théologie Négative*, edited by Marco M. Olivetti, pp. 861–80. Milan: CEDAM, 2002.

——. "Temporal Transcendence: The Very Idea of à-venir in Derrida." In *Transcendence and Beyond: A Postmodern Inquiry*, edited by John D. Caputo and Michael J. Scanlon, pp. 188–203. Bloomington: Indiana University Press, 2007.

——. "The Time of Giving, the Time of Forgiving." In *The Enigma of Gift and Sacrifice*, edited by Edith Wyschogrod, Jean-Joseph Goux, and Eric Boynton, pp. 117–47. New York: Fordham University Press, 2002.

——. "Transcendence and the Transcendental in Husserl's Phenomenology." *Philosophy Today* 23 (1979): 205–16.

——. *The Weakness of God: A Theology of the Event*. Bloomington: Indiana University Press, 2006.

Caputo John D. and Michael J. Scanlon. "Do We Need to Transcend Transcendence?" In *Transcendence and Beyond: A Postmodern Inquiry*, edited by John D. Caputo and Michael J. Scanlon, pp. 1–14. Bloomington: Indiana University Press, 2007.

Carlebach, Elisheva. *Divided Souls: Converts From Judaism in German, 1500–1750*. New Haven: Yale University Press, 2001.

Carlson, Thomas A. *Indiscretion: Finitude and the Naming of God*. Chicago: University of Chicago Press, 1999.

——. "Unlikely Shadows: Transcendence in Image and Immanence." In *Transcendence: Philosophy, Literature, and Theology Approach the Beyond*, edited by Regina Schwartz, pp. 105–25. New York: Routledge, 2004.

Carr, David. *The Paradox of Subjectivity: The Self in the Transcendental Tradition*. New York: Oxford University Press, 1999.

Carrique, Pierre. *Rêve, vérité: Essai sur la philosophie du sommeil et de la veille*. Paris: Éditions Gallimard, 2002.

Casey, Edward S. "Imagination, Fantasy, Hallucination, and Memory." In *Imagination and Its Pathologies*, edited by James Phillips and James Morley, pp. 65–91. Cambridge, MA: The MIT Press, 2003.

——. *Imagining: A Phenomenological Study*. Bloomington: Indiana University Press, 1976.

Caygill, Howard. *Levinas and the Political: Thinking the Political*. London: Routledge, 2002.

Chalier, Catherine. *La trace de l'infini: Emmanuel Levinas et la source hébraïque*. Paris: Cerf, 2002.

Chappell, Vere C. "The Concept of Dreaming." *Philosophical Quarterly* 13 (1963): 193–213. Reprinted in *Philosophical Essays on Dreaming*, edited by Charles E. M. Dunlop, pp. 280–308. Ithaca: Cornell University Press, 1977.

Cheetham, Tom. *The World Turned Inside Out: Henry Corbin and Islamic Mysticism*. Woodstock: Spring Journal Books, 2003.

Chittick, William C. *The Self-Disclosure of God: Principles of Ibn al-'Arabī's Cosmology*. Albany: State University of New York Press, 1998.

——. *The Sufi Path of Knowledge: Ibn al-'Arabi's Metaphysics of Imagination*. Albany: State University of New York Press, 1989.

Cicero, *On Divination: Book 1*. Translated with introduction and commentary by David Wardle. Oxford: Oxford University Press, 2006.

Clark, Christopher M. *The Politics of Conversion: Missionary Protestantism and the Jews in Prussia 1728–1941*. Oxford: Oxford University Press, 1995.

Clements, Ronald E. *Old Testament Prophecy*. Louisville: Westminster Press, 1996.

Cohen, Hermann. *Jüdische Schriften*, Dritter Band. Berlin: C. A. Schwetschke & Sohn, 1924.

Cohen, Mordechai Z. *Three Approaches to Biblical Metaphor From Abraham Ibn Ezra and Maimonides to David Kimhi*. Leiden: Brill, 2003.

Cohen, Richard A. "Against Theology, or 'The Devotion of a Theology without Theodicy': Levinas on Religion." In *The Exorbitant: Emmanuel Levinas between Jews and Christians*, edited by Kevin Hart and Michael A. Signer, pp. 74–89. New York: Fordham University Press, 2010.

The Commentaries to Ezekiel's Chariot of R. Eleazar of Worms and of R. Jacob ben Jacob ha-Kohen, edited and introduced by Asi Farber-Ginat and Daniel Abrams. Los Angeles: Cherub Press, 2004 (Hebrew).

The Complete Works of Chuang Tzu. Translated by Burton Watson. New York: Columbia University Press, 1968.

Cook, Albert. *The Burden of Prophecy: Poetic Utterance in the Prophets of the Old Testament*. Carbondale: Southern Illinois University Press, 1996.

Copjec, Joan. *Read My Desire: Lacan against the Historicists*. Cambridge, MA: The MIT Press, 1994.

Corbin, Henry. *Avicenna and the Visionary Recital*. Translated by Willard R. Trask. New York: Pantheon Books, 1960.

———. *Creative Imagination in the Ṣūfism of Ibn 'Arabī*. Translated by Ralph Manheim. Princeton: Princeton University Press, 1969.

———. *Cyclical Time and Ismaili Gnosis*. London: Kegan Paul International, 1983.

———. *L'imâm caché*. Paris: Éditions de l'Herne, 2003.

———. *Le paradoxe du monothéisme*. Paris: Éditions de L'Herne, 2003.

———. *Temple and Contemplation*. Translated by Philip Sherrard with the assistance of Liadain Sherrard. London: KPI Limited, 1986.

———. "The Visionary Dream in Islamic Spirituality." In *The Dream and Human Societies*, edited by Gustave Edmund von Grunebaum and Roger Caillois, pp. 381–408. Berkeley: University of California Press, 1966.

Cordovero, Moses. *Or Ne'erav*. Jerusalem, 1974.

———. *Pardes Rimmonim*. Jerusalem, 1962.

Corey, Lawrence. "Kabbalah and the Interpretation of Dreams." In *A Modern Jew In Search of a Soul*, edited by J. Marvin Spiegelman and Abraham

Jacobson, pp. 47–84. Phoenix: Falcon Press, 1986.

Covitz, Joel. *Visions in the Night: Jungian and Ancient Dream Interpretation*. Second revised edition. Toronto: Inner City Books, 2000.

Crignon, Philippe. "Figuration: Emmanuel Levinas and the Image." *Yale French Studies* 104 (2004): 100–125.

Critchley, Simon. "*Il y a*—Holding Levinas's Hand to Blanchot's Fire." In *Maurice Blanchot: The Demand of Writing*, edited by Carolyn Bailey Gill, pp. 108–22. London: Routledge, 1996.

Crockett, Clayton. *Interstices of the Sublime: Theology and Psychoanalytic Theory*. New York: Fordham University Press, 2007.

——. "Post-Modernism and Its Secrets: Religion without Religion." *Cross Currents* 52 (2003): 499–515.

Crowell, Steven Galt. *Husserl, Heidegger, and the Space of Meaning: Paths Toward a Transcendental Phenomenology*. Evanston: Northwestern University Press, 2001.

Damiani, Anthony. *Standing in Your Own Way*. Burdett: Larson, 1993.

Dan, Joseph. *Gershom Scholem and the Mystical Dimension of Jewish History*. New York: New York University Press, 1988.

——. "Gershom Scholem's Reconstruction of Early Kabbalah." *Modern Judaism* 5 (1985): 39–66.

——. *On Sanctity: Religion, Ethics and Mysticism in Judaism and Other Religions*. Jerusalem: Magnes Press, 1998 (Hebrew).

——. "On the Teaching Concerning the Dream in Ḥasidei Ashkenaz." *Sinai* 68 (1971): 288–93 (Hebrew).

Daniélou, Alain. *Hindu Polytheism*. New York: Bollingen Foundation, 1964.

Dasgupta, Surendranath. *Indian Idealism*. Cambridge: Cambridge University Press, 1969.

Dastur, Françoise. "Word, Flesh, Vision." In *Chiasms: Merleau-Ponty's Notion of Flesh*, edited by Fred Evans and Leonard Lawlor, pp. 23–49. Albany: State University of New York Press, 2000.

David ben Yehudah he-Ḥasid. *The Book of Mirrors: Sefer Mar'ot ha-Ẓove'ot*, edited by Daniel C. Matt. Chico: Scholars Press, 1982.

Davidson, Herbert A. *Alfarabi, Avicenna, and Averroes, On Intellect: Their Cosmologies, Theories of the Active Intellect, and Theories of Human Intellect*. Oxford: Oxford University Press, 1992.

——. *Moses Maimonides: The Man and His Works*. Oxford: Oxford University Press, 2005.

de Boer, Theodore. *The Rationality of Transcendence: Studies in the Philosophy of Emmanuel Levinas*. Amsterdam: J. C. Gieben, 1997.

De León, Moses. *The Book of the Pomegranate: Moses de León's Sefer ha-Rimmon*, edited by Elliot R. Wolfson. Atlanta: Scholars Press, 1988.

——. *Mishkan ha-Edut*. MS Berlin Or. Quat. 833; MS Vatican 283.

——. *R. Moses de Leon's Commentary to Ezekiel's Chariot*, edited by Asi Farber-Ginat and Daniel Abrams. Los Angeles: Cherub Press, 1998 (Hebrew).

——. *R. Moses de Leon's Sefer Sheqel ha-Qodesh*, critically edited and introduced by Charles Mopsik. Los Angeles: Cherub Press, 1996 (Hebrew).

——. *Sefer Or Zaru'a*, edited by Alexander Altmann, *Qoveṣ al Yad* 9 (1980): 217–93.

——. "Sefer ha-Mishkal: Text and Study." Edited by Jochanan H.A. Wijnhoven, Ph.D. dissertation, Brandeis University, 1964.

——. *She'elot u-Teshuvot le-Rav Moshe di Li'on be-Inyenei Qabbalah*. In Isaiah Tishby, *Studies in Kabbalah and Its Branches: Researches and Sources*, vol. 1, pp. 36–75. Jerusalem: Magnes Press, 1982.

——. *Shushan Edut*, edited by Gershom Scholem, "Shenei Qunṭresim le-R. Moshe di Li'on." *Qoveṣ al Yad* 8 (1976): 330–70.

——. Untitled fragment. MS Munich 47, fols. 335b–404b.

Deleuze, Gilles. *Difference and Repetition*. Translated by Paul Patton. New York: Columbia University Press, 1994.

——. *Expressionism in Philosophy: Spinoza*. Translated by Martin Joughin. New York: Zone Books, 1992.

——. *Pure Immanence: Essays on A Life*, with an introduction by John Rajchman. Translated by Anne Boyman. New York: Zone Books, 2001.

Deleuze, Gilles and Felix Guattari. *What is Philosophy?* Translated by Janis Tomlinson and Graham Burchell. New York: Columbia University Press, 1994.

Dement, William C. *The Promise of Sleep*. New York: Delacorte Press, 1999.

Dennett, Daniel C. "Are Dreams Experiences?" *Philosophical Review* 85 (1976): 151–71. Reprinted in *Philosophical Essays on Dreaming*, edited by Charles E.M. Dunlop, pp. 227–50. Ithaca: Cornell University Press, 1977.

De Nys, Martin J. *Considering Transcendence: Elements of a Philosophical Theology*. Bloomington: Indiana University Press, 2009.

Depoortere, Frederiek. *Badiou and Theology*. New York: Continuum, 2009.

Derksen, Martin. "Dream Interpretation as Test Case for Hermeneutics." *Journal of Phenomenological Psychology* 22 (1991): 134–41.

Derrida, Jacques. *Adieu To Emmanuel Levinas*. Translated by Pascale-Anne Brault and Michael Naas. Stanford: Stanford University Press, 1999.

——. *Dissemination*. Translated, with an introduction and additional notes, by Barbara Johnson. Chicago: University of Chicago Press, 1981.

——. *L'écriture et la différence*. Paris: Seuil, 1967.

——. *Edmund Husserl's Origin of Geometry: An Introduction*. Translated, with a preface and afterword, by John P. Leavey, Jr. Lincoln: University of Nebraska Press, 1989.

——. *On Cosmopolitanism and Forgiveness*. Translated by Mark Dooley and Michael Hughes, with a preface by Simon Critchley and Richard Kearney. London: Routledge, 2001.

——. *Resistances of Psychoanalysis*. Translated by Peggy Kamuf, Pascale-Anne Brault, and Michael Naas. Stanford: Stanford University Press, 1998.

——. *Specters of Marx: The State of the Debt, the Work of Mourning, and the New International*. Translated by Peggy Kamuf, introduction by Bernd Magnus and Stephen Cullenberg. New York: Routledge, 1994.

——. "The *Retrait* of Metaphor." In *The Derrida Reader: Writing Performances*, edited by Julian Wolfreys, pp. 102–29. Lincoln: University of Nebraska Press. 1998.

——. "To Forgive: The Unforgivable and the Imprescriptible." In *Questioning God*, edited by John D. Caputo, Mark Dooley, and Michael J. Scanlon, pp. 21–51. Bloomington: Indiana University Press, 2001.

——. *Writing and Difference*. Translated with introduction and additional notes by Alan Bass. Chicago: The University of Chicago Press, 1978.

Descartes, René. *Meditations on First Philosophy*. In *The Philosophical Writings of Descartes*. Translated by John Cuttingham, Robert Stoothoff, Dugald Murdoch. 2 vols. Cambridge: Cambridge University Press, 1984.

de Beistegui, Miguel. "The Vertigo of Immanence: Deleuze's Spinozism." *Research in Phenomenology* 35 (2005): 77–100.

d'Espagnat, Bernard. *Veiled Reality: An Analysis of Present-Day Quantum Mechanical Concepts*. Boulder: Westview Press, 2003.

Détienne, Marcel. *The Masters of Truth in Ancient Greece*. Translated by Janet Lloyd. New York: Zone Books, 1999.

——. *La notion de* daïmon *dans le pythagorisme ancien*. Paris: Les Belles Lettres, 1963.

Deussen, Paul. *The Philosophy of the Upanishads*. Translated by Alfred S. Geden. New York: Dover Publications, 1966.

——. *The System of Vedânta*. Translated by Charles Johnston. Chicago: Open Court, 1912.

de Vidas, Elijah. *Re'shit Ḥokhmah ha-Shalem*. 3 vols. Jerusalem, 1984.

de Vries, Hent. *Minimal Theologies: Critiques of Secular Reason in Adorno and Levinas*. Translated by Geoffrey Hale. Baltimore: Johns Hopkins University Press, 2005.

——. *Philosophy and the Turn to Religion*. Baltimore: John Hopkins University Press, 1999.

——. "The Theology of the Sign and the Sign of Theology: The Apophatics of Deconstruction." In *Flight of the Gods: Philosophical Perspectives on Negative Theology*, edited by Ilse N. Bulhof and Laurens ten Kate, pp. 166–94. New York: Fordham University Press, 2000.

Diamond, James A. *Maimonides and the Hermeneutics of Concealment: Deciphering Scripture and Midrash in The Guide of the Perplexed.* Albany: State University of New York Press, 2002.

Dobbs-Weinstein, Idit. "The Ambiguity of the Imagination and the Ambivalence of Language in Maimonides and Spinoza." In *Maimonides and His Heritage*, edited by Idit Dobbs-Weinstein, Lenn E. Goodman, and James A. Grady, pp. 95–111. Albany: State University of New York Press, 2009.

Dodd, James. *Crisis and Reflection: An Essay on Husserl's Crisis of the European Sciences.* Dordrecht: Kluwer, 2004.

——. *Idealism and Corporeity: An Essay on the Problem of the Body in Husserl's Phenomenology.* Dordrecht: Kluwer, 1997.

Dodds, Eric R. *The Greeks and the Irrational.* Berkeley: University of California Press, 1951.

Dōgen, Eihei. *The Heart of Dōgen's Shōbōgenzō.* Translated by Norman Waddell and Masao Abe. Albany: State University of New York Press, 2002.

——. *Shōbōgenzō: The True Dharma-Eye Treasury*, vol. 1. Translated by Gudo Wafu Nishijima and Chodo Cross. Berkeley: Numata Center for Buddhist Translation and Research, 2007.

——. *Shōbōgenzō: The True Dharma-Eye Treasury*, vol. 2. Translated by Gudo Wafu Nishijima and Chodo Cross. Berkeley: Numata Center for Buddhist Translation and Research, 2008.

——. *The Wholehearted Way: A Translation of Eihei Dōgen's Bendōwa, with Commentary by Kōshō Uchiyama Roshi.* Translated by Shohaku Okumura and Taigen Daniel Leighton. Tokyo: Tuttle Publishing, 1997.

Domhoff, G. William. *The Scientific Study of Dreams: Neural Networks, Cognitive Development, and Content Analysis.* Washington, D.C.: American Psychological Association, 2003.

Doniger, Wendy. "When a Lingam is Just a Good Cigar: Psychoanalysis and Hindu Sexual Fantasies." In *Vishnu on Freud's Desk: A Reader in Psychoanalysis and Hinduism*, edited by T. G. Vaidyanathan and Jeffrey J. Kripal, pp. 279–303. Delhi: Oxford University Press, 1999.

Dooley, Mark. "Marion's Ambition of Transcendence." In *Givenness and God: Questions of Jean-Luc Marion*, edited by Ian Leask and Eoin Cassidy, pp. 190–98. New York: Fordham University Press, 2005.

Dov Baer of Międzyrzecz. *Or Torah.* Brooklyn: Kehot, 1972.

Dor, Joel. *Introduction to the Reading of Lacan: The Unconscious Structured Like a Language*. New York: Other Press, 1998.

Dorff, Elliot N. *Knowing God: Jewish Journeys to the Unknowable*. Northvale: Jason Aronson, 1992.

Dorje, Rangjung. *Luminous Heart: The Third Karmapa on Consciousness, Wisdom, and Buddha Nature*. Translated and introduced by Karl Brunnhölzl. Ithaca: Snow Lion Publications, 2009.

Dowdey, David. *Jewish-Christian Relations in Eighteenth-Century Germany: Textual Studies on German Archival Holdings, 1729–1742*. Lewiston: Edwin Mellen Press, 2006.

Drabinski, John E. *Sensibility and Singularity: The Problem of Phenomenology in Levinas*. Albany: State University of New York Press, 2001.

The Dream of the Poem: Hebrew Poetry from Muslim and Christian Spain 950–1492. Translated, edited, and introduced by Peter Cole. Princeton: Princeton University Press, 2007.

Drob, Sanford L. *Kabbalistic Visions: C. G. Jung and Jewish Mysticism*. New Orleans: Spring Journal Books, 2010.

———. "'This Is Gold': Freud, Psychotherapy and the Lurianic Kabbalah." Available at http://www.newkabbalah.com.

Dulaey, Martine. *Le rêve dans la vie et la pensée de Saint Augustin*. Paris: Études Augustiniennes, 1973.

Eamon, William. *Science and the Secrets of Nature: Books of Secrets in Medieval and Early Modern Culture*. Princeton: Princeton University Press, 1994.

Ebeling, Florian. *The Secret History of Hermes Trismegistus: Hermeticism from Ancient to Modern Times*. Foreword by Jan Assman. Translated by David Lorton. Ithaca: Cornell University Press, 2007.

Edwards, David, and Michael Jacobs. *Conscious and Unconscious*. Berkshire: Open University Press, 2003.

Edwards, Ian. "Derrida's (I)religion: A Theology (of Différance)." *Janus Head* 6 (2003): 142–53.

Ehrlich, Avrum M. *Leadership in the HaBaD Movement: A Critical Evaluation of HaBaD Leadership, History, and Succession*. Northvale: Jason Aronson, 2000.

———. *The Messiah of Brooklyn: Understanding Lubavitch Hasidism Past and Present*. Jersey City: Ktav, 2004.

Einstein, Gillian, and Owen Flanagan. "Sexual Identities and Narratives of Self." In *Narrative and Consciousness: Literature, Psychology, and the Brain*, edited by Gary D. Fireman, Ted E. McVay, Jr., and Owen J. Flanagan, pp. 209–31. Oxford: Oxford University Press, 2003.

Eleazar ben Judah of Worms. *Ḥokhmat ha-Nefesh*. Jerusalem: Sodei Razayya, 2006.

———. *Sodei Razayya*. Tel-Aviv, 2004.

Ellenberger, Henri. *The Discovery of the Unconscious: The History and Evolution of Dynamic Psychiatry*. New York: Basic Books, 1970.

Elliott, Brian. *Phenomenology and Imagination in Husserl and Heidegger*. London: Routledge, 2005.

Elliott, Neil. "Ideological Closure in the Christ-Event: A Marxist Response to Alain Badiou's Paul." In *Paul, Philosophy, and the Theopolitical Vision*, edited by Douglas Harink, pp. 135–54. Eugene: Cascade Books, 2010.

Elior, Rachel. "Ḥ̣aBaD: The Contemplative Ascent to God." In *Jewish Spirituality From the Sixteenth-Century Revival to the Present*, edited by Arthur Green, pp. 157–205. New York: Crossroad, 1987.

———. *The Mystical Origins of Hasidism*. Oxford: Litman Library of Jewish Civilization, 2006.

———. *The Paradoxical Ascent: The Kabbalistic Theosophy of Habad Hasidism*. Translated by Jeffrey M. Green. Albany: State University of New York Press, 1993.

———. "Reality in the Test of Fiction: Dreams in Mystical Thought—The Freedom of Disassociation and Combination." In *The Spectrum of Opinions and Worldviews about Dreams in Jewish Culture*, edited by Dror Kerem, pp. 63–79. Reḥovot, 1992 (Hebrew).

———. *The Theory of Divinity of Hasidut Habad: Second Generation*. Jerusalem: Magnes Press, 1982 (Hebrew).

Embree, Lester. "The Phenomenology of Representational Awareness." *Human Studies* 15 (1992): 301–11.

Emerson, Ralph Waldo. *Essays and Lectures*. New York: Library of America, 1983.

Endreß, Gerhard. "Al-Kindī über die Wiedererinnerung der Seele: Arabischer Platonismus und die Legitimation der Wissenschaften im Islam." *Oriens* 34 (1994): 174–221.

Ephraim Solomon ben Aaron of Luntshits. *Olelot Efrayim*. Prague, 1619.

Epstein, Yiṣḥaq Aizak. *Ma'amar ha-Shiflut we-ha-Simḥah*. Jerusalem, 1996.

Eran, Amira. "Intuition and Inspiration—The Causes of Jewish Thinkers' Objection to Avicenna's Intellectual Prophecy (Ḥads)." *Jewish Studies Quarterly* 14 (2007): 39–71.

Eribon, Didier. *Michel Foucault*. Translated by Betsy King. Cambridge, MA: Harvard University Press, 1991.

Erlewine, Robert. *Monotheism and Tolerance: Recovering a Religion of Reason*. Bloomington: Indiana University Press, 2010.

———. "Reclaiming the Prophets: Cohen, Heschel, and Crossing the

Theocentric/Neo-Humanist Divide." *Journal of Jewish Thought and Philosophy* 17 (2009): 177–206.

Esudri, Yossi. "Studies on the Philosophy of R. Isaac Ibn Latif: Profile, Knowledge and Prophecy," Ph.D. dissertation, Hebrew University, 2008 (Hebrew).

Etkes, Immanuel. *The Besht: Magician, Mystic, and Leader.* Translated by Saadya Sternberg. Waltham: Brandeis University Press, 2005.

Fagenblat, Michael. *A Covenant of Creatures: Levinas's Philosophy of Judaism.* Stanford: Stanford University Press, 2010.

Fakhry, Majid. *A History of Islamic Philosophy.* 2nd edition. New York: Columbia University Press, 1983.

Farber, Marvin. "Experience and Transcendence." *Philosophy and Phenomenological Research* 12 (1951): 1–23.

Farbman, Herschel. "Blanchot on Dreams and Writing." *SubStance* 34 (2005): 118–40.

Fédida, Pierre. *Le site de l'étranger: La situation psychanalytique.* Paris: Presses Universitaires de France, 1995.

Feldman, Louis H. *Josephus's Interpretation of the Bible.* Berkeley: University of California Press, 1998.

———. "Prophets and Prophecy in Josephus." *Journal of Theological Studies* 41 (1990): 386–422.

Felman, Shoshana. *Jacques Lacan and the Adventure of Insight: Psychoanalysis in Contemporary Culture.* Cambridge, MA: Harvard University Press, 1987.

Felstiner, John. "'*Ziv*, That Light': Translation and Tradition in Paul Celan." In *The Craft of Translation*, edited by John Biguenet and Rainer Schulte, pp. 93–116. Chicago: University of Chicago Press, 1989.

Fenton, Paul B. "The Arabic and Hebrew Versions of the Theology of Aristotle." In *Pseudo-Aristotle in the Middle Ages: The* Theology *and Other Texts*, edited by Jill Kraye, W.F. Ryan, and C.B. Schmitt, pp. 241–64. London: Warburg Institute, 1986.

———. "Henry Corbin et la mystique juive." In *Henry Corbin: Philosophies et sagesses des religions du livre*, edited by Mohammad Ali Amir-Moezzi, Christian Jambet, and Pierre Lory, pp. 151–64. Turnhout: Brepols, 2005.

———. *Philosophie et exégèse dans Le Jardin de la méthaphore de Moïse Ibn 'Ezra, philosophie et poète anadalou du XIIe siècle.* Leiden: E.J. Brill, 1997.

———. "Shem Tov Ibn Falaquera and the Theology of Aristotle." *Da'at* 29 (1992): 27–39 (Hebrew).

Ferguson, Harvie. *The Lure of Dreams: Sigmund Freud and the Construction of Modernity.* London: Routledge, 1996.

Feron, Etienne. *De l'idée de transcendance à la question du langage: L'itinéraire philosophique de Levinas*. Grenoble: J. Millon, 1982.

Fidler, Ruth. *"Dreams Speak Falsely?" Dream Theophanies in the Bible: Their Place in Ancient Israelite Faith and Tradition*. Jerusalem: Magnes Press, 2005 (Hebrew).

Fine, Lawrence. *Physician of the Soul, Healer of the Cosmos: Isaac Luria and His Kabbalistic Fellowship*. Stanford: Stanford University Press, 2003.

Fink, Eugen. "The Phenomenological Philosophy of Edmund Husserl and Contemporary Criticism." In *The Phenomenology of Husserl: Selected Readings*. 2nd edition, edited with an introduction by R. O. Elveton, pp. 70–139. Seattle: Noesis Press, 2000.

———. *Sixth Cartesian Meditation: The Idea of a Transcendental Theory of Method*. With textual notations by Edmund Husserl. Translated with an introduction by Ronald Bruzina. Bloomington: Indiana University Press, 1995.

Fishbane, Eitan P. *As Light Before Dawn: The Inner World of a Medieval Kabbalist*. Stanford: Stanford University Press, 2009.

———. "Mystical Contemplation and the Limits of the Mind: The Case of *Sheqel ha-Qodesh*." *Jewish Quarterly Review* 93 (2002): 1–27.

Fishbane, Michael. *The Exegetical Imagination: On Jewish Thought and Theology*. Cambridge, MA: Harvard University Press, 1998.

———. *Sacred Attunement: A Jewish Theology*. Chicago: University of Chicago Press, 2008.

Fishbane, Simcha. *Deviancy in Early Rabbinic Literature: A Collection of Socio-Anthropological Essays*. Introduction by Nissan Rubin. Leiden: Brill, 2007.

Flannery-Dailey, Frances. *Dreamers, Scribes, and Priests: Jewish Dreams in the Hellenistic and Roman Eras*. Leiden: Brill, 2004.

Fluegel, Maurice. *Philosophy, Qabbala, and Vedānta*. Baltimore: The Sun Printing Office, 1902.

Foshay, Toby. "Introduction: Denegation and Resentment." In *Derrida and Negative Theology*, edited by Howard Coward and Toby Foshay, pp. 1–24. Albany: State University of New York Press, 1992.

Fóti, Véronique M. "Chiasm, Flesh, Figuration: Towards a Non-Objective Ontology." In *Merleau-Ponty and the Possibilities of Philosophy: Transforming the Tradition*, edited by Bernard Flynn, Wayne J. Froman, and Robert Vallier, pp. 183–96. Albany: State University of New York Press, 2009.

Foucault, Michel. *Dits et Écrits 1954–1988*. Edited by Daniel Defert and François Ewald, with the collaboration of Jacques Lagrange. Vol. 1, *1954–1969*. Paris: Gallimard, 1994.

———. "Dream, Imagination and Existence." Translated by Forest Williams.

In Michel Foucault and Ludwig Binswanger, *Dream and Existence*, edited by Keith Hoeller, pp. 29–78. Atlantic Highlands: Humanities Press, 1993.

———. *L'herméneutique du sujet: Cours au Collège de France (1981–1982)*. Edited by Frédéric Gros under the direction of François Ewald and Alessandro Fontana. Gallimard: Le Seuil, 2001.

———. *History of Madness*. Edited by Jean Khalfa. Translated by Jonathan Murphy and Jean Khalfa. London: Routledge, 2006.

———. *The History of Sexuality, Volume 3: The Care of the Self*. Translated by Robert Hurley. New York: Vintage Books, 1988.

———. "Nietzsche, Freud, Marx." In *The Essential Works of Foucault, 1954–1984*. Vol. 2, *Aesthetics, Method, and Epistemology*, edited by James D. Faubion, pp. 269–78. New York: New Press, 1998.

———. *Religion and Culture*. Selected and edited by Jeremy R. Carrette. New York: Routledge, 1999.

———. "Theatrum Philosophicum." In *The Essential Works of Foucault, 1954–1984*. Vol. 2, *Aesthetics, Method, and Epistemology*, edited by James D. Faubion, pp. 343–68. New York: New Press, 1998.

Foulkes, David. *Dreaming: A Cognitive-Psychological Analysis*. Hillsdale: Lawrence Erlbaum Associates, 1985.

Fowl, Stephen. "A Very Particular Universalism: Badiou and Paul." In *Paul, Philosophy, and the Theopolitical Vision*, edited by Douglas Harink, pp. 119–34. Eugene: Cascade Books, 2010.

Fowler, Jeaneane. *Perspectives of Reality: An Introduction to the Philosophy of Hinduism*. Brighton: Sussex Academic Press, 2002.

Franke, William. "Apophasis and the Turn of Philosophy to Religion: From Negative Theology to Postmodern Negation of Theology." *International Journal for Philosophy of Religion* 60 (2006): 61–76.

Frankland, Graham. *Freud's Literary Culture*. Cambridge: Cambridge University Press, 2000.

Frieden, Ken. *Freud's Dream of Interpretation*. Foreword by Harold Bloom. Albany: State University of New York Press, 1990.

———. "Talmudic Dream Interpretation, Freudian Ambivalence, Deconstruction." In *The Dream and the Text: Essays on Literature and Language*, edited by Carol Schreier Rupprecht, pp. 103–11. Albany: State University of New York Press, 1993.

Freud, Sigmund. *An Outline of Psychoanalysis*. Translation by James Strachey. New York: W. W. Norton, 1949.

———. *Collected Papers*. Authorized translation under the supervision of Joan Riviere. Vol. 4. London: Hogarth Press, 1953.

——. *The Complete Letters of Sigmund Freud to Wilhelm Fliess 1887–1904*. Translated and edited by Jeffrey Moussaieff Masson. Cambridge, MA: Harvard University Press, 1985.

——. *The Interpretation of Dreams*. Translated and edited by James Strachey. New York: Basic Books, 1959.

——. *The Interpretation of Dreams*. Translated by Joyce Crick, with an introduction and notes by Ritchie Robertson. Oxford: Oxford University Press, 1999.

——. *Leonardo da Vinci and a Memory of His Childhood*. Translated by Alan Tyson. Edited by James Strachey. New York: W. W. Norton, 1964.

——. *The Standard Edition of the Complete Psychological Works of Sigmund Freud*. Translated and edited by James Strachey, in collaboration with Anna Freud. 24 vols. London: The Hogarth Press, 1958.

——. *Totem and Taboo: Some Points of Agreement between the Mental Lives of Savages and Neurotics*. Translated and edited by James Strachey. New York: W. W. Norton, 1950.

Frith, Chris, Richard Perry, and Erik Lumer. "The Neural Correlates of Conscious Experience: An Experimental Framework." *Trends in Cognitive Sciences* 3 (1999): 105–14.

Frohmann, Heinrich Christian Immanuel. *Evangelium Lucae*. Pars Posterior. Edited by Johann Heinrich Callenberg. Halle: Institutum Judaicum, 1737.

Fromm, Eric. *The Forgotten Language: An Introduction to the Understanding of Dreams, Fairy Tales and Myths*. New York and Toronto: Rinehart, 1951.

Funkenstein, Amos. *Theology and the Scientific Imagination From the Middle Ages to the Seventeenth Century*. Princeton: Princeton University Press, 1986.

Gall, Robert S. "Of/From Theology and Deconstruction." *Journal of the American Academy of Religion* 58 (1990): 413–37.

Gallop, David. "Dreaming and Waking in Plato." In *Essays in Ancient Greek Philosophy*, edited by John P. Anton and George L. Kustas, pp. 187–201. Albany: State University of New York Press, 1971.

Galya Razya. Edited by Rachel Elior. Jerusalem: Hebrew University, 1981.

Galya Razya. Moholov, 1812.

Gamlieli, Dvorah Bat-David. *Psychoanalysis and Kabbalah: The Masculine and Feminine in Lurianic Kabbalah*. Los Angeles: Cherub Press, 2006 (Hebrew).

Ganeri, Jonardon. *The Concealed Art of the Soul: Theories of Self and Practices of Truth in Indian Ethics and Epistemology*. Oxford: Oxford University Press, 2007.

Garb, Jonathan. "Gender and Power in Kabbalah: A Theoretical Investigation." *Kabbalah: Journal for the Study of Jewish Mystical Texts* 13 (2005): 79–107.

——. "Mystics' Critiques of Mystical Experience." *Revue de l'histoire des religions* 221 (2004): 293–325.

Gärdenfors, Peter. "The Detachment of Thought." In *The Mind as a Scientific Object: Between Brain and Culture*, edited by Christina E. Erneling and David Martel Johnson, pp. 323–41. Oxford: Oxford University Press, 2005.

Gasché, Rodolphe. "The Felicities of Paradox: Blanchot on the Null-Space of Literature." In *Maurice Blanchot: The Demand of Writing*, edited by Carolyn Bailey Gill, pp. 34–69. London: Routledge, 1996.

Gätje, Helmut. "Philosophische Traumlehren im Islam." *Zeitschrift der Deutschen Morgenländischen Gesellschaft* 109 (1959): 258–85.

Gay, Peter. *A Godless Jew: Freud, Atheism, and the Masking of Psychoanalysis*. New Haven: Yale University Press, 1987.

Genz, Henning. *Nothingness: The Science of Empty Space*. Cambridge. MA: Perseus Publishing, 1999.

Gershon ben Solomon, *Sha'ar ha-Shamayim*. Rödelheim, 1801.

Gianotti, Timothy J. *Al-Ghazālī's Unspeakable Doctrine of the Soul: Unveiling the Esoteric Psychology and Eschatology of the Iḥyā'*. Leiden: Brill, 2001.

Gibbs, Robert. "The Disincarnation of the Word: The Trace of God in Reading Scripture." In The *Exorbitant: Emmanuel Levinas between Jews and Christians*, edited by Kevin Hart and Michael A. Signer, pp. 32–51. New York: Fordham University Press, 2010.

Gibson. W. R. Boyce. "The Problem of Real and Ideal in the Phenomenology of Husserl." *Mind* 34 (1925): 311–33.

Gieser, Suzanne. *The Innermost Kernel: Depth Psychology and Quantum Physics: Wolfgang Pauli's Dialogue with C. G. Jung*. Berlin: Springer, 2005.

Gikatilla, Joseph. *Ginnat Egoz*. Jerusalem: Yeshivat ha-Ḥayyim we-ha-Shalom, 1989.

——. "Ha-Qeṭa ha-aḥaron shel ha-sefer 'Sha'arei Ṣedeq' le-Rav Yosef Giqaṭilah." In Efraim Gottlieb, *Studies in the Kabbala Literature*, edited by Joseph Hacker, pp. 132–62. Tel-Aviv: Tel-Aviv University Press, 1976 (Hebrew).

——. *Sefer ha-Niqqud*. Jerusalem: Yerid ha-Sefarim, 1994.

——. *Sha'arei Orah*. Edited with introduction and notes by Joseph Ben Shlomo. 2 vols. Jerusalem: Bialik Institute, 1981.

——. *Sha'arei Ṣedeq*. Cracow: Fischer & Deutscher, 1881.

——. *Sod Yod-Gimmel Middot ha-Nov'ot min ha-Keter Elyon we-Niqra'im Ma'yenei ha-Yeshu'ah*. In Gershom Scholem, *Catalogus Codicum Hebraicorum, Pars Prima: Cabbala*, pp. 219–25. Jerusalem: E Prelis Universitatis Hebraicae, 1930.

Giller, Pinchas. *Reading the Zohar: The Sacred Text of the Kabbalah*. Oxford:

Oxford University Press, 2001.

——. *Shalom Shar'abi and the Kabbalists of Beit El.* Oxford: Oxford University Press, 2008.

Gillespie, George. "Dreams and Dreamless Sleep." *Dreaming* 12 (2002): 199–207.

Ginsberg, Allen. *Collected Poems 1947–1977.* New York: HarperCollins, 2006.

Ginsburg, Elliot K. *The Sabbath in the Classical Kabbalah.* Albany: State University of New York Press, 1989.

Ginzberg, Louis. The *Legends of the Jews.* 7 vols. Philadelphia: Jewish Publication Society of America, 1968.

Glasner, Ruth. "The Hebrew Version of De celo et mundo attributed to Ibn Sīnā." *Arabic Sciences and Philosophy* 6 (1996): 89–112.

Gliserman, Martin. *Psychoanalysis, Language, and the Body of the Text.* Gainesville: University Press of Florida, 1996.

Goetschel, Roland. "The Conception of Prophecy in the Works of R. Moses de Leon and R. Joseph Gikatilla." *Jerusalem Studies in Jewish Thought* 8 (1989): 217–37 (Hebrew).

——. "'Ehyeh Asher Ehyeh' in the Works of the Gerona Kabbalists." *Jerusalem Studies in Jewish Thought* 6, nos. 3–4 (1987): 287–98 (Hebrew).

Gohlman, William E. *The Life of Ibn Sina: A Critical Edition and Annotated Translation.* Albany: State of New York University Press, 1974.

Goldish, Matt. *The Sabbatian Prophets.* Cambridge, MA: Harvard University Press, 2004.

Goldziher, Ignaz. "The Appearance of the Prophet in Dreams." *Journal of the Royal Asiatic Society* (1912): 503–506.

Gollnick, James. *Dreams in the Psychology of Religion.* Lewiston: Edwin Mellen Press, 1987.

Gonda, Jan. *Change and Continuity in Indian Religion.* The Hague: Mouton, 1965.

Gordin, Rachel. *Angels Don't Dream: The Teaching of Ibn 'Arabi—the Greatest Sufi Sheikh.* Jerusalem: Carmel, 2007 (Hebrew).

Goshen-Gottstein, Alon. "'The Sage is Superior to the Prophet': The Conception of Torah through the Prism of the History of Jewish Exegesis." In *Study and Knowledge in Jewish Thought*, vol. 2, edited by Howard Kreisel, pp. 37–77. Beer Sheva: Ben-Gurion University of the Negev Press, 2006 (Hebrew).

Gottesmann, Claude. "A Neurobiological History of Dreaming." In *The New Science of Dreaming*, edited by Deirdre Barrett and Patrick McNamara. Vol. 1, *Biological Aspects*, pp. 1–51. Westport: Praeger, 2007.

Gottlieb, Efraim. *The Kabbalah in the Writings of R. Baḥya ben Asher Ibn Ḥalawa*. Jerusalem: Kiryat Sefer, 1970.

———. *Studies in the Kabbala Literature*. Edited by Joseph Hacker. Tel-Aviv: Tel-Aviv University Press, 1976 (Hebrew).

Gourgouris, Stathis. "The Dream-Reality of the Ruin." In *Walter Benjamin and the Arcades Project*, edited by Beatrice Hanssen, pp. 201–24. London: Continuum, 2006.

Gray, Rebecca. *Prophetic Figures in Late Second Temple Jewish Palestine: The Evidence of Josephus*. New York: Oxford University Press, 1993.

The Greek Magical Papyri in Translation. Edited by Hans Dieter Betz. Chicago: University of Chicago Press, 1986.

Green, Arthur. *Devotion and Commandment: The Faith of Abraham in the Hasidic Imagination*. Cincinnati: Hebrew Union College Press, 1989.

———. "Rabbi Isaac Sahula's Commentary on the Song of Songs." *Jerusalem Studies in Jewish Thought* 6, nos. 3–4 (1987): 393–491 (Hebrew).

———. *Radical Judaism: Rethinking God and Tradition*. New Haven: Yale University Press, 2010.

———. *Tormented Master: A Life of Rabbi Nahman of Bratslav*. University: University of Alabama Press, 1979.

Green, Celia E. *Lucid Dreams*. Foreword by H.H. Price. London: Hamish Hamilton, 1968.

Green, Celia E., and Charles McCreery. *Lucid Dreaming: The Paradox of Consciousness During Sleep*. London: Routledge, 1994.

Green, Nile. "The Religious and Cultural Roles of Dreams and Visions in Islam." *Journal of the Royal Asiatic Society* 13 (2003): 287–313.

Griffel, Frank. *Al-Ghazālī's Philosophical Theology*. Oxford: Oxford University Press, 2009.

Griffiths, Paul J. *On Being Mindless: Buddhist Meditation and the Mind-Body Problem*. La Salle: Open Court, 1986.

Grigg, Russell. *Lacan, Language, and Philosophy*. Albany: State University Press of New York, 2008.

Grondin, Jean. "The Task of Hermeneutics in Ancient Philosophy." In *Proceedings of Boston Area Colloquium in Ancient Philosophy, Volume VIII 1992*, edited by John J. Cleary, pp. 211–30. Lanham: University Press of America, 1994.

Grosnick, William H. "The Zen Master Dogen's Understanding of the Buddha-Nature in Light of the Historical Development of the Buddha-Nature Concept in India, China, and Japan." Ph.D. dissertation, University of Wisconsin–Madison, 1979.

Grosz, Elizabeth. *Volatile Bodies: Toward a Corporeal Feminism*. Bloomington: Indiana University Press, 1994.

Gschwandtner, Christina M. *Reading Jean-Luc Marion: Exceeding Metaphysics*. Bloomington: Indiana University Press, 2007.

Guccione, Steven. "Can a Non-Computable Physical Law Be Considered Able to Predict?" In *The Foundations of Quantum Mechanics: Historical Analysis and Open Questions*, edited by Claudio Garola and Arcangelo Rossi, pp. 261–66. Singapore: World Scientific Publishing, 2000.

Guenther, Herbert W. *Wholeness Lost and Wholeness Regained: Forgotten Tales of Individuation from Ancient Tibet*. Albany: State University of New York Press, 1994.

Gutas, Dimitri. *Avicenna and the Aristotelian Tradition*. Leiden: E. J. Brill, 1988.

——. "Imagination and Transcendental Knowledge in Avicenna." In *Arabic Theology, Arabic Philosophy, from the Many to the One: Essays in Celebration of Richard M. Frank*, edited by James E. Montgomery, pp. 337–54. Leuven: Peeters, 2006.

——. "Intellect without Limits: The Absence of Mysticism in Avicenna." In *Intellect et imagination dans la Philosophie Médiévale: Actes du XIe Congrès International de Philosophie Médiévale de la Société Internationale pour l'Étude de la Philosophie Médiévale*, edited by Maria Cândida Pacheco and José Francisco Meirinhos, 1: 351–72. Turnhout: Brepols, 2006.

Gutheil, Emil A. *The Language of the Dream*. New York: Macmillan, 1939.

Habermas, Jürgen. "Transcendence from Within, Transcendence in this World." In *Religion and Rationality: Essays on Reason, God and Modernity*, edited by Eduardo Mendieta, pp. 67–94. Cambridge, MA: The MIT Press, 2002.

Hägglund, Martin. *Radical Atheism: Derrida and the Time of Life*. Stanford: Stanford University Press, 2008.

Halber, Deborah. "Memory Experts Show Sleeping Rats May Have Visual Dreams." Available at http://web.mit.edu/newsoffice/ 2006/visual-cortex.html.

Halbertal, Moshe. *Concealment and Revelation: Esotericism in Jewish Thought and Its Philosophical Implications*. Translated by Jackie Feldman. Princeton: Princeton University Press, 2007.

Halbertal, Moshe, and Avishai Margalit. *Idolatry*. Translated by Naomi Goldblum. Cambridge, MA: Harvard University Press, 1992.

Halbfass, Wilhelm. *India and Europe: An Essay in Understanding*. Albany: State University of New York Press, 1988.

Halevi, Judah. *Sefer ha-Kuzari*. Translated by Yehudah Even Shmuel. Tel-Aviv: Dvir, 1972.

Hallamish, Moshe. "The Theoretical System of R. Shneur Zalman of Liady (Its

Sources in Kabbalah and Hasidism)." Ph.D. dissertation, Hebrew University, 1976 (Hebrew).

Handelman, Susan A. *Fragments of Redemption: Jewish Thought and Literary Theory in Benjamin, Scholem, and Levinas*. Bloomington: Indiana University Press, 1991.

Hanly, Charles. "On Being and Dreaming." In *Psychoanalysis and Philosophy*, edited by Charles Hanly and Morris Lazerowitz, pp. 155–87. New York: International Universities Press, 1970.

Harari, Yuval. *Early Jewish Magic: Research, Method, Sources*. Jerusalem: Bialik Institute, 2010 (Hebrew).

———. "Power and Money: Economic Aspects of the Use of Magic by Jews in Ancient Times and the Early Middle Ages." *Pe'amim: Studies in Oriental Jewry* 85 (2000): 14–42 (Hebrew).

———. "The Sages and the Occult." In *The Literature of the Sages, Second Part: Midrash and Targum, Liturgy, Poetry, Mysticism, Contracts, Inscriptions, Ancient Sciences, and the Languages of Rabbinic Literature*, edited by Shmuel Safrai, Zeev Safrai, Joshua Schwartz, and Peter J. Tomson, pp. 521–64. Assen: Van Gorcum, 2006.

Harris, Monford. "Dreams in Sefer Hasidim." *Proceedings of the American Academy of Jewish Research* 31 (1963): 51–80.

———. *Studies in Jewish Dream Interpretation*. Northvale: Jason Aronson, 1994.

Harris, William V. *Dreams and Experience in Classical Antiquity*. Cambridge, MA: Harvard University Press, 2009.

Har Shefi, Avishar. "Malchin Kadmain: The Myth of the Edomite Kings in the Idrot Literature—The First Appearance." M.A. thesis, Bar-Ilan University, 2006 (Hebrew).

Hart, Kevin. *The Dark Gaze: Maurice Blanchot and the Sacred*. Chicago: University of Chicago Press, 2004.

Hartmann, Ernest. *Dreams and Nightmares: The Origin and Meaning of Dreams*. New York: Perseus Publishing, 2001.

Ḥaver, Yiṣḥaq Isaac. *Beit Olamim*. Warsaw, 1889.

Harvey, Steven. "Shem-Tov Ibn Falaquera's *De'ot ha-Filosofim*: Its Sources and Use of Sources." In *The Medieval Hebrew Encyclopedias of Science and Philosophy: Proceedings of the Bar-Ilan University Conference*, edited by Steven Harvey, pp. 211–47. Dordrecht: Kluwer, 2000.

Harvey, Warren Zev. "Three Theories of the Imagination in 12th-Century Jewish Philosophy." In *Intellect et imagination dans la Philosophie Médiévale: Actes du XIe Congrès International de Philosophie Médiévale de la Société Internationale pour l'Étude de la Philosophie Médiévale*, edited by Maria Cândida

Pacheco and José Francisco Meirinhos, 1:287–302. Turnhout: Brepols, 2006.

Hasan-Rokem, Galit. "'A Dream Amounts to the Sixtieth Part of Prophecy': On Interaction between Textual Establishment and Popular Context in Dream Interpretation by the Jewish Sages." In *Studies in the History of Popular Culture*, edited by Benjamin Z. Kedar, pp. 45–54. Jerusalem: Zalman Shazar Center for Jewish History, 1996 (Hebrew).

———. "Communication with the Dead in Jewish Dream Culture." In *Dream Cultures: Explorations in the Comparative History of Dreaming*, edited by David Shulman and Guy G. Stroumsa, pp. 213–32. New York: Oxford University Press, 1999.

———. *Web of Life: Folklore and Midrash in Rabbinic Literature*. Translated by Batya Stein. Stanford: Stanford University Press, 2000.

Hauser, Marc D. "Minding the Behaviour of Deception." In *Machiavellian Intelligence II: Extensions and Evaluations*, edited by Andrew Whiten and Richard W. Byrne, pp. 112–43. Cambridge: Cambridge University Press, 1997.

Hayes, Richard P. "Principled Atheism in the Buddhist Scholastic Tradition." In *Indian Philosophy: A Collection of Readings*, edited with introductions by Roy W. Perrett, pp. 107–30. New York: Garland Publishing, 2000.

Ḥayyim ben Bezalel, *Sefer ha-Ḥayyim*. Jerusalem, 1993.

Heath, Peter. *Allegory and Philosophy in Avicenna (Ibn Sînâ) with a Translation of the Book of the Prophet Muḥammad's Ascent to Heaven*. Philadelphia: University of Pennsylvania Press, 1992.

The Hebrew Writings of the Author of Tiqqunei Zohar and Ra'aya Mehemna. Edited and annotated by Efraim Gottlieb. Jerusalem: Israel Academy of Sciences, 2003 (Hebrew).

Heck, Paul L. "Mysticism as Morality: The Case of Sufism." *Journal of Religious Ethics* 34 (2006): 253–86.

Hegel, Georg Wilhelm Friedrich. *Lectures on the Philosophy of Spirit 1827–8*. Translated with an introduction by Robert R. Williams. Oxford: Oxford University Press, 2007.

———. *Phenomenology of Spirit*. Translated by Arnold V. Miller with analysis and foreword by John N. Findlay. Oxford: Oxford University Press, 1977.

———. *Philosophy of Mind*. Translated by William Wallace and Arnold V. Miller. Revised with introduction and commentary by Michael Inwood. Oxford: Oxford University Press, 2007.

Heiden, Gerrit Jan van der. *The Truth (and Untruth) of Language: Heidegger, Ricoeur, and Derrida on Disclosure and Displacement*. Pittsburgh: Duquesne University Press, 2010.

Heilman, Samuel, and Menachem Friedman. *The Rebbe: The Life and Afterlife of Menachem Mendel Schneerson*. Princeton: Princeton University Press, 2010.

Heine, Steven. *A Dream within a Dream: Studies in Japanese Thought*. New York: Peter Lang, 1991.

——. *Existential and Ontological Dimensions of Time in Heidegger and Dōgen*. Albany: State University of New York Press, 1985.

Heller-Roazen, Daniel. *The Inner Touch: Archaeology of Sensation*. New York: Zone Books, 2007.

Hellner-Eshed, Melila. *A River Flows from Eden: The Language of Mystical Experience in the Zohar*. Translated by Nathan Wolski. Stanford: Stanford University Press, 2009.

Henry, Michel. *The Essence of Manifestation*. Translated by Girard Etzkorn. The Hague: Martinus Nijhoff, 1973.

——. *Incarnation: Une philosophie de la chair*. Paris: Éditions du Seuil, 2000.

——. *Philosophy and Phenomenology of the Body*. Translated by Girard Etzkorn. The Hague: Martinus Nijhoff, 1975.

Hermansen, Marcia K. "Dreams and Dreaming in Islam." In *Dreams: A Reader on Religious, Cultural and Psychological Dimensions of Dreaming*, edited by Kelly Bulkeley, pp. 73–91. New York: Palgrave, 2001.

——. "Visions as 'Good to Think': A Cognitive Approach to Visionary Experience in Islamic Sufi Thought." *Religion* 27 (1997): 25–43.

Hersch, Edwin L. "Imagination and Its Pathologies: Domain of the Unreal or a Fundamental Dimension of Human Reality?" In *Imagination and Its Pathologies*, edited by James Phillips and James Morley, pp. 37–50. Cambridge, MA: The MIT Press, 2003.

Heschel, Abraham J. *The Circle of the Baal Shem Tov: Studies in Hasidism*. Edited by Samuel H. Dresner. Chicago: University of Chicago Press, 1985.

——. *Heavenly Torah as Refracted through the Generations*. Edited and translated by Gordon Tucker and Leonard Levin. New York: Continuum, 2005.

——. *Prophetic Inspiration After the Prophets: Maimonides and Other Medieval Authorities*. Edited by Morris M. Faierstein. Preface by Moshe Idel. Hoboken: Ktav, 1996.

Heynick, Frank. *Language and Its Disturbances in Dreams: The Pioneering Work of Freud and Kraepelin Updated*. New York: J. Wiley & Sons, 1993.

Hieatt, Constance B. *The Realism of Dream Visions: The Poetic Exploitation of the Dream-Experience in Chaucer and his Contemporaries*. The Hague: Mouton, 1967.

Hillman, James. *The Dream and the Underworld*. New York: Harper & Row, 1979.

———. "Healing Fiction." In *Jungian Literary Criticism*, edited by Richard B. Sugg. pp. 129–38. Evanston: Northwestern University Press, 1993.

———. *Re-Visioning Psychology*. New York: HarperCollins, 1992.

Hobbes, Thomas. *Leviathan*. Edited with an introduction and notes by John Charles Addison Gaskin. Oxford: Oxford University Press, 1996.

Hobson, J. Allan. *The Dream Drugstore: Chemically Altered States of Consciousness*. Cambridge, MA: The MIT Press, 2001.

———. *The Dreaming Brain: How the Brain Creates both the Sense and the Nonsense of Dreams*. New York: Basic Books, 1988.

———. *Dreaming as Delirium: How the Brain Goes Out of Its Mind*. Cambridge, MA: The MIT Press, 1999.

———. *Dreaming: An Introduction to the Science of Sleep*. Oxford: Oxford University Press, 2002.

Hobson, J. Allan, Edward F. Pace-Schott, and Robert Stickgold. "Dreaming and the Brain: Toward a Cognitive Neuroscience of Conscious States." In *Sleep and Dreaming: Scientific Advances and Reconsiderations*, edited by Edward F. Pace-Schitt, Mark Solms, Mark Blagorve, and Stevan Harnad, pp. 1–50. Cambridge: Cambridge University Press, 2003.

Hobson, Marian. *Jacques Derrida: Opening Lines*. London: Routledge, 1998.

Hölderlin, Friedrich. *Essays and Letters on Theory*. Translated and edited by Thomas Pfau. Albany: State University of New York Press, 1988.

Holdrege, Barbara A. *Veda and Torah: Transcending the Textuality of Scripture*. Albany: State University of New York Press, 1996.

Hollander, Dana. "Is the Other My Neighbor?: Reading Levinas Alongside Hermann Cohen." In *The Exorbitant: Emmanuel Levinas between Jews and Christians*, edited by Kevin Hart and Michael A. Signer, pp. 90–107. New York: Fordham University Press, 2010.

Holowchak, M. Andrew. *Ancient Science and Dreams: Oneirology in Greco-Roman Antiquity*. Lanham: University Press of America, 2002.

Holsclaw, Geoffrey. "Subjects between Death and Resurrection: Badiou, Žižek, and St. Paul." In *Paul, Philosophy, and the Theopolitical Vision*, edited by Douglas Harink, pp. 155–76. Eugene: Cascade Books, 2010

Hood Jr., Ralph W. "Mysticism, Reality, Illusion, and the Freudian Critique of Religion." *International Journal for the Psychology of Religion* 2 (1992): 141–59.

Hopkins, Jeffrey. *Tantric Techniques*. Edited by Kevin Vose. Ithaca: Snow Lion Publications, 2008.

Hopper, Stanley R. "Introduction." In *Interpretation: The Poetry of Meanings*, edited by Stanley R. Hopper and David L. Miller, pp. ix–xxii. New York:

Harcourt, Brace and World, 1967.

Horner, Robyn. "The Betrayal of Transcendence." In *Transcendence: Philosophy, Literature, and Theology Approach the Beyond*, edited by Regina Schwartz, pp. 61–79. New York: Routledge, 2004.

——. *Rethinking God as Gift: Marion, Derrida, and the Limits of Phenomenology.* New York: Fordham University Press, 2001.

Horowitz, Aaron Halevi of Staroselye. *Sha'arei Avodah.* Shklov, 1821.

——. *Sha'arei ha-Yiḥud we-ha-Emunah.* Shklov, 1820.

Howells, Christian. *Derrida: Deconstruction from Phenomenology to Ethics.* Cambridge: Polity Press, 1999.

Hoy, Ronald. "The Given and the Self-Presenting." *Noûs* 19 (1985): 347–64.

Hughes, Aaron W. *The Art of Dialogue in Jewish Philosophy.* Bloomington: Indiana University Press, 2008.

——. "Imagining the Divine: Ghazali on Imagination, Dreams, and Dreaming." *Journal of the American Academy of Religion* 70 (2002): 33–53.

——. *The Texture of the Divine: Imagination in Medieval Islamic and Jewish Thought.* Bloomington: Indiana University Press, 2004.

Hundert, Gershon D. *Jews in Poland-Lithuania in the Eighteenth Century: A Genealogy of Modernity*, Berkeley: University of California Press, 2004.

Hurst, Andrea. *Derrida vis-à-vis Lacan: Interweaving Deconstruction and Psychoanalysis.* New York: Fordham University Press, 2008.

Husser, Jean-Marie. *Dreams and Dream Narratives in the Biblical World.* Sheffield: Sheffield Academic Press, 1999.

Husserl, Edmund. *The Basic Problems of Phenomenology From the Lectures, Winter Semester, 1910–1911.* Translated by Ingo Farin and James G. Hart. Dordrecht: Springer, 2006.

——. *Cartesian Meditations: An Introduction to Phenomenology.* Translated by Dorion Cairns. The Hague: Martinus Nijhoff, 1977.

——. *The Crisis of European Sciences and Transcendental Phenomenology.* Translated with an introduction by David Carr. Evanston: Northwestern University Press, 1970.

——. *Ideas Pertaining to a Pure Phenomenology and to a Phenomenological Philosophy. First Book: General Introduction to Pure Phenomenology.* Translated by F. Kersten. Dordrecht: Kluwer, 1983.

——. *Die Krisis der Europäischen Wissenschaften und die Tranzendentale Phänomenologie.* 2nd edition. Edited by Walter Biemel, Husserliana VI. The Hague: Martinus Nijhoff, 1962.

——. *Psychological and Transcendental Phenomenology and the Confrontation with Heidegger (1927–1931).* Translated and edited by Thomas Sheehan and

Richard E. Palmer. Dordrect: Kluwer, 1997.

Huttler, Miriam. "Jewish Origins of Freud's Interpretation of Dreams." *Journal of Psychology and Judaism* 23 (1999): 5–48.

Ibn al-'Arabī, Muḥyīddīn. *The Bezels of Wisdom*. Translation and introduction by Ralph W. J. Austin. Preface by Titus Burckhardt. New York: Paulist Press, 1980.

———. *The Wisdom of the Prophets* (*Fusus al-Hikam*). Translated from Arabic to French with notes by Titus Burckhardt. Translated from French to English by Angela Culme-Seymour. Aldsworth: Beshara, 1975.

Ibn Ezra, Abraham. *Perushei ha-Torah le-Rabbenu Avraham Ibn Ezra*. Edited by Asher Weiser. 3 vols. Jerusaelm: Mosad ha-Rav Kook, 1977.

———. *The Sabbath Epistle of Rabbi Abraham Ibn Ezra* (*'iggeret haShabbat*). Translated and annotated by Mordechai S. Goodman. Jersey City: Ktav, 2009.

Ibn Falaquera, Shem Ṭov ben Joseph. *Moreh ha-Moreh*. Critical Edition, introduction, and commentary by Yair Shiffman. Jerusalem: World Union of Jewish Studies, 2001.

Ibn Gabbai, Meir. *Avodat ha-Qodesh*. Jerusalem: Shevilei Orḥot ha-Ḥayyim, 1992.

Ibn Gaon, Shem Ṭov ben Abraham. *Baddei ha-Aron u-Migdal Ḥananel*. Edited by Samuel Loewinger. Jerusalem: Orient and Occident, 1977.

Ibn Ḥasdai, Abraham. *Ben ha-Melekh we-ha-Nazir*. Jerusalem, 2002.

Ibn Khaldûn. *The Muqaddimah: An Introduction to History*. Translated by Franz Rosenthal. 3 vols. 2nd edition. Princeton: Princeton University Press, 1967.

Ibn Laṭif, Isaac. *Rav Pe'alim*. Edited by Samuel Schoenblum. Lemberg: Anna Wajdowicz, 1885.

———. *Sha'ar ha-Shamayim*. MS Vatican, Biblioteca Apostolica 335.

Ibn Paquda, Baḥya. *Sefer Torat Ḥovot ha-Levavot*. Edited and translated by Joseph Kafiḥ. Jerusalem, 1973.

Idel, Moshe. *Absorbing Perfections: Kabbalah and Interpretation*. New Haven: Yale University Press, 2002.

———. *Ascensions on High in Jewish Mysticism: Pillars, Lines, Ladders*. Budapest: Central European University Press, 2005.

———. "Ashkenazi Esotericism and Kabbalah in Barcelona." *Hispania Judaica Bulletin* 5 (2007): 69–113.

———. "Astral Dreams in Judaism: Twelfth to Fourteenth Centuries." In *Dream Cultures: Explorations in the Comparative History of Dreaming*, edited by David Shulman and Guy G. Stroumsa, pp. 235–51. New York: Oxford University Press, 1999.

———. "Astral Dreams in R. Yohanan Alemanno's Writings." *Accademia: Revue de la Societe Marsile Ficin* 1 (1999): 111–28.

——. "Dream Techniques in Jewish Mysticism." In *Jewish Heritage Online Magazine*. Available at http://www.jhom.com/topics/dreams/techniques.html.

——. "Enoch and Elijah: Some Remarks on Apotheosis, Theophany and Jewish Mysticism." In *The Salt Companion to Harold Bloom*, edited by Roy Sellars and Graham Allen, pp. 347–77. Cambridge: Salt, 2007.

——. "The Function of Symbols in G. G. Scholem." *Jewish Studies* 38 (1998): 43–72 (Hebrew). German translation: "Zur Funktion von Symbolen bei G. G. Scholem." In *Gershom Scholem: Literatur und Rhetorik*, edited by Stéphane Mosès and Sigrid Weigel, pp. 51–92. Köln: Böhlau Verlag, 2000.

——. *Hasidism: Between Ecstasy and Magic*. Albany: State University of New York Press, 1995.

——. "Inquiries in the Doctrine of *Sefer ha-Meshiv*." *Sefunot* 17 (1983): 185–266 (Hebrew).

——. *Kabbalah and Eros*. New Haven: Yale University Press, 2005.

——. *Kabbalah: New Perspectives*. New Haven: Yale University Press, 1988.

——. *Les kabbalistes de la nuit*. Paris: Editions Allia, 2003.

——. *Language, Torah, and Hermeneutics in Abraham Abulafia*. Albany: State University of New York Press, 1989.

——. "Metamorphoses of a Platonic Theme in Jewish Mysticism." *Jewish Studies at the Central European University* 3 (2002–2003): 67–86.

——. *The Mystical Experience in Abraham Abulafia*. Albany: State University of New York Press, 1988.

——. "Nächtliche Kabbalisten." In *Die Wahrheit der Träume*, edited by Gartano Benedetti and Erik Hornung, pp. 85–117. Munich: Wilhelm Fink Verlag, 1997.

——. *Nocturnal Kabbalists*. Jerusalem: Carmel, 2006 (Hebrew).

——. "On Še'elat Ḥalom in Ḥasidei Aškenaz: Sources and Influences." *Materia Giudaica* 10 (2005): 99–109.

——. "Prayer, Ecstasy, and 'Alien Thoughts' in the Religious Experience of the Besht." In *Let the Old Make Way for the New: Studies in the Social and Cultural History of Eastern European Jewry Presented to Immanuel Etkes*, edited by David Assaf and Ada Rapoport-Albert. Vol. 1, *Hasidism and the Musar Movement*, pp. 57–120. Jerusalem: The Zalman Shazar Center for Jewish History, 2009 (Hebrew).

——. "Ta'anug: Erotic Delights From Kabbalah to Hasidism." In *Hidden Intercourse: Eros and Sexuality in the History of Western Esotericism*, edited by Wouter J. Hanegraaff and Jeffrey J. Kripal, pp. 111–51. Leiden: Brill, 2008.

———. "Universalization and Integration: Two Conceptions of Mystical Union in Jewish Mysticism." In *Mystical Union and Monotheistic Faith: An Ecumenical Dialogue*, edited by Moshe Idel and Bernard McGinn, pp. 27–57. New York: Macmillan, 1989.

Indich, William M. *Consciousness in Advaita Vedānta*. Delhi: Motilal Banarsidass, 1980.

In Praise of the Baal Shem Tov [Shivḥei ha-Besht]: The Earliest Collection of Legends about the Founder of Hasidism. Translated and edited by Dan Ben-Amos and Jerome R. Mintz. Bloomington: Indiana University Press, 1970.

Isaac of Acre. *Oṣar Ḥayyim*. MS Günzberg 775.

———. *Sefer Me'irat Einayim: A Critical Edition*. Edited by Amos Goldreich. Jerusalem: Hebrew University, 1981 (Hebrew).

Isayeva, Natalia. *Shankara and Indian Philosophy*. Albany: State University of New York Press, 1993.

Ivry, Alfred L. "The Image of Moses in Maimonides' Thought." In *Maimonides after 800 Years: Essays on Maimonides and His Influence*, edited by Jay M. Harris, pp. 113–34. Cambridge, MA: Harvard University Press, 2007.

———. "Ismāʿīlī Theology and Maimonides' Philosophy." In *The Jews of Medieval Islam: Community, Society, and Identity*, edited by Daniel Frank, pp. 271–99. Leiden: E. J. Brill, 1995.

———. "Maimonides on Possibility." In *Mystics, Philosophers, and Politicians: Essays in Jewish Intellectual History in Honor of Alexander Altmann*, edited by Jehuda Reinharz and Daniel Swetschinski, with the collaboration of Kalman P. Bland, pp. 67–84. Durham: Duke University Press,1982.

———. "Moses Maimonides: An Averroist *Avant la Lettre*?" *Maimonidean Studies* 5 (2008): 121–39.

———. "Providence, Divine Omniscience and Possibility: The Case of Maimonides." In *Divine Omniscience and Omnipotence in Medieval Philosophy*, edited by Tamar Rudavsky, pp. 143–59. Dordrecht: D. Reidel, 1985.

Izutsu, Toshihiko. *Sufism and Taoism: A Comparative Study of Key Philosophical Concepts*. Berkeley: University of California Press, 1983.

Izzi, John. "Proximity in Distance: Levinas and Plotinus." In *Levinas and the Ancients*, edited by Brian Schroeder and Silvia Benso, pp. 196–209. Bloomington: Indiana University Press, 2008.

Jacob bar Asher. *Perush Ba'al ha-Ṭurim al ha-Torah*. Benei Beraq, 1985.

Jacob of Marvège. *She'elot u-Teshuvot min ha-Shamayim*. Edited by Reuven Margaliot. Jerusalem: Mosad ha-Rav Kook, 1957.

Jacob Joseph of Polonnoye. *Ketonet Passim*. Critical edition with introduction and notes by Gedalyah Nigal. Jerusalem: Makhon Peri ha-Areṣ, 1985.

——. *Toledot Ya'aqov Yosef*. Korzec, 1780.

Jacobi, Friedrich Heinrich. *The Main Philosophical Writings and the Novel* Allwill. Translated with an introductory study, notes, and bibliography by George di Giovanni. Montreal: McGill-Queen's University Press, 1994.

Jacobs, Louis. *Seeker of Unity: The Life and Works of Aaron of Starosselje*. London: Vallentine Mitchell, 1966.

——. *Dobh Baer of Lubavitch: Tract on Ecstasy*. Translated with introduction and notes by Louis Jacobs. London: Vallentine Mitchell, 1963.

Jacobson, Yoram. "The Doctrine of Creation in R. Shneur Zalman of Liadi." *Eshel Beer Sheva* 1 (1976): 307–68 (Hebrew).

——. "The Love of God in the Teaching of R. Shneur Zalman of Liadi." *Te'udah* 7 (2001): 353–414 (Hebrew).

Jambet, Christian. *Le caché et l'apparent*. Paris: L'Herne, 2003.

Janicaud, Dominique. "The Theological Turn of French Phenomenology." Translated by Bernard G. Prusak. In *Phenomenology and the "Theological Turn": The French Debate*, pp. 3–106. New York: Fordham University Press, 2000.

Johnston, Sarah Iles. *Ancient Greek Divination*. Chichester: Wiley-Blackwell Publishing, 2008.

Jones, Richard H. *Science and Mysticism: A Comparative Study of Western Natural Science, Theravāda Buddhism, and Advaita Vedānta*. Lewisburg: Bucknell University Press, 1986.

Joseph ben Shalom Ashkenazi. *A Kabbalistic Commentary by Rabbi Yoseph ben Shalom Ashkenazi on Genesis Rabbah*. Edited with an introduction and notes by Moshe Hallamish. Jerusalem: Magnes Press, 1984 (Hebrew).

Joseph, Steven M. "Jung and Kabbalah: Imaginal and Noetic Aspects." *Journal of Analytical Psychology* 52 (2007): 321–41.

Jouvet, Michel. *The Castle of Dreams*. Translated by Laurence Garey. Cambridge, MA : The MIT Press, 2008.

——. *The Paradox of Sleep: The Story of Dreaming*. Translated by Laurence Garey. Cambridge, MA: The MIT Press, 1993.

Judah ben Samuel he-Ḥasid. *Sefer Ḥasidim*. Edited by Jehuda Wistinetzki and Jacob Freimann. Frankfurt am Main: Wahrmann Verlag, 1924.

Jung, Carl G. *Aion: Researches Into the Phenomenology of Self*. Translated by R. F. C. Hull. 2nd edition. Princeton: Princeton University Press, 1969.

——. *Alchemical Studies*. Translated by R. F. C. Hull. Princeton: Princeton University Press, 1967.

——. *The Archetypes and the Collective Unconscious*. Translated by R. F. C. Hull. 2nd edition. Princeton: Princeton University Press, 1969.

——. *C. G. Jung Speaking: Interviews and Encounters*. Edited by William McGuire and R. F. C. Hull. Princeton: Princeton University Press, 1977.

——. *Children's Dreams: Notes from the Seminar Given in 1936–1940*. Edited by Lorenz Jung and Maria Meyer-Grass. Translated by Ernst Falzeder with the collaboration of Tony Woolfson. Princeton: Princeton University Press, 2008.

——. *Dream Analysis: Notes of the Seminar Given in 1928–1930*. Edited by William McGuire. Princeton: Princeton University Press, 1984.

——. *Memories, Dreams, Reflections*. Recorded and edited by Aniela Jaffé. Translated by Richard and Clara Winston. New York: Vintage Books, 1965.

——. *Mysterium Coniunctionis: An Inquiry into the Separation and Synthesis of Psychic Opposites in Alchemy*. Translated by R. F. C. Hull. Princeton: Princeton University Press, 1970.

——. *The Practice of Psychotherapy: Essays on the Psychology of the Transference and Other Subjects*. Translated by R. F. C. Hull. 2nd edition. Princeton: Princeton University Press, 1966.

——. *The Psychogenesis of Mental Disease*. Translated by R. F. C. Hull. Princeton: Princeton University Press, 1960.

——. *Psychology and Alchemy*. Translated by R. F. C. Hull. 2nd edition. Princeton: Princeton University Press, 1968.

——. *Psychology and Religion: East and West*. Translated by R. F. C. Hull. 2nd edition. Princeton: Princeton University Press, 1969.

——. *Psychology of the Unconscious: A Study of the Transformations and Symbolisms of the Libido*. With a new foreword by Eugene Taylor. Princeton: Princeton University Press, 2001.

——. *The Structure and Dynamics of the Psyche*. Translated by R. F. C. Hull. 2nd edition. Princeton: Princeton University Press, 1969.

Kafka, Franz. *Parables and Paradoxes*. New York: Schocken Books, 1971.

Kahan, Tracey, Raania Moshen, Jeanette Tandez, and Jennifer McDonald. "Discriminating Memories for Actual and Imagined Taste Experiences: A Reality Monitoring Approach." *American Journal of Psychology* 112 (1999): 97–112.

Kahan, Tracey L. "Consciousness in Dreaming: A Metacognitive Approach." In *Dreams: A Reader on the Religious, Cultural, and Psychological Dimensions of Dreaming*, edited by Kelley Bulkeley, pp. 333–60. New York: Palgrave, 2001.

Kahan, Tracey L., and Stephen LaBerge. "Cognition and Metacognition in Dreaming and Waking: Comparisons of First and Third-Person Ratings." *Dreaming* 6 (1996): 235–49.

——. "Lucid Dreaming as Metacognition: Implications for Cognitive Science."

Consciousness and Cognition 3 (1994): 246–64.

Kahana-Smilansky, Hagar. "Aristotle on Sleep and Wakefulness: A Medieval Hebrew Adaptation of an Unknown Latin Treatise." *Aleph* 10 (2010): 67–118.

Kahn, Charles H. *The Art and Thought of Heraclitus: An Edition of the Fragments with Translation and Commentary.* Cambridge: Cambridge University Press, 1979.

Kaidonover, Ṣevi Hirsch. *Qav ha-Yashar.* New York: Beit Sefer, 1974.

Kakar, Sudhir. *Shamans, Mystics, and Doctors: A Psychological Inquiry into India and Its Healing Traditions.* Chicago: University of Chicago Press, 1991.

Kalmin, Richard. *Sages, Stories, Authors, and Editors in Rabbinic Babylonia.* Atlanta: Scholars Press, 1994.

———. "Talmudic Attitudes toward Dream Interpreters: Preliminary Thoughts on their Iranian Cultural Context." In *The Talmud in Its Iranian Context*, edited by Carol Bakhos and M. Rahim Shayegan, pp. 83–99. Tübingen: Mohr Siebeck, 2010.

Kalupahana, David J. *A History of Buddhist Philosophy: Continuities and Discontinuities.* Honolulu: University of Hawaii Press, 1992.

Kamenetz, Rodger. *The History of Last Night's Dream: Discovering the Hidden Path to the Soul.* New York: HarperCollins, 2007.

Kandel, Eric R. *Psychiatry, Psychoanalysis, and the New Biology of Mind.* Washington, D.C.: American Psychiatric Publishing, 2005.

Kasher, Hannah. "On the Terms Kabbalah and Kabbalist in Laṭif's Treatises." *Da'at* 41 (1999): 5–12 (Hebrew).

———. "The *Rav Pe'alim* by Isaac Ibn Laṭif." M.A. thesis, Bar Ilan University, 1974 (Hebrew).

Katz, Jonathan G. *Dreams, Sufism and Sainthood: The Visionary Career of Muhammad Al-Zawâwî*. Leiden: E. J. Brill, 1996.

Katz, Steven T. "Language, Epistemology, and Mysticism." In *Mysticism and Philosophical Analysis*, edited by Steven T. Katz, pp. 22–74. Oxford: Oxford University Press, 1978.

Kauffman, Tsippi. *In All Your Ways Know Him: The Concept of God and Avodah be-Gashmiyut in the Early Stages of Hasidism.* Ramat-Gan: Bar-Ilan University Press, 2009 (Hebrew).

Kavka, Martin. "Levinas between Monotheism and Cosmotheism." In *Levinas Studies: An Annual Review* 2 (2007): 79–103.

Kearney, Richard. "Enabling God." In *After God: Richard Kearney and the Religious Turn in Continental Philosophy*, edited by John Panteleimon Manoussakis, pp. 39–54. New York: Fordham University Press, 2006.

——. *The God Who May Be: A Hermeneutics of Religion*. Bloomington: Indiana University Press, 2001.

——. "In Place of a Response." In *After God: Richard Kearney and the Religious Turn in Continental Philosophy*, edited by John Panteleimon Manoussakis, pp. 365–87. New York: Fordham University Press, 2006

——. "On the Gift: A Discussion between Jacques Derrida and Jean-Luc Marion." In *God, the Gift, and Postmodernism*, edited by John D. Caputo and Michael J. Scanlon, pp. 54–78. Bloomington: Indiana University Press, 1999.

——. *The Wake of Imagination: Toward a Postmodern Culture*. Minneapolis: University of Minnesota Press, 1988.

Keller, Catherine. "The Apophasis of Gender: A Fourfold Unsaying of Feminist Theology." *Journal of the American Academy of Religion* 76 (2008): 905–33.

——. *The Face of the Deep: A Theology of Becoming*. London: Routledge, 2003.

——. "The Flesh of God: A Metaphor in the Wild." In *Theology That Matters: Ecology, Economy, and God*, edited by Darby Kathleen Ray, pp. 91–107. Minneapolis: Fortress Press, 2006.

——. *God and Power: Counter-Apocalyptic Journeys*. Minneapolis: Fortress Press, 2005.

——. *On the Mystery: Discerning Divinity in Process*. Minneapolis: Fortress Press, 2008.

——. "Rumors of Transcendence: The Movement, State, and Sex of 'Beyond.'" In *Transcendence and Beyond: A Postmodern Inquiry*, edited by John D. Caputo and Michael J. Scanlon, pp. 129–50. Bloomington: Indiana University Press, 2007.

Kellner, Menachem. "Maimonides and Gersonides on Mosaic Prophecy." *Speculum* 52 (1977): 62–79.

Kelly, Edward F., Emily Williams Kelly, Adam Crabtree, Alan Gauld, Michael Grosso, and Bruce Greyson. *Irreducible Mind: Toward a Psychology for the 21st Century*. Lanham: Rowman & Littlefield, 2007.

Kenaan, Vered Lev. "Delusion and Dream in Apuleius' *Metamorphoses*." *Classical Antiquity* 23 (2004): 247–84.

Kierkegaard, Søren. *Philosophical Fragments*; *Johannes Climacus*. Edited and translated with introduction and notes by Howard V. Hong and Edna H. Hong. Princeton: Princeton University Press, 1987.

——. *Søren Kierkegaard's Journals and Papers*. Vol. 2, *F–K*. Edited by and translated by Howard V. Hong and Edna H. Hong. Bloomington: Indiana University Press, 1970.

Kilroe, Patricia A. "The Dream as Text, The Dream as Narrative." *Dreaming* 10 (2000): 125–37.

Kim, Chin-Tai. "Transcendence and Immanence." *Journal of the American Academy of Religion* 55 (1987): 537–49.

Kimḥi, David. *Perush al Yirmeyahu*. In *Miqra'ot Gedolot*. New York: Abraham Isaac Friedman, 1961.

——. *Sefer ha-Shorashim im ha-Nimmuqim me-R'abbi Eliyahu ha-Levi ha-Ashkenazi*. Edited by Johann Heinrich Biesenthal and Fürchtegott Lebrecht. Berlin: Impensis G. Bethge, 1847.

Kinberg, Leah. *Morality in the Guide of Dreams: A Critical Edition of* Kitāb al-Manām *with Introduction*. Leiden: E. J. Brill, 1994.

Kings, Steven. "Jung's Hermeneutics of Scripture." *Journal of Religion* 77 (1997): 233–51.

Kister, Menahem J. "The Interpretation of Dreams: An Unknown Manuscript of Ibn Qutayba's 'Ibârât al-Ru'yâ.'" *Israel Oriental Studies* 4 (1974): 67–103.

Klaassen, Frank. "Magical Dream Provocation in the Later Middle Ages." *Esoterica* 8 (2006): 111–35.

Klein, Dennis B. *Jewish Origins of the Psychoanalytic Movement*. Chicago: University of Chicago Press, 1985.

Klemm, David E. "Open Secrets: Derrida and Negative Theology." In *Negation and Theology*, edited by Robert P. Scharlemann, pp. 8–24. Charlottesville: University Press of Virginia, 1992.

Kofman, Sarah. *Nietzsche and Metaphor*. Translated by Duncan Large. Stanford: Stanford University Press, 1993.

Kojima, Hiroshi. "The Vertical Intentionality of Time-Consciousness and Sense-Giving." In *Husserl in Contemporary Context: Prospects and Projects for Phenomenology*, edited by Burt C. Hopkins, pp. 79–93. Dordrecht: Kluwer, 1997.

Komem, Aharon. "Between Poetry and Prophecy: Studies in the Poetry of Judah Halevi." *Molad* 2 (1969): 676–98 (Hebrew).

Kongtrul, Jamgön. *The Treasury of Knowledge: Esoteric Instructions*. Translated and annotated by Sarah Harding. Ithaca: Snow Lion Publications, 2007.

Kook, Abraham Isaac. *Ein Ayah al Aggadot Ḥazal she-be-Ein Ya'aqov: Berakhot*. 2 vols. Jerusalem: Makhon al shem ha-Rav Ṣevi Yehudah Quq, 1995–2000.

Kordela, A. Kiarina. "Marx, Condensed and Displaced." In *The Dreams of Interpretation: A Century down the Royal Road*, edited by Catherine Liu, John Mowitt, Thomas Pepper, and Jakki Spicer, pp. 303–19. Minneapolis: University of Minnesota Press, 2007.

Kraemer, Joel L. "Is There a Text in this Class?" *Aleph* 8 (2008): 247–99.

——. *Maimonides: The Life and World of One of Civilization's Greatest Minds*. New York: Doubleday, 2008.

———. "Maimonides' Use of Aristotelian Dialectic." In *Maimonides and the Sciences*, edited by Robert S. Cohen and Hillel Levine, pp. 111–30. Dordrecht: Kluwer, 2000.

Kramer, Milton. *The Dreamer Experience: A Systematic Exploration*. New York: Routledge, 2007.

Kriegel, Uriah. "Is Intentionality Dependent Upon Consciousness?" *Philosophical Studies* 116 (2003): 271–307.

Kreisel, Howard. *Maimonides' Political Thought: Studies in Ethics, Law, and the Human Ideal*. Albany: State University of New York Press, 1999.

———. *Prophecy: The History of an Idea in Medieval Jewish Philosophy*. Dordrecht: Kluwer, 2001.

Kripal, Jeffrey J. *Esalen: America and the Religion of No Religion*. Chicago: University of Chicago Press, 2007.

———. *Roads of Excess, Palaces of Wisdom: Eroticism and Reflexivity in the Study of Mysticism*. Chicago: University of Chicago Press, 2001.

Kruger, Steven F. *Dreaming in the Middle Ages*. Cambridge: Cambridge University Press, 1992.

Kuspit, Donald B. "Fiction and Phenomenology." *Philosophy and Phenomenological Research* 29 (1968): 16–33.

Kuyt, Annelies. "Hasidut Ashkenaz on the Angel of Dreams: A Heavenly Messenger Reflecting or Exchanging Man's Thoughts." In *Creation and Re-Creation in Jewish Thought: Festschrift in Honor of Joseph Dan on the Occasion of his Seventieth Birthday*, edited by Rachel Elior and Peter Schäfer, pp. 147–63. Tübingen: Mohr Siebeck, 2005.

———. "With One Foot in the Renaissance: Shlomoh Almoli and his Dream Interpretation." *Jewish Studies Quarterly* 6 (1999): 205–17.

Kwant, Remy C. *Phenomenology of Language*. Pittsburgh: Duquesne University Press, 1965.

LaBerge, Stephen. *Lucid Dreaming*. Foreword by Robert Ornstein. Los Angeles: Jeremy P. Tarcher, 1985.

———. "Lucid Dreaming and the Yoga of the Dream State: A Psychophysiological Perspective." In *Buddhism and Science: Breaking New Ground*, edited by B. Alan Wallace, pp. 233–58. New York: Columbia University Press, 2003.

Lacan, Jacques. *The Seminar of Jacques Lacan, Book I: Freud's Papers on Technique 1953–1954*. Edited by Jacques-Alain Miller. Translated with notes by John Forrester. New York: W. W. Norton, 1991.

———. *The Seminar of Jacques Lacan, Book II: The Ego in Freud's Theory and in the Technique of Psychoanalysis 1954–1955*. Edited by Jacques-Alain Miller. Translated by Sylvana Tomaselli with notes by John Forrester. New York:

W. W. Norton, 1988.

——. *The Seminar of Jacques Lacan, Book XI: The Four Fundamental Concepts of Psychoanalysis*. Edited by Jacques-Alain Miller. Translated by Alan Sheridan. New York: W. W. Norton, 1981.

Lamoreaux, John C. *The Early Muslim Tradition of Dream Interpretation*. Albany: State University of New York Press, 2002.

Lancaster, Irene. *Deconstructing the Bible: Abraham ibn Ezra's Introduction to the Torah*. London: RoutledgeCurzon, 2003.

Lang, Hermann. *Language and the Unconscious: Lacan's Hermeneutics of Psychoanalysis*. Atlantic Highlands: Humanities Press, 1997.

Langermann, T. Zvi. "A New Hebrew Passage from the *Theology of Aristotle* and Its Significance." *Arabic Sciences and Philosophy* 9 (1999): 247–59.

Lapide, Pinchas E. *Hebrew in the Church: The Foundations of Jewish-Christian Dialogue*. Grand Rapids: William B. Eerdmans, 1984.

Lavi, Simeon. *Ketem Paz*. Livorno, 1795.

Lecerf, Jean. "The Dream in Popular Culture: Arabic and Islamic." In *The Dream and Human Societies*, edited by Gustave Edmund von Grunebaum and Roger Caillois, pp. 365–79. Berkeley: University of California Press, 1966.

Ledbetter, Grace M. *Poetics before Plato: Interpretation and Authority in Early Greek Theories of Poetry*. Princeton: Princeton University Press, 2003.

Lederberg, Netanel. *Sod ha-Da'at: Rabbi Israel Ba'al Shem Tov, His Spiritual Character and Social Leadership*. Jerusaelm: Rubin Mass, 2007 (Hebrew).

Le Goff, Jacques. *The Medieval Imagination*. Translated by Arthur Goldhammer. Chicago: University of Chicago Press, 1988.

Leighton, Taigen Dan. *Visions of Awakening Space and Time: Dōgen and the Lotus Sutra*. Oxford: Oxford University Press, 2007.

Levene, Nancy K. *Spinoza's Revelation: Religion, Democracy, and Reason*. Cambridge: Cambridge University Press, 2004.

Levi ben Gershom (Gersonides). *Milḥamot ha-Shem*. Riva di Trento, 1560.

——. *The Wars of the Lord*. 3 vols. Translated with an appendix and notes by Seymour Feldman. Philadelphia: Jewish Publication Society, 1987–1999.

Levinas, Emmanuel. *Alterity and Transcendence*. Translated by Michael B. Smith. New York: Columbia University Press, 1999.

——. *Autrement qu'être ou au-delà de l'essence*. The Hague: Martinus Nijhoff, 1974.

——. *Beyond the Verse: Talmudic Readings and Lectures*. Translated by Gary D. Mole. London: Athlone, 1994.

——. *Collected Philosophical Papers*. Translated by Alphonso Lingis. Dordrecht: Martinus Nijhoff, 1987.

——. *Entre Nous: On Thinking-of-the-Other*. Translated by Michael B. Smith and Barbara Harshav. New York: Columbia University Press, 1998.

——. *Ethics and Infinity: Conversations with Philippe Nemo*. Translated by Richard A. Cohen. Pittsburgh: Duquesne University Press, 1985.

——. *Existence and Existents*. Translated by Alphonso Lingis. Foreword by Robert Bernasconi. Pittsburgh: Duquesne University Press, 2001.

——. *In the Time of the Nations*. Translated by Michael B. Smith. London: Athlone, 1994.

——. "Jean Wahl et le sentiment." *Cahiers du Sud* 42 (1955): 453–59.

——. "Jean Wahl: Sans avoir ni être." In *Jean Wahl et Gabriel Marcel*, edited by Jeanne Hersch, pp. 13–31. Paris: Editions Beauchesne, 1976.

——. "The Jewish Understanding of Scripture." *Cross Currents* 44 (1994): 488–505.

——. *The Levinas Reader*. Edited by Seán Hand. Oxford: Blackwell, 1989.

——. *Of God Who Comes to Mind*. Translated by Bettina Bergo. Stanford: Stanford University Press, 1998.

——. *Otherwise Than Being or Beyond Essence*. Translated by Alphonso Lingis. Dordrecht: Kluwer, 1991.

——. *Outside the Subject*. Translated by Michael B. Smith. Stanford: Stanford University Press, 1993.

——. *Proper Names*. Translated by Michael B. Smith. Stanford: Stanford University Press, 1996.

——. *Time and the Other*. Translated by Richard A. Cohen. Pittsburgh: Duquesne University Press, 1987.

——. *Totalité et infini: Essai sur l'extériorité*. The Hague: Martinus Nijhoff, 1961.

——. *Totality and Infinity: An Essay on Exteriority*. Translated by Alphonso Lingis. Dordrecht: Kluwer, 1969.

Levison, John R. "The Prophetic Spirit as an Angel According to Philo." *Harvard Theological Review* 88 (1995): 189–207.

Lewin, Isaac, Dror Schlezinger, and Danny Derby. "The Personality of R. Nahman of Bratslav: Comparing Dream Content Analysis and Biography." *Journal of Psychology and Judaism* 22 (1998): 33–50.

Libet, Benjamin. *Mind Time: The Temporal Factor in Consciousness*. Cambridge, MA : Harvard University Press, 2004.

Lieberman, Saul. *Greek in Jewish Palestine: Studies on the Life and Manners of Jewish Palestine in the II–IV Centuries C.E.* New York: Philip Feldheim, 1965.

——. *Hellenism in Jewish Palestine: Studies in the Literary Transmission, Beliefs, and Manners of Palestine in the I Century B.C.E.–IV Century C.E.* New York: Jewish Theological Seminary of America, 1962.

——. *Tosefta Ki-Fshuṭah: A Comprehensive Commentary on the Tosefta, Order Zera'im, Part 1*. 2nd augmented edition. Jerusalem: Jewish Theological Seminary of America, 1992 (Hebrew).

Liebes, Yehuda. "Zohar and Eros." *Alpayyim* 9 (1994): 67–115 (Hebrew).

——. *Studies in the Zohar*. Translated by Arnold Schwartz, Stephanie Nakache, and Penina Peli. Albany: State University of New York Press, 1993.

Lindorff, David. *Pauli and Jung: The Meeting of Two Great Minds*. Wheaton: Quest Books, 2004.

Lingis, Alphonso. "Imperatives." In *Merleau-Ponty Vivant*, edited by Martin C. Dillon, pp. 91–115. Albany: State University of New York Press,1991.

Liphshitz, Ya'aqov Qoppel. *Sha'arei Gan ha-Eden*. 2 vols. Jerusalem: Yerid ha-Sefarim, 2004.

Llewelyn, John. "Am I Obsessed by Bobby? (Humanism of the Other Animal)." In *Re-Reading Levinas*, edited by Robert Bernasconi and Simon Critchley, pp. 234–45. Bloomington: Indiana University Press, 1991.

——. *Derrida on the Threshold of Sense*. New York: St. Martin's Press, 1986.

Lloyd, Alan T. "Evolution and the Interpretation of (REM Sleep) Dreams." In *The New Science of Dreaming*, edited by Deirdre Barrett and Patrick McNamara. Vol. 3, *Cultural and Theoretical Perspectives*, pp. 249–75. Westport: Praeger, 2007.

Lobel, Diane. *A Sufi-Jewish Dialogue: Philosophy and Mysticism in Baḥya Ibn Paqūda's Duties of the Heart*. Philadelphia: University of Pennsylvania Press, 2007.

Locke, John. *An Essay Concerning Human Understanding*. New York: Prometheus Books, 1994.

Loewe, Raphael. "The 'Plain' Meaning of Scripture in Early Jewish Exegesis." *Papers of the Institute of Jewish Studies* 1 (1964): 140–85.

Loewenthal, Naftali. "The Baal Shem Tov's Iggeret ha-Kodesh and Contemporary Habad 'Outreach'." In *Let the Old Make Way for the New: Studies in the Social and Cultural History of Eastern European Jewry Presented to Immanuel Etkes*, edited by David Assaf and Ada Rapoport-Albert. Vol. 1, *Hasidism and the Musar Movement*, pp. 69–101. Jerusalem: The Zalman Shazar Center for Jewish History, 2009 (English section).

——. *Communicating the Infinite: The Emergence of the Habad School*. Chicago: University of Chicago Press, 1990.

Lorberbaum, Yair. "Changes in Maimonides' Approach to Aggadah." *Tarbiz* 78 (2009): 81–122 (Hebrew).

——. "'Incline Thy Ear, and Hear the Words of the Wise, and Apply Thy Heart unto My Knowledge': Criticism of Aggadah in *The Guide of the Perplexed*."

Tarbiz 78 (2009): 203–30 (Hebrew).

Lory, Pierre. *Le rêve et ses interpretations en Islam*. Paris: Albin Michel, 2003.

Love, Jane. "Appetite and Violability: Questioning a Platonic Metaphor." In *Crises in Continental Philosophy*, edited by Arleen B. Dallery, Charles E. Scott, with P. Holley Roberts, pp. 175–85. Albany: State University of New York Press, 1990.

Lowry, Atherton C. "The Invisible World of Merleau-Ponty." *Philosophy Today* 23 (1979): 294–303.

Loy, David R. *Awareness Bound and Unbound: Buddhist Essays*. Albany: State University of New York Press, 2009.

Luzzatto, Moses Ḥayyim. *Adir ba-Marom*, part 2. Jerusalem, 1988.

———. *Derekh ha-Shem*. Jerusalem, 1996.

———. *Oṣerot Ramḥal*. Edited by Ḥayyim Friedlander. Benei Beraq, 1986.

———. *Qelaḥ Pitḥei Ḥokhmah*. Edited by Ḥayyim Friedlander. Benei Beraq, 1992.

MacKendrick, Karmen. *Fragmentation and Memory: Meditations on Christian Doctrine*. New York: Fordham University Press, 2008.

Mackinlay, Shane. "Exceeding Truth: Jean-Luc Marion's Saturated Phenomena." *Pacifica* 20 (2007): 40–51.

———. *Interpreting Excess: Jean-Luc Marion, Saturated Phenomenon, and Hermeneutics*. New York: Fordham University Press, 2009.

Macy, Jeffrey. "Prophecy in al-Farabi and Maimonides." In *Maimonides and Philosophy*, edited by Shlomo Pines and Yirmiyahu Yovel, pp. 185–201. Dordrecht: Martinus Nijhoff, 1986.

Mageo, Jeannette Marie. "Subjectivity and Identity in Dreams." In *Dreaming and the Self: New Perspectives on Subjectivity, Identity, and Emotion*, edited by Jeannette Marie Mageo, pp. 23–40. Albany: State University of New York Press, 2003.

Magid, Shaul. *From Metaphysics to Midrash: Myth, History, and the Interpretation of Scripture in Lurianic Kabbala*. Bloomington: Indiana University Press, 2008.

———. *Hasidism on the Margin: Reconciliation, Antinomianism, and Messianism in Izbica/Radzin Hasidism*. Madison: University of Wisconsin Press, 2003.

Mahāparinirvāṇa Sūtra. Translated by Kosho Yamamoto. Edited, revised, and copyrighted by Tony Page. London: Nirvana Publications, 1999–2000. Available at http://www.nirvanasutra.net .

Maḥazor la-Yamim ha-Nora'im. Edited and annotated by Ernst Daniel Goldschmidt. Vol. 1, *Rosh ha-Shanah*. Jerusalem: Qoren, 1970.

Mahdi, Muhsin S. *Alfarabi and the Foundation of Islamic Political Philosophy*. Chicago: University of Chicago Press, 2001.

Maimonides, Moses. *The Guide of the Perplexed*. Translated with an introduction and notes by Shlomo Pines. With an introductory essay by Leo Strauss. 2 vols. Chicago: University of Chicago Press, 1963.

——. *Introduction to Logic in the Hebrew Version of Moses Ibn Tibbon*. Edited by Leon Roth, collated with the manuscript fragments in Arabic by David H. Baneth. 2nd edition. Jerusalem: Magnes Press, 1965 (Hebrew).

——. *Ma'amar Teḥiyyat ha-Metim*. In *Iggerot ha-Rambam*, edited, translated, and annotated by Isaac Shilat, pp. 319–74. Jerusalem: Ma'aliyyot, 1987.

——. *Mishnah im Perush Rabbenu Moshe ben Maimon: Seder Neziqin*. Translated and edited by Joseph Kafiḥ, Jerusalem: Mosad ha-Rav Kook, 1965.

——. *Mishnah im Perush Rabbenu Moshe ben Maimon: Seder Ṭaharot*. Translated and edited by Joseph Kafiḥ, Jerusalem: Mosad ha-Rav Kook, 1968.

——. *Mishneh Torah*. New York: Schlusinger, 1947.

——. *Shemoneh Peraqim le-ha-Rambam im Perush Ḥesed Avraham*. Jerusalem: Yesodi, 1998.

Main, Roderick. *Revelations of Chance: Synchronicity as Spiritual Experience*. Albany: State University of New York, 2007.

——. *The Rupture of Time: Synchronicity and Jung's Critique of Modern Western Culture*. New York: Brunner-Routledge, 2004.

Malcolm, Norman. *Dreaming*. London: Routledge & Kegan Paul Ltd, 1959.

Malin, Shimon. *Nature Loves to Hide: Quantum Physics and Reality, a Western Perspective*. Oxford: Oxford University Press, 2001.

Malinowski, Bronislaw. *The Sexual Life of Savages*. With a new introduction by Annette B. Weiner. Boston: Beacon Press, 1987.

Malka, Salomon. *Emmanuel Levinas: His Life and Legacy*. Foreword by Philippe Nemo. Translated by Michael Kigel and Sara M. Embree. Pittsburgh: Duquesne University Press, 2006.

Maltby, Michael. "Wordless Words: Poetry and the Symmetry of Being." In *Acquainted with the Night: Psychoanalysis and the Poetic Imagination*, edited by Hamish Canham and Carole Satyamurti, pp. 49–70. London: Karnac, 2003.

Malter, Henry. "Shem Tob ben Joseph Palquera: His Treatise of the Dream." *Jewish Quarterly Review* 1 (1910–1911): 451–550.

Mancuso, Piergabriele. *Shabbatai Donnolo's Sefer Ḥakhmoni: Introduction, Critical Text, and Annotated Translation*. Leiden: Brill, 2010.

Manolopoulos, Mark. *If Creation Is a Gift*. Albany: State University of New York Press, 2009.

Mansfield, Victor. "Time and Impermanence in Middle Way Buddhism and Modern Physics." In *Buddhism and Science: Breaking New Ground*, edited by B. Alan Wallace, pp. 305–21. New York: Columbia University Press, 2003.

Marcus, Laura. "Introduction: Histories, Representations, Autobiographics in *The Interpretation of Dreams*." In *Sigmund Freud's The Interpretation of Dreams: New Interdisciplinary Essays*, edited by Laura Marcus, pp. 1–65. Manchester: Manchester University Press, 1999.

Marder, Elissa. "Walter Benjamin's Dream of 'Happiness.'" In *Walter Benjamin and the Arcades Project*, edited by Beatrice Hanssen, pp. 184–200. London: Continuum, 2006.

Margolin, Ron. *The Human Temple: Religious Interiorization and the Structuring of Inner Life in Early Hasidism*. Jerusalem: Magnes Press, 2005 (Hebrew).

Marinelli, Lydia, and Andreas Mayer. *Dreaming by the Book: Freud's The Interpretation of Dreams and the History of the Psychoanalytic Movement*. Translated by Susan Fairfield. New York: Other Press, 2003.

Marion, Jean-Luc. *Being Given: Toward a Phenomenology of Givenness*. Translated by Jeffrey L. Kosky. Stanford: Stanford University Press, 2002.

———. "The Event, the Phenomenon, and the Revealed." In *Transcendence in Philosophy and Religion*, edited by James E. Faulconer, pp. 87–105. Bloomington: Indiana University Press, 2003.

———. *God without Being: Hors-Texte*. Translated by Thomas A. Carlson. With a foreword by David Tracy. Chicago: University of Chicago Press, 1991.

———. *In Excess: Studies in Saturated Phenomena*. Translated by Robyn Horner and Vincent Berraud. New York: Fordham University Press, 2002.

———. "In the Name: How to Avoid Speaking of 'Negative Theology'." In *God, the Gift, and Postmodernism*, edited by John D. Caputo and Michael J. Scanlon, pp. 20–53. Bloomington: Indiana University Press, 1999.

———. "The Reason of the Gift." In *Givenness and God: Questions of Jean-Luc Marion*, edited by Ian Leask and Eoin Cassidy, pp. 101–34. New York: Fordham University Press, 2005.

———. *Reduction and Givenness: Investigations of Husserl, Heidegger, and Phenomenology*. Translated by Thomas A. Carlson. Evanston: Northwestern University Press, 1998.

———. "The Saturated Phenomenon." *Philosophy Today* 40 (1996): 103–24.

Marion, Jean-Luc, and Richard Kearney. "Hermeneutics of Revelation." In *After God: Richard Kearney and the Religious Turn in Continental Philosophy*, edited by John Panteleimon Manoussakis, pp. 318–39. New York: Fordham University Press, 2006.

Marrati, Paola. *Genesis and Trace: Derrida Reading Husserl and Heidegger*. Stanford: Stanford University Press, 2005.

Martin, Paul C. "The Erotic Imaginary of Divine Realization in Kabbalistic and Tantric Metaphysics." Available at http://espace.library.uq.edu.au/eserv/

UQ:179374/Kabbalah_and_Tantra_wpv2.pdf.

Masuzawa, Tomoko. *In Search of Dreamtime: The Quest for the Origins of Religion*. Chicago: University of Chicago Press, 1993.

Matt, Daniel C. "Ayin: The Concept of Nothingness in Jewish Mysticism." In *The Problem of Pure Consciousness: Mysticism and Philosophy*, edited by Robert K. C. Forman, pp. 121–59. New York: Oxford University Press, 1990.

Matthews, Gareth B. *Socratic Perplexity and the Nature of Philosophy*. Oxford: Oxford University Press, 1999.

Maudlin, Tim. *The Metaphysics within Physics*. Oxford: Oxford University Press, 2007.

Mavroudi, Maria. *A Byzantine Book on Dream Interpretation: The Oneirocriticon of Achmet and Its Arabic Sources*. Leiden: Brill, 2002.

May, Todd. *Reconsidering Difference: Nancy, Derrida, Levinas, and Deleuze*. University Park: Pennsylvania State University Press, 1997.

Mazis, Glen A. *Emotion and Embodiment: Fragile Ontology*. New York: Peter Lang, 1993.

———. "The Flesh of the World Is Emptiness and Emptiness is the Flesh of the World, and Their Ethical Implications." In *Merleau-Ponty and Buddhism*, edited by Jin Y. Park and Gereon Kopf, pp. 183–208. Lanham: Rowman & Littlefield, 2009.

McCallum, Donald. *Maimonides' Guide for the Perplexed: Silence and Salvation*. London: Routledge, 2007.

McClintock, Sara L. "The Role of the 'Given' in the Classification of Śaṅkarakṣita and Kamalaśīla as Svātantrika-Mādhyamikas." In *The Svātantrika-Prāsaṅgika Distinction: What Difference a Difference Make?* edited by George B. J. Dreyfus and Sara L. McClintock, pp. 125–71. Boston: Wisdom Publications, 2003.

McGhee, Michael. *Transformations of Mind: Philosophy as Spiritual Practice*. Cambridge: Cambridge University Press, 2000.

McGushin, Edward F. *Foucault's Askēsis: An Introduction to Philosophical Life*. Evanston: Northwestern University Press, 2007.

McKenna, Terence. *The Archaic Revival: Speculations on Psychedelic Mushrooms, the Amazon, Virtual Reality, UFOs, Evolution, Shamanism, the Rebirth of the Goddess, and the End of History*. New York: HarperCollins, 1991.

McMahan, David L. *Empty Vision: Metaphor and Visionary Imagery in Mahāyāna Buddhism*. London: RoutledgeCurzon, 2002.

McNamara, Patrick. "Counterfactual Thought in Dreams." *Dreaming* 10 (2000): 237–46.

Megill, Allan. *Prophets of Extremity: Nietzsche, Heidegger, Foucault, Derrida*.

Berkeley: University of California Press, 1987.

Meillassoux, Quentin. *After Finitude: An Essay on the Necessity of Contingency.* Translated by Ray Brassier. New York: Continuum, 2008.

Mekhilta de-Rabbi Ishmael. Edited by Ḥayyim S. Horovitz and Israel A. Rabin. Jerusalem: Wahrmann, 1970.

Melamed, Abraham. "The Image of India in Medieval Jewish Culture: Between Adoration and Rejection." *Jewish History* 20 (2006): 299–314.

———. "Ibn Laṭif and Falaquera on the Characteristics of the Philosopher-King." *Tura: Studies in Jewish Thought* 2 (1992): 162–77 (Hebrew).

———. *The Philosopher-King in Medieval and Renaissance Jewish Political Thought.* Edited with a foreword by Lenn E. Goodman. Albany: State University of New York Press, 2003.

Menaḥem Mendel of Viṭebsk. *Liqquṭei Amarim.* Lemberg, 1911.

Menasseh ben Israel, *Nishmat Ḥayyim.* Amsterdam, 1652.

Mensch, James R. "Manifestation and the Paradox of Subjectivity." *Husserl Studies* 21 (2005): 35–53.

———. *Postfoundational Phenomenology: Husserlian Reflections on Presence and Embodiment.* University Park: Pennsylvania State University Press, 2001.

Merleau-Ponty, Maurice. *The Incarnate Subject: Malebranche, Biran, and Bergson on the Union of Body and Soul.* Preface by Jacques Taminiaux. Translation by Paul B. Milan. Edited by Andrew G. Bjelland Jr. and Patrick Burke. Amherst: Humanity Books, 2001.

———. *Nature: Course Notes from the Collège de France.* Compiled and with notes by Dominique Séglard. Translated by Robert Vallier. Evanston: Northwestern University Press, 2003.

———. *The Visible and the Invisible.* Edited by Claude Lefort. Translated by Alphonso Lingis. Evanston: Northwestern University Press, 1968.

———. *Phenomenology of Perception.* Translated by Colin Smith. New York: Humanities Press, 1962.

Meroz, Ronit. "The Resplendent Light is in the East: On the Time and Place of the *Sefer Bahir.*" *Da'at* 49 (2002): 137–80 (Hebrew).

———. "Redemption in the Lurianic Teaching." Ph.D. dissertation, Hebrew University, 1988 (Hebrew).

———. "Zoharic Narratives and Their Adaptations." *Hispania Judaica* 3 (2000): 3–63.

Midrash Bere'shit Rabba. Edited by Julius Theodor and Chanoch Albeck. Jerusalem: Wahrmann Books, 1965.

Midrash ha-Gadol on Genesis. Edited by Mordecai Margulies. Jerusalem: Mosad ha-Rav Kook, 1975.

Midrash Shir ha-Shirim Rabbah. Edited by Shimon Dunaski. Jerusalem: Dvir, 1980.

Midrash Tanḥuma. Jerusalem: Eshkol, 1972.

Midrash Tanḥuma. Edited by Solomon Buber. Vilna: Rom, 1885.

Midrash Tehillim. Edited by Solomon Buber. Vilna: Rom, 1891.

Midrash Wayyikra Rabbah. Edited by Mordecai Margulies. New York: Jewish Theological Seminary of America, 1993.

Miedema, Siebren and Gert J. J. Biesta. "Jacque Derrida's Religion without Religion and the Im/Possibility of Religious Education." *Religious Education* 99 (2004): 23–37.

Miller, David L. "The Body Is No Body." In *Apophatic Bodies: Infinity, Ethics, and Incarnation*, edited by Christopher Boesel and Catherine Keller, pp. 137–46. New York: Fordham University Press, 2009.

——. "The Brokenness of Beauty and the 'Beauty' of Brokenness: Toward a Postmodern Theopoetics." Drew Tripple-Vosburgh Lecture, October 2009.

——. *Christs: Meditations on Archetypal Images in Christian Theology*. New Orleans: Spring Journal Books, 2005.

——. *Hells and Holy Ghosts: A Theopoetics of Christian Belief*. Nashville: Abingdon Press, 1989.

——. "Theologia Imaginalis." In *The Archaeology of the Imagination*, edited by Charles E. Winquist, *Journal of the American Academy of Religion Thematic Studies* 48/2 (1981): 1–18.

——. "Theopoiesis." In Stanley R. Hopper, *Why Permissions and Other Poems: Transformations of Theology in Poetry*, pp. 1–12. Atlanta: Scholars Press, 1987.

Miller, Justin. "Interpretations of Freud's Jewishness, 1924–1974." *Journal of the History of the Behavioral Sciences* 17 (1981): 357–74.

Miller, Melvin E. "No-Self and the Emptying God: Dwelling in the Emptying Place." In *Self and No-Self: Continuing the Dialogue between Buddhism and Psychotherapy*, edited by Dale Mathers, Melvin E. Miller, and Osamu Ando, pp. 79–91. London: Routledge, 2009.

Miller, Patricia Cox. *Dreams in Late Antiquity: Studies in the Imagination of a Culture*. Princeton: Princeton University Press, 1994.

Miller, Tyrus. "'Glass Before Its Time, Premature Iron': Architecture, Temporality, and Dream in Benjamin's Arcades Project." In *Walter Benjamin and the Arcades Project*, edited by Beatrice Hanssen, pp. 240–58. London: Continuum, 2006.

Min, Anslem K. "Naming the Unnameable God: Levinas, Derrida, and Marion." *International Journal for Philosophy of Religion* 60 (2006): 99–116.

Mittermaier, Amira. "The Book of Visions: Dreams, Poetry, and Prophecy in Contemporary Egypt." *International Journal of Middle Eastern Studies* 39 (2007): 229–47.

——. "(Re)Imagining Space: Dreams and Saint Shrines in Egypt." In *Dimensions of Locality: Muslim Saints, Their Place and Space*, edited by Georg Stauth and Samuli Schielke, pp. 47–66. Bielefeld: Transcript, 2008.

Mooij, Jan Johann Albinn. *Time and Mind: The History of a Philosophical Problem*. Leiden: Boston, 2005.

Moosa, Ebrahim. *Ghazālī and the Poetics of Imagination*. Chapel Hill: University of North Carolina Press, 2005.

Mopsik, Charles. *Sex of the Soul: The Vicissitudes of Sexual Difference in Kabbalah*. Edited with a foreword by Daniel Abrams. Los Angeles: Cherub Press, 2005.

Moran, Dermot. *An Introduction to Phenomenology*. London: Routledge, 2000.

Morgan, Michael L. *Discovering Levinas*. Cambridge: Cambridge University Press, 2007.

——. *Platonic Piety: Philosophy and Ritual in Fourth-Century Athens*. New Haven: Yale University Press,1990.

Morgenstern, Isaac Meir. *Yam ha-Ḥokhmah Erev Rosh ha-Shanah 5766*. Jerusalem: Makhon Yam ha-Ḥokhmah, 2005.

——. *Yam ha-Ḥokhmah 5769*. Jerusalem: Makhon Yam ha-Ḥokhmah, 2009.

Morley, James. "The Texture of the Real: Merleau-Ponty on Imagination and Psychopathology." In *Imagination and Its Pathologies*, edited by James Phillips and James Morley, pp. 93–108. Cambridge, MA: The MIT Press, 2003.

Morrison, Roy D. II. *Science, Theology and the Transcendental Horizon: Einstein, Kant and Tillich*. Atlanta: Scholars Press, 1994.

Moses Ḥayyim Ephraim of Sudlykow. *Degel Maḥaneh Efrayim*. Jerusalem: Mir, 1995.

Moss, Robert. *The Secret History of Dreaming*. Novato: New World Library, 2009.

Moyn, Samuel. *Origins of the Other: Emmanuel Levinas between Revelation and Ethics*. Ithaca: Cornell University Press, 2005.

Munk, Salomon. *Mélanges de philosophie juive et arabe*. Paris: A. Franck, 1857.

Murata, Junichi. "The Indeterminacy of Images: An Approach to a Phenomenology of the Imagination." In *Phenomenology: Japanese and American Perspectives*, edited by Burt C. Hopkins, pp. 169–83. Dordrecht: Kluwer, 1999.

Murchadha, Felix Ó. "Glory, Idolatry, Kairos: Revelation and the Ontological Difference in Marion." In *Givenness and God: Questions of Jean-Luc Marion*, edited by Ian Leask and Eoin Cassidy, pp. 69–86. New York: Fordham University Press, 2005.

Murphy, Tim. *Nietzsche, Metaphor, Religion*. Albany: State University of New York Press, 2001.

Myers, Frederic W. H. *Science and the Future Life with Other Essays*. 2nd edition. London: Macmillan, 1901.

Naddaff, Ramona A. *Exiling the Poets: The Production of Censorship in Plato's Republic*. Chicago: University of Chicago Press, 2002.

Nāgārjuna's Reason Sixty with Chandrakīrti's Commentary. Translated with an introduction by Joseph Loizzo. New York: American Institute of Buddhist Studies, 2007.

Naḥman of Bratslav. *Liqquṭei MoHaRaN*. Benei Beraq, 1972.

Naḥmanides, Moses. *Perushei ha-Torah le-Rabbenu Moshe ben Naḥman*. Edited by Ḥayyim D. Chavel. 2 vols. Jerusalem: Mosad ha-Rav Kook, 1984.

Nakamura, Katsuhiro. *Quantum versus Chaos: Questions Emerging from Mesoscopic Cosmos*. Dordrecht: Kluwer, 1997.

Nanay, Bence. "Is Twofoldness Necessary for Representational Seeing?" *British Journal of Aesthetics* 45 (2005): 248–57.

Nancy, Jean-Luc. "A Deconstruction of Monotheism." In *Religion: Beyond a Concept*, edited by Hent de Vries, pp. 380–91. New York: Fordham University Press, 2008.

———. *Dis-Enclosure: The Deconstruction of Christianity*. Translated by Bettina Bego, Gabriel Malenfant, and Michael B. Smith. New York: Fordham University Press, 2008.

Narbonne, Jean-Marc. *Levinas and the Greek Heritage*. Leuven: Peeters, 2006.

Nasio, Juan-David. *Le silence en psychanalyse*. Paris: Désir/Payot, 1998.

Nesteruk, Alexei V. "From the Unknowability of the Universe to the Teleology of Reason: A Phenomenological Insight into Apophatic Cosmology." In *Knowing the Unknowable: Science and Religions on God and the Universe*, edited by John Bowker, pp. 63–86. London: I. B. Tauris, 2009.

Neusner, Jacob. "Science and Magic, Miracle and Magic in Formative Judaism: The System and the Difference." In *Religion, Science, and Magic: In Concert and in Conflict*, edited by Jacob Neusner, Ernest S. Frerichs, and Paul Virgil McCracken Flesher, pp. 61–81. New York: Oxford University Press, 1989.

Nicholson, Reynold A. *Studies in Islamic Mysticism*. Cambridge: Cambridge University Press, 1921.

Niehoff, Maren R. "A Dream Which Is Not Interpreted Is Like a Letter Which Is Not Read." *Journal of Jewish Studies* 43 (1992): 58–84.

Niekerk, Anton A. van. "Postmetaphysical versus Postmodern Thinking: Retaining the Baby without the Bathwater." *Philosophy Today* 39 (1995): 171–84.

Nietzsche, Friedrich. *Beyond Good and Evil*. In *Basic Writings of Nietzsche*. Translated and edited, with commentaries, by Walter Kaufmann, pp. 192–435. New York: Modern Library, 1968.

——. *The Birth of Tragedy*. In *Basic Writings of Nietzsche*. Translated and edited, with commentaries, by Walter Kaufmann, pp. 17–144. New York: Modern Library, 1968.

——. *Humanity, All Too Human, I*. Translated, with an Afterword, by Gary Handwerk. Stanford: Stanford University Press, 1995.

——. *On Truth and Lying in a Non-Moral* Sense. In *The Birth of Tragedy and Other Writings*. Edited by Raymond Geuss and Ronald Speirs. Translated by Ronald Speirs. Cambridge: Cambridge University Press, 1999.

——. *Sämtliche Werke: Kritische Studienausgabe*. Edited by Giorgio Colli and Mazzino Montinari. 15 vols. Berlin: Walter de Gruyter, 1999.

——. *Unpublished Writings from the Period of Unfashionable Observations*. Translated, with an Afterword, by Richard T. Gray. Stanford: Stanford University Press, 1995.

Nissim ben Moses of Marseilles, *Ma'aseh Nissim: Perush la-Torah*. Edited by Howard Kreisel. Jerusalem: Mekize Nirdamim, 2000.

Nobus, Dany. "Lacan's Science of the Subject: Between Linguistics and Topology." In *The Cambridge Companion to Lacan*, edited by Jean-Michel Rabaté, pp. 50–68. Cambridge: Cambridge University Press, 2003.

Noegel, Scott B. *Nocturnal Ciphers: The Allusive Language of Dreams in the Ancient Near East*. New Haven: American Oriental Society, 2007.

Novalis. *Notes for a Romantic Encyclopaedia: Das Allgemeine Brouillon*. Translated, edited, and with an introduction by David W. Wood. Albany: State University of New York Press, 2007.

——. *Novalis: Philosophical Writings*. Translated and edited by Margaret Mahony Stoljar. Albany: State University of New York Press, 1997.

Nuki, Shigeto. "Phenomenology as Calculus?" In *Phenomenology: Japanese and American Perspectives*, edited by Burt C. Hopkins, pp. 1–14. Dordrecht: Kluwer, 1999.

Oakes, Robert. "Life, Death, and the Hiddenness of God." *International Journal for Philosophy of Religion* 64 (2008): 155–60.

Oberhelman, Steven M. "Dreams in Graeco-Roman Medicine." *Aufstieg und Niedergang der römischen Welt* II.37.1 (1993): 121–56.

O'Donovan-Anderson, Michael. *Content and Comportment: On Embodiment and the Epistemic Availability of the World*. Lanham: Rowman & Littlefield, 1997.

——. "Merleau-Ponty and the Fourth Dogma of Empiricism." Available at http://www.cs.umd.edu/~anderson/papers/apa2000pdf.

O'Flaherty, Wendy Doniger. *Dreams, Illusion and Other Realities*. Chicago: University of Chicago Press, 1984.

Oppenheim, A. Leo. "The Interpretation of Dreams in the Ancient Near East, with a Translation of an Assyrian Dream-Book." *Transactions of the American Philosophical Society* 46 (1956): 179–373.

——. "Mantic Dreams in the Ancient Near East." In *The Dream and Human Societies*, edited by Gustave Edmund von Grunebaum and Roger Caillois, pp. 341–50. Berkeley: University of California Press, 1966.

Ornet, Leah. "Expressions of Mystical Union in R. Shneur Zalman of Liadi." *Tarbiz* 74 (2004): 585–611 (Hebrew).

——. *"Ratso va-shov, Running and Returning": Ethical and Mystical Perspectives in the Teaching of R. Shneur Zalman of Liadi—A Comparative Study*. Tel-Aviv: Hakibbutz Hameuchad, 2007 (Hebrew).

Ornstein, Robert. *The Evolution of Consciousness: Of Darwin, Freud, and Cranial Fire—The Origins of the Way We Think*. New York: Prentice-Hall, 1991.

Oron, Michal. "Dream, Vision, and Reality in Ḥayyim Viṭal's *Book of Visions*." *Jerusalem Studies in Jewish Thought* 10 (1992): 299–309 (Hebrew).

O'Sullivan, Michael. *The Incarnation of Language: Joyce, Proust and a Philosophy of the Flesh*. New York: Continuum, 2008.

——. *Michel Henry: Incarnation, Barbarism, and Belief*. Oxford: Peter Lang, 2006.

Oubré, Alondra Yvette. *Instinct and Revelation: Reflections on the Origins of Numinous Perception*. Amsterdam: Gordon and Breach, 1997.

Overgaard, Søren. *Husserl and Heidegger on Being in the World*. Dordrecht: Kluwer, 2004.

Pace-Schott, Edward F. "Postscript: Recent Findings on the Neurobiology of Sleep and Dreaming." In *Sleep and Dreaming: Scientific Advances and Reconsiderations*, edited by Edward F. Pace-Schitt, Mark Solms, Mark Blagorve, and Stevan Harnad, pp. 335–50. Cambridge: Cambridge University Press, 2003.

Pachter, Mordecai. *Roots of Faith and Devequt: Studies in the History of Kabbalistic Ideas*. Los Angeles: Cherub Press, 2004.

Parkes, Graham. *Composing the Soul: Reaches of Nietzsche's Psychology*. Chicago: University of Chicago Press, 1994.

Parman, Susan. *Dream and Culture: An Anthropological Study of the Western Intellectual Tradition*. New York: Praeger, 1991.

Parsons, William B. *The Enigma of the Oceanic Feeling: Revisioning the Psychoanalytic Theory of Mysticism*. New York: Oxford University Press, 1999.

Patai, Raphael. *The Hebrew Goddess*. New York: Ktav, 1967.

Patton, Kimberley C. "'A Great and Strange Correction': Intentionality, Locality, and Epiphany in the Category of Dream Incubation." *History of Religions* 43 (2004): 194–223.

Pedaya, Ḥaviva. "The Baal Shem Tov, R. Jacob Joseph of Polonnoye, and the Maggid of Mezhirech: Outlines for a Religious Typology." *Da'at* 45 (2000): 25–73 (Hebrew).

——. "The Baal Shem Tov's Iggeret Hakodesh Toward a Critique of the Textual Versions and an Exploration of Its Convergence with the World Picture: Messianism, Revelation, Ecstasy, and the Sabbatean Background." *Zion* 70 (2005): 311–54 (Hebrew).

——. *Nahmanides: Cyclical Times and Holy Text*. Tel-Aviv: Am Oved, 2003 (Hebrew).

Pedaya, Yehudah. *Minḥat Yehudah*. Jerusalem, 1990.

Peperzak, Adriaan T. *Beyond: The Philosophy of Emmanuel Levinas*. Evanston: Northwestern University Press, 1997.

The Perfection of Wisdom in Eight Thousand Lines and Its Verse Summary. Translated by Edward Conze. Bolinas: Four Seasons Foundation, 1973.

Philo. *On Dreams*. Translated by Francis H. Colson and George H. Whitaker. Cambridge, MA: Harvard University Press, 1968.

——. *The Special Laws*. Translated by Francis H. Colson. Cambridge, MA: Harvard University Press, 1968.

Phineḥas of Korzec. *Imrei Pinḥas ha-Shalem*. Edited by Elimelekh Eleazar Frankel. 2 vols. Benei Beraq: Yeḥezqel Shraga Frankel, 2003.

Piekarz, Mendel. *Between Ideology and Reality: Humility, Ayin, Self-Negation, and Devekut in the Hasidic Thought*. Jerusalem: Bialik Institute, 1994 (Hebrew).

Pieper, Josef. "*Divine Madness*": *Plato's Case against Secular Humanism*. Translated by Lothar Krauth. San Francisco: Ignatius Press, 1995.

——. *Enthusiasm and Divine Madness: On the Platonic Dialogue Phaedrus*. Translated by Richard and Clara Winston. New York: Harcourt, Brace & World, 1964.

Pihlström, Sami. *Naturalizing the Transcendental: A Pragmatic View*. Amherst: Humanity Books, 2003.

Pines, Shlomo. "The Arabic Recension of *Parva Naturalia* and the Philosophical Doctrine concerning Veridical Dreams according to *al-Risāla al-Manāmiyya* and Other Sources." *Israel Oriental Studies* 4 (1974): 104–53.

——. *The Collected Works of Shlomo Pines: Studies in the History of Jewish Thought*, vol. 5. Edited by Warren Zev Harvey and Moshe Idel. Jerusalem: Magnes Press, 1997.

——. "Dieu et l'être selon Maïmonide: Exégèse d'Exode 3, 14 et doctrine connexe." In *Celui qui est: Interprétations juives et chrétiennes d'Exode 3, 14*, edited by Alain de Libera and Emile Zum Brunn, pp. 15–24. Paris: Cerf, 1986.

——. "The Limitations of Human Knowledge according to Al-Farabi, Ibn Bajja, and Maimonides." In *Studies in Medieval Jewish History and Literature*, edited by Isadore Twersky, pp. 82–109. Cambridge, MA: Harvard University Press, 1979.

——. "Les limites de la métaphysique selon al-Farrabi, Ibn Bajja, et Maïmonide: Sources et antitheses de ces doctrines chez Alexandre d'Aprodise et chez Themistius." *Miscellanea Mediaevalia* 13 (1981): 211–25.

——. "Truth and Falsehood Versus Good and Evil: A Study in Jewish and General Philosophy in Connection with The Guide of the Perplexed, 1.2." In *Studies in Maimonides*, edited by Isadore Twersky, pp. 95–157. Cambridge, MA: Harvard University Press, 1990.

Pines, Shlomo, and Tuvia Gelblum. "Al-Bīrūnī's Arabic Version of Patañjali's *Yogasūtra*: A Translation of His First Chapter and a Comparison with Related Sanskrit Texts." *Bulletin of the School of Oriental and African Studies* 29 (1966): 302–25.

Pirqei Rabbi Eli'ezer. Warsaw, 1852.

Plato. *The Collected Dialogues of Plato Including the Letters*. Edited by Edith Hamilton and Huntington Cairns. Princeton: Princeton University Press, 1980.

Polansky, Ronald M. *Philosophy and Knowledge: A Commentary on Plato's Theaetetus*. Lewisburg: Bucknell University Press, 1992.

Popovics, Zoltán. "'Counter-time': A Non-dialectical Temporality in the Works of Maurice Blanchot." *Colloquy: Text Theory Critique* 10 (2005): 42–56.

Poppers, Meir. *Me'orot Natan*. Frankfurt am Main, 1709.

The Practice of the Six Yogas of Naropa. Translated, edited, and introduced by Glenn H. Mullin. Ithaca: Snow Lion Publications, 1997.

Pratt, Louise. "*Odyssey* 19.535–50: On the Interpretation of Dreams and Signs in Homer." *Classical Philology* 19 (1994): 147–52.

Price, S. R. F. "The Future of Dreams: From Freud to Artemidorus." *Past and Present* 113 (1986): 3–37.

Price-Williams, Douglass. "The Waking Dream in Ethnographic Perspective." In *Dreaming: Anthropological and Psychological Interpretations*, edited by Barbara Tedlock, pp. 246–62. Cambridge: Cambridge University Press, 1987.

Purcell, Michael. *Levinas and Theology*. Cambridge: Cambridge University Press, 2006.

Putt, B. Keith. "Theopoetics of the Possible." In *After God: Richard Kearney and the Religious Turn in Continental Philosophy*, edited by John Panteleimon Manoussakis, pp. 241–69. New York: Fordham University Press, 2006.

Radhakrishnan, Sarvepalli. *Indian Philosophy*. 2 vols. Oxford: Oxford University Press, 1929.

Raffel, Charles M. "Providence as Consequent upon Intellect: Maimonides' Theory of Providence." *Association for Jewish Studies Review* 12 (1987): 25–71.

Rahman, Fazlur. *Avicenna's Psychology*. London: Oxford University Press, 1952.

——. "Dream, Imagination, and 'Ālam al-mithāl." In *The Dream and Human Societies*, edited by Gustave Edmund von Grunebaum and Roger Caillois, pp. 409–19. Berkeley: University of California Press, 1966.

Rainey, Reuben M. *Freud as Student of Religion: Perspectives on the Background and Development of His Thought*. Missoula: Scholars Press, 1975.

Ravitzky, Aviezer. "Hebrew Quotations from the Lost Arabic Recension of *Parva Naturalia*." *Jerusalem Studies in Arabic and Islam* 3 (1981–1982): 191–202.

——. *History and Faith: Studies in Jewish Philosophy*. Amsterdam: J. C. Gieben, 1996.

——. "The Secrets of The Guide of the Perplexed: Between the Thirteenth and Twentieth Centuries." In *Studies in Maimonides*, edited by Isadore Twersky, pp. 159–207. Cambridge, MA: Harvard University Press, 1990.

Ravven, Heidi M. "Some Thoughts on What Spinoza Learned from Maimonides about the Prophetic Imagination, Part One: Maimonides on Prophecy and Imagination." *Journal of the History of Philosophy* 39 (2001): 193–214.

——. "Some Thoughts on What Spinoza Learned from Maimonides about the Prophetic Imagination, Part Two: Spinoza's Maimonideanism." *Journal of the History of Philosophy* 39 (2001): 385–406.

Raz, Shoey. "Isaac Ibn Laṭif and the Guide of the Perplexed." M.A. thesis, Bar-Ilan University, 2004 (Hebrew).

——. "Metaphysics and the Account of the Chariot: Maimonides and Iṣḥaq Ibn Laṭif." In *Maimonides and Mysticism: Presented to Moshe Hallamish On the Occasion of his Retirement*, edited by Avraham Elqayam and Dov Schwartz, pp. 133–64 [*Da'at* 64–66]. Ramat-Gan: Bar-Ilan University Press, 2009 (Hebrew).

Reines, Alvin. "Maimonides' Concept of Mosaic Prophecy." *Hebrew Union College Annual* 40–41 (1969–70): 325–62.

Renard, John. *Friends of God: Islamic Images of Piety, Commitment, and Servanthood*. Berkeley: University of California Press, 2008.

Renberg, Gil H. "'Commanded By the Gods': An Epigraphical Study of Dreams and Visions in Greek and Roman Religious Life." Ph.D. dissertation, Duke University, 2003.

Rice, Emanuel. *Freud and Moses: The Long Journey Home*. Albany: State of New York Press, 1990.

Richardson, John. "Nietzsche Contra Darwin." *Philosophy and Phenomenological Research* 65 (2002): 537–75.

Richir, Marc. "Le sensible dans le rêve." In *Merleau-Ponty: Notes de cours sur l'origine de la géométrie de Husserl; suivi de Récherches sur la phénoménologie de Merleau-Ponty*, edited by Renaud Barbaras, pp. 239–54. Paris: Presses Universitaires de France, 1998.

Ricklin, Thomas. *Der Traum der Philosophie im 12. Jahrhundert: Traumtheorien zwischen Constantinus Africanus und Aristoteles*. Leiden: Brill, 1998.

Ricoeur, Paul. *Freud and Philosophy: An Essay on Interpretation*. Translated by Denis Savage. New Haven: Yale University Press, 1970.

———. *Interpretation Theory: Discourse and the Surplus of Meaning*. Fort Worth: Texas Christian Press, 1976.

Riffaterre, Michael. *Fictional Truth*. Baltimore: Johns Hopkins University Press, 1990.

Rizo-Patron, Eileen. "On the Role of the Oneiric in Testimonial Narrative." In *Traversing the Imaginary: Richard Kearney and the Postmodern Challenge*, edited by Peter Gratton and John Panteleimon Manoussakis, foreword by Richard Kearney, pp. 152–64. Evanston: Northwestern University Press, 2007.

Rizvi, Ali Muhammed. "Habermas' Conception of 'Transcendence from Within': An Interpretation." Ph.D. dissertation, La Trobe University, Melbourne, 2007.

Robert, Marthe. *From Oedipus to Moses: Freud's Jewish Identity*. London: Routledge & Kegan Paul, 1977.

Robinson, James T. "Gershom ben Solomon's *Sha'ar ha-Shamayim*: Its Sources and Use of Sources." In *The Medieval Hebrew Encyclopedias of Science and Philosophy: Proceedings of the Bar-Ilan University Conference*, edited by Steven Harvey, pp. 248–74. Dordrecht: Kluwer, 2000.

Roodurmun, Pulasth Soobah. *Bhāmatī and Vivaraṇa Schools of Advaita Vedānta: A Critical Approach*. Delhi: Motilal Banarsidaas, 2002.

Rosenzweig, Franz. *The Star of Redemption*. Translated by Barbara E. Galli. Madison: University of Wisconsin Press, 2005.

Rosman, Moshe. *Founder of Hasidism: A Quest for the Historical Ba'al Shem Tov*. Berkeley: University of California Press, 1996.

Rotenstreich, Nathan. "Symbolism and Transcendence: On Some Philosophical Aspects of Gershom Scholem's Opus." *The Review of Metaphysics* 31 (1978): 604–14.

Rubenstein, Jeffrey L. *The Culture of the Babylonian Talmud*. Baltimore: Johns Hopkins University Press, 2003.

Rubenstein, Mary-Jane. "Of Ghosts and Angels: Derrida, Kushner, and the Impossibility of Forgiveness." *Journal for Cultural and Religious Theory* 9 (2008): 79–95.

———. *Strange Wonder: The Closure of Metaphysics and the Opening of Awe*. New York: Columbia University Press, 2008.

———. "Unknow Thyself: Apophaticism, Deconstruction, and Theology after Ontotheology." *Modern Theology* 19 (2003): 387–417.

Rudd, Anthony. *Expressing the World: Skepticism, Wittgenstein, and Heidegger*. La Salle: Open Court, 2003.

Rūmī, Jalal al-Din. *The Mathnawí of Jalálu'ddin Rúmí*. Edited and translated by Reynold A. Nicholson. London: Luzac, 1926–1940.

Rupprecht, Carol Schreier. "Divinity, Insanity, Creativity: A Renaissance Contribution to the History and Theory of Dream/Text(s)." In *The Dream and the Text: Essays on Literature and Language*, edited by Carol Schreier Rupprecht, pp. 112–32. Albany: State University of New York Press, 1993.

———. "Dreaming, Language, Literature." In *The New Science of Dreaming*, edited by Deirdre Barrett and Patrick McNamara. Vol. 3, *Cultural and Theoretical Perspectives*, pp. 1–34. Westport: Praeger, 2007.

Rupprecht, Carol Schreier, and Kelly Bulkeley, "Reading Yourself to Sleep: Dreams in/and/as Texts." In *The Dream and the Text: Essays on Literature and Language*, edited by Carol Schreier Rupprecht, pp. 1–12. Albany: State University of New York Press, 1993.

Russell, James R. *Armenian and Iranian Studies*. Cambridge, MA: Harvard University Press, 2004.

———. "'Sleep' and 'Dreaming' in Armenian." In *Proceedings of the Fourth International Conference on Armenian Linguistics*, edited by John A. C. Greppin, pp. 147–69. Delmar: Caravan Books, 1992.

Russo, Richard A. "Dream Poetry as Dream Work." *Dreaming* 13 (2003): 13–27.

Rymatzki, Christoph. *Hallischer Pietismus und Judenmission: Johann Heinrich Callenbergs Institutum Judaicum und dessen Freundeskreis*. Tübingen: Niemeyer, 2004.

Sachs, Hanns. *The Creative Unconscious: Studies in the Psychoanalysis of Art*. Edited by Abraham A. Roback. 2nd edition. Cambridge, MA: Sci-Art Publishers, 1951.

Sack, Bracha. *The Kabbalah of Rabbi Moshe Cordovero*. Jerusalem: Bialik Institute, 1995 (Hebrew).

Ṣadoq ha-Kohen of Lublin. *Dover Ṣedeq*. Jerusalem: Makhon Har Berakhah, 2008.

———. *Liqquṭei Ma'amarim*. Jerusalem: Makhon Har Berakhah, 2008.

———. *Maḥashavot Ḥaruṣ*. Jerusalem: Makhon Har Berakhah, 2006.

———. *Resisei Laylah*. Jerusalem: Makhon Har Berakhah, 2003.

———. *Ṣidqat ha-Ṣaddiq*. Jerusalem: Makhon Har Berakhah, 2005.

Saghafi, Kas. *Apparitions—Of Derrida's Other*. New York: Fordham University Press, 2010.

Sallis, John. *Chorology: On Beginning in Plato's Timaeus*. Bloomington: Indiana University Press, 1999.

———. *Delimitations: Phenomenology and the End of Metaphysics*. Bloomington: Indiana University Press, 1986.

———. *The Gathering of Reason*. 2nd edition. Albany: State University of New York Press, 2005.

Samely, Alexander. *Rabbinic Interpretation of Scripture in the Mishnah*. Oxford: Oxford University Press, 2002.

Sandford, Stella. *The Metaphysics of Love: Gender and Transcendence in Levinas*. London: Athlone, 2000.

Sartre, Jean-Paul. *Being and Nothingness: An Essay on Phenomenological Ontology*. Translated and with an introduction by Hazel E. Barnes. New York: Philosophical Library, 1956.

———. *The Imaginary: A Phenomenological Psychology of the Imagination*. Revisions and historical introduction by Arlette Elkaïm-Sartre. Translation and philosophical introduction by Jonathan Webber. London: Routledge, 2004.

———. *The Psychology of Imagination*. Secaucus: Citadel Press, 1972.

Savage-Rumbaugh, Sue, and Kevin McDonald. "Deception and Social Manipulation in Symbol-Using Apes." In *Machiavellian Intelligence: Social Expertise and the Evolution of Intellect in Monkeys, Apes and Humans*, edited by Richard W. Byrne and Andrew Whitten, pp. 224–37. Oxford: Oxford University Press. 1988.

Sawai, Yoshitsugu. "The Structure of Consciousness in Śaṅkara's Philosophy." In *Consciousness and Reality: Studies in Memory of Toshihiko Izutsu*, edited by Sayyid Jalāl al-Dīn Āshtiyānī, Hideichi Matsubara, Takashi Iwami, and Akiro Matsumoto, pp. 323–40. Leiden: Brill, 2000.

Ṣawwa'at ha-Ribash. Brooklyn: Kehot, 1998.

Scarry, Elaine. *Dreaming by the Book*. New York: Farrar, Straus and Giroux, 1999.

———. *Resisting Representation*. New York: Oxford University Press, 1994.

Schäfer, Peter. "Magic and Religion in Ancient Judaism." In *Envisioning Magic: A Princeton Seminar and Symposium*, edited by Peter Schäfer and Hans G. Kippenberg, pp. 19–43. Leiden: Brill, 1997.

Schatz, Rivka. "Contemplative Prayer in Hasidism." In *Studies in Mysticism and Religion Presented to Gershom G. Scholem on His Seventieth Birthday*, pp. 209–26. Jerusalem: Magnes Press, 1967.

Schatz-Uffenheimer, Rivka. *Hasidism as Mysticism: Quietistic Elements in Eighteenth Century Hasidic Thought*. Translated by Jonathan Chipman. Princeton: Princeton University Press, 1993.

Schaub, Uta Liebmann. "Foucault's Oriental Subtext." *Proceedings of the Modern Language Association* 104 (1989): 306–16. Reprinted in *Critical Essays on Michel Foucault*, edited by Karlis Racevskis, pp. 101–17. New York: G.K. Hall, 1999.

Schechterman, Deborah. "Studies in the Short Version of *Sha'ar ha-Shamayim* of Isaac Ibn Laṭif." M.A. thesis, University of Haifa, 1980 (Hebrew).

Scheindlin, Raymond P. *The Gazelle: Medieval Hebrew Poems on God, Israel, and the Soul*. Philadelphia: Jewish Publication Society, 1991.

Schimmel, Annemarie. *Die Träume des Kalifen: Träume und ihre Deutung in der islamischen Kultur*. Munich: Verlag C.H. Beck, 1998.

Schlüter, Margarte. "The Creative Force of a Hermeneutic Rule: The Principle 'There Is No Earlier and Later in the Torah' in Midrashic and Talmudic Literature." In *Creation and Re-Creation in Jewish Thought: Festschrift in Honor of Joseph Dan on the Occasion of His Seventieth Birthday*, edited by Rachel Elior and Peter Schäfer, pp. 59–84. Tübingen: Mohr Siebeck, 2005.

Schmitt, Jean-Claude. *The Conversion of Herman the Jew: Autobiography, History, and Fiction in the Twelfth Century*. Translated by Alex J. Novikoff. Philadelphia: University of Pennsylvania Press, 2010.

Schneersohn, Dov Baer. *Derushei Ḥatunah*, vol. 2. Brooklyn: Kehot, 1991.

——. *Ma'amerei Admor ha-Emṣa'i: Hanaḥot*. Brooklyn: Kehot, 1994.

——. *Ner Miṣwah we-Torah Or*. Brooklyn: Kehot, 1995.

——. *Perush ha-Millot*. Brooklyn: Kehot, 1993.

——. *Sha'arei Orah*. Brooklyn: Kehot, 1979.

——. *Sha'arei Teshuvah*. Brooklyn: Kehot, 1995.

——. *Torat Ḥayyim: Bere'shit*. Brooklyn: Kehot, 1993.

——. *Torat Ḥayyim: Shemot*. Brooklyn: Kehot, 2003.

Schneersohn, Menaḥem Mendel. *Ma'amerei Admur ha-Ṣemaḥ Ṣedeq 5614–5615*. Brooklyn: Kehot, 1997.

——. *Or ha-Torah: Bemidbar*. 4 vols. Brooklyn: Kehot, 1995–2000.

——. *Or ha-Torah: Bere'shit*, vol. 5. Brooklyn: Kehot, 1971.

——. *Or ha-Torah: Devarim*, vol. 6. Brooklyn: Kehot, 1984.

——. *Or ha-Torah: Siddur Tefillah*. Brooklyn: Kehot, 1984.

Schneersohn, Shalom Dovber. *Be-Sha'ah she-Hiqdimu 5672*. Brooklyn: Kehot, 1991.

——. *Sefer ha-Ma'amarim 5678*. Brooklyn: Kehot, 1984.

Schneersohn, Shmuel. *Liqquṭei Torah: Torat Shmu'el 5627*. Brooklyn: Kehot, 2000.

——. *Liqquṭei Torah: Torat Shmu'el 5632*, vol. 1. Brooklyn: Kehot, 1999.

——. *Liqquṭei Torah: Torat Shmu'el 5633*, vol. 2. Brooklyn: Kehot, 1994.

Schneersohn, Yosef Yiṣḥaq. *Sefer ha-Ma'amarim 5689*. Brooklyn: Kehot, 1990.

——. *Sefer ha-Ma'amarim 5692–5693*. Brooklyn: Kehot, 2004.

——. *Sefer ha-Ma'amarim 5710–5711*. Brooklyn: Kehot, 1986.

——. *Sefer ha-Siḥot 5696 – Ḥoref 5700*. Brooklyn: Kehot, 1989.

Schneerson, Menaḥem Mendel. *Liqquṭei Siḥot*. 39 vols. Brooklyn: Kehot, 1962–2001.

——. *Sefer ha-Ma'amarim 5732–5733*. Brooklyn: Wa'ad Kitvei Qodesh, 1989.

——. *Sefer ha-Ma'amarim 5734–5735*. Brooklyn: Wa'ad Kitvei Qodesh, 1989.

——. *Torat Menaḥem: Hitwwa'aduyyot 5711*, vol. 1. Brooklyn: Lahak Hanochos, 1994.

——. *Torat Menaḥem: Hitwwa'aduyyot 5712*, vol. 1. Brooklyn: Lahak Hanochos, 1995.

——. *Torat Menaḥem: Hitwwa'aduyyot 5712*, vol. 2. Brooklyn: Lahak Hanochos, 1997.

——. *Torat Menaḥem: Hitwwa'aduyot 5712*, vol. 3. Brooklyn: Lahak Hanochos, 1996.

——. *Torat Menaḥem: Hitwwa'aduyyot 5713*, vol. 1. Brooklyn: Lahak Hanochos, 1997.

——. *Torat Menaḥem: Hitwwa'aduyyot 5713*, vol. 2. Brooklyn: Lahak Hanochos, 1997.

——. *Torat Menaḥem: Hitwwa'aduyyot 5713*, vol. 3. Brooklyn: Lahak Hanochos, 1998.

——. *Torat Menaḥem: Hitwwa'aduyyot 5714*, vol. 1. Brooklyn: Lahak Hanochos, 1998.

——. *Torat Menaḥem: Hitwwa'aduyyot 5723*, vol. 1. Brooklyn: Lahak Hanochos, 2007.

——. *Torat Menaḥem: Hitwwa'aduyyot 5742*, vol. 1. Brooklyn: Lahak Hanochos, 1990.

——. *Torat Menaḥem: Hitwwa'aduyyot 5742*, vol. 3. Brooklyn: Lahak Hanochos, 1990.

——. *Torat Menaḥem: Hitwwa'aduyyot 5743*, vol. 1. Brooklyn: Lahak Hanochos, 1990.

——. *Torat Menaḥem: Hitwwa'aduyyot 5743*, vol. 2. Brooklyn: Lahak Hanochos, 1993.

——. *Torat Menaḥem: Hitwwa'aduyyot 5746*, vol. 1. Brooklyn: Lahak Hanochos, 1990.

——. *Torat Menaḥem: Hitwwa'aduyyot 5748*, vol. 1. Brooklyn: Lahak Hanochos, 1990.

——. *Torat Menaḥem: Hitwwa'aduyyot 5751*, vol. 3. Brooklyn: Lahak Hanochos, 1993.

——. *Torat Menaḥem: Sefer ha-Ma'amarim 5714*. Brooklyn: Vaad Hanochos BLahak, 2006.

——. *Torat Menaḥem: Sefer ha-Ma'amarim 5722*. Brooklyn: Vaad Hanochos BLahak, 2001.

——. *Torat Menaḥem: Sefer ha-Ma'amarim 5724*. Brooklyn: Lahak Hanochos, 2010.

Schoenfeld, Devorah. "Madness and Prophecy: Dreams, Texts, and the Power of Rabbinic Interpretation." *Pastoral Psychology* 56 (2007): 223–35.

Scholem, Gerhard. *Das Buch Bahir: Ein Schriftdenkmal aus der Frühzeit der Kabbala auf Grund der kritischen Neuausgabe.* Leipzig: W. Druglin, 1923.

Scholem, Gershom. *Devils, Demons, and Souls: Essays on Demonology by Gershom Scholem*. Edited by Esther Liebes. Jerusalem: Ben-Zvi Institute, 2004 (Hebrew).

——. "Did Rabbi Moses de León Compose the Book of the Zohar?" *Madda'ei ha-Yahadut* 1 (1926): 26–27 (Hebrew).

——. *The Dreams of R. Mordecai Ashkenazi: A Follower of Shabbetai Zevi*. Jerusalem: Schocken, 1938 (Hebrew).

——. "The First Citation from the Midrash ha-Ne'lam." *Tarbiz* 3 (1932): 181–83 (Hebrew).

——. *Lurianic Kabbalah: Collected Studies by Gershom Scholem*. Edited by Daniel Abrams. Los Angeles: Cherub Press, 2008 (Hebrew).

——. "The Maggid of R. Joseph Taitatzak." *Sefunot* 11 (1968): 47–112 (Hebrew).

——. *Major Trends in Jewish Mysticism*. New York: Schocken Books, 1954.

——. *The Messianic Idea in Judaism and Other Essays on Jewish Spirituality*. New York: Schocken Books, 1971.

——. "The Name of God and the Linguistic Theory of the Kabbala." *Diogenes* 79 (1972): 59–80; 80 (1972): 164–94.

——. *On Jews and Judaism in Crisis: Selected Essays*. Edited by Werner J. Dannhauser. New York: Schocken Books, 1976.

——. *On the Kabbalah and Its Symbolism*. Translated by Ralph Manheim. New York: Schocken Books, 1969.

——. *On the Possibility of Jewish Mysticism in Our Time and Other Essays*. Edited and with an introduction by Avraham Shapira. Translated by Jonathan

Chipman. Philadelphia: Jewish Publication Society of America, 1997.
——. *Origins of the Kabbalah*. Edited by R. J. W. Werblowsky. Translated by Allan Arkush. Princeton: Princeton University Press, 1987.
——. "Schöpfung aus Nichts und Selbstverschränkung Gottes." *Eranos Jahrbuch* 25 (1956): 87–119.
Schopenhauer, Arthur. *The World as Will and Representation*. Translated by E. F. J. Payne. 2 vols. Indian Hills: Falcon's Wing Press, 1958.
Schrag, Calvin O. *God as Otherwise Than Being: Toward a Semantics of the Gift*. Evanston: Northwestern University Press, 2002.
Schroeder, Brian. "A Trace of the Eternal Return? Levinas and Neoplatonism." In *Levinas and the Ancients*, edited by Brian Schroeder and Silvia Benso, pp. 210–29. Bloomington: Indiana University Press, 2008.
Schwartz, Dov. "The Quadripartite Division of the Intellect in Medieval Jewish Thought." *Jewish Quarterly Review* 84 (1993–94): 227–36.
Schwarzschild, Steven. *The Pursuit of the Ideal: Jewish Writings of Steven Schwarzschild*. Edited by Menachem Kellner. Albany: State University of New York Press, 1990.
Schweid, Eliezer. *Judaism and Mysticism According to Gershom Scholem: A Critical Analysis and Programmatic Discussion*. Translated with an introduction by David Avraham Weiner. Atlanta: Scholars Press, 1985.
Seder Avodat Yisra'el. Edited by Seligman Baer. Berlin: Schocken, 1937.
Sefer ha-Peli'ah. Przemysl: Zupnik, Knoller, and Hammerschmidt, 1883.
Sefer ha-Zohar. Edited and annotated by Reuven Margaliot. 3 vols. Jerusalem: Mosad ha- Rav Kook, 1960.
Sefer Yeṣirah. Jerusalem: Yeshivat Kol Yehuda, 1990.
Sefer Yezirah with Commentary by Dunash Ben Tamim. Edited by Menasche Grossberg. London: R. W. Rabinowicz, 1902.
Seidel, Jonathan L. "Charming Criminals: Classification of Magic in the Babylonian Talmud." In *Ancient Magic and Ritual Power*, edited by Marvin Meyer and Paul Mirecki, pp. 145–66. Leiden: E. J. Brill, 1995.
——. "Studies in Ancient Jewish Magic." Ph.D. dissertation, University of California, Berkeley, 1996.
Seifert, Josef. *Back to Things Themselves: A Phenomenological Foundation for Classical Realism*. New York: Routledge & Kegan Paul, 1987.
Sellars, Roy Wood. "Referential Transcendence." *Philosophy and Phenomenological Research* 22 (1961): 1–15.
Sellars, Wilfrid. *Empiricism and the Philosophy of Mind*. With an introduction by Richard Rorty and a study guide by Robert Brandom. Cambridge, MA: Harvard University Press, 1997.

Shafton, Anthony. *Dream Reader: Contemporary Approaches to the Understanding of Dreams*. Albany: State University of New York Press, 1995.

Shainberg, Catherine. *Kabbalah and the Power of Dreaming: Awakening the Visionary Life*. Rochester: Inner Traditions, 2005.

Shamdasani, Sonu. *Jung and the Making of Modern Psychology: The Dream of a Science*. Cambridge: Cambridge University Press, 2003.

Shapiro, Kam. *Carl Schmitt and the Intensification of Politics*. Lanham: Rowman & Littlefield, 2008

———. "Politics Is a Mushroom: Worldly Sources of Rule and Exception in Carl Schmitt and Walter Benjamin." *Diacritics* 37 (2007): 121–34.

Sharma, Arvind. *The Philosophy of Religion and Advaita Vedānta: A Comparative Study in Religion and Reason*. University Park: Pennsylvania State University Press, 1995.

———. *Sleep as a State of Consciousness in Advaita Vedānta*. Albany: State University of New York Press, 2004.

———. *The World as Dream*. New Delhi: D. K. Printworld, 2006.

Sharpe, Ella Freeman. *Dream Analysis: A Practical Handbook for Psycho-Analysts*. London: Hogarth, 1937.

Shaviv, Yehuda. "The Words of Dreams Do Not Raise Up or Bring Down." *Sinai* 111 (1993): 174–77 (Hebrew).

Shayegan, Daryush. *Henry Corbin: La topographie spirituelle de l'islam iranien*. Paris: Éditions de la Différence, 1990.

Shefi, Avishar Har. "Malchin Kadmain: The Myth of the Edomite Kings in the Idrot Literature—The First Appearance." M.A. thesis, Bar-Ilan University, 2006 (Hebrew).

Shields, Philip. "Dreaming and Interpretation: A Treatment of the Interpretation of Dreams as a Dream." *Psychoanalysis and Contemporary Thought* 13 (1990): 79–105.

Shinan, Avigdor. "The Dream in Midrash and the Midrash of the Dream." In *The Spectrum of Opinions and Worldviews about Dreams in Jewish Culture*, edited by Dror Kerem, pp. 43–61. Reḥovot, 1995 (Hebrew).

Shneur Zalman of Liadi, *Liqquṭei Amarim: Tanya*. Brooklyn: Kehot, 1984.

———. *Liqquṭei Torah*. 2 vols. Brooklyn: Kehot, 1996–1998.

———. *Ma'amerei Admor ha-Zaqen 5562*. Brooklyn: Kehot, 1975.

———. *Ma'amerei Admur ha-Zaqen 5565*, vol. 1. Brooklyn: Kehot, 1980.

———. *Ma'amerei Admor ha-Zaqen: Ketuvim*, vol. 1. Brooklyn: Kehot, 1985.

———. *Ma'amerei Admor ha-Zaqen: Al Ma'amerei Razal*. Brooklyn: Kehot, 1984.

———. *Seder Tefillot mi-kol ha-Shanah*. Brooklyn: Kehot, 1986.

———. *Torah Or*. Brooklyn: Kehot, 1991.

Shulman, David. "Dreaming the Self in South India." In *Dream Cultures: Explorations in the Comparative History of Dreaming*, edited by David Shulman and Guy G. Stroumsa, pp. 43–73. New York: Oxford University Press, 1999.

Shwartz, Itamar. *Qol Demamah Daqqah* [*Bilevavi Mishkan Evneh*, vol. 10]. Jerusalem, n.d.

Sifre on Deuteronomy. Edited by Louis Finkelstein. New York: Jewish Theological Seminary of America, 1969.

Sikka, Sonya. *Forms of Transcendence: Heidegger and Medieval Mystical Theology*. Albany: State University of New York Press, 1997.

Silman, Yochanan. *Philosopher and Poet: Judah Halevi, the Kuzari, and the Evolution of His Thought*. Translated by Lenn J. Schramm. Albany: State University of New York Press, 1995.

Sinha, Debabrata. *Metaphysic of Experience in Advaita Vedānta: A Phenomenological Approach*. Delhi: Motilal Banarsidass, 1983.

Sirat, Colette. *Les théories des visions surnaturelles dans la pensée juive du moyen-âge*. Leiden: E. J. Brill, 1969.

Skrbina, David. *Panpsychism in the West*. Cambridge, MA: The MIT Press, 2005.

Smith, Daniel W. "Deleuze and Derrida, Immanence and Transcendence: Two Directions in Recent French Thought." In *Between Deleuze and Derrida*, edited by Paul Patton and John Protevi, pp. 46–66. New York: Continuum, 2003.

Snyder, Holly. "A Tree with Two Different Fruits: The Jewish Encounter with German Pietists in the Eighteenth Century Atlantic World." *The William and Mary Quarterly* 58 (2001): 855–82.

Solms, Mark. "Dreaming and REM Sleep Are Controlled By Different Brain Mechanisms." In *Sleep and Dreaming: Scientific Advances and Reconsiderations*, edited by Edward F. Pace-Schitt, Mark Solms, Mark Blagorve, and Stevan Harnad, pp. 51–58. Cambridge: Cambridge University Press, 2003.

——. *The Neuropsychology of Dreams: A Clinico-Anatomical Study*. Mahwah: Lawrence Erlbaum Associates, 1997.

Solms, Mark, and Oliver Turnbull. *The Brain and the Inner World: An Introduction to the Neuroscience of Subjective Experience*. New York: Other Press, 2002.

A Sourcebook in Indian Philosophy. Edited by Sarvepalli Radhakrishnan and Charles E. Moore. Princeton: Princeton University Press, 1957.

Sperber, Daniel. *Magic and Folklore in Rabbinic Literature*. Ramat-Gan: Bar-Ilan University Press. 1994.

Srajek, Martin C. *In the Margins of Deconstruction: Jewish Conceptions of Ethics in Emmanuel Levinas and Jacques Derrida*. Dordrecht: Kluwer, 1997.

Staehler, Tanja. *Plato and Levinas: The Ambiguous Out-Side of Ethics.* New York: Routledge, 2010.

Stambaugh, Joan. *The Formless Self.* Albany: State University of New York Press, 1999.

Stapp, Henry P. "Quantum Interactive Dualism: An Alternative to Materialism."Available at http://www-physics.lbl.gov/~stapp/QID.pdf.

States, Bert O. "Bizarreness in Dreams and Other Fictions." In *The Dream and the Text: Essays on Literature and Language*, edited by Carol Schreier Rupprecht, pp. 13–31. Albany: State University of New York Press, 1993.

——. "Dream Bizarreness and Inner Thought." *Dreaming* 10 (2000): 179–92.

——. "Dreaming and Storytelling." *Hudson Review* 43 (1990): 571–86.

——. *Dreaming and Storytelling*. Ithaca: Cornell University Press, 1993.

——. *The Rhetoric of Dreams*. Ithaca: Cornell University Press, 1988.

——. *Seeing in the Dark: Reflections on Dreams and Dreaming*. New Haven: Yale University Press, 1997.

Steeves, James B. *Imagining Bodies: Merleau-Ponty's Philosophy of Imagination.* Pittsburgh: Duquesne University Press, 2004.

Steinbock, Anthony J. "Face and Revelation: Levinas on Teaching as Way-Faring." In *Addressing Levinas*, edited by Eric Sean Nelson, Antje Kapust, and Kent Still, pp. 119–37. Evanston: Northwestern University Press, 2005.

Steinschneider, Moritz. *Die hebräischen übersetzungen des mittelalters und die Juden als dolmetscher: Ein Beitrag zur literaturgeschichte des mittelalters, meist nach handschriftlichen quellen*. Berlin: Kommissionsverlag des Bibliographischen Bureaus, 1893.

Stekel, Wilhelm. *Sex and Dreams: The Language of Dreams*. Translated by James S. Van Teslaar. Boston: Gorham Press, 1922.

Stellardi, Giuseppe. *Heidegger and Derrida on Philosophy and Metaphor*. Amherst: Humanity Books, 2000.

Stemberger, Brigitte. "Der Traum in der rabbinischen Literatur." *Kairos: Zeitschrift für Religionswissenschaft und Theologie* 18 (1976): 1–42.

Stephen, Michele. "Memory, Emotion, and the Imaginal Mind." In *Dreaming and the Self: New Perspectives on Subjectivity, Identity, and Emotion*, edited by Jeannette Marie Mageo, pp. 97–129. Albany: State University of New York Press, 2003.

Stern, Josef. "The Enigma of the *Guide of the Perplexed* I, 68." In *Maimonides: Conservatism, Originality, Revolution*, 2 vols., edited by Aviezer Ravitzky, 2:437–51. Jerusalem: Zalman Shazar Center for Jewish History, 2008 (Hebrew).

——. "Maimonides on the Growth of Knowledge and the Limitations of the

Intellect." In *Maïmonide, philosophie et savant (1138–1204)*, edited by Tony Lévy and Roshdi Rashed, pp. 143–91. Leuven: Peters, 2004.

——. Maimonides on Language and the Science of Language." In *Maimonides and the Sciences*, edited by Robert S. Cohen and Hillel Levine, pp. 173–226. Dordrecht: Kluwer, 2000.

Stern, Samuel M. "Ibn Ḥasdāy's Neoplatonist: A Neoplatonic Treatise and Its Influence on Isaac Israeli and the Longer Version of the Theology of Aristotle." *Oriens* 13–14 (1960–61): 58–120.

——. "Rationalists and Kabbalists in Medieval Allegory." *Journal of Jewish Studies* 6 (1955): 73–86.

Stevens, Anthony. "Jungian Psychology, the Body, and the Future." *Journal of Analytic Psychology* 40 (1995): 353–64.

——. *Private Myths: Dreams and Dreaming*. Cambridge, MA: Harvard University Press, 1995.

Stokes, Douglas M. *The Nature of Mind: Parapsychology and the Role of Consciousness in the Physical World.* Jefferson: McFarland, 1997.

Straight From the Heart: Buddhist Pith Instructions. Translated and introduced by Karl Brunnhölzl. Ithaca: Snow Lion Productions, 2007.

Strawser, Michael. *Both/And: Reading Kierkegaard From Irony to Edification*. New York: Fordham University Press, 1997.

Stroumsa, Guy G. "Madness and Divinization in Early Christian Monasticism." In *Self and Self-Transformation in the History of Religions*, edited by David Shulman and Guy G. Stroumsa, pp. 73–88. Oxford: Oxford University Press, 2002.

Stroumsa, Sarah. *Maimonides in His World: Portrait of a Mediterranean Thinker.* Princeton: Princeton University Press, 2009.

——. "The Literary Corpus of Maimonides and Averroes." *Maimonidean Studies* 5 (2008): 223–41.

Struck, Peter. *Birth of the Symbol: Ancient Readers at the Limits of Their Texts.* Princeton: Princeton University Press, 2004.

——. "The Self in Artemidorus' *Interpretation of Dreams*." In *Religion and the Self in Antiquity*, edited by David Brakke, Michael L. Satlow, and Steven Weitzman, pp. 109–22. Bloomington: Indiana University Press, 2005.

——. "Viscera and the Divine: Dreams as the Divinatory Bridge between the Corporeal and the Incorporeal." In *Prayer, Magic, and the Stars in Ancient and Late Antique World*, edited by Scott Noegel, Joel Walker and Brannon Wheeler, pp. 125–36. University Park: Pennsylvania State University Press, 2003.

Subtelny, Maria E. "Le motif du trône et les rapports entre mystique islamique et mystique juive." In *Henry Corbin: Philosophies et sagesses des religions du livre*, edited by Mohammad Ali Amir-Moezzi, Christian Jambet, and Pierre Lory, pp. 195–212. Turnhout: Brepols, 2005.

——. "The Traces of the Traces: Reflections of the Garden in the Persian Mystical Imagination." In *Gardens and Imagination: Cultural History and Agency*, Dumbarton Oaks Colloquium on the History of Landscape Architecture, edited by Michael Conan, pp. 19–39. Washington, D.C.: Dumbarton Oaks Research Library and Collection, 2008.

Sumegi, Angela. *Dreamworlds of Shamanism and Tibetan Buddhism: The Third Place.* Albany: State University of New York Press, 2008.

Suzuki, Daisetz T. *The Zen Doctrine of No Mind: The Significance of the Sūtra of Hui-neng (Wei-Lang).* Edited by Christmas Humphreys. New York: Samuel Weiser, 1972.

Sviri, Sara. "Dreaming Analyzed and Recorded: Dreams in the World of Medieval Islam." In *Dream Cultures: Explorations in the Comparative History of Dreaming*, edited by David Shulman and Guy G. Stroumsa, pp. 252–73. New York: Oxford University Press, 1999.

——. "Fear and Hope: On the Coincidence of Opposites in Islamic Mysticism." *Jerusalem Studies in Arabic and Islam* 9 (1987): 316–49.

Taber, John. "Reason, Revelation and Idealism in Śaṅkara's Vedānta." In *Indian Philosophy: A Collection of Readings*, edited with introductions by Roy W. Perrett, pp. 161–85. New York: Garland Publishing, 2000.

Tacey, David. "Imagining Transcendence at the End of Modernity: Jung and Derrida." In *Dreaming the Myth Onwards: New Directions in Jungian Therapy and Thought*, edited by Lucy Huskinson, pp. 58–68. London: Routledge, 2008.

Talbot, Michael. *Mysticism and the New Physics.* London: Penguin Books, 1993.

Tamar, David. "The Messianic Dreams and Visions of R. Ḥayyim Viṭal." *Shalem* 4 (1984): 211–29 (Hebrew).

Taylor, Mark C. *Altarity.* Chicago: University of Chicago Press, 1987.

——. *Erring: A Postmodern A/theology.* Chicago: University of Chicago Press, 1984.

——. *Nots.* Chicago: University of Chicago, 1993.

——. *Tears.* Albany: State University of New York Press, 1990.

Tibetan Yoga and Secret Doctrines. Edited by Walter Y. Evans-Wentz. Oxford: Oxford University Press, 1958.

Theunissen, Michael. *The Other: Studies in the Social Ontology of Husserl, Heidegger, Sartre, and Buber.* Translated by Christopher Macann, with an introduction by Fred R. Dallmayr. Cambridge, MA: The MIT Press, 1984.

Thomas, R. R. "The Narrative of Theory: The Novel in the 'Interpretation of Dreams.'" *Psychohistory Review* 18 (1989): 1–31.

Thurman, Robert A. E. "Transcendence and the Sacred in the Mahāyāna Middle Way." In *Transcendence and the Sacred*, edited by Alan M. Olson and Leroy S. Rouner, pp. 100–14. Notre Dame: University of Notre Dame Press, 1981.

Tigner, Steven S. "Plato's Philosophical Uses of the Dream Metaphor." *American Journal of Philology* 91 (1970): 204–12.

Tillich, Paul. *The Courage to Be*. New Haven: Yale University Press, 1952.

Timalsina, Sthaneshwar. *Consciousness in Indian Philosophy: The Advaita Doctrine of "Awareness Only."* London: Routledge, 2009.

Tiqqunei Zohar. Edited by Reuven Margaliot. Jerusalem: Mosad ha-Rav Kook, 1978.

Tishby, Isaiah. *The Doctrine of Evil and the 'Kelippah' in Lurianic Kabbalism*. Jerusalem: Schocken, 1942 (Hebrew).

———. "Gnostic Doctrines in Sixteenth-Century Jewish Mysticism." *Journal of Jewish Studies* 6 (1955): 146–52.

———. *Messianic Mysticism: Moses Hayim Luzzatto and the Padua School*. Translated by Morris Hoffman. Oxford: Litman Library of Jewish Civilization, 2008.

———. *Paths of Faith and Heresy: Essays in Kabbalah and Sabbateanism*. Jerusalem: Magnes Press, 1982 (Hebrew).

———. *The Wisdom of the Zohar: An Anthology of Texts*. Translated by David Goldstein. Oxford: Oxford University Press, 1989.

Tosafot ha-Shalem: Commentary on the Bible, vol. 9. Edited by Jacob Gellis. Jerusalem: Harry Fischel Institute, 1993 (Hebrew).

Touati, Charles. *La pensée philosophique et théologique de Gersonide*. Paris: Les Éditions de minuit, 1973.

Toumayan, Alain P. *Encountering the Other: The Artwork and the Problem of Difference in Blanchot and Levinas*. Pittsburgh: Duquesne University Press, 2004.

Trachtenberg, Joshua. *Jewish Magic and Superstition: A Study in Folk Religion*. New York: Behrman's Jewish Book House, 1939.

Turner, Donald L., and Ford Turrell. "The Non-Existent God: Transcendence, Humanity, and Ethics in the Philosophy of Emmanuel Levinas." *Philosophia* 35 (2007): 375–82.

Twersky, Isadore. "Did R. Abraham Ibn Ezra Influence Maimonides?" In *Rabbi Abraham Ibn Ezra: Studies in the Writings of a Twelfth-Century Jewish Polymath*, edited by Isadore Twersky and Jay M. Harris, pp. 21–48. Cambridge, MA: Harvard University Press, 1993 (Hebrew section).

Ulrich, Moses. "Paper Clips and Black Cows: On Poetry and Dreams." *The Psychoanalytic Quarterly* 69 (2000): 28–49.

Urbach, Ephraim E. *The Sages: Their Concepts and Beliefs*. Translated by Israel Abrams. Jerusalem: Magnes Press, 1975.

Ur-Rahman, Mu'tazid Wali. "Al- Fârâbî and his Theory of Dreams." *Islamic Culture* 10 (1936): 137–51.

Vajda, Georges. *Le commentaire sur le "Livre de la création" de Dūnaš ben Tāmīm de Kairouan (Xe siècle)*. New edition. Edited and augmented by Paul B. Fenton. Paris-Louvain: Peeters, 2002.

Valabregue-Perry, Sandra. *Concealed and Revealed: 'Ein Sof' in Theosophic Kabbalah*. Los Angeles: Cherub Press, 2010 (Hebrew).

Valle, Moses David. *Sefer Megalleh Amuqot: Be'ur Sefer Iyyov al Derekh Pardes*. Jerusalem, 2009.

———. *Sefer Or Olam: Be'ur Sefer Bere'shit*, vol. 2. Jerusalem, 1994.

Van Peursen, C.A. "Metaphor and Reality." *Man and World* 25 (1992): 165–80.

Vasubandhu. *Wei Shih Er Shih Lun: The Treatise in Twenty Stanzas on Representation-Only*. Translated by Clarence H. Hamilton. New Haven: American Oriental Society, 1938.

The Vedānta Sutras of Bādarāyana with the Commentary of Śaṅkara. Translated by George Thibaut. 2 vols. New York: Dover Publications, 1962.

Veltri, Giuseppe. *Magie und Halakha: Ansätze zu einem empirischen Wissenschaftsbegriff im spätantiken und frühmiitelalterlichen Judentum*. Tübingen: J. C. B. Mohr, 1997.

Ver Eecke, Wilfried. *Denial, Negation, and the Forces of the Negative: Freud, Hegel, Lacan, Spitz, and Sophocles*. Albany: State University of New York Press, 2006.

Verhack, Ignace. "Immanent Transcendence as Way to 'God': Between Heidegger and Marion." In *Religious Experience and the End of Metaphysics*, edited by Jeffrey Bloechl, pp. 106–18. Bloomington: Indiana University Press, 2003.

Verhaeghe, Paul. "The Dream between Drive and Desire: A Question of Representability." In *The Dreams of Interpretation: A Century down the Royal Road*, edited by Catherine Liu, John Mowitt, Thomas Pepper, and Jakki Spicer, pp. 135–45. Mineapolis: University of Minnesota Press, 2007.

Viṭal, Ḥayyim. *The "Book of Visions": The Diary of Rabbi Hayyim Vital*. Edited with notes and an introduction by Morris M. Faierstein. Jerusalem: Ben-Zvi Institute, 2005 (Hebrew).

———. *Eṣ Ḥayyim*. Jerusalem, 1963.

———. *Jewish Mystical Autobiographies: Book of Visions and Book of Secrets*. Translated and introduced by Morris M. Faierstein. Preface by Moshe Idel. New York: Paulist Press, 1999.

——. *Liqquṭei Torah*. Jerusalem: Yeshivat Kol Yehuda, 1995.

——. *Sefer ha-Pe'ulot: Refu'ot, Segullot, Qabbalah Ma'asit, Kimeyah*. Jerusalem, 2010.

——. *Sha'ar ha-Pesuqim*. Jerusalem: Yeshivat Qol Yehudah, 1995.

——. *Sha'arei Qedushshah*. Jerusalem: Mishor, 2005.

Von Franz, Marie Louise. *Dreams*. Foreword by Robert Hinshaw. Boston: Shambhala, 1991.

Von Grunebaum, Gustav E. "Introduction: The Cultural Function of the Dream as Illustrated by Classical Islam." In *The Dream and Human Societies*, edited by Gustave Edmund von Grunebaum and Roger Caillois, pp. 4–21. Berkeley: University of California Press, 1966.

Wagner, Hans. "Critical Observations Concerning Husserl's Posthumous Writings." In *The Phenomenology of Husserl: Selected Readings*, 2nd edition, edited with an introduction by R. O. Elveton, pp. 192–242. Seattle: Noesis Press, 2000.

Wahl, Jean. *Existence humaine et transcendance*. Neuchatel: Éditions de la Baconnière, 1944.

——. "Realism, Dialectic, and the Transcendent." *Philosophy and Phenomenological Research* 4 (1944): 496–506.

Wallace, B. Alan. *Contemplative Science: Where Buddhism and Neuroscience Converge*. New York: Columbia University Press, 2007.

——. *Hidden Dimensions: The Unification of Physics and Consciousness*. New York: Columbia University Press, 2007.

Walde, Christine. "Dream Interpretation in a Prosperous Age?: Artemidorus, the Greek Interpreter of Dreams." In *Dream Cultures: Explorations in the Comparative History of Dreaming*, edited by David Shulman and Guy G. Stroumsa, pp. 121–42. New York: Oxford University Press, 1999.

Waldenfels, Bernhard. "Levinas on the Saying and the Said." In *Addressing Levinas*, edited by Eric Sean Nelson, Antje Kapust, and Kent Still, pp. 86–97. Evanston: Northwestern University Press, 2005.

Walfish, Barry D. "Typology, Narrative, and History: Isaac ben Joseph ha-Kohen on the Book of Ruth." In *With Reverence for the Word: Medieval Scriptural Exegesis in Judaism, Christianity, and Islam*, edited by Jane Dammen McAuliffe, Barry D. Walfish, and Joseph W. Goering, pp. 119–32. Oxford: Oxford University Press, 2003.

Wallace, Edwin R. "Freud's Mysticism and Its Psychodynamic Determinants." *Bulletin of the Menninger Clinic* 42 (1978): 203–22.

Walton, Kendall L. *Mimesis as Make-Believe: On the Foundations of the Representational Arts*. Cambridge, MA: Harvard University Press, 1990.

Walzer, Richard. "Al-Fārābī's Theory of Prophecy and Divination." *Journal of Hellenic Studies* 77 (1957): 142–48.

——. *Greek into Arabic*. Cambridge, MA: Harvard University Press, 1962.

Ward, Graham. "On Time and Salvation: The Eschatology of Emmanuel Levinas." In *Facing the Other: The Ethics of Emmanuel Levinas*, edited by Seán Hand, pp. 153–72. Surrey: Curzon, 1996.

——. "Transcendence and Representation." In *Transcendence: Philosophy, Literature, and Theology Approach the Beyond*, edited by Regina Schwartz, pp. 127–47. New York: Routledge, 2004.

Warrack, John. *Richard Wagner: Die Meistersinger von Nürnberg*. Cambridge: Cambridge University Press, 1994.

Wasserstrom, Steven M. *Religion After Religion: Gershom Scholem, Mircea Eliade, and Henry Corbin at Eranos*. Princeton: Princeton University Press, 1999.

——. "Sharing Secrets: Inter-Confessional Philosophy as Dialogical Practice." In *New Directions in Jewish Philosophy*, edited by Aaron W. Hughes and Elliot R. Wolfson, pp. 205–28. Bloomington: Indiana University Press, 2010.

Wax, Murray L. "Interpreting Dreams: Joseph, Freud and the Judaic Tradition." *Journal of Psychology and Judaism* 22 (1998): 21–32.

——. *Western Rationality and the Angel of Dreams: Self, Psyche, Dreaming*. Lanham: Rowman & Littlefield, 1999.

Webb, Stephen H. *The Gifting God: A Trinitarian Ethics of Excess*. New York: Oxford University Press, 1996.

Wegner, Daniel M. *The Illusion of Conscious Will*. Cambridge, MA: The MIT Press, 2002.

Weidner, Daniel. *Gershom Scholem: Politisches, esoterisches und historiographisches Schreiben*. Munich: Wilhelm Fink Verlag, 2003.

Weineck, Silke-Maria. *The Abyss Above: Philosophy and Poetic Madness in Plato, Hölderlin, and Nietzsche*. Albany: State University of New York Press, 2002.

Weiss, Ḥayyim. "'Twenty-Four Dream-Interpreters Were in Jerusalem...': On Dream-Interpreters and the Approaches to Dream-Interpretation in the 'Treatise on Dreams' in the Babylonian Talmud." *Madda'ei ha-Yahadut* 44 (2007): 37–77 (Hebrew).

——. "'What This One Interpreted for Me That One Did Not Interpret for Me': A Cultural and Literary Reading of the 'Treatise on Dreams' in the Babylonian Talmud." Ph.D. dissertation, Hebrew University, 2007 (Hebrew).

Weiss, Joseph. *Studies in Eastern European Jewish Mysticism*. Edited by David Goldstein. Oxford: Oxford University Press, 1985.

Werblowsky, R. J. Zwi. *Joseph Karo: Lawyer and Mystic*. Philadelphia: Jewish

Publication Society of America, 1977.

———. "Kabbalistische Buchstabenmystik und der Traum (Joseph ben Abraham Gikatilas Exkurs über Herkunft und Bedeutung der Träume)." *Zeitschrift für Religion und Geistesgeschichte* 8 (1956): 164–69.

Westerkamp, Dirk. *Via Negativa: Sprache und Methode der negativen Theologie.* Munich: Wilhelm Fink Verlag, 2006.

Westphal, Merold. *Levinas and Kierkegaard in Dialogue.* Bloomington: Indiana University Press, 2008.

Wheeler, Samuel C. III. *Deconstruction as Analytic Philosophy.* Stanford: Stanford University Press, 2000.

Whitehead, Alfred North. *Science and the Modern World.* New York: Free Press, 1967.

Wicks, Robert. "Foucault." In *The Blackwell Guide to Continental Philosophy*, edited by Robert C. Solomon and David Sherman, pp. 243–64. Oxford: Blackwell Publishing Ltd, 2003.

Wider, Kathleen V. *The Bodily Nature of Consciousness: Sartre and Contemporary Philosophy of Mind.* Ithaca: Cornell University Press, 1997.

Wikse, John R. "Night Rule: Dreams as Social Intelligence." In *The Variety of Dream Experience: Expanding Our Ways of Working with Dreams*, 2nd edition, edited by Montague Ullman and Claire Limmer, pp. 141–59. Albany: State University of New York Press, 1999.

Wilder, Amos N. *Theopoetic: Theology and the Religious Imagination.* Philadelphia: Fortress Press, 1976.

Wilensky, Sara O. Heller. "The 'First Created Being' in Early Kabbalah and its Philosophical Sources." In *Studies in Jewish Thought*, edited by Sara O. Heller Wilensky, pp. 261–76. Jerusalem: Magnes Press, 1989 (Hebrew). English translation in *Jewish Intellectual History in the Middle Ages* [*Binah: Studies in Jewish History, Thought, and Culture*, volume 3], edited by Joseph Dan, pp. 65–77. Westport: Praeger, 1994.

———. "The Guide and the Gate: The Dialectical Influence of Maimonides on Isaac Ibn Latif and Early Spanish Kabbalah." In *A Straight Path—Studies in Medieval Philosophy and Culture: Essays in Honor of Arthur Hyman*, edited by Ruth Link Salinger, pp. 266–78. Washington, D.C.: Catholic University of America Press, 1988.

———. "Isaac Ibn Laṭif—Philosopher or Kabbalist?" In *Jewish Medieval and Renaissance Studies*, edited by Alexander Altmann, pp. 185–223. Cambridge, MA: Harvard University Press, 1967.

———. "Isaac Ibn Latif's 'The Gate of Heaven': A Mystical Guide of the Perplexed." In *Perspectives in Jewish Learning*, vol. 2, edited by Moses A. Shulvass, pp. 17–25. Chicago: Spertus College of Judaica, 1966.

———. "Messianism, Eschatology, and Utopia in the Philosophic-Mystical Current of Kabbalah in the Thirteenth Century." In *Messianism and Eschatology: A Collection of Essays*, edited by Zvi Baras, pp. 221–37. Jerusalem: Zalman Shazar Centre, 1983 (Hebrew).

———. "The Relations between Mysticism and Philosophy in the Teachings of Rabbi Isaac Ibn Latif." *Jerusalem Studies in Jewish Thought* 6, nos. 3–4 (1987): 367–82 (Hebrew).

Williams, Paul. *Mahāyāna Buddhism: The Doctrinal Foundations*. 2nd edition. London: Routledge, 2009.

Wilson, Robert R. *Prophecy and Society in Ancient Israel*. Philadelphia: Fortress Press, 1980.

Windt, Jennifer Michelle, and Thomas Metzinger. "The Philosophy of Dreaming and Self-Consciousness: What Happens to the Experiential Subject during the Dream State?" In *The New Science of Dreaming*, edited by Deirdre Barrett and Patrick McNamara. Vol. 3, *Cultural and Theoretical Perspectives*, pp. 193–247. Westport: Praeger, 2007.

Winson, Jonathan. *Brain and Psyche: The Biology of the Unconscious*. Garden City: Anchor Press, 1985.

———. "The Meaning of Dreams." *Scientific American* 243 (1990): 86–96.

Withers, Robert. "Descartes' Dreams." *Journal of Analytic Psychology* 53 (2008): 691–709.

Wittgenstein, Ludwig. *The Big Typescript: TS 213*. Edited and translated by C. Grant Luckhardt and Maximilian A. E. Aue. Oxford: Blackwell, 2005.

———. *Lectures and Conversations on Aesthetics, Psychology and Religious Belief*. Compiled from notes taken by Yorick Smythies, Rush Rhees, and James Taylor. Edited by Cyril Barrett. Oxford: Blackwell, 1966.

———. *Philosophical Grammar*. Edited by Rush Rees. Translated by Anthony Kenny. Berkeley: University of California Press, 1974.

———. *Remarks on the Philosophy of Psychology*. 2 vols. Edited by Gertrude E. M. Anscombe and Georg H. Wright. Translated by Gertrude E. M. Anscombe. Oxford: Basil Blackwell, 1980.

Wolf, Fred Alan. *The Dreaming Universe: A Mind-Expanding Journey Into the Realm Where Psyche and Physics Meet*. New York: Simon & Schuster, 1994.

———. "The Quantum Mechanics of Dreams and the Emergence of Self-Awareness." In *Toward a Scientific Basis for Consciousness*, edited by S. R. Hameroff, A. W. Kaszniak, and A. C. Scott, pp. 451–67. Cambridge, MA: The MIT Press, 1996.

Wolfson, Elliot R. *Abraham Abulafia—Kabbalist and Prophet: Hermeneutics,*

Theosophy, and Theurgy. Los Angeles: Cherub Press, 2000.

——. *Alef, Mem, Tau: Kabbalistic Musings on Time, Truth, and Death*. Berkeley: University of California Press 2005.

——. "The Anonymous Chapters of the Elderly Master of Secrets: New Evidence for the Early Activity of the Zoharic Circle." *Kabbalah: Journal for the Study of Jewish Mystical Texts* 19 (2009): 143–278.

——. "Beyond Good and Evil: Hypernomianism, Transmorality, and Kabbalistic Ethics." In *Crossing Boundaries: Ethics, Antinomianism and the History of Mysticism*, edited by G. William Barnard and Jeffrey J. Kripal, pp. 103–56. New York : Seven Bridges Press, 2002.

——. *Circle in the Square: Studies in the Use of Gender in Kabbalistic Symbolism*. Albany: State University of New York Press, 1995.

——. "Circumcision, Vision of God, and Textual Interpretation: From Midrashic Trope to Mystical Symbol." *History of Religions* 27 (1987): 189–215.

——. "Coronation of the Sabbath Bride: Kabbalistic Myth and the Ritual of Androgynisation." *Journal of Jewish Thought and Philosophy* 6 (1997): 301–44.

——. "The Cut That Binds: Time, Memory, and the Ascetic Impulse." In *God's Voice from the Void: Old and New Studies in Bratslav Hasidism*, edited by Shaul Magid, pp. 103–54. Albany: State University of New York Press, 2002.

——. "Divine Suffering and the Hermeneutics of Reading: Philosophical Reflections on Lurianic Mythology." In *Suffering Religion*, edited by Robert Gibbs and Elliot R. Wolfson, pp. 101–62. London: Routledge, 2002.

——. "Eunuchs Who Keep the Sabbath: Becoming Male and the Ascetic Ideal in Thirteenth-Century Jewish Mysticism." In *Becoming Male in the Middle Ages*, edited by Jeffrey J. Cohen and Bonnie Wheeler, pp. 151–85. New York: Garland, 1997.

——. *Footdreams and Treetales: 92 Poems*. New York: Fordham University Press, 2007.

——. "*Imago Templi* and the Meeting of the Two Seas: Liturgical Time-Space and the Feminine Imaginary in Zoharic Kabbalah." *Res: Anthropology and Aesthetics* 51 (2007): 121–35.

——. "Kenotic Overflow and Temporal Transcendence: Angelic Embodiment and the Alterity of Time in Abraham Abulafia." *Kabbalah: Journal for the Study of Jewish Mystical Texts* 18 (2008): 133–90.

——. *Language, Eros, Being: Kabbalistic Hermeneutics and Poetic Imagination*. New York: Fordham University Press, 2005.

——. "Light Does Not Talk But Shines: Apophasis and Vision in Rosenzweig's

Theopoetic Temporality." In *New Directions in Jewish Philosophy*, edited by Aaron W. Hughes and Elliot R. Wolfson, pp. 87–148. Bloomington: Indiana University Press, 2010.

———. *Luminal Darkness: Imaginal Gleanings From Zoharic Literature*. London: Oneworld Publications, 2007.

———. "Murmuring Secrets: Eroticism and Esotericism in Medieval Kabbalah." In *Hidden Intercourse: Eros and Sexuality in the History of Western Esotericism*, edited by Wouter J. Hanegraaff and Jeffrey J. Kripal, pp. 65–109. Leiden: Brill, 2008.

———. "Mystical Rationalization of the Commandments in the Prophetic Kabbalah of Abraham Abulafia." In *Perspectives on Jewish Thought and Mysticism*, edited by Alfred Ivry, Allan Arkush, and Elliot R. Wolfson, pp. 311–60. Reading: Harwood, 1998.

———. "Negative Theology and Positive Assertion in the Early Kabbalah." *Da'at* 32–33 (1994): v–xxii.

———. "Occultation of the Feminine and the Body of Secrecy in Medieval Kabbalah." In *Rending the Veil: Concealment and Revelation of Secrets in the History of Religions*, edited by Elliot R. Wolfson, pp. 113–54. New York: Seven Bridges Press, 1999.

———. *Open Secret: Postmessianic Messianism and the Mystical Revision of Menaḥem Mendel Schneerson*. New York: Columbia University Press, 2009.

———. "Revisioning the Body Apophatically: Incarnation and the Acosmic Naturalism of Habad Hasidism." In *Apophatic Bodies: Infinity, Ethics, and Incarnation*, edited by Christopher Boesel and Catherine Keller, pp. 147–99. New York: Fordham University Press, 2009.

———. "Sacred Space and Mental Iconography: *Imago Templi* and Contemplation in Rhineland Jewish Pietism." In *Ki Baruch Hu: Ancient Near Eastern, Biblical, and Judaic Studies in Honor of Baruch A. Levine*, edited by Robert Chazan, William Hallo, and Lawrence H. Schiffman, pp. 593–634. Winona Lake: Eisenbrauns, 1999.

———. "'Sage is Preferable to Prophet': Revisioning Midrashic Imagination." In *Scriptural Exegesis: The Shapes of Culture and the Religious Imagination: A Festschrift in Honor of Michael Fishbane*, edited by Deborah A. Green and Laura S. Lieber, pp. 186–210. Oxford: Oxford University Press, 2008.

———. "Secrecy, Modesty, and the Feminine: Kabbalistic Traces in the Thought of Levinas." In *The Exorbitant: Emmanuel Levinas between Jews and Christians*, edited by Kevin Hart and Michael A. Signer, pp. 52–73. New York: Fordham University Press, 2010.

———. "Seven Mysteries of Knowledge: Qumran E/sotericism Reconsidered."

In *The Idea of Biblical Interpretation: Essays in Honor of James L. Kugel*, edited by Hindy Najman and Judith H. Newman, pp. 173–213. Leiden: Brill, 2003.

———. "Structure, Innovation, and Diremptive Temporality: The Use of Models to Study Continuity and Discontinuity in Kabbalistic Tradition." *Journal for the Study of Religions and Ideologies* 18 (2007): 141–65.

———. "Suffering Eros and Textual Incarnation: A Kristevan Reading of Kabbalistic Poetics." In *Toward a Theology of Eros: Transfiguring Passion at the Limits of Discipline*, edited by Virginia Burrus and Catherine Keller, pp. 341–65. New York: Fordham University Press, 2006.

———. *Through a Speculum That Shines: Vision and Imagination in Medieval Jewish Mysticism*. Princeton: Princeton University Press, 1994.

———. *Venturing Beyond—Law and Morality in Kabbalistic Mysticism*. Oxford: Oxford University Press, 2006.

———. "*Via Negativa* in Maimonides and Its Impact on Thirteenth-Century Kabbalah." *Maimonidean Studies* 5 (2008): 393–442.

———. "Woman—The Feminine as Other in Theosophic Kabbalah: Some Philosophical Observations on the Divine Androgyne." In *The Other in Jewish Thought and History: Constructions of Jewish Culture and Identity*, edited by Laurence J. Silberstein and Robert L. Cohn, pp. 166–204. New York: New York University Press, 1994.

———. "Yeridah la-Merkavah: Typology of Ecstasy and Enthronement in Ancient Jewish Mysticism." In *Mystics of the Book: Themes, Topics, and Typologies*, edited and with an introduction by Robert A. Herrera, pp. 13–44. New York: Peter Lang, 1993.

Wolfson, Harry A. *Philo: Foundations of Religious Philosophy in Judaism, Christianity, and Islam*. 2 vols. Cambridge, MA: Harvard University Press, 1947.

———. *Studies in the History of Philosophy and Religion*. Edited by Isadore Twersky and George H. Williams. 2 vols. Cambridge, MA: Harvard University Press, 1973–1977.

Wolosky, Shira. "An 'Other' Negative Theology: On Derrida's 'How To Avoid Speaking: Denials.'" *Poetics Today* 19 (1998): 261–80.

Wood, Thomas E. *The Māṇḍūkya Upaniṣad and the Āgama Śāstra: An Investigation into the Meaning of the Vedānta*. Honolulu: University of Hawaii Press, 1992.

Woodman, Ross. *Sanity, Madness, Transformation: The Psyche in Romanticism*. Edited and with an afterword by Joel Faflak. Toronto: University of Toronto Press, 2005.

Wyschogrod, Edith. *An Ethics of Remembering: History, Heterology, and the Nameless Others*. Chicago: University of Chicago Press, 1998.

———. "Between Phenomenology and the Negative's Power." In *Portraits of*

American Continental Philosophers, edited by James R. Watson, pp. 221–28. Bloomington: Indiana University Press, 1999.

——. "The Civilizational Perspective in Comparative Studies of Transcendence." In *Transcendence and the Sacred*, edited by Alan M. Olson and Leroy S. Rouner, pp. 58–79. Notre Dame: University of Notre Dame Press, 1981.

——. "Corporeality and the Glory of the Infinite in the Philosophy of Emmanuel Levinas." *Incarnation: Proceedings of the Conference of the Instituto di Studi Filosofici Enrico Castelli* 63 (1998): 113–26.

——. *Crossover Queries: Dwelling with Negatives, Embodying Philosophy's Others*. New York: Fordham University Press, 2006.

——. *Emmanuel Levinas: The Problem of Ethical Metaphysics*. 2nd edition. New York: Fordham University Press, 2000.

——. "Intending Transcendence: Desiring God." In *Companion to Postmodern Theology*, edited by Graham Ward, pp. 349–65. London: Blackwell, 2001.

——. "Language and Alterity in the Thought of Levinas." In *The Cambridge Companion to Levinas*, edited by Simon Critchley and Robert Bernasconi, pp. 188–205. Cambridge: Cambridge University Press, 2002.

——. "Repentance and Forgiveness: The Undoing of Time." *International Journal for Philosophy of Religion* 60 (2006): 157–68.

Yalles, Ya'aqov Ṣevi. *Qehillat Ya'aqov*. Lemberg, 1870.

Yao, Zhihua. *The Buddhist Theory of Self-Cognition*. London: Routledge, 2005.

Yerushalmi, Yosef H. *Freud's Moses: Judaism Terminable and Interminable*. New Haven: Yale University Press, 1991.

The Yoga-system of Patañjali; or, The Ancient Hindu Doctrine of Concentration of Mind, Embracing the Mnemonic Rules, Called Yoga-sūtras of Patañjali, and the Comment, Called Yoga-bhāshya, Attributed to Veda-Vyāsa, and the Explanation, Called Tattva-vāiçāradī, of Vāchaspati-Miçra. Translated by James Haughton Woods. Cambridge, MA: Harvard University Press, 1927.

Yosef Ḥayyim of Baghdad, *Da'at u-Tevunah*. Jerusalem, 2001.

——. *Sod Yesharim*. Jerusalem, 1994.

Yost, Robert M., Jr., and Donald Kalish. "Miss MacDonald on Sleeping and Waking." *Philosophical Quarterly* 5 (1955): 109–24.

Young, Robert J. C. "Freud's Secret: *The Interpretation of Dreams* Was a Gothic Novel." In *Sigmund Freud's The Interpretation of Dreams: New Interdisciplinary Essays*, edited by Laura Marcus, pp. 206–31. Manchester: Manchester University Press, 1999.

Young, Serinity. *Dreaming in the Lotus: Buddhist Dream Narrative, Imagery, and Practice*. Foreword by Carol Schreier Rupprecht. Boston: Wisdom Publications, 1999.

Zabolotnaya, Natasha Esther. "Cosmology and Color Symbolism in R. Eleazar of Worms." *Kabbalah: Journal for the Study of Jewish Mystical Texts* 12 (2004): 45–80.

Zahavi, Dan. *Husserl's Phenomenology*. Stanford: Stanford University Press, 2003.

Zarader, Marlène. "Phenomenality and Transcendence." In *Transcendence in Philosophy and Religion*, edited by James E. Faulconer, pp. 106–19. Bloomington: Indiana University Press, 2003.

Zeitlin, Solomon. "Dreams and Their Interpretation From the Biblical Period to the Tannaitic Time: An Historical Study." *Jewish Quarterly Review* 66 (1975): 1–18.

Zellentin, Holger M. "Late Antiquity Upside-Down: Rabbinic Parodies of Jewish and Christian Literature." Ph.D. dissertation, Princeton University, 2007.

Zimmer, Heinrich. *Myth and Symbols in Indian Art and Civilization*. Edited by Joseph Campbell. New York: Pantheon Books, 1946.

——. *Philosophies of India*. Edited by Joseph Campbell. Cleveland: Meridian Books, 1956.

Žižek, Slavoj. *In Defense of Lost Causes*. London: Verso, 2008.

——. *The Parallax View*. Cambridge, MA: The MIT Press, 2006.

Zohar, Danah. *The Quantum Self: Human Nature and Consciousness Defined by the New Physics*. New York: Quill, 1990.

Zohar Ḥadash. Edited by Reuven Margaliot. Jerusalem: Mosad ha-Rav Kook, 1978.

Index

Zone Books series design by Bruce Mau
Typesetting by Meighan Gale
Printed and bound by Thompson-Shore